Signs, Syndromes, and Eponyms: Our Legacy

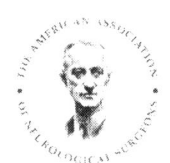

Timir Banerjee, MD,
and
Alvaro Augusto Domingues da Silva, MD,
Editors

Signs, Syndromes and Eponyms: Our Legacy
Timir Banerjee, MD, and Alvaro Augusto Domingues da Silva, MD, Editors

Library of Congress Catalog
ISBN: 1-879284-68-5

Warren R. Selman, MD, Chairman
AANS Publications Committee

Gay L. Palazzo, AANS Editor

AANS 0.5M599
.2M899
.2M200

DEDICATION

To Dr. William E. Hunt, my professor

To Dr. K. Chatterjee, my grandfather

INTRODUCTION

The authors present in this volume an extremely complete description of the eponyms in the fields of neurosurgery, neurology, medicine, and surgery. The signs and symptoms associated with these disorders are described in a very thorough manner. The alphabetical arrangement of the material enables the reader to use this book as a quickly available resource for information concerning any eponym.

Dr. Banerjee has had wide clinical experience as an extremely well-trained neurosurgeon. He served for three years on the neurosurgical faculty at the University of North Carolina School of Medicine at Chapel Hill. He is widely known for his teaching and his clinical research as well as his extensive clinical practice in neurosurgery.

This monumental work provides a valuable source of information to practitioners in all fields of medicine as well as to medical students and residents in all fields of medicine.

Thomas W. Farmer, MD
Chapel Hill, North Carolina

PREFACE

Dr. Banerjee and Dr. da Silva are to be congratulated for completing a monumental task and for providing a valuable gift to the medical community. *Signs, Syndromes, and Eponyms: Our Legacy* is a compilation of thousands of descriptions of these entities. Such a comprehensive collection enhances, refines, and improves the categorization of terms required for medical record-keeping and patient care.

Eponyms are wonderful memory aids for understanding cumbersome descriptions of diseases. Indeed, it is important to realize that eponyms seldom identify a discoverer or an inventor, more often bearing the name of the individual responsible for popularizing a given observation. Eponyms often are considered an aggravation to neophytes in medicine, and interestingly enough, are a tremendous solace to more senior practitioners. Many of us are accustomed to using an eponym such as Down's syndrome instead of the longer, more descriptive definition. The popularity of these familiar terms is also evident in the amount of material that the authors have presented. While other books about medical eponyms have traced the historical paths of diseases and syndromes, Drs. Banerjee and da Silva focus more on common definitions and noting misunderstandings associated with these terms.

This meticulously prepared encyclopedic volume is intended to be a ready resource for the curious scientist and a briefly informative guide for the maturing young clinician. The book is alphabetized and serves as a useful tool for easily locating the definitions for each eponym, disease, operation, phenomenon, sign, syndrome, and test.

Dr. Banerjee is a respected neurological surgeon who has long been interested in medical education. This book is a tremendous achievement for an active surgeon as well as a testimonial to his dedication to the student and practitioner. Generous in his support of research at his adopted medical school, the University of Louisville, Dr. Banerjee's scientific interest in surgery and medicine is obvious from this scholarly effort.

Hiram C. Polk, Jr., MD
Louisville, Kentucky

3-M SYNDROME, characterized by low birth weight at full term and proportionate small size.
1. Callaghan KA: Asymmetrical dwarfism, or Silver syndrome in two male siblings. Med J Aust 2:789-792, 1970
2. Gorlin RJ, Cohen MM Jr, Levin LS: Syndromes of the Head and Neck. 3rd ed. New York: Oxford University Press, 1990

4P SYNDROME, ocular hypertelorism with a broad or beaked nose, microcephaly, and/or cranial asymmetry, and low-set, simple ears with preauricular dimple.
1. Guthrie RD, et al: The 4p-syndrome. Am J Dis Child 122:421, 1971
2. Smith DW, Jones KL: Recognizable Patterns of Human Malformations: Genetic, Embryologic, and Clinical Aspects. 3rd ed. Philadelphia: WB Saunders, 1982

9P SYNDROME, craniostenosis with trigonocephaly, upward slanting palpebral fissures, and hypoplastic supraorbital ridges.
1. Alfi OS, et al: The 9p-syndrome. Ann Genet 19:11, 1976
2. Smith DW, Jones KL: Recognizable Patterns of Human Malformations: Genetic, Embryologic, and Clinical Aspects. 3rd ed. Philadelphia: WB Saunders, 1982

17-α-HYDROXYLASE DEFICIENCY SYNDROME, congenital adrenocortical hyperplasia resulting from a deficiency of the enzyme 17-α-hydroxylase, with resultant deficiency of estrogen and androgen and consequent sexual infantilism; the compensatory increase in secretion of deoxycorticosterone and corticosterone results in hypokalemic alkalosis and hypertension.
1. Schinzel A, Schmid U, Lüscher U, et al: The 18p-syndrome. Arch Genetik 47:1, 1974
2. Smith DW, Jones KL: Recognizable Patterns of Human Malformations: Genetic, Embryologic, and Clinical Aspects. 3rd ed. Philadelphia: WB Saunders, 1982

18Q SYNDROME, midfacial hypoplasia, prominent anthelix, and whorl digital pattern are features.
1. Smith DW, Jones KL: Recognizable Patterns of Human Malformations: Genetic, Embryologic, and Clinical Aspects. 3rd ed. Philadelphia: WB Saunders, 1982
2. Wertelecki W, Gerald PS: Clinical and chromosomal studies of the 18q-syndrome. J Pediatr 78:44, 1971

AARON SIGN, a pressing at the McBurney point that produces epigastric pain; seen in acute appendicitis. (Charles D. Aaron, Norwegian pediatrician)
1. Casas EC: Diccionario Terminologico de Ciencias Medicas. 5th ed. Salvat Editores, SA, 1954

AARSKOG SYNDROME, AARSKOG-SCOTT SYNDROME, a congenital growth deficiency with mild degrees of mental retardation, reduced fertility in males, and a peculiar "scrotal shawl" above the penis. X-linked semidominant inheritance, with the carrier female often showing minor manifestations, especially in the facies and hands. Cross-reference: Facial-digital-genital syndrome. (Dagfinn C. Aarskog, Norwegian pediatrician; Charles I. Scott, Jr., U.S. pediatrician)
1. Aarskog D: J Pediatr 77:856-861, 1970
2. Gorlin RJ, Cohen MM Jr, Levin LS: Syndromes of the Head and Neck. 3rd ed. New York: Oxford University Press, 1990
3. Smith DW, Jones KL: Recognizable Patterns of Human Malformation: Genetic, Embryologic, and Clinical Aspects. 3rd ed. Philadelphia: WB Saunders, 1982

AASE-SMITH SYNDROME II, congenital hypoplastic anemia, triphalangeal thumbs, hypoplastic radii, and cleft lip are features. Other features include somatic and mental retardation, narrow shoulders, abnormal pigmentation of the skin, and a short, webbed neck. Cross-references: Blackfan-Diamond syndrome; Diamond-Blackfan syndrome. (John M. Aase; David W. Smith, 1926-1981, U.S. pediatrician)
1. Aase JM, Smith DW: Congenital anemia and triphalangeal thumbs: a new syndrome. J Pediatr 74:471-474, 1969
2. Diamond LK, Blackfan KD: Am J Dis Child 56:464-467, 1938

ABADIE SIGN, insensibility of the Achilles tendon to pressure; often seen in the patient with neurosyphilis. (Charles A. Abadie, 1842-1932, French ophthalmologist)
1. Grinker RR, Sahs AL: Neurology. 6th ed. Springfield: Charles C Thomas, 1966

ABBÉ OPERATION, intracranial resection (or section) of the second and third trigeminal branches. (Robert Abbé, 1851-1928, U.S. surgeon)
1. Maffei WE: Os Fundamentos da Medicina. 2nd ed. Livraria Editora Artes Medicas Ltd, 1978

ABBÉ-ESTLANDER OPERATION, the transfer of a full-thickness flap from one lip to fill a defect in the other. (Jakob A. Estlander, 1831-1881, Finnish surgeon)
1. Maffei WE: Os Fundamentos da Medicina. 2nd ed. Livraria Editora Artes Medicas Ltd, 1978

ABERCROMBIE SYNDROME, amyloidosis. (John Abercrombie, 1780-1844, British)

1. Casas EC: Diccionario Terminologico de Ciencias Medicas. 5th ed. Salvat Editores, SA, 1954

ABERNETHY OPERATION, ligation of the external iliac artery through an incision from a point 2.5 cm inward and above the anterosuperior iliac spine to a point 3.0 cm outward and above the center of the Poupart ligament.

1. Maffei WE: Os Fundamentos da Medicina. 2nd ed. Livraria Editora Artes Medicas Ltd, 1978

ABLEPHARON-MACROSTOMIA SYNDROME, a congenital syndrome of triangular facies, hypertelorism, internal strabismus, late development of sparse, thin hair, absence of upper and lower eyelids, eyebrows, and eyelashes. Intelligence may be moderately affected.

1. Gorlin RJ, Cohen MM Jr, Levin LS: Syndromes of the Head and Neck. 3rd ed. New York: Oxford University Press, 1990
2. Hornblass A, Reifler DM: Ablepharon macrostomia syndrome. Am J Ophthalmol 99:552-556, 1985

ABRAHAMS SIGN, 1) a dull sound heard on percussion over the acromial process; seen in tuberculosis of the lung; 2) when pressure is applied between the umbilicus and the 9th right costal cartilage, pain in vesical lithiasis is acute. (Robert Abrahams, 1861-1935, U.S.)

1. Dorland's Medical Dictionary. 28th ed. Philadelphia: WB Saunders, 1994

ABRAMI DISEASE, hemolytic jaundice. Cross-reference: Widal-Abrami disease. (Pierre Abrami, 1879-1943, French)

1. Casas EC: Diccionario Terminologico de Ciencias Medicas. 5th ed. Salvat Editores, SA, 1954

ABRASHANOFF OPERATION, closure of abdominal or other fistulae using pediculated flaps.

1. Maffei WE: Os Fundamentos da Medicina. 2nd ed. Livraria Editora Artes Medicas Ltd, 1978

ABRUZZO-ERICKSON SYNDROME, an X-linked inherited disorder of a cleft palate in association with short stature, hypospadias, hearing loss, eye coloboma, and radial synostosis. Intelligence is normal. Stature is below the 3rd percentile.

1. Abruzzo MA, Erickson RP: A new syndrome of cleft palate associated with coloboma, hypospadias, deafness, short stature and radial synostosis. J Med Genet 14:76-80, 1977
2. Abruzzo MA, Erickson RP: Re-evaluation of new X-linked syndrome for evidence of CHARGE syndrome or association. Am J Med Genet 34:397-400, 1989
3. Gorlin RJ, Cohen MM Jr, Levin LS: Syndromes of the Head and Neck. 3rd ed. New York: Oxford University Press, 1990

ABSTINENCE SYNDROME, see Withdrawal syndrome.

ACHARD SYNDROME, arachnodactyly with mandibulofacial dysostosis, particularly a receding lower jaw. A Marfan variant. (Emile Charles Achard, 1860-1944, French)

1. Achard C: Arachnodactylie. Bull Med Soc Med Hosp (Par) 19:834-840, 1902
2. McKusick VA: Heritable Disorders of Connective Tissue. 4th ed. St Louis: CV Mosby, 1972

ACHARD-THIERS SYNDROME, the constellation of diabetes, hirsutism, and other masculinizing features in postmenopausal women resulting from overproduction of adrenocortical androgens. (Emile Charles Achard; Joseph T. Thiers, French)

1. Achard C, Thiers J: Le virilisme pilaire et son association à l'insufficance glycolytique. Bull Acad Natl Med (Par) 86:51-66, 1921

ACHONDROGENESIS SYNDROME, extremely small stature with a normal to large cranium, severe macromelia, large liver, hydrops, and polyhydramnios are features. An early death is often indicated. Autosomal recessive inheritance. Cross-reference: Saldino syndrome.

1. Saldino RM: Lethal short-limbed dwarfism: achondrogenesis and thanatophoric dwarfism. Am J Roentgenol 112:185-197, 1971
2. Smith DW, Jones KL: Recognizable Patterns of Human Malformation: Genetic, Embryologic, and Clinical Aspects. 3rd ed. Philadelphia: WB Saunders, 1982

ACHRONDROPLASIA SYNDROME, chondrodysplasia foetalis; small stature, megalocephaly, and skeletal disorders including a short neck, short hands and fingers, short tubular bones, small iliac wings, and lumbar lordosis are features. Older parent age is a contributing factor. Autosomal dominant inheritance.

1. Maroteaux P, Lamy M: Achondroplasia in man and animals. Clin Orthop 33:91-103, 1964
2. Smith DW, Jones KL: Recognizable Patterns of Human Malformation: Genetic, Embryologic, and Clinical Aspects. 3rd ed. Philadelphia: WB Saunders, 1982

ACKERLUND SIGN, a radiological sign of duodenal ulcer (asymmetry of the pylorus).

1. Casas EC: Diccionario Terminologico de Ciencias Medicas. 5th ed. Salvat Editores, SA, 1954

ACKERMAN SYNDROME, a familial syndrome of pyramidal, taurodont, and fused molar roots with a single root canal; sparse body hair, full upper lip without a cupid's bow, and thickening and widening of the philtrum are also features. (James L. Ackerman, U.S. orthodontist)

1. Ackerman JL: Taurodont, pyramidal, and fused molar roots associated with other anomalies in a kindred. Am J Phys Anthropol 38:681-694, 1973
2. Gorlin RJ, Cohen MM Jr, Levin LS: Syndromes of the Head and Neck. 3rd ed. New York: Oxford University Press, 1990

ACQUIRED IMMUNODEFICIENCY SYNDROME, defined by the occurrence of a disease predictive of a deficit in cell-mediated immunity in a person with no known cause for diminished resistance to that disease. Often associated with Kaposi sarcoma. The incidence has increased dramatically since first reported in 1978. Blood examination is positive for human immunodeficiency virus, and there is T cell reduction and pulmonary involvement.

1. Campbell MF, Walsh PC: Campbell's Urology. 5th ed. Philadelphia: WB Saunders, 1986
2. Curran JW, Morgan WM, Hardy AM, et al: The epidemiology of AIDS: current status and future prospects. Science 229:1352-1357, 1985
3. Rowland LP (ed): Merritt's Textbook of Neurology. 9th ed. Baltimore: Williams & Wilkins, 1995

ACROCALLOSAL SYNDROME, characterized by post- and/or preaxial polydactyly and syndactyly of the fingers or toes, severe mental retardation, agenesis or hypoplasia of the corpus callosum, and growth retardation.

1. Casamassima AC, Beneck D, Gewitz MH: Acrocallosal syndrome: additional manifestations. Am J Med Genet 32:311-317, 1989
2. Gorlin RJ, Cohen MM Jr, Levin LS: Syndromes of the Head and Neck. 3rd ed. New York: Oxford University Press, 1990
3. Nelson MM, Thompson AJ: The acrocallosal syndrome. Am J Med Genet 12:195-199, 1982

ACROCEPHALO-SYNANKIE SYNDROME, craniosynostosis, radiohumeral synostosis, and fusion of the cuboid and third cuneiform bones are features. May represent atypical Apert syndrome. Cross-reference: Multiple synostoses syndrome.

1. Gorlin RJ, Cohen MM Jr, Levin LS: Syndromes of the Head and Neck. 3rd ed. New York: Oxford University Press, 1990

ACROCRANIOFACIAL SYNDROME, short stature, craniosynostosis involving the corneal suture, ocular hypertelorism, ocular proptosis, ptosis of the eyelids, down-slanting palpebral fissures, a high nasal bridge, anteverted nostrils, a short philtrum, cleft palate, micrognathia, mixed hearing loss, proximally placed thumbs and great toes, bulbous digits, metatarsus adductus, and other abnormalities are features. Autosomal recessive inheritance.

1. Gorlin RJ, Cohen MM Jr, Levin LS: Syndromes of the Head and Neck. 3rd ed. New York: Oxford University Press, 1990

ACRODYSOSTOSIS SYNDROME, short hands with peripheral dysostosis, a small nose, and mental deficiency are features. Occurs sporadically, and etiology is uncertain. Cross-reference: Maroteaux-Malamut syndrome.

1. Maroteaux P, Malamut GL: L'acrodyostose. Presse Med 76:2189-2192, 1968
2. Smith DW, Jones KL: Recognizable Patterns of Human Malformation: Genetic, Embryologic, and Clinical Aspects. 3rd ed. Philadelphia: WB Saunders, 1982

ACRO-OSTEOLYSIS SYNDROME, see Hajdu syndrome.

ACRO-RENAL-MANDIBULAR SYNDROME, a syndrome featuring severe split hand and foot malformations, renal (polycystic kidneys, renal agenesis, or absent ureters) and genital (septate uterus, unicornuate uterus, or a single fallopian tube) abnormalities, and very severe micrognathia.

1. Gorlin RJ, Cohen MM Jr, Levin LS: Syndromes of the Head and Neck. 3rd ed. New York: Oxford University Press, 1990
2. Halal F, Desgranges MF, Leduc B, et al: Acro-renal-mandibular syndrome. Am J Med Genet 5:277-284, 1980

ACUTE BRAIN-ACUTE ORGANIC SYNDROME, see Organic mental syndrome.

ACUTE RADIATION SYNDROME, results from exposure to a whole-body dose >1 Gy of ionizing radiation. Symptoms and signs include erythema, nausea, vomiting, diarrhea, fever, petechiae, and fatigue.

1. Bennett JC, Plum F (eds): Cecil Textbook of Medicine. 20th ed. Philadelphia: WB Saunders, 1996

ADAIR-DIGHTON SYNDROME, see Osteogenesis imperfecta syndrome type I.

ADAM SIGN, the standing Adam position motion is most restricted and most painful, extension may be almost as restricted and painful but never more, lateral bending is freer, and rotation is the freest and least painful of all motions. Present in acute low back pain.

1. Mazion JM: Illustrated Manual of Orthopedic Signs/Tests/Maneuvers for Office Procedure. 2nd ed. Orlando: Daniels Publishing, 1980

ADAMS OPERATION, 1) intrascapular division of the femur in ankylosis of the hip; 2) subcutaneous palmar fasciotomy in the Dupuytren contraction; 3) surgery for ectropion using a cuneiform incision of the eyelid. (William Adams, 1810-1900, British surgeon)

1. Maffei WE: Os Fundamentos da Medicina. 2nd ed. Livraria Editora Artes Medicas Ltd, 1978

ADAMS-STOKES SYNDROME, complete heart block; seizures may occur during the course of cardiovascular dysfunction in the form of cerebral anoxia or appear as a manifestation of hypertensive encephalopathy, embolism, and much less often as an accompaniment of vascular malformations of the brain also associated with cerebral arteriosclerosis. Cross-references: Morgagni disease; Spens syndrome; Stokes-Adams syndrome. (Robert Adams, 1791-1875, Irish surgeon; William Stokes, 1804-1878, Irish)

1. Adams R: Dublin Hosp Rep 4:353, 1827
2. Grinker RR, Sahs AL: Neurology. 6th ed. Springfield: Charles C Thomas, 1966
3. Stokes W: Dublin QJ Med Sci 2:73-85, 1846

ADDISON DISEASE, adrenocortical hypofunction or postcortisone adrenocortical insufficiency. Characterized by weakness and loss of weight, peculiar bronze pigmentation of skin, low blood pressure, nausea, abdominal pain, vomiting, diarrhea, hypoglycemia, anemia, and severe mental symptoms (depression). Cross-reference: Schaumberg disease. (Thomas Addison, 1793-1860, British)

1. Addison T: Lond Hosp Gaz 43:517-518, 1849
2. Grinker RR, Sahs AL: Neurology. 6th ed. Springfield: Charles C Thomas, 1966
3. Moschella SL, Hurley HJ: Dermatology. 2nd ed. Philadelphia: WB Saunders, 1985

ADDISON-BIERMER DISEASE, see Biermer-Addison-Castle disease. (Thomas Addison)

ADDISONIAN SYNDROME, see Nelson syndrome. (Thomas Addison)

ADDUCTED THUMBS SYNDROME, see Christian syndrome.

ADELMANN OPERATION, disarticulation of a finger together with the head of the corresponding metacarpal joint.

1. Maffei WE: Os Fundamentos da Medicina. 2nd ed. Livraria Editora Artes Medicas Ltd, 1978

ADEN DISEASE, dengue.

1. Casas EC: Diccionario Terminologico de Ciencias Medicas. 5th ed. Salvat Editores, SA, 1954

ADHERENCE SYNDROME, Type I: adhesions between the sheaths of the lateral rectus and inferior oblique muscles that make it impossible to abduct the eye. Type II: adhesions between the sheaths of the superior rectus and the superior oblique muscles, preventing elevation of the involved eye.

1. Walsh FB, Hoyt EF, Miller NR: Clinical Neuro-Ophthalmology. 4th ed. Baltimore: Williams & Wilkins, 1982

ADIE SYNDROME, ADIE TONIC PUPIL, characterized by a tonic pupillary reaction and absence of one or more tendon reflexes; both pupils are large or one pupil is large and the other is normal size. Most cases occur in women. Cross-references: Holmes-Adie syndrome; Ross syndrome; Sweat retention syndrome. (William J. Adie, 1886-1935, British neurologist)

1. Adie WJ: Pseudo-Argyll Robertson pupils with absent tendon reflexes. Br Med J 1:928-930, 1931
2. Ross AT: Progressive selective sudomotor denervation. Neurology 8:809-817, 1958

ADIE-CRITCHLEY SYNDROME, forced grasping and inability to release as well as groping by the hand contralateral to a tumor of the superior part of the frontal lobe. (William J. Adie)

1. Adie WJ, Critchley M: Forced grasping and groping. Brain 50:142-170, 1927

ADIPOSOGENITAL SYNDROME, see Fröhlich syndrome.

ADRENOGENITAL SYNDROME, congenital adrenal hyperplasia. A clinical manifestation of hypofunction of the adrenal cortex, associated with virilism in females and precocious sexual development. There may be excessive feminization in men. Pseudohermaphroditism may develop as a result of androgenic hyperplasia of the adrenal cortex before birth.

1. Campbell WC, Walsh PC: Campbell's Urology. 5th ed. Philadelphia: WB Saunders, 1986
2. Rowland LP (ed): Merritt's Textbook of Neurology. 9th ed. Baltimore: Williams & Wilkins, 1995

ADSON MANEUVER, ADSON TEST, coolness and pallor of the forearm and hand and a decrease in strength of the radial pulse, especially while tilting the head back and turning the head to the affected side. Considered diagnostic for thoracic outlet syndrome. Present in about 15%-40% of normal individuals. (Alfred W. Adson, 1887-1951, U.S. neurosurgeon)

    1. Campbell WC, Crenshaw AH: Campbell's Operative Orthopaedics. 7th ed. St Louis: CV Mosby, 1987

ADSON SYNDROME, see Zellweger syndrome. (Alfred W. Adson)

ADULT RESPIRATORY DISTRESS SYNDROME, adult hyaline membrane disease; acute clinical, physiological, and pathological events found as a complication of many otherwise unrelated conditions. The common feature is the presence of diffuse injury to the alveolar capillary membrane of the lungs.

    1. Ashbaugh DG, et al: Lancet 2:319-323, 1967
    2. Bennett JC, Plum F (eds): Cecil Textbook of Medicine. 20th ed. Philadelphia: WB Saunders, 1996
    3. Cheitlin MD, Sokolow M: Clinical Cardiology. 5th ed. Norwalk, Conn: Appleton & Lange, 1993

ADVANCED-SLEEP-PHASE SYNDROME, a sleep-wake disorder; a person with this syndrome would complain of undesirably early sleep onset and wake times. Aging leads to such a characteristic change in the timing of sleep. Syndrome is not yet clearly identified.

    1. Association of Sleep Centers: Diagnostic classification of sleep and arousal disorders. Sleep 2:1-154, 1979
    2. Rowland LP (ed): Merritt's Textbook of Neurology. 9th ed. Baltimore: Williams & Wilkins, 1995

ADYNAMIC BOWEL SYNDROME, congenital intestinal obstruction in newborn infants; the rare occurrence of a child with a megacolon like that seen in Hirschsprung disease, but biopsy of the narrow segment of the colon shows a normal complement of neurons or, sometimes, enlargement of the myenteric ganglia. These children may have a more subtle fault in the innervation of the colon.

    1. Kapila L, et al: J Pediatr Surg 10:885-892, 1975
    2. Ritchie AC: Boyd's Textbook of Pathology. 9th ed. Philadelphia: Lea & Febiger, 1990

AEC SYNDROME, ankyloblepharon-ectodermal dysplasia-cleft lip/palate (AEC); see Hay-Wells syndrome.

AFFERENT LOOP SYNDROME, chronic partial obstruction of the proximal loop of the duodenum and jejunum after partial gastrectomy and gastrojejunostomy, leading to duodenal distention. Cross-references: Jejenal syndrome; Postgastrectomy syndrome.

    1. Haymaker W: Bing's Local Diagnosis in Neurological Diseases. 15th ed. St Louis: CV Mosby, 1969

AFFLECK OPERATION, rachiotomy of the fetus followed by podalic version.

    1. Maffei WE: Os Fundamentos da Medicina. 2nd ed. Livraria Editora Artes Medicas Ltd, 1978

AGNEW OPERATION, vertical incision of the lacrimal sac and cauterization of its interior.

    1. Maffei WE: Os Fundamentos da Medicina. 2nd ed. Livraria Editora Artes Medicas Ltd, 1978

AHLFELD SIGN, uterine spasms occurring after the first trimester of pregnancy.

    1. Casas EC: Diccionario Terminologico de Ciencias Medicas. 5th ed. Salvat Editores, SA, 1954

AHUMADA-DEL CASTILLO SYNDROME, a nonpuerperal triad of galactorrhea, amenorrhea, and low gonadotropin secretion. (Juan C. Ahumada, Argentine; E.B. del Castillo, Argentine endocrinologist)

    1. Ahumada J, del Castillo EB: J Clin Endocrinol 13:79-87, 1953

AICARDI SYNDROME, agenesis of the corpus callosum, with mental retardation, seizures, and characteristic retinal patches of pigment and epithelial and choroidal atrophy; affects female infants. (J. Aicardi, French neurologist)

    1. Aicardi J, Chevrie JJ, Rousselie F: Arch Fr Pediatr 26:1103-1120, 1969
    2. Gorlin RJ, Cohen MM Jr, Levin LS: Syndromes of the Head and Neck. 3rd ed. New York: Oxford University Press, 1990
    3. Rowland LP (ed): Merritt's Textbook of Neurology. 9th ed. Baltimore: Williams & Wilkins, 1995

AIRD TEST, while standing, the patient is asked to touch the toes with the knees straight. If flexion of the spine is greatly reduced, the patient is then asked to sit down and touch the toes. If pain is of a nonorganic basis, the patient is able to do so with ease (spinal flexion is identical to that required to touch the toes when standing). (Ian Aird, 1905-1962, British surgeon)

    1. Lumley JS, Clain A: Hamilton Bailey's Demonstration of Physical Signs in Clinical Surgery. 18th ed. London: Butterworth-Heinemann, 1997

AITKEN OPERATION, double pelviotomy for narrow pelvis.
1. Maffei WE: Os Fundamentos da Medicina. 2nd ed. Livraria Editora Artes Medicas Ltd, 1978

AKUREYRI DISEASE, see Iceland disease. (Town in Iceland where more than 1000 cases occurred in 1948)

ALAGILLE SYNDROME, arteriohepatic dysplasia; patient has a triangular face with a broad forehead, narrow chin, and bulbous tip of the nose. (Daniel Alagille, French)
1. Alagille D: J Pediatr 86:63-71, 1915
2. Fowler NO: Cardiac Diagnosis and Treatment. 3rd ed. Cambridge: Harper & Row, 1980

ALAJOUANINE SYNDROME, bilateral facial paralysis and lateral rectus palsy of the eyeball owing to lesions of the 6th and 7th cranial nerves associated with bilateral clubfoot. (Théophile Alajouanine, 1890-1980, French neurologist)
1. Alajouanine T, Huc G, Gopcevitch M, et al: Rev Neurol 2:501-511, 1930
2. Bordas LB (ed): Neurologia Fundamental. 2nd ed. Toray, 1968

ALBARRÁN DISEASE, colibacilluria.
1. Casas EC: Diccionario Terminologico de Ciencias Medicas. 5th ed. Salvat Editores, SA, 1954

ALBARRÁN OPERATION, resection of a portion of a dilated renal pelvis, followed by suturing.
1. Maffei WE: Os Fundamentos da Medicina. 2nd ed. Livraria Editora Artes Medicas Ltd, 1978

ALBATROSS SYNDROME, lack of correlation between objective signs and symptoms of antisocial behavior, abdominal pain, and vomiting in a patient with personality defects after gastrectomy.
1. Johnstone FR, et al: Post-gastrectomy problems in patients with personality defects: the "albatross" syndrome. Can Med Assoc J 96:1559-1564, 1967

ALBEAUX-FERNET SYNDROME, obesity in a young woman related to psychological factors such as emotional stress and also occurring during pregnancy.
1. Maffei WE: Os Fundamentos da Medicina. 2nd ed. Livraria Editora Artes Medicas Ltd, 1978

ALBEE OPERATION, an operation for ankylosis of the hip. (Fred Albee, 1876-1945, U.S. surgeon)
1. Maffei WE: Os Fundamentos da Medicina. 2nd ed. Livraria Editora Artes Medicas Ltd, 1978

ALBEE-DELBET OPERATION, surgery for fracture of the neck of the femur using bone grafting.
1. Maffei WE: Os Fundamentos da Medicina. 2nd ed. Livraria Editora Artes Medicas Ltd, 1978

ALBERS-SCHÖNBERG SYNDROME, osteopetrosis or marble bone disease; a heterogeneous group of disorders characterized by increased bone mineral content. There are three distinct forms: adult benign dominant, malignant recessive, and clinically intermediate. (Heinrich E. Albers-Schönberg, 1865-1921, German radiologist)
1. Albers-Schönberg HE: Munch Med Wochenschr 51:365, 1904
2. McKusick VA: Heritable Disorders of Connective Tissue. 4th ed. St Louis: CV Mosby, 1972
3. Wilson JD, Foster DW, Kronenberg HM, et al (eds): Williams Textbook of Endocrinology. 9th ed. Philadelphia: WB Saunders, 1998

ALBERT DISEASE, achillobursitis; inflammation of the bursa around the Achilles tendon. (Eduard Albert, 1841-1900, Austrian surgeon)
1. Albert E: Achillodynie. Wien Med Presse 34:41-43, 1893

ALBERT OPERATION, resection of the patella to obtain ankylosis of the knee. (Eduard Albert)
1. Maffei WE: Os Fundamentos da Medicina. 2nd ed. Livraria Editora Artes Medicas Ltd, 1978

ALBRIGHT SYNDROME, ALBRIGHT-McCUNE-STERNBERG SYNDROME, polyostotic fibrous dysplasia, irregular brown pigmentation, and sexual precocity in girls. Hypercalcemia, diabetes, and pituitary anomalies also occur. The cause of bone lesions and their relationship to the reported endocrine abnormalities remain unexplained. Cross-references: McCune-Albright syndrome; Seabright bantam syndrome. (Fuller Albright, 1900-1969, U.S. endocrinologist; Donovan J. McCune, 1902-1976, U.S. pediatrician)
1. Albright F: Endocrinology 30:92, 1942
2. Albright F, Butler AM, Hampton AO, et al: N Engl J Med 216:727-746, 1937
3. Farmer TW: Pediatric Neurology. 2nd ed. Hagerstown: Harper & Row, 1975
4. McCune DJ: Osteodystrophia fibrosa. Am J Dis Child 54:806-848, 1937

ALCOHOL WITHDRAWAL SYNDROME, the organic brain syndrome that occurs in steady drinkers from whom alcohol has been withdrawn for some reason; also observed in binge or periodic drinkers.

1. Baker AB, Baker LH: Clinical Neurology. Revised ed. Philadelphia: Harper & Row, 1982
2. Ritchie AC: Boyd's Textbook of Pathology. 9th ed. Philadelphia: Lea & Febiger, 1990

ALDRICH SYNDROME, see Wiskott-Aldrich syndrome.

ALEXANDER DISEASE, a disorder of uncertain pathogenesis resembling spongy leukodystrophy with regard to early onset and enlargement of the head. Autosomal recessive inheritance transmission. (W. Stewart Alexander, New Zealand pathologist)

1. Alexander WS: Progressive fibrinoid degeneration of fibrillary astrocytes associated with mental retardation in a hydrocephalic infant. Brain 72:373-381, 1949
2. Grinker RR, Sahs AL: Neurology. 6th ed. Springfield: Charles C Thomas, 1969

ALEXANDER OPERATION, ALEXANDER-ADAMS OPERATION, 1) surgery for shortening the round ligaments of the uterus in cases of uterus dislocation (Alquié operation); 2) prostatectomy through a suprapubic and perineal incision; 3) ligature of the vertebral arteries to treat epilepsy (Alexander-Adams operation). (William Alexander, 1844-1919, British surgeon; James Adams, 1857-1930, Scottish gynecologist)

1. Maffei WE: Os Fundamentos da Medicina. 2nd ed. Livraria Editora Artes Medicas Ltd, 1978

ALEZZANDRINI SYNDROME, an oculocutaneous, probably pigmentary, sensitization syndrome; features are unilateral tapetoretinal degeneration followed by facial vitiligo and poliosis on the same side. Perceptual deafness was reported in two cases, and poliosis of the eyelashes, which is very rare in vitiligo, may also occur. Cross-reference: Pigment dispersion syndrome. (A.A. Alezzandrini, Argentine ophthalmologist)

1. Alezzandrini AA: Ophthalmologica 147:409-419, 1964
2. Moschella SL, Hurley HJ: Dermatology. 2nd ed. Philadelphia: WB Saunders, 1985

ALIBERT DISEASE, ALIBERT-BAZIN DISEASE, mycosis fungoides; a chronic disease of the reticuloendothelial system. Usually fatal. (Jean Louis Alibert, 1768-1837, French; Antoine P.E. Bazin, 1807-1877, French)

1. Alibert JL: Descriptions des Maladies de la Peau. Bruxelles: Wahlen, 1806
2. Bazin A: Affections Cutanees Artificialles. Paris, 1852

ALICE IN WONDERLAND SYNDROME, a delusional state; may present itself by depersonalization, disturbance of body image, and alteration in the sense of the passage of time associated with schizophrenia, epilepsy, migraine, or diseases of the parietal lobe. Cross-reference: Todd syndrome. (Named after a young girl in the Lewis Carroll story "Alice in Wonderland" who experienced feelings of depersonalization.)

1. Todd J: Syndrome of Alice in Wonderland. Can Med Assoc J 73:701-705, 1955

ALLAN-CUSWORTH-DENT-WILSON SYNDROME, accumulation of arginine succinate acid in the urine, blood, and cerebrospinal fluid. Symptoms and signs similar to many other aminoacidurias.

1. Bordas LB: Neurologia Fundamental. 2nd ed. Toray, 1968

ALLARTON OPERATION, perineal cystotomy.

1. Maffei WE: Os Fundamentos da Medicina. 2nd ed. Livraria Editora Artes Medicas Ltd, 1978

ALLEMANN SYNDROME, the association of clubbed fingers and double kidney; facial asymmetry and degeneration of various motor nerves may occur as well. (Richard Allemann, 1893-1958, Swiss)

1. Allemann R: Die Klinische Bedentung familiarer Heredopatie und Mutation füo die Urologie. Z Urol 80:641-649, 1936

ALLEN SIGN, ALLEN-CLECKLEY SIGN, 1) a sign elicited by a forceful downward stretching or snapping of the distal phalanx of either the second or fourth toe; 2) a sign produced by a sharp upward flick of the second toe or by pressure applied to the ball of the toe. Cross-reference: Gonda sign. (Alfred H. Allen, 1846-1943, British chemist)

1. Baker AB, Baker LH: Clinical Neurology. Revised ed. Philadelphia: Harper & Row, 1982

ALLEN TEST, a measurement of arterial supply to the hand; compression and release of radial and ulnar vessels to check for color change. (Edgar V. Allen, 1900-1961, U.S.)

1 Dorland's Medical Dictionary. 28th ed. Philadelphia: WB Saunders, 1994

ALLINGHAM OPERATION, 1) ablation of the rectum through an incision from the ischiorectal fossa to the coccyx. (William Allingham, 1829-1908, British); 2) inguinal colotomy through an incision parallel to the Poupart ligament. (H. Allingham)

1. Maffei WE: Os Fundamentos da Medicina. 2nd ed. Livraria Editora Artes Medicas Ltd, 1978

ALLIS SIGN, the aponeurosis between the iliac crest and the greater trochanter is relaxed; seen in the patient with fracture of the femoral neck. (Oscar H. Allis, 1836-1921, U.S. surgeon)
1. Casas EC: Diccionario Terminologico de Ciencias Medicas. 5th ed. Salvat Editores, SA, 1954

ALMEIDA DISEASE, paracoccidioidomycosis. (Floriano Paula de Almeida, Brazilian)
1. Casas EC: Diccionario Terminologico de Ciencias Medicas. 5th ed. Salvat Editores, SA, 1954

ALPERS DISEASE, progressive poliodystrophy; severe degeneration of the cerebral cortex developing in infancy. Not certain whether this constitutes one or multiple entities. Some cases have been attributed to severe anoxia or status epilepticus. (Bernard J. Alpers, U.S. neurologist)
1. Alpers BJ: Arch Neurol Psychiatr 25:469-505, 1931
2. Farmer TW: Pediatric Neurology. 2nd ed. Hagerstown: Harper & Row, 1975
3. Rowland LP (ed): Merritt's Textbook of Neurology. 9th ed. Baltimore: Williams & Wilkins, 1995

ALPORT SYNDROME, hereditary nephropathy and progressive sensorineural hearing loss. (Arthur Alport, 1880-1959, South African)
1. Alport AC: Br Med J 1:504-506, 1927
2. Campbell MF, Walsh PC: Campbell's Urology. 5th ed. Philadelphia: WB Saunders, 1986

ALQUIÉ OPERATION, see Alexander operation.

ALSTRÖM SYNDROME, a distinct entity associated with retinal dystrophy and obesity. The affected patient usually becomes blind in early childhood and develops moderately severe deafness before the age of 10 years. Autosomal recessive inheritance. Cross-reference: Retino-otodiabetic syndrome. (Carl H. Alström, Swedish geneticist)
1. Alström CH, Hallgren B, Nielson LB, et al: Acta Psychiatr Neurol Scand 34 (Suppl 129):1-35, 1959
2. Campbell MF, Walsh PC: Campbell's Urology. 5th ed. Philadelphia: WB Saunders, 1986
3. Wilson JD, Foster DW, Kronenberg HM, et al (eds): Williams Textbook of Endocrinology. 9th ed. Philadelphia: WB Saunders, 1998

ALTAMIRA SYNDROME, hemorrhages of the skin preceded by low-grade fever subsequent to a bite by blackflies called *Simulium* in Brazil.
1. Pinheiro FP, et al: Hemorrhagic syndrome of Altamira. Lancet 1:639-642, 1974

ALVEOLAR CAPILLARY BLOCK SYNDROME, abnormalities of gas transfer resulting from thickening of the air-blood barrier by a pathological process that lengthens the pathway for diffusion of gases.
1. Bennett JC, Plum F (eds): Cecil Textbook of Medicine. 20th ed. Philadelphia: WB Saunders, 1996

ALZHEIMER DISEASE, classified as one of the presenile dementias; a disabling degenerative disease of the nervous system. Usually appears initially in the 5th and 6th decades of life. Onset is insidious and disease is usually fatal. (Alois Alzheimer, 1864-1915, German neurologist)
1. Alzheimer A: Zentralbl Nervenkheilkd 25:1134, 1906; 30:177-179, 1907
2. Alzheimer A: Zschr Ges Neurol Psychiatr 4:356-385, 1911
3. Rowland LP (ed): Merritt's Textbook of Neurology. 9th ed. Baltimore: Williams & Wilkins, 1995

AMENORRHEA-GALACTORRHEA SYNDROME, see Chiari-Frommel syndrome.

AMERICAN MOUNTAIN DISEASE, AMERICAN MOUNTAIN FEVER, see Colorado tick fever.

AMMON OPERATION, dacryocystotomy. (Friedrich von Ammon, 1799-1861, German ophthalmologist)
1. Maffei WE: Os Fundamentos da Medicina. 2nd ed. Livraria Editora Artes Medicas Ltd, 1978

AMNESIA SYNDROME, AMNESTIC SYNDROME, altered psychic states in which a memory defect is prominent.
1. Baker AB, Baker LH: Clinical Neurology. Revised ed. Philadelphia: Harper & Row, 1982

AMNIOTIC INFECTION SYNDROME OF BLANE, a syndrome of fetal sepsis following swallowing and/or aspiration of contaminated amniotic fluid.
1. Dorland's Medical Dictionary. 28th ed. Philadelphia: WB Saunders, 1994

AMOSS SIGN, painful flexion of the spine; when rising to a sitting position in a bed, the patient supports himself with his hands placed far behind him on the bed. Seen in vertebral tuberculosis. (Harold L. Amoss, 1886-1956, U.S.)
1. Evans RC: Illustrated Essentials in Orthopedic Physical Assessment. St Louis: Mosby Yearbook, 1994

AMUSSAT OPERATION, a transverse incision for exposing the colon. (Jean Z. Amussat, 1796-1856, French surgeon)
1. Maffei WE: Os Fundamentos da Medicina. 2nd ed. Livraria Editora Artes Medicas Ltd, 1978

ANAGNOSTAKIS OPERATION, surgery for correction of entropion through an incision parallel to the tarsus, with resection of the fibers of the orbicular muscle and suturing. Cross-reference: Holt operation. (Andrei Anagnostakis, Cretan ophthalmologist)
1. Maffei WE: Os Fundamentos da Medicina. 2nd ed. Livraria Editora Artes Medicas Ltd, 1978

ANDERMANN SYNDROME, dyskinesia of the corpus callosum with progressive neuropathy and mental retardation. Cross-reference: Charlevoix disease. (Frederick Andermann, Canadian)
1. Andermann F: Trans Am Neurol Assoc 97:242-244, 1972
2. Rowland LP (ed): Merritt's Textbook of Neurology. 9th ed. Baltimore: Williams & Wilkins, 1995

ANDERS DISEASE, adipogenic tuberoses. (James M. Anders, 1854-1936, U.S.)
1. Casas EC: Diccionario Terminologico de Ciencias Medicas. 5th ed. Salvat Editores, SA, 1954

ANDERSEN DISEASE, glycogen storage disease type IV; a branching enzyme disorder characterized by failure to thrive and progressive liver cirrhosis. Death from hepatic failure or gastrointestinal bleeding usually occurs before 4 years of age. (Dorothy H. Andersen, 1901-1963, U.S. pediatrician)
1. Andersen DH: Lab Invest 5:11-20, 1956

ANDERSEN TRIAD, see Clarke-Hadfield syndrome. (Dorothy H. Andersen)

ANDERSON OPERATION, widening of a tendon through a longitudinal incision and sliding of the sectioned surfaces.
1. Maffei WE: Os Fundamentos da Medicina. 2nd ed. Livraria Editora Artes Medicas Ltd, 1978

ANDERSON PHENOMENON, clumps of red blood cells are seen in the stools of amebic dysentery.
1. Dorland's Medical Dictionary. 28th ed. Philadelphia: WB Saunders, 1994

ANDERSON SYNDROME, familial osteodysplasia; an autosomal recessive syndrome consisting of characteristic facies, paddle-shaped feet, and bone abnormalities. (L.G. Anderson; U.S.)
1. Anderson LG, Cook AJ, Coccato PJ, et al: Familial osteodysplasia. JAMA 220:1687-1693, 1972
2. Gorlin RJ, Cohen MM Jr, Levin LS: Syndromes of the Head and Neck. 3rd ed. New York: Oxford University Press, 1990

ANDERSON-HYNES OPERATION, pyeloureteroplasty to achieve anastomosis (1949).
1. Campbell MF, Walsh PC: Campbell's Urology. 5th ed. Philadelphia: WB Saunders, 1986

ANDRAL SIGN, the patient tends to lie on the unaffected side; seen in the early stages of pleurisy. (Gabriel Andral, 1797-1876, French)
1. Casas EC: Diccionario Terminologico de Ciencias Medicas. 5th ed. Salvat Editores, SA, 1954

ANDRÉ THOMAS SIGN, the patient's arm rebounds if asked to raise one arm over the head and then let it fall suddenly; seen in the patient with cerebellar disease. Cross-reference: Pende sign. (André A.H. Thomas, 1867-1963, French neurologist)
1. Casas EC: Diccionario Terminologico de Ciencias Medicas. 5th ed. Salvat Editores, SA, 1954

ANDREWS DISEASE, pyoderma of the plantar region or palm of the hand. (George C. Andrews, U.S.)
1. Casas EC: Diccionario Terminologico de Ciencias Medicas. 5th ed. Salvat Editores, SA, 1954

ANDREWS OPERATION, surgery for hydrocele.
1. Maffei WE: Os Fundamentos da Medicina. 2nd ed. Livraria Editora Artes Medicas Ltd, 1978

ANDY CRUMP DEFORMITY, the most difficult head and neck cancer defect to reconstruct; maneuvers to avoid creating it include completely "degloving" the symphysis while leaving a 1-cm rim interiorly to support a myocutaneous flap.
1. Ballenger JJ: Diseases of the Nose, Throat, Ear, Head and Neck. 12th ed. Philadelphia: Lea & Febiger, 1977

ANEL OPERATION, 1) arterial ligature for the treatment of an aortic aneurysm; 2) dilatation of the lacrimal duct using an appropriate bougie. (Dominique Anel, 1679-1725, French surgeon)
1. Maffei WE: Os Fundamentos da Medicina. 2nd ed. Livraria Editora Artes Medicas Ltd, 1978

ANGELL SIGN, found in torsion of the testis. If the patient is examined standing, the unaffected testis is found to lie horizontally instead of in the normal vertical position. The sign is usually obscured on the affected side. Cross-reference: Gonda sign. (James C. Angell, British urologist)
1. Bailey H: Physical Signs in Clinical Surgery. 16th ed. Baltimore: Williams & Wilkins, 1983

ANGELMAN SYNDROME, facial hair, prognathism, midfacial retrusion, frequent extrusion of the tongue with drooling, and macrostomia are characteristics. Severe mental retardation with an IQ below 40, no speech, and delayed motor development are features as well as decreased muscular tone producing an awkward gait. Also exhibited is unprovoked and prolonged bursts of laughter. Cross-reference: Happy puppet syndrome. (Harry Angelman, British)

1. Angelman H: "Puppet" children. Dev Med Child Neurol 7:681-688, 1965
2. Baraitser M, Patton M, Lam STS, et al: The Angelman (happy puppet) syndrome: is it autosomal recessive? Clin Genet 3:323-330, 1987
3. Gorlin RJ, Cohen MM Jr, Levin LS: Syndromes of the Head and Neck. 3rd ed. New York: Oxford University Press, 1990
4. Knoll JH, Nicholls RD, Magenis RE, et al: Angelman and Prader-Willi syndromes share a common chromosome 15 deletion but differ in parental origin of the deletions. Am J Med Genet 32:285-290, 1989

ANGELUCCI SYNDROME, periodic allergic conjunctivitis; excitable temperament, rapid heart rate, and vasomotor disturbance in the patient with vernal conjunctivitis affecting young adults with allergic history in family. (Arnaldo Angelucci, 1854-1933, Italian ophthalmologist)

1. Angelucci A: D'una sindrome sconosciuta negli infermidicatarro Primaverile. Arch Ottol (Palermo) 5:270-267, 1897/98

ANGHELESCU SIGN, difficulty with flexion of the neck when the patient attempts to rest weight on the heels and occiput; an indication of spinal tuberculosis. (Constantin Anghelescu, 1869-1948, Romanian surgeon)

1. Casas EC: Diccionario Terminologico de Ciencias Medicas. 5th ed. Salvat Editores, SA, 1954

ANHIDROTIC ECTODERMAL DYSPLASIA SYNDROME, see Christ-Siemens-Touraine syndrome.

ANKYLOBLEPHARON-ECTODERMAL SYNDROME, see Hay-Wells syndrome.

ANNANDALE OPERATION, 1) resection of the femoral condyle for correction of genu valgus; 2) fixation of dislocated patellar cartilage by suturing.

1. Maffei WE: Os Fundamentos da Medicina. 2nd ed. Livraria Editora Artes Medicas Ltd, 1978

ANOREXIA-CACHEXIA SYNDROME, a systemic response to cancer manifested by malnutrition, weight loss, muscular weakness, acidosis, and toxemia.

1. Dorland's Medical Dictionary. 28th ed. Philadelphia: WB Saunders, 1994

ANOTHER SYNDROME, hypohidrotic ectodermal dysplasia, freckling, enteropathy, onychodystrophy, and hypothyroidism are features; pulmonary and upper respiratory infection due to a ciliary defect has been found.

1. Gorlin RJ, Cohen MM Jr, Levin LS: Syndromes of the Head and Neck. 3rd ed. New York: Oxford University Press, 1990

ANTALGIA SIGN, a patient with a disc protrusion or disc lesion assumes an antalgic, leaning gait.

1. Evans RC: Illustrated Essentials in Orthopedic Physical Assessment. St Louis: Mosby Yearbook, 1994

ANTERIOR ABDOMINAL WALL SYNDROME, unexplained continuous pain in the anterior abdominal wall, affecting any quadrant.

1. Dorland's Medical Dictionary. 28th ed. Philadelphia: WB Saunders, 1994

ANTERIOR CEREBELLAR SYNDROME, gait ataxia; disturbed gait and postural reflexes are characteristics. May appear in an early phase of olivopontocerebellar ataxia or may be caused by a tumor of the anterior lobe.

1. Baker AB, Baker LH: Clinical Neurology. Revised ed. Philadelphia: Harper & Row, 1982

ANTERIOR CHAMBER CLEAVAGE SYNDROME, see Rieger syndrome.

ANTERIOR CHEST WALL SYNDROME, see Prinzmetal angina.

ANTERIOR CORD SYNDROME, compression of the anterior column of the spinal cord or lesions of the anterior spinal artery; voluntary motor function and pain and temperature sensation are absent, but distal position senses, light touch, and vibratory sensation remain.

1. Bennett JC, Plum F (eds): Cecil Textbook of Medicine. 20th ed. Philadelphia: WB Saunders, 1996
2. Rowland LP (ed): Merritt's Textbook of Neurology. 9th ed. Baltimore: Williams & Wilkins, 1995

ANTERIOR CORNUAL SYNDROME, muscular atrophy due to lesions of the anterior horns of the spinal cord.

1. Dorland's Medical Dictionary. 28th ed. Philadelphia: WB Saunders, 1994

ANTERIOR DRAWER SIGN OF THE ANKLE, while pushing the tibia posteriorly and anteriorly drawing the calcaneus and talus, the talus slides anteriorly under the ankle mortise; an indication of anterior talofibular ligament instability.

1. Evans RC: Illustrated Essentials in Orthopedic Physical Assessment. St Louis: Mosby Yearbook, 1994

ANTERIOR DRAWER SIGN OF THE FOOT, with legs of the patient dangling and feet in plantar flexion, the examiner grips just above the ankle with one hand and the calcaneus in the other hand. The examiner then pushes the tibia posteriorly and the calcaneus is drawn anteriorly. Normally there is no other movement due to this action. When the talus slides anteriorly from under the ankle mortise, the sign is positive for anterior talofibular ligament instability.

1. Mazion JM: Illustrated Manual of Orthopedic Signs/Tests/Maneuvers for Office Procedure. 2nd ed. Orlando: Daniels Publishing, 1980

ANTERIOR ETHMOIDAL NERVE SYNDROME, believed to be due to injury of the nerve consequent to pressure from prolonged swelling of the nasal mucosa.

1. Haymaker W: Bing's Local Diagnosis in Neurological Diseases. 15th ed. St Louis: CV Mosby, 1969

ANTERIOR INFERIOR CEREBELLAR ARTERY SYNDROME, consists of ipsilateral deafness and incoordination.

1. Baker AB, Baker LH: Clinical Neurology. Revised ed. Philadelphia: Harper & Row, 1982

ANTERIOR INTEROSSEOUS NERVE SYNDROME, see Kiloh-Nevin syndrome.

ANTERIOR TIBIAL COMPARTMENT SYNDROME, traumatic necrosis of pretibial muscles; the muscle of one or both lower extremities becomes acutely swollen, painful, and paralyzed after vigorous exercise. Etiology unknown.

1. Campbell WC, Crenshaw AH: Campbell's Operative Orthopaedics. 7th ed. St Louis: CV Mosby, 1987
2. Farmer TW: Pediatric Neurology. 2nd ed. Hagerstown: Harper & Row, 1975

ANTICHOLINERGIC SYNDROME, anticholinergic intoxication; delirium, disorientation, or hallucination produced by overdosage or abnormal reaction to a clinical dosage of anticholinergic drugs.

1. Dorland's Medical Dictionary. 28th ed. Philadelphia: WB Saunders, 1994

ANTIMONGOLISM SYNDROME, associated with a partial deletion of the long arm of chromosome 21; round face and mental retardation are features.

1. Baker AB, Baker LH: Clinical Neurology. Revised ed. Philadelphia: Harper & Row, 1982

ANTLEY SYNDROME, ANTLEY-BIXLER SYNDROME, consists of craniosynostosis, dysplastic ears, arachnodactyly, radiohumeral synostosis, femoral bowing, and joint contractures. Autosomal recessive or sporadic inheritance. Cross-reference: Bixler-Antley syndrome. (Ray M. Antley, U.S. geneticist; David Bixler, U.S. dentist)

1. Antley R, Bixler D: Trapezoidocephaly, midfacial hypoplasia and cartilage abnormalities with multiple synostoses and skeletal fractures. Birth Defects 11(2):397-401, 1975
2. Bixler D, Antley RM: Familial aortic dissection with iris anomalies: a new connective tissue disease syndrome? Birth Defects 12(5):229-234, 1976
3. Gorlin RJ, Cohen MM Jr, Levin LS: Syndromes of the Head and Neck. 3rd ed. New York: Oxford University Press, 1990
4. Robinson LK, et al: The Antley-Bixler syndrome. J Pediatr 101:201-205, 1982

ANTON SYNDROME, ANTON-BABINSKI SYNDROME, denial of clinically demonstrable blindness; visual anosognosia associated with post cerebral artery infarction confabulation and allocheiria (reference of sensation to opposite site from stimulus application). (Gabriel Anton, 1858-1933, Austrian neurologist; Joseph F.F. Babinski, 1857-1932, French neurologist)

1. Anton G: Ueber die Selbstwahrnehmung der Herderkrankungen des Gehirns durch den Krauken bei Rindenblindheit und Rindentaubheit. Arch Psychiatr Nervenkr 32:86, 1899
2. Rowland LP (ed): Merritt's Textbook of Neurology. 9th ed. Baltimore: Williams & Wilkins, 1995

ANXIETY SYNDROME, ANXIETY NEUROSIS, term describing the physical symptoms that accompany anxiety, including heart palpitation, sweating, rapid and shallow respiration, pallor, and a panic disorder.

1. Dorland's Medical Dictionary. 28th ed. Philadelphia: WB Saunders, 1994

AORTIC ARCH SYNDROME, aortic arch arteritis or idiopathic aortopathy. Often called pulseless disease because involvement of the arch of the aorta can reduce the pulses in the arms or neck, although narrowing of the great arteries arising from the arch of the aorta sufficient to cause reduction in the pulse is more like to be due to atherosclerosis than to idiopathic aortopathy. Cross-references:

Martorell syndrome; Pulseless disease.

1. Haymaker W: Bing's Local Diagnosis in Neurological Diseases. 15th ed. St Louis: CV Mosby, 1969
2. Martorell F, Fabré Tersol J: Med Clin Barcelona 2:26-30, 1944
3. Nakao K, Ikeda M, Kimata S, et al: Takayasu's arteritis. Clinical report of eighty-four cases and immunological studies of seven cases. Circulation 35:1141-1155, 1967

AORTIC OCCLUSION SYNDROME, see Leriche syndrome.

APALLIC SYNDROME, a condition that may develop during recovery from a deep coma due to traumatic or nontraumatic acute brain damage. Patient is mute and immobile. Cross-references: Coma vigile syndrome; Kretschmer syndrome.

1. Kretschmer E: Das appallische Syndrome. Zschr Ges Neurol Psychiatr 169:576-579, 1940
2. Stanley J: Illustrated Dictionary of Eponymic Syndromes and Diseases and Their Synonyms. Philadelphia: WB Saunders, 1969

APERT SYNDROME, acrocephaly syndactyly type I; craniofacial abnormalities may accompany premature craniosynostosis. (Eugene Apert, 1868-1940, French pediatrician)

1. Apert E: De l'acrocephalosyndactyly. Bull Soc Med Hop (Par) 23:1310-1330, 1906
2. Baker AB, Baker LH: Clinical Neurology. Revised ed. Philadelphia: Harper & Row, 1982
3. Farmer TW: Pediatric Neurology. 2nd ed. Hagerstown: Harper & Row, 1975

APLEY TEST, with the patient lying on the stomach, the clinician stands on the side of the affected knee. Grasping the foot of the affected side with both hands, the physician flexes the knee to a right angle. Lateral rotation of the foot is performed; normally this should cause only slight discomfort. The clinician then places his/her knee on the patient's hamstring muscles and pulls the leg upward while performing lateral rotation. If on distraction, pain on rotation is produced, a lesion of the medial collateral ligament is diagnosed. The clinician then leans over the patient and repeats the test while his or her body weight compresses the tibial plateau onto the condyles of the femur. If lateral rotation with the addition of compression produces increased pain, then the grinding test is positive and a tear of the medial meniscus is diagnosed. To test the lateral meniscus a reverse test is performed, the foot being rotated medially instead of laterally.

1. Bailey H: Physical Signs in Clinical Surgery. 16th ed. Baltimore: Williams & Wilkins, 1983

APOSTOLI OPERATION, electrolysis of uterine fibromas.

1. Maffei WE: Os Fundamentos da Medicina. 2nd ed. Livraria Editora Artes Medicas Ltd, 1978

APPOLITO OPERATION, enterorrhaphy using uninterrupted suturing on a right angle.

1. Maffei WE: Os Fundamentos da Medicina. 2nd ed. Livraria Editora Artes Medicas Ltd, 1978

AQUEOUS-INFLUX PHENOMENON, clear liquid enters conjunctival or subconjunctival vessels; derived from an aqueous vein during compression of the recipient vessel via a glass rod. Cross-reference: Ascher positive glass-rod phenomenon.

1. Dorland's Medical Dictionary. 28th ed. Philadelphia: WB Saunders, 1994

ARAN-DUCHENNE SYNDROME, a spinal form of progressive muscular atrophy that most often begins in the small muscles of the hands. The process is usually symmetrical. (François A. Aran, 1817-1861, French; Guillaume B.A. Duchenne, 1806-1875, French neurologist)

1. Aran F: Recherchés sur une maladie non encore décrite du système musculaire (atrophie musculaire progressive). Arch Gen Med Paris (4th ser) 24:1-35, 172-214, 1850

ARBUTHNOT-LANE DISEASE, see Lane disease.

ARCE SIGN, a radiological sign in the patient with pneumothorax associated with lung tumor.

1. Casas EC: Diccionario Terminologico de Ciencias Medicas. 5th ed. Salvat Editores, SA, 1954

ARCHIBALD DISEASE, fever observed in the Sudan, caused by a micro-organism from the group *Bacillus cloacae.*

1. Casas EC: Diccionario Terminologico de Ciencias Medicas. 5th ed. Salvat Editores, SA, 1954

ARGENTAFFINOMA SYNDROME, see Carcinoid syndrome.

ARGYLL ROBERTSON PUPIL, small (1- to 2-mm), unequal, irregular pupils that are fixed to light and constrict to accommodation. The principal cause is tertiary neurosyphilis, although partial Argyll Robertson changes occur with diabetes and certain of the autonomic neuropathies. Cross-reference: Vincent sign. (Douglas Argyll Robertson, 1837-1909, Scottish ophthalmologist)

1. Argyll Robertson D: Bull Soc Fr Derm Syph 10:347-352, 1899
2. Grinker RR, Sahs AL: Neurology. 6th ed. Springfield: Charles C Thomas, 1969

ARIAS-STELLA PHENOMENON, swollen, vacuolated epithelial gland cells with large irregular and hyperchromic nuclei that give the endometrial epithelium a hobnail appearance; occurs in association with pregnancy, but examples have been encountered in patients taking oral contraceptives. (Janvier Arias-Stella, Peruvian pathologist)
   1. Gold JJ, Josimovich JB: Gynecologic Endocrinology. 3rd ed. New York: Plenum Medical, 1980

ARIES-PITANGUY OPERATION, surgery to reduce mild ptosis of the breast.
   1. Schwartz SI: Principles of Surgery. 4th ed. New York: McGraw-Hill, 1983

ARLT OPERATION, ARLT-JAESCHE OPERATION, surgery for correction of entropion; transplantation of ciliary bulbs from the eyelid edge in distichiasis. Name given to many operations for blepharoplasty, entropion, eye enucleation, and tarsorrhaphy. Cross-reference: Jaesche-Arlt operation. (Carl F. von Arlt, 1812-1887, Austrian ophthalmologist)
   1. Maffei WE: Os Fundamentos da Medicina. 2nd ed. Livraria Editora Artes Medicas Ltd, 1978

ARMANNI-EHRLICH DISEASE, hyaline degeneration of the Henle ansa cells in diabetes. (Luciano Armanni, 1839-1903, Italian pathologist)
   1. Casas EC: Diccionario Terminologico de Ciencias Medicas. 5th ed. Salvat Editores, SA, 1954

ARMENDARES SYNDROME, a heritable disorder consisting of growth hormone deficiency, craniosynostosis, retinitis pigmentosa, and other anomalies.
   1. Armendares S, Antillon F, Del Castillo EB: J Pediatr 85:872-873, 1974. Birth Defects 11:49-53, 1975
   2. Gorlin RJ, Cohen MM Jr, Levin LS: Syndromes of the Head and Neck. 3rd ed. New York: Oxford University Press, 1990

ARMSBY OPERATION, surgery for an inguinal hernia.
   1. Maffei WE: Os Fundamentos da Medicina. 2nd ed. Livraria Editora Artes Medicas Ltd, 1978

ARMSTRONG DISEASE, lymphocytic meningitis.
   1. Casas EC: Diccionario Terminologico de Ciencias Medicas. 5th ed. Salvat Editores, SA, 1954

ARNOLD NERVE REFLEX COUGH SYNDROME, a reflex cough that occurs following irritation of the external ear supplied by the Arnold nerve; this area is the posterior and inferior portions of the external auditory canal and the posterior half of the tympanic membrane.
   1. Dorland's Medical Dictionary. 28th ed. Philadelphia: WB Saunders, 1994

ARNOLD-CHIARI SYNDROME, a congenital anomaly characterized by downward displacement of the cerebellum through the foramen magnum of the skull and by caudal elongation of the medulla. Often associated with a small posterior fossa and a variety of neurological findings ranging from deafness to evidence of compression of medulla. Cross-reference: Chiari syndrome. (Julius Arnold, 1835-1915, German pathologist; Hans Chiari, 1851-1916, Austrian pathologist)
   1. Arnold J: Myelocyste. Transposition von Gewebskeimen und Sympodie. Beitr Pathol Anat Pathol 16:1-28, 1894
   2. Chiari H: Ueber Veranderungen des Kleinhirns, des Pons und der medulla oblongata in Folge von congenitaler Hydrocephalie des Grosshirns. Denkschr Akad Wissen Wien 63:71-116, 1895
   3. Grinker RR, Sahs AL: Neurology. 6th ed. Springfield: Charles C Thomas, 1966
   4. Krayenbühl HA, Yasargil MG: Cerebral Angiography. 2nd ed. Philadelphia: JB Lippincott, 1968

ARNOSS SIGN, the patient with meningismus cannot sit up with arms crossed in front of the chest. Cross-reference: Dreifuss sign.
   1. Pedro-Pons A: Patologia-y-Clinica Medicus. Salvat Editores, SA, 1952

ARNOUX SIGN, fetal cardiac murmur in the patient pregnant with twins.
   1. Casas EC: Diccionario Terminologico de Ciencias Medicas. 5th ed. Salvat Editores, SA, 1954

ARROYO SIGN, asthenocoria; lost or diminished pupillary reflex seen in the patient with hypoadrenalism. (Carlos F. Arroyo, 1892-1928, U.S.)
   1. Casas EC: Diccionario Terminologico de Ciencias Medicas. 5th ed. Salvat Editores, SA, 1954

ARRUGA OPERATION, dacryocystostomy.
   1. Maffei WE: Os Fundamentos da Medicina. 2nd ed. Livraria Editora Artes Medicas Ltd, 1978

ASCH OPERATION, surgery for correction of nasal septum deviation. (Morris Asch, 1833-1902, U.S. laryngologist)
   1. Maffei WE: Os Fundamentos da Medicina. 2nd ed. Livraria Editora Artes Medicas Ltd, 1978

ASCHER POSITIVE GLASS-ROD PHENOMENON, see Aqueous-influx phenomenon. (Karl W. Ascher, 1887-1971, Czech-born U.S. ophthalmologist)

ASCHER SYNDROME, progressive enlargement of the upper eyelid due to inflammation of the labial salivary glands within the first decade of life. (Karl W. Ascher)
1. Ascher KW: Blepharochalasis mit Struma und Doppellippe. Klin Monatsbl Augenheilkd 65:86-97, 1920
2. McKusick VA: Heritable Disorders of Connective Tissue. 4th ed. St Louis: CV Mosby, 1972
3. Moschella SL, Hurley HJ: Dermatology. 2nd ed. Philadelphia: WB Saunders, 1985

ASCHNER PHENOMENON, oculocardiac reflex; the pulse slows with pressure on the eyeball. An indication of cardiac vagus irritability. (Bernard Aschner, 1883-1960, Austrian gynecologist)
1. Dorland's Medical Dictionary. 28th ed. Philadelphia: WB Saunders, 1994

ASHERMAN SYNDROME, traumatic amenorrhea associated with postpartum endometritis or vigorous dilatation and curettage. (Joseph G. Asherman, 1885-1968, Israeli)
1. Asherman JG: Amenorrhea traumatica (atretica). J Obstet Gynaecol Br Emp 55:25-30, 1948
2. Gold JJ, Josimovich JB: Gynecologic Endocrinology. 3rd ed. New York: Plenum Medical, 1980
3. Kase NG, Weingold AB: Principles and Practice of Clinical Gynecology. New York: John Wiley & Sons, 1983

ASHERSON SYNDROME, dysphagia followed by coughing due to neuromuscular imbalance and achalasia of the cricopharyngeal sphincter with failure of relaxation of the cricopharyngeal muscle during the third stage of swallowing. Cross-reference: Cricopharyngeal achalasia syndrome. (N. Asherson, British)
1. Asherson N: Achalasia of the cricopharyngeal sphincter. J Laryngol Otol 64:747-758, 1950

ASHMAN PHENOMENON, aberrant ventricular beat ending a short cycle preceded by a longer cycle; most commonly seen with atrial fibrillation. (R. Ashman, U.S. physiologist)
1. Dorland's Medical Dictionary. 28th ed. Philadelphia: WB Saunders, 1994

ASKANAZY CELL, see Hürthle cell.

ASK-UPMARK KIDNEY, segmental atrophy arising in association with vesicoureteral reflux. (Erik Ask-Upmark, Swedish pathologist)
1. Ask-Upmark E: Acta Pathol Microbiol Scand 7:383-345, 1929
2. Campbell MF, Walsh PC: Campbell's Urology. 5th ed. Philadelphia: WB Saunders, 1986

ASPERGER SYNDROME, see Kanner syndrome.

ASPLENIA SYNDROME, see Ivemark syndrome.

ASSAM DISEASE, kala azar.
1. Casas EC: Diccionario Terminologico de Ciencias Medicas. 5th ed. Salvat Editores, SA, 1954

ATKINSON OPERATION, a block causing paralysis of the orbicularis muscle that intercepts the facial nerve fibers as they cross the zygomatic arch.
1. Spaeth GL: Ophthalmic Surgery. Principles and Practice. Philadelphia: WB Saunders, 1982

AUBERT PHENOMENON, an optical illusion; in a dark room, a bright vertical line tilts to one side when the patient's head tilts to the opposite side. (Hermann Aubert, 1826-1892, German physiologist)

AUENBRUGGER SIGN, epigastric distention seen in the patient with pericardial effusion. (Leopold J. von Auenbrugger, 1722-1809, Austrian)
1. Casas EC: Diccionario Terminologico de Ciencias Medicas. 5th ed. Salvat Editores, SA, 1954

AUJESZKY DISEASE, pseudorabies. (Aládár Aujeszky, 1869-1933, Hungarian pathologist)
1. Casas EC: Diccionario Terminologico de Ciencias Medicas. 5th ed. Salvat Editores, SA, 1954

AURALCEPHALOSYNDACTYLY SYNDROME, consists of craniosynostosis involving the coronal suture, unusual ears shaped like question marks, cutaneous syndactyly of the fourth and fifth toes, and a hearing deficit. Autosomal dominant inheritance.
1. Gorlin RJ, Cohen MM Jr, Levin LS: Syndromes of the Head and Neck. 3rd ed. New York: Oxford University Press, 1990

AURICULOTEMPORAL NERVE SYNDROME, see Frey syndrome.

AURO-DIGITAL-ANAL SYNDROME, consists of sensorineural hearing loss, bifid and/or triphalangeal thumbs, and either an imperforate or anteriorly placed anus. Autosomal dominant inheritance.
1. Gorlin RJ, Cohen MM Jr, Levin LS: Syndromes of the Head and Neck. 3rd ed. New York: Oxford University Press, 1990

AUSPITZ SIGN, when the scab of a papule is removed by scratching, a bloody spot is seen; occurs in the patient with syphilis.
1. Casas EC: Diccionario Terminologico de Ciencias Medicas. 5th ed. Salvat Editores, SA, 1954

AUSTIN FLINT DISEASE, hepatosplenomegaly, facial deformity, and ichthyosis are features. Aryl sulfatase deficiency A, B, and C. (Austin Flint, 1812-1886, U.S.)
1. Rosenberg S: Neuropediatria. Sarvier,1992

AUSTIN FLINT MURMUR, described as a blubbering murmur that may appear or become louder at the time of atrial systole and thus be confused with murmur of the mitral valve. (Austin Flint)
1. Cheitlin MD, Sokolow M: Clinical Cardiology. 5th ed. Norwalk, Conn: Appleton & Lange, 1993
2. Flint A: Am J Med Sci 44:29-54, 1862

AUSTIN SYNDROME, mucosulfatidosis; the features are those found in steroid sulfate sulfatase deficiency, mucopolysaccharidoses, and late infantile metachromatic leukodystrophy. Autosomal recessive inheritance.
1. Austin J: Studies in metachromatic leukodystrophy. XII. Multiple sulfatase deficiency. Arch Neurol 28:258-264, 1973
2. Gorlin RJ, Cohen MM Jr, Levin LS: Syndromes of the Head and Neck. 3rd ed. New York: Oxford University Press, 1990
3. Soong BW, Casamassima AC, Fink JK, et al: Multiple sulfatase deficiency. Neurology 38:1273-1275, 1988

AUSTRALIAN TICK TYPHUS, see Queensland tick typhus.

AUSTRIAN SYNDROME, a triad of pneumonia, meningitis, and endocarditis usually seen in the alcoholic. The patient is bacteremic and the prognosis is very grave; about 80% die despite treatment.
1. Austrian R: Random gleanings from a life with the pneumococcus. J Infect Dis 131:474-484, 1975
2. Bennett JC, Plum F (eds): Cecil Textbook of Medicine. 20th ed. Philadelphia: WB Saunders, 1996

AUTOERYTHROCYTE SENSITIZATION SYNDROME, see Gardner-Diamond syndrome.

AUTOKINETIC VISIBLE LIGHT PHENOMENON, the apparently spontaneous movement of a pinpoint source of light as seen by susceptible persons after gazing at it in a completely dark room.
1. Dorland's Medical Dictionary. 28th ed. Philadelphia: WB Saunders, 1994

AVELLIS SYNDROME, combined cranial nerve palsies characterized by vagus nerve paralysis with loss of pain and temperature sensation in the contralateral extremities. (Georg Avellis, 1864-1916, German otolaryngologist)
1. Avellis G: Berl Klin 40:1-26, 1891
2. Gorlin RJ, Cohen MM Jr, Levin LS: Syndromes of the Head and Neck. 3rd ed. New York: Oxford University Press, 1990
3. Grinker RR, Sahs AL: Neurology. 6th ed. Springfield: Charles C Thomas, 1966

AVIRAGNET SIGN, a white ring around syphilitic spots; seen in the patient with syphilis.
1. Casas EC: Diccionario Terminologico de Ciencias Medicas. 5th ed. Salvat Editores, SA, 1954

AXENFELD ANOMALY, AXENFELD SYNDROME, consists of glaucoma and the anomalous development of the corneoscleral trabecular meshwork and other angle structures. There is increased visibility of the Schwalbe line. (Theodor Axenfeld, 1867-1930, German ophthalmologist)
1. Axenfeld T: Embryotoxon corneae posterius. Berl Dtsch Ophthalmol Ges 42:301, 1920

AYALA DISEASE, congenital absence of the pectoralis major muscle.
1. Casas EC: Diccionario Terminologico de Ciencias Medicas. 5th ed. Salvat Editores, SA, 1954

AYERZA SYNDROME, AYERZA-ARILLAGA SYNDROME, cardiopathy nigra; erythremia characterized by chronic cyanosis, dyspnea, hypertrophy and spasm of the liver, hyperplasia of bone marrow, and sclerosis of the pulmonary artery. (Abel Ayerza, 1861-1918, Argentine; F.C. Arillaga, Argentine)
1. Ayerza L: Sem Med Buenos Aires 32:43-44, 1925

AZUA DISEASE, pyodermatitis with vegetations.
1. Casas EC: Diccionario Terminologico de Ciencias Medicas. 5th ed. Salvat Editores, SA, 1954

BAASTRUP DISEASE, pseudoarthrosis of a spinous process of the cervical spine causing pain in the shoulder. Cross-reference: Kissing spine disease. (Christian I. Baastrup, 1885-1950, Danish)
1. Baastrup C: Fortschr Roentgenstr 48:430-435, 1933

BABCOCK OPERATION, a technique for eradication of varicose veins by extirpation of the saphenous vein. (William Babcock, 1872-1963, U.S. surgeon)
1. Maffei WE: Os Fundamentos da Medicina. 2nd ed. Livraria Editora Artes Medicas Ltd, 1978

BABES SIGN, muscular rigidity caused by an abdominal aneurysm near the anterior spinal artery.
1. Casas EC: Diccionario Terminologico de Ciencias Medicas. 5th ed. Salvat Editores, SA, 1954

BABINSKI REFLEX, BABINSKI SIGN, a plantar reflex; stroking the sole of the foot results in dorsiflexion of the big toe and fanning of the other toes. A sign of a pyramidal tract lesion. (Joseph F.F. Babinski)

1. Farmer TW: Pediatric Neurology. 2nd ed. Hagerstown: Harper & Row, 1975
2. Grinker RR, Sahs AL: Neurology. 6th ed. Springfield: Charles C Thomas, 1966

BABINSKI REINFORCEMENT SIGN, when the patient is seated with the legs hanging free from the examining table, forceful pulling of the flexed fingers of one side against those of the other side is followed by extension of the leg on the paretic side. (Joseph F.F. Babinski, 1857-1932, French neurologist)

1. Baker AB, Baker LH: Clinical Neurology. Revised ed. Philadelphia: Harper & Row, 1982

BABINSKI SIGN OF TRUNK-THIGH, a combined flexion phenomenon; while lying recumbent with the legs abducted, the patient attempts to rise to a sitting position holding the arms crossed in front of the chest. Normally the legs remain motionless and the heels are kept down. With pyramidal hemiplegia, there is flexion of the thigh in association with flexion of the trunk. In paraplegia, both legs are raised. In hysteria, the normal leg is elevated or neither leg is raised. (Joseph F.F. Babinski)

1. Baker AB, Baker LH: Clinical Neurology. Revised ed. Philadelphia: Harper & Row, 1982

BABINSKI SYNDROME, BABINSKI-VAQUEZ SYNDROME, the association of cardiovascular disorders with chronic syphilitic meningitis, paralytic dementia, tabes dorsalis, and other late manifestations of syphilis. (Joseph F.F. Babinski)

1. Babinski JFF: Bull Soc Hop Paris 18:1121-1124, 1901

BABINSKI-FRÖHLICH SYNDROME, see Fröhlich syndrome. (Joseph F.F. Babinski; Alfred Fröhlich, 1871-1953, Austrian-born U.S. neurologist)

BABINSKI-NAGEOTTE SYNDROME, medullary paralysis; includes cerebellar hemiataxia with lateropulsion, nystagmus, and Horner syndrome on the same side as the lesion and hemiparesis and sensory loss of a variable nature on the contralateral side. (Joseph F.F. Babinski; Jean N. Nageotte, 1866-1948, French)

1. Babinski JFF, Nageotte J: Hémiasynergie, latéropulsion et myosis bulbaires avec hémianethésie et hémiplégie croisées. Rev Neurol 10:358-365, 1902
2. Baker AB, Baker LH: Clinical Neurology. Revised ed. Philadelphia: Harper & Row, 1982

BACCELLI SIGN, a "whisper" heard in the chest of a patient with pleural effusion. (Guido Baccelli, 1832-1916, Italian)

1. Dorland's Medical Dictionary. 28th ed. Philadelphia: WB Saunders, 1994

BACELLI OPERATION, introduction of a wire into an aneurysmal sac.

1. Maffei WE: Os Fundamentos da Medicina. 2nd ed. Livraria Editora Artes Medicas Ltd, 1978

BACHTIAROW SIGN, stroking downward along the radius with the thumb and index finger is followed by extension and slight abduction of the thumb. It has been said to indicate lesions of the pyramidal system, but there is evidence of reflex hyperactivity; this may suggest pyramidal tract involvement only if it is unilateral or associated with other reflex changes.

1. Baker AB, Baker LH: Clinical Neurology. Revised ed. Philadelphia: Harper & Row, 1982

BACILLUS CALMETTE-GUÉRIN, a preparation of killed or attenuated tubercle bacillus, introduced as a means of treating superficial bladder cancers by recruitment of immune response mechanisms. (Léon C.A. Calmette, 1863-1933, French bacteriologist; Camille Guérin, 1982-1961, French veterinarian)

1. Campbell MF, Walsh PC: Campbell's Urology. 5th ed. Philadelphia: WB Saunders, 1986

BACON OPERATION, laterolateral anastomosis between the colon and rectum in cases of rectal stenosis. (Harry E. Bacon, U.S. proctologist)

1. Maffei WE: Os Fundamentos da Medicina. 2nd ed. Livraria Editora Artes Medicas Ltd, 1978

BADAL OPERATION, dilaceration of the infratrochlear nerve for alleviation of pain in glaucoma.

1. Maffei WE: Os Fundamentos da Medicina. 2nd ed. Livraria Editora Artes Medicas Ltd, 1978

BADS SYNDROME, oculocutaneous albinism; *b*lack locks, oculocutaneous *a*lbinism, and *d*eafness of the *s*ensorineural type (BADS).

1. Dorland's Medical Dictionary. 28th ed. Philadelphia: WB Saunders, 1994

BAEHR-SCHIFFRIN SYNDROME, see Moschcowitz syndrome. (George Baehr, U.S.)

BAELZ DISEASE, papular formation on the lip mucosa. (Erwin von Baelz, 1849-1913, German)

1. Casas EC: Diccionario Terminologico de Ciencias Medicas. 5th ed. Salvat Editores, SA, 1954

BÄFVERSTEDT SYNDROME, lymphocytoma benigna cutis; a rare form of benign recurring tumor of the tent lymphoreticular tissue. (Bo Erik Bäfverstedt, Swedish)

1. Bäfverstedt BE: Acta Dermvener 24 (Suppl 11):1-202, 1943

BAILEY OPERATION, named for surgeon who was active in research on surgery of intracranial neoplasms and the more highly invasive gliomas associated with poor survival rates. (Percival Bailey, 1892-1973, U.S. neurosurgeon)

BAILLARGER SIGN, anisocoria; seen in general paresis. (Jules G.F. Baillarger, 1809-1890, French neurologist)

1. Baillarger JGF: Mem Acad R Med Paris 8:149-183, 1840

BAILLARGER SYNDROME, see Frey syndrome. (Jules G.F. Baillarger)

BAKER CYST, medial gastrocnemius bursitis; when a swelling in the popliteal space is situated centrally and the patient is over 40 years of age, the swelling is likely to be a Baker cyst, which sometimes is bilateral and is a pressure diverticulum of the synovial membrane through a hiatus in the capsule of the knee joint. (William M. Baker, 1839-1896, British surgeon)

1. Baker WM: St Bartholomews Hosp Rep 21:177-190, 1885
2. Lumley JS, Clain A: Hamilton Bailey's Demonstration of Physical Signs in Clinical Surgery. 18th ed. London: Butterworth-Heinemann, 1997

BAKER OPERATION, transverse cuneiform incision of the neck wall of the posterior uterus for treating uterus anteflexion.

1. Maffei WE: Os Fundamentos da Medicina. 2nd ed. Livraria Editora Artes Medicas Ltd, 1978

BAKODY SIGN, in the patient with cervical radicular pain, the patient places the hand of the affected side on top of the head, raising the elbow level with the head. The sign is positive when the radicular pain is lessened or relieved by this maneuver.

1. Evans RC: Illustrated Essentials in Orthopedic Physical Assessment. St Louis: Mosby Yearbook, 1994
2. Mazion JM: Illustrated Manual of Orthopedic Signs/Tests/Maneuvers for Office Procedure. 2nd ed. Orlando: Daniels Publishing, 1980

BALDWIN OPERATION, creation of an artificial vagina by transplantation of a portion of the ileum.

1. Maffei WE: Os Fundamentos da Medicina. 2nd ed. Livraria Editora Artes Medicas Ltd, 1978

BALDY OPERATION, BALDY-WEBSTER OPERATION, operation for retrodisplacement of the uterus. Cross-reference: Webster operation. (John M. Baldy, 1860-1934, U.S. gynecologist; John Webster, 1863-1950, U.S. gynecologist)

1. Maffei WE: Os Fundamentos da Medicina. 2nd ed. Livraria Editora Artes Medicas Ltd, 1978

BALFOUR DISEASE, chloroma. (George W. Balfour, 1822-1903, British)

1. Balfour GW: Br Med Surg J 43:319-325, 1935

BALINT SYNDROME, psychic paralysis of visual fixation, optic ataxia, and a disturbance of visual attention. (Rudolf Balint, 1874-1929, Hungarian neurologist and psychiatrist)

1. Balint R: Monatsschr Psych Neurol 25:51-81, 1909
2. Rowland LP (ed): Merritt's Textbook of Neurology. 9th ed. Baltimore: Williams & Wilkins, 1995

BALL OPERATION, 1) formation of an artificial anus by incision of the left semilunar line; 2) section of the sensitive nerves of the anal region for treating anal itching; 3) surgery for an inguinal hernia using obliteration, torsion, and fixation of the sac to the inguinal ring. (Sir Charles Ball, 1851-1916, Irish surgeon)

1. Maffei WE: Os Fundamentos da Medicina. 2nd ed. Livraria Editora Artes Medicas Ltd, 1978

BALLANCE OPERATION, facial-hypoglossal-accessory nerve anastomosis in facial paralysis. Cross-reference: Koerte-Ballance operation. (Charles A. Ballance, 1856-1936, British surgeon)

1. Maffei WE: Os Fundamentos da Medicina. 2nd ed. Livraria Editora Artes Medicas Ltd, 1978

BALLER-GEROLD SYNDROME, a syndrome of craniosynostosis and radial reduction defects, growth hormone deficiency, abnormal ears, palatal defects, imperforate or anteriorly placed anus, various skeletal defects, and other anomalies. Autosomal recessive inheritance. (Fredrich Baller, German; M. Gerold, German)

1. Baller F: Z Menschl Vererb Konstit Lehre 29:782-790, 1950
2. Gerold M: Zbl Chir 84:831-843, 1959
3. Volpe J: Neurology of the Newborn. Philadelphia: WB Saunders, 1995

BALLET SIGN, external ophthalmoplegia with normal pupils; suggests hysteria or external goiter. (Louis G. Ballet, 1853-1916, French neurologist)
1. Casas EC: Diccionario Terminologico de Ciencias Medicas. 5th ed. Salvat Editores, SA, 1954

BALLINGALL DISEASE, mycetoma or maduromycosis. Cross-reference: Madura foot disease. (Sir George Ballingall, 1780-1855, British)
1. Ballinghall G: Practical Observations on Fever, Dysentery, and Liver Complaints.... Edinburgh: Brown and Constable, 1818

BALÓ DISEASE, a variant of diffuse sclerosis; areas of demyelination are arranged concentrically, thus accounting for the term "encephalitis, periaxialis concentrica." (Jozsef Baló, Hungarian)
1. Baló J: Arch Psychiatr 98:457-461, 1933
2. Courville CB: Concentric sclerosis, in Vinken PJ, Bruyn GW (eds): Handbook of Clinical Neurology, Vol 9. Disorders of the Spinal Cord. New York: North-Holland, 1970, pp 437-451
3. Itoyama Y, Tateishi J, Kuroiwa Y: Atypical multiple sclerosis with concentric or lamellar demyelinated lesions: two Japanese patients studied post mortem. Ann Neurol 17:481-487, 1985

BAMATTER SYNDROME, geroderma osteodysplastica; a characteristic facies, hyperlaxity of the skin and joints, and growth retardation are features. (Fred Bamatter, Swiss)
1. Franceschetti A, Klein D, et al: Confin Neurol 9:397, 1949
2. Gorlin RJ, Cohen MM Jr, Levin LS: Syndromes of the Head and Neck. 3rd ed. New York: Oxford University Press, 1990
3. Patton MA, Tolmie J, Ruthnum P, et al: Congenital cutis laxa with retardation of growth and development. J Med Genet 24:556-561, 1987

BAMBERGER SIGN, an indication of pericardial effusion when scapular angle percussion becomes more tympanic. (Eugene Bamberger, 1853-1940, Austrian)
1. Casas EC: Diccionario Terminologico de Ciencias Medicas. 5th ed. Salvat Editores, SA, 1954

BAMBERGER-MARIE DISEASE, see Marie-Bamberger disease. (Eugene Bamberger; Pierre Marie)

BAMBLE DISEASE, epidemic diaphragmatic pleurodynia.
1. Casas EC: Diccionario Terminologico de Ciencias Medicas. 5th ed. Salvat Editores, SA, 1954

BANERJEE SIGN, when the toes are pointed down and the knee reflex is tested, the knee reflex is elicited and reinforcement is not necessary. (Timir Banerjee, b. 1943, U.S., neurosurgeon)

BANG DISEASE, infection with *Brucella*, which is transmissible to man and involves the reticuloendothelial system. Polyneuritis, encephalomyelitis, and aseptic meningitis caused by brucellosis. Cross-reference: Neapolitan fever. (Bernhard L.F. Bang, 1848-1932, Danish veterinarian)
1. Bang B: Zschr Tiermed 1:241-278, 1897
2. Moschella SL, Hurley HJ: Dermatology. 2nd ed. Philadelphia: WB Saunders, 1985

BANNAYAN-RILEY-RUVALCABA SYNDROME, BANNAYAN-ZONANA SYNDROME, familial megalencephaly with mesodermal hamartomas; symmetrical macrocephaly without ventricular enlargement, mild neurological dysfunction, growth retardation, and mesodermal hamartomas are present. Cross-reference: Riley-Smith syndrome. (George A. Bannayan, U.S.; Harris D. Riley, Jr., U.S. pediatrician; R.H. Ruvalcaba, U.S.)
1. Bannayan GA: Arch Pathol 92:1-5, 1971
2. Riley HD Jr, Smith WR: Pediatrics 526:293-300, 1960
3. Volpe J: Neurology of the Newborn. 3rd ed. Philadelphia: WB Saunders, 1995

BANNISTER DISEASE, angioneurotic edema. (Henry Bannister, 1844-1920, U.S.)
1. Bannister HM: J Nerve Ment Dis 21:627-631, 1894

BANNWARTH SYNDROME, a tick-transmitted meningopolyneuritis; manifestations include myeloradiculitis and facial paralysis. Cross-reference: Lyme disease. (Alfred Bannwarth, 1903-1970, German neurologist)
1. Ackermann R, et al: Tick-borne meningopolyneuritis (Garin-Bujadoux, Bannwarth). Yale J Biol Med 57:485-490, 1984
2. Bannwarth A: Arch Psychiatr Nervenkr 113:284-376, 1941
3. Rowland LP (ed): Merritt's Textbook of Neurology. 9th ed. Baltimore: Williams & Wilkins, 1995

BANTI SYNDROME, nonfamilial splenic anemia; portal hypertension with congestive splenomegaly and a patent portal vein are features. Liver biopsy may be normal. Cross-reference: Klemperer disease. (Guido Banti, 1852-1925, Italian pathologist)

1. Bennett JC, Plum F (eds): Cecil Textbook of Medicine. 20th ed. Philadelphia: WB Saunders, 1996
2. Ritchie AC: Boyd's Textbook of Pathology. 9th ed. Philadelphia: Lea & Febiger, 1990

BANTU HYPOKINETIC HEAT DISEASE, occurs in adults in Bantu, Africa, with a poor nutritional background, due to lack of essential amino acids and protein.

1. Bennett JC, Plum F (eds): Cecil Textbook of Medicine. 20th ed. Philadelphia: WB Saunders, 1996

BAPAT TEST, see Bed-shaking test.

BARACZ OPERATION, surgery to free the sciatic nerve from adherents in cases of chronic and persistent sciatic pain.

1. Maffei WE: Os Fundamentos da Medicina. 2nd ed. Livraria Editora Artes Medicas Ltd, 1978

BARAITSER SYNDROME, craniosynostosis involving the coronal suture, mental retardation, seizures, choroidal colobomas, mild hypertelorism, beaked nose, cleft lip/palate, protuberant ears, mild mesomelic shortening of the upper and lower extremities, short broad fingers, and cystic dysplastic kidneys. Presumed autosomal recessive inheritance.

1. Gorlin RJ, Cohen MM Jr, Levin LS: Syndromes of the Head and Neck. 3rd ed. New York: Oxford University Press, 1990

BÁRÁNY SIGN, when the head is moved, the entire body tends to veer to that side; a sign of vestibular dysfunction. (Robert Bárány, 1876-1936, Austrian)

1. Casas EC: Diccionario Terminologico de Ciencias Medicas. 5th ed. Salvat Editores, SA, 1954

BARBADOS DISEASE, Arabian elephantiasis.

1. Casas EC: Diccionario Terminologico de Ciencias Medicas. 5th ed. Salvat Editores, SA, 1954

BARCLAY SIGN, quick emptying of the stomach; a radiological sign of duodenal ulcer.

1. Casas EC: Diccionario Terminologico de Ciencias Medicas. 5th ed. Salvat Editores, SA, 1954

BARD SIGN, organic nystagmus where the oscillations of the eye increase as a target is moved. (Louis Bard, 1857-1930, French)

1. Casas EC: Diccionario Terminologico de Ciencias Medicas. 5th ed. Salvat Editores, SA, 1954

BARD-PIC SYNDROME, chronic jaundice with dilatation of the biliary tree in carcinoma of the pancreas. Cross-reference: Courvoisier syndrome. (Louis Bard; Adrien Pic, French)

1. Bard L, Pic A: Rev Med (Par) 8:257-282, 363-405, 1888

BARDENHEUER OPERATION, ligature of the brachiocephalic trunk with partial osseous resection.

1. Maffei WE: Os Fundamentos da Medicina. 2nd ed. Livraria Editora Artes Medicas Ltd, 1978

BARDET-BIEDL SYNDROME, see Laurence-Moon-Bardet-Biedl syndrome.

BARE LYMPHOCYTE SYNDROME, a rare immunodeficiency syndrome in which lymphocytes are devoid of surface HLA antigens at the A and B loci. The syndrome is clinically similar to the Nezelof syndrome; severe mucocutaneous candidiasis is often noted.

1. Moschella SL, Hurley HJ: Dermatology. 2nd ed. Philadelphia: WB Saunders, 1985

BARKAN OPERATION, goniotomy. (Otto Barkan, 1887-1958, U.S. ophthalmologist)

1. Maffei WE: Os Fundamentos da Medicina. 2nd ed. Livraria Editora Artes Medicas Ltd, 1978

BARKER OPERATION, 1) anterior resection of the hip joint; 2) resection of the astragalus through an incision from the lateral malleolus to the dorsum of the foot.

1. Maffei WE: Os Fundamentos da Medicina. 2nd ed. Livraria Editora Artes Medicas Ltd, 1978

BARLOW SYNDROME, see Mitral valve prolapse syndrome. (John Barlow, South African cardiologist)

BARME-BIRMANIA-BURMA DISEASE, see Tsutsugamushi disease.

BARNARD-SCHOLZ SYNDROME, see Kearns-Sayre syndrome.

BARON SIGN, in chronic appendicitis, pain on pressing the psoas muscle.

1. Casas EC: Diccionario Terminologico de Ciencias Medicas. 5th ed. Salvat Editores, SA, 1954

BARR OPERATION, see Mixter-Barr operation. (Jason S. Barr, U.S.)

BARRAQUER DISEASE, BARRAQUER-SIMONS DISEASE, progressive lipodystrophy of the face, arms, and upper half of the body, sometimes with excessive fat accumulation in the legs. Cross-reference: Morquio-Barraquer-Simons disease. (José A.R. Barraquer, 1855-1928, Spanish; Arthur Simons, German)

1. Barraquer J: Histoire Clinique d'un Case d'Atrophie du Tissue Cellulo-adipeux. Barcelona, 1906
2. Simons A: Eine seltene trophoneurosis (lipodystrophy progressiva). Zschr Ges Neurol Psychiatr 5:29-38, 1911

BARRAQUER OPERATION, phacoerysis. (Ignacio Barraquer, 1884-1965, Spanish ophthalmologist)
1. Maffei WE: Os Fundamentos da Medicina. 2nd ed. Livraria Editora Artes Medicas Ltd, 1978

BARRÉ PYRAMIDAL SIGN, the patient is unable to keep the legs flexed when in the prone position; an indication of a pyramidal lesion. (Jean A. Barré, 1880-1971, French neurologist)
1. Casas EC: Diccionario Terminologico de Ciencias Medicas. 5th ed. Salvat Editores, SA, 1954

BARRÉ SIGN, slow contraction of the iris in mental deterioration. (Jean A. Barré)
1. Casas EC: Diccionario Terminologico de Ciencias Medicas. 5th ed. Salvat Editores, SA, 1954

BARRÉ-LIÉOU SYNDROME, ischemic dysfunction of the brain stem caused by vertebral compression in cervical spondylosis. Buckling of the ipsilateral vertebral artery is indicated if the patient experiences vertigo, dizziness, visual disturbances, nausea, syncope, and nystagmus. (Jean A. Barré; Yong C. Liéou, French-Chinese)
1. Barré JA: Rev Neurol 1:1246-1248, 1926
2. Evans RC: Illustrated Essentials in Orthopedic Physical Assessment. St Louis: Mosby Yearbook, 1994

BARRETT SYNDROME, BARRETT ESOPHAGUS, ulcerative disease of the lower esophagus, often with stricture due to the presence of columnar-lined epithelium, which may contain functional mucous cells, parietal cells, or chief cells. (Norman Barrett, 1903-1979, British surgeon)
1. Barrett NR: Br J Surg 38:175-182, 1950

BARRY-PERKINS-YOUNG SYNDROME, see Young syndrome.

BART SYNDROME, epidermolysis bullosa dystrophica; characterized by congenital localized absence of the skin with blister formation as a result of mechanical trauma and nail dystrophy. Autosomal dominant inheritance. (Bruce J. Bart, U.S. dermatologist)
1. Bart BJ, Gorlin RJ, Anderson VE, et al: Congenital localized absence of skin and associated abnormalities resembling epidermolysis bulosa: a new syndrome. Arch Dermatol 93:296-304, 1966

BARTHÉLEMY DISEASE, bromide acne. (P. Toussant Barthélemy, French)
1. Barthélemy PT: Arch Derm Syph 2:2-38, 1891

BARTHOLIN DUCT, the sublingual gland is situated beneath the mucous membrane of the floor of the mouth, at the point where the frenulum of the tongue is in contact with sublingual depression on the inner surface of the mandible close to the symphysis. Has multiple excretory ducts; the larger one (Bartholin duct) opens into the submandibular duct. (Casper Bartholin, 1655-1738, Danish anatomist)
1. Ballenger JJ: Diseases of the Nose, Throat, Ear, Head and Neck. 12th ed. Philadelphia: Lea & Febiger, 1977
2. Lumley JS, Clain A: Hamilton Bailey's Demonstration of Physical Signs in Clinical Surgery. 18th ed. London: Butterworth-Heinemann, 1997

BARTON OPERATION, see Rhea Barton operation. (John Rhea Barton, 1794-1871, U.S. surgeon)

BARTTER SYNDROME, hypokalemic alkalosis; possibly due to a loop of Henlé defect that has not been elucidated, although this disorder appears to include profound salt wasting, potassium wasting, and compensatory hypertrophy of the juxtaglomerular apparatus with hyperreninemia and may be the result of a salt-absorption defect in the thick ascending limb of the loop of Henlé. (Frederick C. Bartter, 1919-1983, U.S.)
1. Bartter FC, Pronove P, Gill JR: Am J Med 33:811-828, 1962
2. Bennett JC, Plum F (eds): Cecil Textbook of Medicine. 20th ed. Philadelphia: WB Saunders, 1996
3. Ritchie AC: Boyd's Textbook of Pathology. 9th ed. Philadelphia: Lea & Febiger, 1990

BARUCH SIGN, an indication of typhoid fever if the patient maintains a high fever even following a bath with 24°C water.
1. Casas EC: Diccionario Terminologico de Ciencias Medicas. 5th ed. Salvat Editores, SA, 1954

BARWELL OPERATION, procedure for genu valgus.
1. Maffei WE: Os Fundamentos da Medicina. 2nd ed. Livraria Editora Artes Medicas Ltd, 1978

BASAL CELL NEVUS SYNDROME, characterized by the development of numerous basal cell carcinomas in early life, often associated with abnormalities of the skin, bone, nervous system, eyes, and reproductive tract. Autosomal dominant inheritance. Cross-references: Gorlin syndrome; Nevoid basal cell epithelioma syndrome.
1. Gorlin RJ, Cohen MM Jr: Syndromes of the Head and Neck. 3rd ed. New York: Oxford University Press, 1990
2. Gorlin RJ, Goltz RW: N Engl J Med 262:908-912, 1960

3. Smith DW, Jones KL: Recognizable Patterns of Human Malformation: Genetic, Embryologic, and Clinical Aspects. 3rd ed. Philadelphia: WB Saunders, 1982

BASAL CEREBELLAR SYNDROME, truncal ataxia with disturbed equilibrium; seen in diseases of the vestibular complex. Vestibular nystagmus is common.

1. Baker AB, Baker LH: Clinical Neurology. Revised ed. Philadelphia: Harper & Row, 1982

BASEDOW DISEASE, see Graves disease. (Karl A. von Basedow, 1799-1854, German)

BASEX SYNDROME, see Bazex syndrome.

BASIS PEDUNCULI SYNDROME, Weber syndrome caused by arterial occlusion. The lateral half or more of the basis pedunculi is supplied by branches of the circumferential arteries that arise from the posterior cerebral artery. At low midbrain levels, the superior cerebellar artery sends feeding arteries to this area; the field of irrigation includes the corticospinal tract.

1. Haymaker W: Bing's Local Diagnosis in Neurological Diseases. 15th ed. St Louis: CV Mosby, 1969

BASSEN-KORNZWEIG SYNDROME, abetalipoproteinemia; characterized by the complete absence of low and very low density lipoproteins and chylomicrons. The absence of the B protein appears to be accompanied by a virtually complete loss of triglyceride transport in the blood, resulting in malabsorption with steatorrhea, retinitis pigmentosa, and findings similar to Friedreich ataxia. Autosomal recessive inheritance. (Frank A. Bassen, U.S.; Abraham Kornzweig, U.S. ophthalmologist)

1. Bassen FA, Kornzweig AL: Blood 5:381-387, 1950
2. Fowler NO: Cardiac Diagnosis and Treatment. 3rd ed. Cambridge: Harper & Row, 1980
3. Rowland LP (ed): Merritt's Textbook of Neurology. 9th ed. Baltimore: Williams & Wilkins, 1995

BASSET OPERATION, resection of inguinal lymph nodes for treating vulval carcinoma.

1. Maffei WE: Os Fundamentos da Medicina. 2nd ed. Livraria Editora Artes Medicas Ltd, 1978

BASSETT OPERATION, a technique that uses an electromagnetic field to induce a weak electric current in bones by the application of external coils across a fracture site. (Antoine Bassett, 1882-1951, French surgeon)

1. Schwartz SI: Principles of Surgery. 4th ed. New York: McGraw-Hill, 1983

BASSINI OPERATION, plastic repair of an inguinal hernia; the cord lies on top of the repaired canal floor. (Edoardo Bassini, 1844-1924, Italian surgeon)

1. Maffei WE: Os Fundamentos da Medicina. 2nd ed. Livraria Editora Artes Medicas Ltd, 1978
2. Schwartz SI: Principles of Surgery. 4th ed. New York: McGraw-Hill, 1983

BASSLER SIGN, pain caused by compression of the appendix between the thumb and the iliac crest. (Anthony Bassler, 1874-1959, U.S.)

1. Casas EC: Diccionario Terminologico de Ciencias Medicas. 5th ed. Salvat Editores, SA, 1954

BASTEDO SIGN, pain is provoked in the right iliac crest fossa by insufflation of air in the colon; seen in chronic appendicitis. (Walter A. Bastedo, 1873-1952, U.S.)

1. Casas EC: Diccionario Terminologico de Ciencias Medicas. 5th ed. Salvat Editores, SA, 1954

BASTIAN SYNDROME, complete, acute transverse myelitis. (Henry C. Bastian, 1837-1915, British)

1. Pedro-Pons A: Patologia-y-Clinica Medicus. Salvat Editores, SA, 1952

BATEMAN DISEASE, molluscum contagiosum. (Thomas Bateman, 1778-1821, British)

1. Bateman T: Delineation of Cutaneous Diseases. London: Longman, 1817

BATTEN DISEASE, BATTEN-MAYOU DISEASE, late juvenile-type ceroid lipofuscinosis. Autosomal recessive trait inheritance in most patients. (Frederick E. Batten, 1865-1918, British ophthalmologist; Marmaduke S. Mayou, British)

1. Batten FE: Trans Ophthalmol Soc UK 23:386-390, 1903
2. Mayou MS: Trans Ophthalmol Soc UK 24:142-145, 1904

BATTERED CHILD SYNDROME, see Whiplash shake syndrome.

BATTEY OPERATION, oophorectomy.

1. Maffei WE: Os Fundamentos da Medicina. 2nd ed. Livraria Editora Artes Medicas Ltd, 1978

BATTLE OPERATION, appendectomy in which the rectus muscle is temporarily retracted. (William H. Battle, 1855-1936, British surgeon)

1. Maffei WE: Os Fundamentos da Medicina. 2nd ed. Livraria Editora Artes Medicas Ltd, 1978

BATTLE SIGN, ecchymosis over the mastoid process; an indication of a basal temporal fracture. (William H. Battle)

1. Farmer TW: Pediatric Neurology. 2nd ed. Hagerstown: Harper & Row, 1975

BAUDELOCQUE OPERATION, in extrauterine pregnancy, extirpation of the ovum by an incision through the posterior vaginal cul-de-sac. (Louis A. Baudelocque, 1800-1864, French obstetrician)

1. Maffei WE: Os Fundamentos da Medicina. 2nd ed. Livraria Editora Artes Medicas Ltd, 1978

BAUDRON DISEASE, post-hysterectomy decubitus ulcer.

1. Casas EC: Diccionario Terminologico de Ciencias Medicas. 5th ed. Salvat Editores, SA, 1954

BAUM OPERATION, lengthening of the facial nerve through an incision beneath the ear.

1. Maffei WE: Os Fundamentos da Medicina. 2nd ed. Livraria Editora Artes Medicas Ltd, 1978

BAUMÉS SIGN, retrosternal pain in angina pectoris.

1. Casas EC: Diccionario Terminologico de Ciencias Medicas. 5th ed. Salvat Editores, SA, 1954

BAYLE DISEASE, paralysis agitans or general paralysis of the insane caused by syphilis. (Antoine L.J. Bayle, 1799-1858, French)

1. Bayle ALJ: Recherchés sur la Maladie Mentale. Paris, 1822 (Thesis)
2. Pedro-Pons A: Patologia-y-Clinica Medicus. Salvat Editores, SA, 1952

BAZEX SYNDROME, acrokeratosis paraneoplastica; eczematous and psoriasiform lesions on the ears, nose, cheeks, hands, feet, and knees in a patient often associated with carcinomas of the upper respiratory and digestive tracts. Multiple "ice pick" marks affect the dorsum of hands and feet. (André Bazex [Basex], 1911-1988, French dermatologist)

1. Bazex A, Dupe A, Chirstol B: Bull Soc Fr Dermatol Syph 71:206, 1964
2. Moschella SL, Hurley HJ: Dermatology. 2nd ed. Philadelphia: WB Saunders, 1985

BAZIN DISEASE, erythema induratum. (Antoine P.E. Bazin, 1807-1878, French dermatologist)

1. Bazin APE: Leçons sur la Scrofule. Paris, 1861

BEALS SYNDROME, auriculo-osteodysplasia; joint contractures, "crumpled ear," and short stature are features. Autosomal dominant inheritance. (Rodney K. Beals, U.S. orthopedic surgeon)

1. Beals RK: Auriculo-osteodysplasia: a syndrome of multiple osseous dysplasia, ear anomaly, and short stature. J Bone Joint Surg (Am) 49:1541-1550, 1967
2. Smith DW, Jones KL: Recognizable Patterns of Human Malformation: Genetic, Embryologic, and Clinical Aspects. 3rd ed. Philadelphia: WB Saunders, 1982

BEAN SYNDROME, see Blue rubber bleb nevus syndrome.

BEARD DISEASE, nervous exhaustion; sometimes classified with neurasthenia. (George M. Beard, U.S.)

1. Beard GM: Bost Med Surg J 80:217-221, 1869
2. Pedro-Pons A: Patologia-y-Clinica Medicus. Salvat Editores, SA, 1952

BEARE-STEVENSON CUTIS GYRATUM SYNDROME, characterized by cutis gyratum, acanthosis nigricans, hypertelorism, cleft palate, bifid scrotum, large umbilical stump, and other anomalies. (J. Martin Beare, Irish)

1. Beare JM, Dodge JA, Nevin NC: Br J Dermatol 81:241-247, 1969
2. Gorlin RJ, Cohen MM Jr, Levin LS: Syndromes of the Head and Neck. 3rd ed. New York: Oxford University Press, 1990

BEARN-KÜNKEL SYNDROME, BEARN-KÜNKEL-SLATER SYNDROME, hepatitis associated with lupus; hirsutism, acne, hepatomegaly, and recurrent idiopathic fever are features. Cross-reference: Künkel syndrome. (Alexander G. Bearn, U.S.; Henry G. Künkel, 1916-1983, U.S.; Robert J. Slater, U.S. pediatrician)

1. Bearn AG, Künkel HG, Slater RJ: The problem of chronic liver disease in young women. Am J Med 21:3-15, 1956

BEATSON OPERATION, oophorectomy in cases of breast cancer.

1. Maffei WE: Os Fundamentos da Medicina. 2nd ed. Livraria Editora Artes Medicas Ltd, 1978

BEAU LINES, transverse grooves on fingernails and toenails that occur as a result of defective nail plate formation. Reported in association with a variety of infectious diseases, cardiopulmonary conditions, dermatitides, metabolic disorders, drug therapies, and traumatic disorders involving the extremities. First described by Johann C. Reil in 1792 and subsequently by Beau in 1846. (Honore S. Beau, 1806-1865, French)

1. Colvett KL, Patel D, Smith JK: Multiple Beau's lines in a patient with fever of unknown origin. South Med J 86:1424-1426, 1993

BEAU SYNDROME, cardiac insufficiency and asystole. (Honore S. Beau)

1. Beau HS: Arch Gen Med (Par), 1836, pp 425-427

BEAUVAIS DISEASE, chronic arthritis.
1. Casas EC: Diccionario Terminologico de Ciencias Medicas. 5th ed. Salvat Editores, SA, 1954

BECCARIA SIGN, pulsating pain in the occiput during pregnancy.
1. Casas EC: Diccionario Terminologico de Ciencias Medicas. 5th ed. Salvat Editores, SA, 1954

BECHTEREW DISEASE, see Marie-Strümpell spondylitis. (Vladimir M. von Bechterew, 1857-1927, Russian neurologist)

BECHTEREW SIGN, see Bekhterev sign. (Vladimir M. von Bechterew)

BECHTEREW SYNDROME, see Von Bechterew syndrome. (Vladimir M. von Bechterew)

BECHTEREW-MENDEL REFLEX, see Mendel reflex. (Vladimir M. von Bechterew)

BECK OPERATION, a one-stage (Beck I) or two-stage (Beck II) operation for supplying collateral circulation to the heart.
1. Maffei WE: Os Fundamentos da Medicina. 2nd ed. Livraria Editora Artes Medicas Ltd, 1978

BECK-KASHIN DISEASE, see Bek-Kashin disease.

BECKER MUSCULAR DYSTROPHY, manifestations are similar to those of Duchenne dystrophy, including an X-linked distribution pattern of nevus unius lateris and a tendency to favor the pectoral area. Usually appears in otherwise normal males in their teens or 20s as segmental, uniform, light tan hyperpigmentation. (Peter E. Becker, German geneticist)
1. Becker PE: Acta Psychiatr Neurol Scand 193:427, 1955

BECKER PHENOMENON, an increase in pulsation of the retinal arteries; seen in Graves disease. (Otto H.E. Becker, 1828-1890, German oculist)
1. Braunwald E: Heart Disease: A Textbook of Cardiovascular Medicine. 4th ed. Philadelphia: WB Saunders, 1992

BECKWITH SYNDROME, BECKWITH-WIEDEMANN SYNDROME, newborns exhibiting marked macrosomia, macroglossia, omphalocele, and hypoglycemia. Cross-references: Exomphalos-macroglossia-gigantism syndrome; Wiedemann-Beckwith syndrome. (John B. Beckwith, U.S. pediatrician/pathologist; Hans R. Wiedemann, German pediatrician)
1. Beckwith JB, Wang CI, Donnell GN, et al: Proceedings of the American Pediatrician Society. Seattle, 1964
2. Volpe J: Neurology of the Newborn. Philadelphia: WB Saunders, 1995
3. Wiedemann HR: J Hum Genet 13:223-363, 1964
4. Wilson JD, Foster DW, Kronenberg HM, et al (eds): Williams Textbook of Endocrinology. 9th ed. Philadelphia: WB Saunders, 1998

BÉCLARD SIGN, a radiological sign of a mature fetus; the center of ossification is recognized in the distal end of the femur. (Pierre A. Béclard, 1785-1825, French anatomist)
1. Casas EC: Diccionario Terminologico de Ciencias Medicas. 5th ed. Salvat Editores, SA, 1954

BED-SHAKING TEST, if doubt persists whether early peritonitis is present, shake the foot of the patient's bed. This causes pain at the site of the inflammation if pain is present. Cross-reference: Bapat test. (S.D. Bapat, Indian general practitioner)
1. Bailey H: Physical Signs in Clinical Surgery. 16th ed. Baltimore: Williams & Wilkins, 1983

BEER OPERATION, a flap method for cataract treatment. (Georg J. Beer, 1763-1821, Austrian ophthalmologist)
1. Maffei WE: Os Fundamentos da Medicina. 2nd ed. Livraria Editora Artes Medicas Ltd, 1978

BEEVOR SIGN, upward displacement of the umbilicus due to paralysis of the lower recti abdominis muscles. (Charles E. Beevor, 1854-1908, British neurologist)
1. Grinker RR, Sahs AL: Neurology. 6th ed. Springfield: Charles C Thomas, 1966
2. Pedro-Pons A: Patologia-y-Clinica Medicus. Salvat Editores, SA, 1952
3. Rowland LP (ed): Merritt's Textbook of Neurology. 9th ed. Baltimore: Williams & Wilkins, 1995

BEGBIE DISEASE, see Graves disease. (James Begbie, 1798-1869, Scottish)

BEHÇET DISEASE, an inflammatory disorder characterized by recurrent aphthous ulcers in the oral and genital areas and inflammatory disease of the eye. Common in northern Japan, Korea, China, and the Middle East, but rare in the U.S. Cause unknown, although a viral etiology is implicated. (Hulusi Behçet, 1889-1948, Turkish dermatologist)
1. Behçet H: Dermatol Wochenschr 104:1152-1157, 1937
2. Farmer TW: Pediatric Neurology. 2nd ed. Hagerstown: Harper & Row, 1975

3. Rowland LP (ed): Merritt's Textbook of Neurology. 9th ed. Baltimore: Williams & Wilkins, 1995

BEHIER-HARDY SIGN, when aphonia develops prior to gangrene of the lung.
    1. Casas EC: Diccionario Terminologico de Ciencias Medicas. 5th ed. Salvat Editores, SA, 1954

BEHR SIGN, a lesion in the optic tract causing contralateral pupillary dilatation. (Carl Behr, 1874-1943, German ophthalmologist)
    1. Bordas LB (ed): Neurologia Fundamental. 2nd ed. Barcelona: Ed. Toray, 1968

BEHR SYNDROME, see Pterygopalatine syndrome. (Carl Behr)

BEIGEL DISEASE, hysterical chorea. (Hermann Beigel, 1830-1879, German)
    1. Casas EC: Diccionario Terminologico de Ciencias Medicas. 5th ed. Salvat Editores, SA, 1954

BEK-KASHIN DISEASE, disabling degenerative disease of the peripheral joints and spine, endemic in eastern Siberia, northern China, and Korea; believed to be caused by ingestion of cereal grains infected with the fungus *Fusarium sporotrichiella*. Cross-reference: Kashin-Bek disease. (E.V. Beck [Bek], Russian; Nikolai Kashin, 1825-1872, Russian orthopedist)
    1. Casas EC: Diccionario Terminologico de Ciencias Medicas. 5th ed. Salvat Editores, SA, 1954

BEKHTEREV SIGN, see Bechterew sign. (Vladimir M. von Bechterew, 1857-1927, Russian neurologist)

BELFIELD OPERATION, vasectomy.
    1. Maffei WE: Os Fundamentos da Medicina. 2nd ed. Livraria Editora Artes Medicas Ltd, 1978

BELL PALSY, unilateral facial paralysis. (Sir Charles Bell, 1774-1842, Scottish surgeon/anatomist/ physiologist)
    1. Bell C: Philos Trans R Soc Lond 111:398-424, 1821

BELL PHENOMENON, when a patient with Bell's palsy attempts to close the eye on the affected side, the eye rolls upward and outward. Cross-reference: Bordier-Fränkel sign. (Sir Charles Bell)
    1. Bodechtel G: Diagnostico Diferencial de las Enfermedades Neurologicas. Madrid, 1967

BELSEY OPERATION, a transthoracic procedure that creates a segment of intra-abdominal esophagus held in place by a buttress of plicated stomach which surrounds approximately 280 degrees of the distal esophagus. (Ronald Belsey, British surgeon)
    1. Schwartz SI: Principles of Surgery. 4th ed. New York: McGraw-Hill, 1983

BELT-FUQUA OPERATION, two-stage repair and chordee release (orthoplasty; 1955, 1973)
    1. Campbell MF, Walsh PC: Campbell's Urology. 5th ed. Philadelphia: WB Saunders, 1986

BENCZE SYNDROME, mild facial asymmetry, esotropia, amblyopia, and submucous cleft palate are features. Autosomal dominant inheritance with variable expression. (J. Bencze, Hungarian)
    1. Bencze J, Schnitzler A, Walawska J, et al: Dominant inheritance of hemifacial hypoplasia associated with strabismus. Oral Surg 35:489-500, 1973
    2. Gorlin RJ, Cohen MM Jr, Levin LS: Syndromes of the Head and Neck. 3rd ed. New York: Oxford University Press, 1990
    3. Kurnit D, Hall JG, Shurtleff DB, et al: An autosomal dominantly inherited syndrome of facial asymmetry, esotropia, and amblyopia, and submucous cleft palate (Bencze syndrome). Clin Genet 16:301-304, 1979

BENEDIKT SYNDROME, tegmental mesencephalic paralysis; degeneration of the fibers of the 3rd cranial nerve and the tegmentum through which they course. The pyramidal tracts are spared, giving rise to paralysis of the ipsilateral extraocular muscles and to hyperkinesis of the contralateral limbs. In some instances there is also contralateral hemiataxia. Cross-reference: Tegmental syndrome. (Moritz Benedikt, 1835-1920, Austrian)
    1. Benedikt M: Tremblement avec paralysie crosiée du moteur oculaire common. Bull Med Par 3:547-548, 1889
    2. Grinker RR, Sahs AL: Neurology. 6th ed. Springfield: Charles C Thomas, 1966
    3. Haymaker W: Bing's Local Diagnosis in Neurological Diseases. 15th ed. St Louis: CV Mosby, 1969

BENNETT DISEASE, leukemia. (John H. Bennett, 1812-1875, British)
    1. Bennett JH: Edinb Med Sci J 64:413-423, 1845

BENNETT FRACTURE, an oblique fracture through the articular surface of the first metacarpal joint that allows subluxation of the joint. (Edward H. Bennett, 1837-1907, Irish surgeon)
    1. Bennett EH: Dublin J Med Sci 73:72, 1882

BENNETT OPERATION, surgery for a varicocele consisting of partial excision of the pampiniform plexus followed by suturing the cut endings.

1. Maffei WE: Os Fundamentos da Medicina. 2nd ed. Livraria Editora Artes Medicas Ltd, 1978

BENSON DISEASE, asteroid hyalitis. (Arthur H. Benson, 1852-1912, British ophthalmologist)
1. Benson AH: Trans Ophthalmol Soc UK 14:101-104, 1894

BENT OPERATION, resection of the shoulder joint and utilization of a flap from the deltoid muscle.
1. Maffei WE: Os Fundamentos da Medicina. 2nd ed. Livraria Editora Artes Medicas Ltd, 1978

BENZADON SIGN, squeezing the nipple causes retraction of the areola; a sign of breast cancer. (Austrian ophthalmologist)
1. Casas EC: Diccionario Terminologico de Ciencias Medicas. 5th ed. Salvat Editores, SA, 1954

BERANT SYNDROME, consists of craniosynostosis involving the sagittal suture and radioulnar synostosis. Autosomal dominant inheritance with variable expressivity likely.
1. Berant W, Berant N: J Pediatr 83:88-90, 1923
2. Gorlin RJ, Cohen MM Jr, Levin LS: Syndromes of the Head and Neck. 3rd ed. New York: Oxford University Press, 1990

BERARDINELLI SYNDROME, lipodystrophic diabetes; features include the generalized disappearance of body fat, an increased rate of skeletal growth, acanthosis nigricans, enlarged external genitalia, hepatomegaly, and insulin-resistant diabetes. Cross-references: Lawrence syndrome; Seip syndrome. (Waldemar Berardinelli, 1903-1956, Argentine)
1. Berardinelli W: An undiagnosed endocrinometabolic syndrome: report of 2 cases. J Clin Endocrinol Metab 14:193-204, 1954
2. Gorlin RJ, Cohen MM Jr, Levin LS: Syndromes of the Head and Neck. 3rd ed. New York: Oxford University Press, 1990
3. Seip M: Lipodystrophy and gigantism with associated endocrine manifestations. A new diencephalic syndrome? Acta Paediatr Scand 48:555-574, 1959

BERAUD SIGN, a tic involving constant touching of the genitals.
1. Casas EC: Diccionario Terminologico de Ciencias Medicas. 5th ed. Salvat Editores, SA, 1954

BERGARA-WARTENBERG SIGN, the diminution or absence of vibrations in the eyelid as the examiner attempts to open the closed eye against resistance. An early sign of facial palsy.
1. Baker AB, Baker LH: Clinical Neurology. Revised ed. Philadelphia: Harper & Row, 1982

BERGENHEIM OPERATION, implantation of the ureter in the rectum.
1. Maffei WE: Os Fundamentos da Medicina. 2nd ed. Livraria Editora Artes Medicas Ltd, 1978

BERGER DISEASE, immunoglobulin A nephropathy; typical presentation is recurrent gross hematuria after an upper respiratory tract infection or exercise. (Jean Berger, French nephrologist)
1. Berger J, Hinglais N: J Nephrol Paris 74:694-695, 1968
2. Haymaker W: Bing's Local Diagnosis in Neurological Diseases. 15th ed. St Louis: CV Mosby, 1969
3. Southwest Pediatric Nephrology Study Group: A multicenter study of IgA neuropathy in children. A report of the Southwest Pediatric Nephrology Study Group. Kidney Int 22:643-652, 1982

BERGER OPERATION, interscapulothoracic amputation. (Paul Berger, 1845-1908, French surgeon)
1. Maffei WE: Os Fundamentos da Medicina. 2nd ed. Livraria Editora Artes Medicas Ltd, 1978

BERGER SIGN, elliptical or otherwise irregularly shaped pupil in the early stages of tabes dorsalis. (Emil Berger, 1855-1926, Austrian ophthalmologist)
1. Casas EC: Diccionario Terminologico de Ciencias Medicas. 5th ed. Salvat Editores, SA, 1954

BERGERON DISEASE, electric chorea; a disease of childhood characterized by violent, but short, benign spasms. Cross-reference: Dubini disease.
1. Casas EC: Diccionario Terminologico de Ciencias Medicas. 5th ed. Salvat Editores, SA, 1954

BERGMAN SIGN, the ureter is dilated (not collapsed) just below a neoplasm, and the ureteral catheter coils in this portion of the ureter. (Harry Bergman, U.S. urologist)
1. Dorland's Medical Dictionary. 28th ed. Philadelphia: WB Saunders, 1994

BERI-BERI SYNDROME, the most common nutritional deficiency disease in the world related to vitamin B1 deficiency presenting as polyneuropathy, cardiac disease, and/or edema of the lower extremities. (Singhalese for "I cannot"—a person too ill to do anything.)
1. Bennett JC, Plum F (eds): Cecil Textbook of Medicine. 20th ed. Philadelphia: WB Saunders, 1996

BERLIN DISEASE, retinal traumatic edema. (Rudolph Berlin, 1833-1897, German ophthalmologist)
1. Berlin R: Klin Mbl Augenheilkd 11:43-78, 1873

BERMAN SYNDROME, mucolipidosis type IV; a rare lysosomal storage disease characterized by bilateral corneal opacities in infancy, full facial features, and progressive psychomotor retardation. About one half of patients are Jews of Ashkenazi origin, probably from southern Poland. Autosomal recessive inheritance.

1. Gorlin RJ, Cohen MM Jr, Levin LS: Syndromes of the Head and Neck. 3rd ed. New York, NY: Oxford University Press, 1990
2. Lake BD, Milla PJ, Taylor DS, et al: A mild variant of mucolipidosis type 4 (MLA4). Birth Defects 18:391-404, 1982

BERNARD-HORNER SYNDROME, see Horner syndrome. (Claude Bernard, 1813-1878, French physiologist; Johann F. Horner, 1831-1886, Swiss ophthalmologist)

BERNARD-SERGENT SYNDROME, diarrhea, vomiting, and collapse associated with Addison disease. (Claude Bernard; Emile Sergent, 1867-1943, French)

1. Casas EC: Diccionario Terminologico de Ciencias Medicas. 5th ed. Salvat Editores, SA, 19

BERNARD-SOULIER SYNDROME, a rare, inherited bleeding disorder of unusual severity, transmitted as an autosomal recessive trait and characterized by the presence of platelets with an unusually wide variation in size and morphology. Cross-reference: Giant platelet syndrome. (Jean B. Bernard, French; Jean P. Soulier, French hematologist)

1. Bennett JC, Plum F (eds): Cecil Textbook of Medicine. 20th ed. Philadelphia: WB Saunders, 1996
2. Bernard J, Soulier JP: Bull Mem Soc Med Hop (Par) 64:969-974, 1948
3. Ritchie AC: Boyd's Textbook of Pathology. 9th ed. Philadelphia: Lea & Febiger, 1990

BERNHARDT SIGN, paresthetica meralgia. (Martin B. Bernhardt, 1844-1915, German neurologist)

1. Casas EC: Diccionario Terminologico de Ciencias Medicas. 5th ed. Salvat Editores, SA, 1954

BERNHARDT SYNDROME, BERNHARDT-ROTH [ROT] SYNDROME, paresthetica meralgia. (Martin B. Bernhardt; Vladimir K. Roth [Rot], 1848-1916, Russian neurologist)

1. Bernhardt M: Paraesthesien. Neurol Centralbl 14:242-244, 1895
2. Dyck PJ: Peripheral Neuropathy. 3rd ed. Philadelphia: WB Saunders, 1993
3. Roth VK: Neurol Zbl 28:1126-1127, 1909

BERNHEIM SYNDROME, progressive insufficiency of the right ventricle with a hypertrophied left ventricle. (Hippolyte Bernheim, 1837-1919, French)

1. Bernheim H: Rev Med (Par) 30:785-800, 1910

BERRY SIGN, when the thyroid gland enlarges, it displaces the carotid tree posteriorly and distally. Consequently, in many cases of large goiter the pulsation of the carotid artery can be felt behind the posterior edge of the swelling. (Sir James Berry, 1860-1946, British surgeon)

1. Bailey H: Physical Signs in Clinical Surgery. 16th ed. Baltimore: Williams & Wilkins, 1983

BERRY-DEDRICK PHENOMENON, the transformation of fibroma viruses into myxoma viruses.

BERTOLOTTI SYNDROME, sacralization of the 5th lumbar vertebra with sciatica and scoliosis. (Mario Bertolotti, Italian)

1. Bertolotti M: Les syndromes lombo-ischialgiques d'origine vertebrale. Rev Neurol 29:1125, 1922

BESNIER-BOECK-SCHAUMANN DISEASE, sarcoidosis; a generalized disease of unknown etiology, perhaps infectious, that is characterized by the development of small nodules (follicles or tubercles). Numerous clinical syndromes result, depending on the organ involved in the granulomatous process. Cross-reference: Boeck sarcoidosis. (Ernest Besnier, 1831-1909, French dermatologist; Caesar P.M. Boeck, 1845-1917, Norwegian dermatologist; Jörgen Schaumann, 1879-1953, Swedish)

1. Besnier E: Ann Derm Syph 10:333-336, 1889
2. Delaney P: Neurologic manifestations in sarcoidosis. Review of the literature, with a report of 23 cases. Ann Intern Med 87:336-345, 1977
3. Jabs DA, Johns CJ: Ocular involvement in chronic sarcoidosis. Am J Ophthalmol 102:297-301, 1986

BESPALOFL SIGN, otitis and nasal catarrh at the onset of measles.

1. Casas EC: Diccionario Terminologico de Ciencias Medicas. 5th ed. Salvat Editores, SA, 1954

BEST DISEASE, atrophic degeneration of the macula in children. (Franz Best, 1878-1920, German pathologist)

1. Best F: Zschr Augenheilkd 13:199-212, 1905

BEST OPERATION, subcutaneous suture of the inguinal ring in a case of hernia.

1. Maffei WE: Os Fundamentos da Medicina. 2nd ed. Livraria Editora Artes Medicas Ltd, 1978

BETHEA SIGN, a test to distinguish dysfunction of lung expansion by standing behind the patient and placing the examiner's thumb under the patient's, while the patient's arms are elevated behind the head. (Oscar W. Bethea, 1878-1963, U.S.)

1. Casas EC: Diccionario Terminologico de Ciencias Medicas. 5th ed. Salvat Editores, SA, 1954

BEUERMANN DISEASE, disseminated sporotrichosis. Cross-reference: Schenck disease. (Charles L. de Beuermann, 1851-1923, French)

1. De Beuermann CL, Gougerot H: Les Sporotrichoses. Paris, 1912
2. Schenck BR: Bull Johns Hopkins Hosp 9:286-290, 1898

BEUTTNER OPERATION, resection of the fundus of the uterus together with bilateral salpingostomy.

1. Maffei WE: Os Fundamentos da Medicina. 2nd ed. Livraria Editora Artes Medicas Ltd, 1978

BEVAN OPERATION, fixation of an ectopic testis to the scrotum. (Arthur Bevan, 1861-1943, U.S. surgeon)

1. Maffei WE: Os Fundamentos da Medicina. 2nd ed. Livraria Editora Artes Medicas Ltd, 1978

BEYEA OPERATION, gastroplication.

1. Maffei WE: Os Fundamentos da Medicina. 2nd ed. Livraria Editora Artes Medicas Ltd, 1978

BEZOLD SIGN, inflammatory swelling below the apex of the mastoid process; an indication of mastoiditis. (Friedrich Bezold, 1842-1908, German otologist)

1. Dorland's Medical Dictionary. 28th ed. Philadelphia: WB Saunders, 1994

BHATTACHARYA-CONNOR SYDROME, features include tendon xanthomas, xanthelasma, recurrent arthralgia, hemolytic anemia, and atherosclerosis owing to increased absorption of sitosterol and accumulation in tissues.

1. Bhattacharya AK, Connor WE: Sitosterolemia and xanthomatosis: a newly described lipid storage disease in two sisters. J Clin Invest 53:1033-1043, 1974

BIANCHI SYNDROME, the combination of aphasia, apraxia, alexia, and right hand and foot hemianesthesia in lesions of the right parietal lobe. (Leonard Bianchi, 1848-1927, Italian psychiatrist)

1. Bianchi L: Med Ital 9:187, 1911

BIBER-HAAB-DIMMER SYNDROME, see Meretoja syndrome.

BICIPITAL SYNDROME, dislocation of the biceps tendon.

1. Campbell WC, Crenshaw AH: Campbell's Operative Orthopaedics. 7th ed. St Louis: CV Mosby, 1987
2. Gilcreest EL: Dislocation and elongation of the long head of the biceps brachii. An analysis of six cases. Ann Surg 104:118-138, 1936

BICKERS-ADAMS DISEASE, a hereditary syndrome characterized by hydrocephalus, mental retardation, and thumbs opposed. Occurs in males only. (D.S. Bickers, U.S.; R.D. Adams, U.S.)

1. Bickers DS, Adams RD: Brain 72:246-262, 1949

BIEDERMAN SIGN, molar discoloration in the patient with syphilis. (Joseph Biederman, U.S.)

1. Casas EC: Diccionario Terminologico de Ciencias Medicas. 5th ed. Salvat Editores, SA, 1954

BIEG SIGN, if the patient can hear with "acoustic trump," an indication of disease of the malleus.

1. Casas EC: Diccionario Terminologico de Ciencias Medicas. 5th ed. Salvat Editores, SA, 1954

BIELSCHOWSKY DISEASE, BIELSCHOWSKY-JANSKY DISEASE, gangliosidosis G_{M2} type III or late infantile amaurotic idiocy; a glycogen storage disorder in which the patient presents between the ages of 2-1/2 and 4 years with generalized seizures. This is followed by atypical absence and akinetic spells. Myoclonus appears within a few months, beginning as spontaneous asymmetrical segmental myoclonus; death usually occurs by ages 4 to 8. Cross-reference: Jansky-Bielschowsky disease. (Max Bielschowsky, 1869-1940, German neuropathologist; Jan Jansky, 1873-1921, Czech)

1. Bielschowsky M: Dtsch Zschr Nervenheilkd 50:7-29, 1914
2. Rowland LP (ed): Merritt's Textbook of Neurology. 9th ed. Baltimore: Williams & Wilkins, 1995

BIELSCHOWSKY-LUTZ-COGAN SYNDROME, internuclear ophthalmoplegia. Cross-reference: Unilateral internuclear ophthalmoplegia syndrome. (Alfred Bielschowsky, 1871-1940, German ophthalmogist; Adolfo Lutz, 1855-1940, Brazilian; David G. Cogan, U.S. neuro-ophthalmologist)

1. Bielschowsky A: Berl Dtsch Ophthalmol Ges 30:164-171, 1902
2. Bordas LB (ed): Neurologia Fundamental. 2nd ed. Barcelona: Ed. Toray, 1968
3. Cogan DG, Kuoik GS, Smith L: Unilateral internuclear ophthalmoplegia: report of eight clinical cases with one postmortem study. Arch Ophthalmol 44:783-796, 1950
4. Lutz A: Graefes Arch Ophthalmol 115:692-717, 1924

BIEMOND SYNDROME, a syndrome identified by the features of iris coloboma, obesity, mental insufficiency, postaxial polydactyly, and hypogonadism. An autosomal recessive disorder. (A. Biemond, French)
  1. Biemond A: Het Syndroom van Lawrence-Biedle en een aarverwant, nieuw syndroom. Ned Tijdschr Geneeskd 78:1801-1834, 1934
  2. Rowland LP (ed): Merritt's Textbook of Neurology. 9th ed. Baltimore: Williams & Wilkins, 1995

BIERMER-ADDISON-CASTLE DISEASE, pernicious anemia; a gastric disease associated with intrinsic factor deficiency leading to deficiency of vitamin B12. Cross-reference: Addison-Biermer syndrome. (Anton Biermer, 1827-1892, German; Thomas Addison, 1793-1860, British)
  1. Addison T: Lond Hosp Gaz 43:517-518, 1849
  2. Biermer A: Korresp Bl Schweiz Arzt 2:15-18, 1872

BIERMER-GERHARDT SIGN, 1) a change in the percussion sound of the chest; seen in the patient with hydropneumothorax; 2) an aortic artery aneurysm causing fixation of the larynx and dyspnea. Cross-reference: Gerhardt sign. (Anton Biermer; Carl A.C.J. Gerhardt, 1833-1902, German)
  1. Casas EC: Diccionario Terminologico de Ciencias Medicas. 5th ed. Salvat Editores, SA, 1954

BIERNACKI SIGN, 1) the absence of pain on squeezing or pressing the ulnar nerve in the olecranon fossa; 2) anesthesia of the ulnar nerve in syphilis. (Edmund A. Biernacki, 1866-1912, Polish pathologist)
  1. Pedro-Pons A: Patologia-y-Clinica Medicus. Salvat Editores, SA, 1952
  2. Grinker RR, Sahs AL: Neurology. 6th ed. Springfield: Charles C Thomas, 1966

BIGELOW OPERATION, lithotripsy. (Henry Bigelow, 1818-1890, U.S. surgeon)
  1. Maffei WE: Os Fundamentos da Medicina. 2nd ed. Livraria Editora Artes Medicas Ltd, 1978

BIKELE SIGN, with the patient seated, the forearm is flexed at the elbow and the arm is abducted, elevated, extended, and externally rotated, or it is moved upward and backward at the shoulder to a maximum degree. The examiner then attempts to passively extend the forearm at the elbow. Similar to the Kernig sign in that it is positive when irritated nerve roots are stretched.
  1. Baker AB, Baker LH: Clinical Neurology. Revised ed. Philadelphia: Harper & Row, 1982

BILLROTH DISEASE, false meningocele; the accumulation of cerebrospinal fluid under the scalp. Associated with skull fracture and arachnoid tear. (C.A. Theodor Billroth, 1829-1894, Austrian surgeon)
  1. Billroth CAT: Arch Klin Chir Berl 3:398-412, 1862

BILLROTH OPERATION, partial resection of the stomach with anastomosis to the duodenum (Billroth I) or to the jejunum (Billroth II). (C.A. Theodor Billroth)
  1. Maffei WE: Os Fundamentos da Medicina. 2nd ed. Livraria Editora Artes Medicas Ltd, 1978

BINDA SIGN, a sudden movement of the shoulder when the head is firmly turned in the opposite direction; an indication of tuberculous meningitis. (Luigi Binda, Italian)
  1. Pedro-Pons A: Patologia-y-Clinica Medicus. Salvat Editores, SA, 1952

BINDER SYNDROME, facies scaphoidea or maxillonasal dysplasia; a form of rhinencephaly. Cervical vertebral anomalies, skeletal defects, cardiac anomalies, orofacial clefting, strabismus, mental retardation, and other abnormalities are features. Cross-reference: Congenital flat nose syndrome. (K.H. Binder, German dentist)
  1. Binder KH: Dtsch Zschr 17:438-444, 1962
  2. Gorlin RJ, Cohen MM Jr, Levin LS: Syndromes of the Head and Neck. 3rd ed. New York: Oxford University Press, 1990

BING-SIEBENMANN DISEASE, congenital hereditary hearing loss; the bony labyrinth is well formed but the membrane labyrinth is not.
  1. Ballenger JJ: Diseases of the Nose, Throat, Ear, Head and Neck. 12th ed. Philadelphia: Lea & Febiger, 1977

BINSWANGER DISEASE, presenile dementia; chronic progressive subcortical encephalopathy that appears in the 5th and 6th decades. Memory and judgment deteriorate and abnormal psychic symptoms appear. (Otto L. Binswanger, 1852-1929, German neurologist)
  1. Binswanger OL: Berl Klin Wochenschr 31:1103-1105, 1894
  2. Rowland LP (ed): Merritt's Textbook of Neurology. 9th ed. Baltimore: Williams & Wilkins, 1995

BIOT SIGN, abrupt and irregular respiration in the patient with meningitis. (Camille Biot, French)
  1. Casas EC: Diccionario Terminologico de Ciencias Medicas. 5th ed. Salvat Editores, SA, 1954

BIRCHER OPERATION, suturing the anterior wall of the stomach to the posterior wall in cases of

stomach dilation.
   1. Maffei WE: Os Fundamentos da Medicina. 2nd ed. Livraria Editora Artes Medicas Ltd, 1978

BIRD SIGN, an area of absence of sound on auscultation in a hydatid cyst. Cross-reference: Duncan-Bird sign. (Samuel D. Bird, 1832-1904, Australian)
   1. Casas EC: Diccionario Terminologico de Ciencias Medicas. 5th ed. Salvat Editores, SA, 1954

BISSELL OPERATION, ablation of a part of the teres uteri and the ligamentum latum uteri in cases of uterine retroversion.
   1. Maffei WE: Os Fundamentos da Medicina. 2nd ed. Livraria Editora Artes Medicas Ltd, 1978

BIXLER SYNDROME, see Hypertelorism-microtia-clefting syndrome.

BIXLER-ANTLEY SYNDROME, see Antley syndrome.

BJERRUM SIGN, a semilunar-shaped scotoma near a blind spot; occurs in glaucoma. (Jannik P. Bjerrum, 1827-1892, Danish ophthalmologist)
   1. Casas EC: Diccionario Terminologico de Ciencias Medicas. 5th ed. Salvat Editores, SA, 1954

BJÖRNSTAD SYNDROME, BJÖRNSTAD-CRANDALL SYNDROME, identified by findings of congenital sensorineural deafness and pili torti. An autosomal recessive disorder. Cross-reference: Crandall syndrome. (R. Björnstad, Swedish)
   1. Crandall BF, et al: A familial syndrome of deafness, alopecia and hypogonadism. J Pediatr 82:461-465, 1973

BK MOLE SYNDROME, characterized by myriad heritable melanocytic nevi and a grave risk of multiple primary melanomas. Cross-reference: Dysplastic nevus syndrome.
   1. Bennett JC, Plum F (eds): Cecil Textbook of Medicine. 20th ed. Philadelphia: WB Saunders, 1996

BLACKFAN-DIAMOND SYNDROME, see Aase-Smith syndrome II. (Kenneth Blackfan, 1883-1941, U.S.; Louis Diamond, U.S.)

BLACKWATER FEVER, see Uriolla sign.

BLALOCK OPERATION, subclavian-pulmonary artery anastomosis; occurs more frequently in older children with cardiac malformations. (Alfred Blalock, 1899-1965, U.S. surgeon)
   1. Schwartz SI: Principles of Surgery. 4th ed. New York: McGraw-Hill, 1983

BLALOCK-HANLON OPERATION, a technique for treating cardiac enlargement or congestive heart failure which creates an atrial septal defect. (Alfred Blalock; C. Rollins Hanlon, U.S. cardiovascular and thoracic surgeon)
   1. Schwartz SI: Principles of Surgery. 4th ed. New York: McGraw-Hill, 1983

BLALOCK-TAUSSIG OPERATION, surgical anastomosis of the carotid or subclavian arteries to the pulmonary artery in the Fallot tetralogy and other congenital cardiopathies. A milestone in cardiac surgery, especially in infants. Cross-reference: Taussig operation. (Alfred Blalock; Helen B. Taussig, 1898-1986, U.S. pediatrician)
   1. Maffei WE: Os Fundamentos da Medicina. 2nd ed. Livraria Editora Artes Medicas Ltd, 1978
   2. Schwartz SI: Principles of Surgery. 4th ed. New York: McGraw-Hill, 1983

BLASKOVICS OPERATION, correction of the epicanthus by resection of a cutaneous semilunar flap from the internal angle of the eye. (Laszlo de Blaskovics, 1869-1938, Hungarian ophthalmologist)
   1. Maffei WE: Os Fundamentos da Medicina. 2nd ed. Livraria Editora Artes Medicas Ltd, 1978

BLATIN SIGN, hydatid thrill. (Marc Blatin, 1878-1943, French)
   1. Dorland's Medical Dictionary. 28th ed. Philadelphia: WB Saunders, 1994

BLATIN SYNDROME, hydatid fremitus; tremor felt on the palm of the hand when placed on a cyst with hydatidosis (echinococcus). (Marc Blatin)
   1. Casas EC: Diccionario Terminologico de Ciencias Medicas. 5th ed. Salvat Editores, SA, 19544

BLEPHARONASOFACIAL SYNDROME, telecanthus, bulky nose with broad nasal bridge, midfacial hypoplasia, lateral displacement and stenosis of lacrimal puncta, longitudinal cheek furrows, trapezoidal upper lip, mask-like facies, and hyperextensible joints are characteristics. Autosomal dominant inheritance.
   1. Gorlin RJ, Cohen MM Jr, Levin LS: Syndromes of the Head and Neck. 3rd ed. New York: Oxford University Press, 1990
   2. Pashayan H, Pruzansky S, Putterman A: A family with blepharo-naso-facial malformations. Am J Dis Child 125:389-393, 1973
   3. Putterman AM, Pashayan H, Pruzansky S: Eye findings in the blepharo-naso-facial malformation syndrome. Am J

Ophthalmol 76:825 831, 1973

BLEPHAROPHIMOSIS SYNDROME, lateral displacement of the inner canthi and ptosis of the inner canthal fold. Autosomal dominant inheritance.

1. Smith DW, Jones KL: Recognizable Patterns of Human Malformation: Genetic, Embryologic, and Clinical Aspects. 3rd ed. Philadelphia: WB Saunders, 1982
2. Vignes: Epicanthus héréditaire. Rev Gen Opthalmol 8:438, 1889

BLIND LOOP SYNDROME, malabsorption, stasis, and bacterial overgrowth in the jejunal diverticula are features.

1. Bennett JC, Plum F (eds): Cecil Textbook of Medicine. 20th ed. Philadelphia: WB Saunders, 1996

BLOCH-SIEMENS-SULZBERGER SYNDROME, BLOCH-SULZBERGER SYNDROME, incontinentia pigmenti; a distinctive genodermatosis that eventuates in macular hyperpigmentation in bizarre irregular patterns of striae, whorls, polyangular flecks, and fountain-spray splatters, in no known anatomic or neural line segmental or band pattern. Most often seen in female infants. (Bruno Bloch, 1878-1933, Swiss dermatologist; Hermann N. Siemens, 1891-1969, German; Marion B. Sulzberger, 1895-1983, U.S. dermatologist)

1. Morgan JD: Incontinentia pigmenti (Bloch-Sulzberger syndrome). Am J Dis Child 122:294-300, 1971
2. Moschella SL, Hurley HJ: Dermatology. 2nd ed. Philadelphia: WB Saunders, 1985

BLOCK SYNDROME, irritability, crying, melancholy, sexual dysfunction, pigmentata of the skin are characteristics; seen in premenopausal women.

1. Casas EC: Diccionario Terminologico de Ciencias Medicas. 5th ed. Salvat Editores, SA, 1954

BLOODGOOD DISEASE, benign cystic disease of the breast. Cross-reference: Cheatle disease. (Joseph C. Bloodgood, 1866-1935, U.S.)

1. Bloodgood JC: Bull Soc Anat Paris 8:428-433, 1883

BLOOM SYNDROME, facial telangiectatic erythema, photosensitivity, and dwarfism are features. Although cutaneous features similar to lupus erythematosus were noted in the original patients, the condition was recognized as a distinct heritable entity. (David Bloom, U.S. dermatologist)

1. Bloom D: Am J Dis Child 88:754-758, 1954
2. Bloom D: Hereditary lymphedema (Nonne-Milroy-Meige): report of a family with hereditary lymphedema associated with ptosis of the eyelids in several generations. NY State J Med 41:856-863, 1941
3. Moschella SL, Hurley HJ: Dermatology. 2nd ed. Philadelphia: WB Saunders, 1985

BLOUNT DISEASE, a genetic disease consisting of bowed legs, tibial torsion, and obesity. (Walter P. Blount, U.S. orthopedic surgeon)

1. Wilson JD, Foster DW, Kronenberg HM, et al (eds): Williams Textbook of Endocrinology. 9th ed. Philadelphia: WB Saunders, 1998

BLUE DIAPER SYNDROME, hypercalcemia with nephrocalcinosis indicanuria; a defect in intestinal transport of tryptophan leads to excessive indole production by intestinal bacteria. Conversion of indican to indigo blue appears to account for the syndrome's name.

1. McKusick VA: Heritable Disorders of Connective Tissue. 4th ed. St Louis: CV Mosby, 1972

BLUE DRUM SYNDROME, hemorrhage into the middle ear that may result from otitis media or may be idiopathic.

1. Ritchie AC: Boyd's Textbook of Pathology. 9th ed. Philadelphia: Lea & Febiger, 1990

BLUE RUBBER-BLEB NEVUS SYNDROME, cavernous hemangiomas of subcutaneous tissue and submucosa of the bowel, with gastrointestinal bleeding. Cross-reference: Bean syndrome.

1. Bean WW: Vascular Spiders and Related Lesions of the Skin. Springfield: Charles C Thomas, 1958
2. Moschella SL, Hurley HJ: Dermatology. 2nd ed. Philadelphia: WB Saunders, 1985

BLUE VALVE SYNDROME, see Mitral valve prolapse syndrome.

BLUM SYNDROME, hypochloremic azotemia.

1. Casas EC: Diccionario Terminologico de Ciencias Medicas. 5th ed. Salvat Editores, SA, 1954

BLUMBERG SIGN, rebound tenderness in the abdomen; an indication of peritonitis. Cross-reference: Release sign. (J. Moritz Blumberg, 1873-1955, German general practitioner/surgeon)

1. Casas EC: Diccionario Terminologico de Ciencias Medicas. 5th ed. Salvat Editores, SA, 1954

BLUMENTHAL DISEASE, erythroleukemia.

1. Casas EC: Diccionario Terminologico de Ciencias Medicas. 5th ed. Salvat Editores, SA, 1954

BLUMER SIGN, horizontal bulging in the colon due to inflammation or tumor. (George Blumer,

1858-1940, U.S.)
  1. Casas EC: Diccionario Terminologico de Ciencias Medicas. 5th ed. Salvat Editores, SA, 1954

BOARI OPERATION, transplantation of the deferent duct to the urethra.
  1. Maffei WE: Os Fundamentos da Medicina. 2nd ed. Livraria Editora Artes Medicas Ltd, 1978

BOAS SIGN, the presence of lactic acid in gastric juice; seen in the patient with stomach cancer. (Ismar I. Boas, 1858-1938, German gastroenterologist)
  1. Bailey H, Love M: A Short Practice of Surgery. 12th ed. London: HK Lewis & Co, 1962

BOBBS OPERATION, cholecystectomy.
  1. Maffei WE: Os Fundamentos da Medicina. 2nd ed. Livraria Editora Artes Medicas Ltd, 1978

BOBROFF OPERATION, osteoplastic surgery for spina bifida; excision of a hydatid cyst membrane of the liver followed by suture of the abdominal walls without drainage.
  1. Maffei WE: Os Fundamentos da Medicina. 2nd ed. Livraria Editora Artes Medicas Ltd, 1978

BODER-SEDGWICK SYNDROME, see Louis-Bar syndrome.

BODY OF LUYS SYNDROME, corpus Luysii; hemiballismus of unknown etiology.
  1. Dorland's Medical Dictionary. 28th ed. Philadelphia: WB Saunders, 1994

BOECK SARCOIDOSIS, see Besnier-Boeck-Schaumann disease.

BOERHAAVE SYNDROME, spontaneous rupture of the esophagus; a variant of the Mallory-Weiss syndrome. (Hermann Boerhaave, 1668-1738, Dutch)
  1. Ballenger JJ: Diseases of the Nose, Throat, Ear, Head and Neck. 12th ed. Philadelphia: Lea & Febiger, 1977

BOERI SIGN, pain when the superior part of the trapezius muscle is compressed; seen in the patient with tuberculosis.
  1. Casas EC: Diccionario Terminologico de Ciencias Medicas. 5th ed. Salvat Editores, SA, 1954

BOGORAD SYNDROME, gustatory lacrimation; a syndrome of lacrimation that accompanies eating or drinking. Cross-reference: Crocodile tears syndrome. (F.A. Bogorad, Russian)
  1. Axelsson A, Laage-Hellman JE: The gusto-lachrymal reflex. The syndrome of crocodile tears. Acta Otolaryngol 54:239-254, 1962
  2. Biedner B, Geltman C, Rothkoff L: Bilateral Duane's syndrome associated with crocodile tears. J Pediatr Ophthalmol 16:113-114, 1979
  3. Bogorad FA: Syndrome of crocodile tears. Vrach Delo 11:1328-1330, 1928
  4. Gorlin RJ, Cohen MM Jr, Levin LS: Syndromes of the Head and Neck. 3rd ed. New York: Oxford University Press, 1990

BOGUE OPERATION, use of catgut suture for ligation of multiple veins in the treatment of varicocele.
  1. Maffei WE: Os Fundamentos da Medicina. 2nd ed. Livraria Editora Artes Medicas Ltd, 1978

BÖHM OPERATION, ocular tenotomy for treating strabismus.
  1. Maffei WE: Os Fundamentos da Medicina. 2nd ed. Livraria Editora Artes Medicas Ltd, 1978

BOIFFIN OPERATION, resection of the lowest six ribs in the treatment of posterior empyema.
  1. Maffei WE: Os Fundamentos da Medicina. 2nd ed. Livraria Editora Artes Medicas Ltd, 1978

BOISSOM SIGN, a change in the color of the nails that precedes a malaria attack.
  1. Casas EC: Diccionario Terminologico de Ciencias Medicas. 5th ed. Salvat Editores, SA, 1954

BOLOGNINI SIGN, alternating pressure on the stomach produces a feeling of crepitation; seen in the patient with measles. (Amédée Bolognini, 1802-1858, French surgeon)
  1. Casas EC: Diccionario Terminologico de Ciencias Medicas. 5th ed. Salvat Editores, SA, 1954

BONA-JÄGER OPERATION, disarticulation of the navicular and cuneiform bones.
  1. Maffei WE: Os Fundamentos da Medicina. 2nd ed. Livraria Editora Artes Medicas Ltd, 1978

BONFILS DISEASE, see Hodgkin disease. (Emil A. Bonfils, French)

BONNET SYNDROME, BONNET-deCHAUME-BLANC SYNDROME, nevus flammeus of the face, retinal angiomatosis, and intracranial angiomas in the region of the thalamus and mesencephalon are characteristics. (Paul Bonnet, French; Jean deChaume, 1896-1968, French; Emile Blanc, 1901-1952, French)
  1. Bonnet P, deChaume J, Blanc E: J Med Lyon 18:163-178, 1937
  2. Krayenbühl HA, Yasargil MG: Cerebral Angiography. 2nd ed. Philadelphia: JB Lippincott, 1968
  3. Moschella SL, Hurley HJ: Dermatology. 2nd ed. Philadelphia: WB Saunders, 1985

BONNEVIE-ULLRICH SYNDROME, hyperplastic joints and skin, dwarfism, webbing of the neck, gonadal dysgenesis, and an XO chromosome pattern are features. (Kristin Bonnevie, 1872-1950, Norwegian zoologist; Otto Ullrich, 1894-1957, German pediatrician)

1. Bonnevie K: J Exp Zool 67:443-520, 1934
2. Krayenbühl HA, Yasargil MG: Cerebral Angiography. 2nd ed. Philadelphia: JB Lippincott, 1968
3. Ullrich O: Z Kinderheilkd 49:271-276, 1930

BONNIER SYNDROME, a cluster of symptoms due to a lesion of Deiters nucleus (lateral nucleus of the vestibular nerve) or of the vestibular tracts. Consists of vertigo, pallor, and various aural and ocular dysfunctions. (Pierre Bonnier, 1861-1918, French)

1. Bonnier P: Syndrome du noyau de Deiters. Compt Rendu Soc Biol (Par) 4:1525-1528, 1902

BONZEL OPERATION, iridodialysis through a corneal incision.

1. Maffei WE: Os Fundamentos da Medicina. 2nd ed. Livraria Editora Artes Medicas Ltd, 1978

BÖÖK SYNDROME, see Premolar aplasia-hyperhidrosis-premature canities syndrome. (Jan Arvid Böök, Swedish geneticist)

BORDIER-FRÄNKEL SIGN, see Bell phenomenon.

BÖRJESON-FORSSMAN-LEHMANN SYNDROME, short stature, moderate obesity, microcephaly, nystagmus, ptosis, poor vision, and hypogonadism are features. Variable radiographic abnormalities are present. X-linked recessive inheritance. (Mats G. Börjeson, Swedish; Hans A. Forssman, Swedish; Orla Lehmann, Swedish)

1. Börjeson MG, Forssman HA, Lehmann O: Acta Med Scand 171:13-21, 1962
2. Smith DW, Jones KL: Recognizable Patterns of Human Malformation: Genetic, Embryologic, and Clinical Aspects. 3rd ed. Philadelphia: WB Saunders, 1982
3. Weber FT, Frias JL, Julius RL, et al: Primary hypogonadism in the Börjeson-Forssman-Lehmann syndrome. J Med Genet 15:63-66, 1978

BORNHOLM DISEASE epidemic pleurodynia or epidemic myalgia; an acute febrile disease characterized by sudden, sharp chest pain or abdominal pain. An inflammatory muscle disorder caused by a virus. Relates to the Danish Island of Bornholm, where an outbreak of myositis occurred. Cross-references: Devil's grip; Sylvest disease.

1. Bennett JC, Plum F (eds): Cecil Textbook of Medicine. 20th ed. Philadelphia: WB Saunders, 1996
2. Farmer TW: Pediatric Neurology. 2nd ed. Hagerstown: Harper & Row, 1975
3. Sylvest E: Ugeskr Laeger 92:798-801, 1930

BORRAS DISEASE, endemic disease of South America believed to be an attenuated form of yellow fever.

1. Casas EC: Diccionario Terminologico de Ciencias Medicas. 5th ed. Salvat Editores, SA, 1954

BORSIERI SIGN, blanched skin becomes pink very quickly; seen in the early stages of scarlet fever. (Giovanni Borsieri, 1725-1785, Italian)

1. Casas EC: Diccionario Terminologico de Ciencias Medicas. 5th ed. Salvat Editores, SA, 1954

BORTHEN OPERATION, iridotasis.

1. Maffei WE: Os Fundamentos da Medicina. 2nd ed. Livraria Editora Artes Medicas Ltd, 1978

BOSE OPERATION, tracheostomy.

1. Maffei WE: Os Fundamentos da Medicina. 2nd ed. Livraria Editora Artes Medicas Ltd, 1978

BOSTOCK DISEASE, hay fever. (John Bostock, 1773-1846, British)

1. Bostock J: Med Chir Trans Lond 10:161-165, 1819

BOSTON SIGN, when the patient looks down, the upper lid lags behind; occurs in exophthalmic goiter. (Leonard N. Boston, 1871-1931, U.S.)

1. Casas EC: Diccionario Terminologico de Ciencias Medicas. 5th ed. Salvat Editores, SA, 1954

BOTTINI OPERATION, the use of electrocautery for making an artificial duct in the hypertrophied prostate.

1. Maffei WE: Os Fundamentos da Medicina. 2nd ed. Livraria Editora Artes Medicas Ltd, 1978

BOUCHARD NODES, see Heberden nodes. (Charles J. Bouchard, 1837-1915, French)

BOUCHARD SIGN, Fehling solution (an alkaline copper sulfate solution) dropped in infected urine brings the pus to the top. (Charles J. Bouchard)

1. Casas EC: Diccionario Terminologico de Ciencias Medicas. 5th ed. Salvat Editores, SA, 1954

BOUCHET DISEASE, cysticercosis.

    1. Casas EC: Diccionario Terminologico de Ciencias Medicas. 5th ed. Salvat Editores, SA, 1954

BOUILLAUD SIGN, a sound heard at the cardiac apex; found in the patient with myocardial hypertrophy. (Jean B. Bouillaud, 1796-1881, French)

    1. Casas EC: Diccionario Terminologico de Ciencias Medicas. 5th ed. Salvat Editores, SA, 1954

BOUILLAUD SYNDROME, concomitant pericarditis and endocarditis in acute inflammation of joints. (Jean B. Bouillaud)

    1. Bouillaud JB: Traité Clinique des Maladies due Coeur, Vol. 2. 1835

BOUILLY OPERATION, excision of the central part of the mucous membrane of the uterine neck in atresia of the uterus.

    1. Maffei WE: Os Fundamentos da Medicina. 2nd ed. Livraria Editora Artes Medicas Ltd, 1978

BOURNEVILLE DISEASE, BOURNEVILLE-PRINGLE DISEASE, tuberous sclerosis characterized clinically by the triad of mental retardation, epileptic seizures, and cutaneous lesions (so-called sebaceous adenomas). Cross-references: Pringle disease; Tuberous sclerosis syndrome. (Desiré-Magliore Bourneville, 1840-1909, French; John J. Pringle, 1855-1922, British dermatologist)

    1. Bourneville DM: Arch Neurol Paris 1:69-91, 1880

    2. Cooper JR: Brain tumors in hereditary multiple system hamartomatosis (tuberous sclerosis). J Neurosurg 34:194-202, 1971

    3. Kenishi Y, et al: Tuberous sclerosis. Early neurological manifestations and CT features in 18 patients. Brain Dev 1:31, 1979

BOUVERET SIGN, the cecum and the right iliac fossa are distended; seen in the patient with bowel obstruction.

    1. Casas EC: Diccionario Terminologico de Ciencias Medicas. 5th ed. Salvat Editores, SA, 1954

BOUVERET SYNDROME, paroxysmal supraventricular tachycardia. (Léon Bouveret, 1850-1929, French)

    1. Bouveret L: Rev Med (Par) 9:753-793, 837-855, 1889

BOWEL BYPASS SYNDROME, intestinal bypass surgery for the treatment of morbid obesity complicated by a constellation of medical complications, including asymmetric polyarthritis, tenosynovitis, sterile skin pustules, mucous membrane ulcerations, retinal vasculitis, and thrombophlebitis.

    1. Moschella SL, Hurley HJ: Dermatology. 2nd ed. Philadelphia: WB Saunders, 1985

BOWEN DISEASE, precancerous dermatitis; in itself a squamous cell carcinoma in situ, but at the same time may be an indicator of underlying malignancy. A variant of a usually noninvasive squamous cell carcinoma, found more frequently in patients with a history of prolonged exposure to or ingestion of arsenic. (John T.B. Bowen, 1857-1941, U.S. dermatologist)

    1. Bennett JC, Plum F (eds): Cecil Textbook of Medicine. 20th ed. Philadelphia: WB Saunders, 1996

    2. Bowen JTB: J Cutan Dis 30:241-255, 1912

    3. Campbell MF, Walsh PC: Campbell's Urology. 5th ed. Philadelphia: WB Saunders, 1986

BOWEN-ARMSTRONG SYNDROME, consists of mild to moderate mental retardation, ectodermal dysplasia, and cleft lip and/or palate.

    1. Bowen P, Armstrong HB: Ectodermal dysplasia, mental retardation, cleft lip/palate and other anomalies in three sibs. Clin Genet 9:35-42, 1976

    2. Gorlin RJ, Cohen MM Jr, Levin LS: Syndromes of the Head and Neck. 3rd ed. New York: Oxford University Press, 1990

BOWSTRING SIGN, while lying down, the patient performs straight leg raising to the point of some discomfort. The knee is then flexed and the examiner applies pressure to the hamstrings. If this does not produce pain, pressure is applied to the popliteal nerve. The sign is present when there is reproduction of pain, which signifies nerve root compression and/or a ruptured intervertebral disc.

    1. Evans RC: Illustrated Essentials in Orthopedic Physical Assessment. St Louis: Mosby Yearbook, 1994

    2. Mazion JM: Illustrated Manual of Orthopedic Signs/Tests/Maneuvers for Office Procedure. 2nd ed. Orlando: Daniels Publishing, 1980

BOYCE SIGN, pressure of the hand on the side of the neck elicits a gurgling sound in the pharyngoesophageal diverticulum. (Frederick F. Boyce, U.S.)

    1. Dorland's Medical Dictionary. 28th ed. Philadelphia: WB Saunders, 1994

BOZEMAN OPERATION, hysterocystocleisis in cases of vesicouterine fistula. Surgery consists of suturing the neck of the uterus to the lips of the fistula. (Nathan Bozeman, 1825-1905, U.S. surgeon)

1. Maffei WE: Os Fundamentos da Medicina. 2nd ed. Livraria Editora Artes Medicas Ltd, 1978

BOZZOLO SIGN, visible pulsation of the nasal fossa; seen at times in the patient with thoracic aortic aneurysm. (Camillo Bozzolo, 1845-1920, Italian)

1. Casas EC: Diccionario Terminologico de Ciencias Medicas. 5th ed. Salvat Editores, SA, 1954

BRACHIAL PLEXUS COMPRESSION SYNDROME, neurovascular structures passing from the thorax may be compressed by the pectoralis minor muscle at its coracoid attachment. The symptoms of aching pain in the arm and shoulder referred to the anterior chest and periscapular area may be reproduced by abduction of the arm or by pressure in the region of the coracoid process.

1. Campbell WC, Crenshaw AH: Campbell's Operative Orthopaedics. 7th ed. St Louis: CV Mosby, 1987

BRACHMANN-DE LANGE SYNDROME, see De Lange syndrome. (W. Brachmann, German; Cornelia de Lange, 1871-1950, Dutch pediatrician)

BRACHYDACTYLY SYNDROME TYPE C, various anomalies of the digits; frequently seen in Mormon families.

1. Baritser M, Burn J: Recessively inherited brachydactyly type C. J Med Genet 20:128-129, 1983

BRACHYDACTYLY SYNDROME TYPE E, mild to moderate shortness of stature with short limbs, hands, and feet with short metacarpals and metatarsals, especially the fourth and fifth. Autosomal dominant inheritance.

1. Riccardi VM, Holmes LB: Brachydactyly, type E: hereditary shortening digits, metacarpals, and long bones. J Pediatr 84:251-259, 1974
2. Smith DW, Jones KL: Recognizable Patterns of Human Malformation: Genetic, Embryologic, and Clinical Aspects. 3rd ed. Philadelphia: WB Saunders, 1982

BRADBURNE SIGN, a characteristic upper limb position of abduction of the arms, flexion of the forearms, and external rotation. A sign of bilateral spinal cord damage between the 5th and 6th cervical segments.

1. Mazion JM: Illustrated Manual of Neurological Reflexes/Signs/Tests For Office Procedure. 2nd ed. Arizona City: Daniels Publishing, 1980

BRADBURY-EGGLESTON SYNDROME, the gradual onset of postural hypotension, anhidrosis, and impotence; due possibly to autonomic failure among middle-aged males. (Samuel Bradbury, U.S.; Cary Eggleston, U.S.)

1. Bannister R: Clinical Autonomic Disorders: Evaluation and Management. Boston: Little, Brown & Co., 1993, pp 517-526
2. Bradbury S, Eggleston C: Postural hypotension: report of three cases. Am Heart J 1:73-86, 1925
3. Low PA, Gilder JL, Freeman R, et al: Efficacy of midodrine vs. placebo in neurogenic orthostatic hypotension. JAMA 277:1046-1051, 1997

BRADLEY DISEASE, epidemic nausea and vomiting. Cross-reference: Spencer disease. (William H. Bradley, British)

1. Casas EC: Diccionario Terminologico de Ciencias Medicas. 5th ed. Salvat Editores, SA, 1954

BRADYCARDIA SYNDROME, BRADYCARDIA-TACHYCARDIA SYNDROME, bursts of ectopic atrial tachycardia or atrial fibrillation alternate with inappropriate suppression of the sinus node as well as subsidiary pacemaker activity. Cross-reference: Sick sinus syndrome.

1. Bennett JC, Plum F (eds): Cecil Textbook of Medicine. 20th ed. Philadelphia: WB Saunders, 1996
2. Cheitlin MD, Sokolow M: Clinical Cardiology. 5th ed. Norwalk, Conn: Appleton & Lange, 1993
3. Ferrer MI: The sick sinus syndrome in atrial disease. JAMA 206:645-646, 1968

BRAGARD SIGN, a sciatic nerve compression phenomenon; dorsiflexion of the foot until the patient experiences pain during the Lasègue test. (Karl Bragard, German orthopedist)

1. Baker AB, Baker LH: Clinical Neurology. Revised ed. Philadelphia: Harper & Row, 1982

BRAILEY OPERATION, lengthening of the supratrochlear nerve to alleviate pain in glaucoma.

1. Maffei WE: Os Fundamentos da Medicina. 2nd ed. Livraria Editora Artes Medicas Ltd, 1978

BRAILSFORD-MORQUIO SYNDROME, see Morquio syndrome.

BRAKE PHENOMENON, the tendency of a muscle to maintain itself in its normal resting position. Cross-reference: Rieger phenomenon.

1. Dorland's Medical Dictionary. 28th ed. Philadelphia: WB Saunders, 1994

BRANCH-ROMBERG SIGN, see Romberg sign.

BRANCHIO-OCULO-FACIAL SYNDROME, a syndrome of branchial clefts, pseudocleft of the upper lip, and congenital nasolacrimal duct obstruction; reduced fertility is likely. Autosomal dominant inheritance has been noted.

1. Fujimoto A, Liposon M, Larco RV, et al: A new autosomal dominant branchio-oculo-facial syndrome. Am J Med Genet 27:943-951, 1987
2. Gorlin RJ, Cohen MM Jr, Levin LS: Syndromes of the Head and Neck. 3rd ed. New York: Oxford University Press, 1990
3. Hall BD, de Lorimeir A, Foster LH: A new syndrome of hemangiomatous branchial clefts, lip pseudoclefts, and unusual facial appearance. Am J Med Genet 14:135-138, 1983

BRANCHIO-OTO-RENAL SYNDROME, an autosomal dominant disorder with a pattern of malformations that includes malformed ears, preauricular tags, preauricular sinus, and branchial cleft sinus. Cross-reference: Melnick-Fraser syndrome.

1. Bennett JC, Plum F (eds): Cecil Textbook of Medicine. 20th ed. Philadelphia: WB Saunders, 1996
2. Fraser FC, et al: Genetic aspects of the BOR syndrome—branchial fistulas, ear pits, hearing loss, and renal abnormalities. Am J Med Genet 2:241-252, 1978
3. Gorlin RJ, Cohen MM Jr, Levin LS: Syndromes of the Head and Neck. 3rd ed. New York: Oxford University Press, 1990

BRANCHIO-SKELETON SYNDROME, BRANCHIO-SKELETO-GENITAL SYNDROME, seizures, moderate mental retardation (IQ 45-60), pectus excavatum, and penoscrotal hypospadias are features. Cross-reference: Elsahy-Waters syndrome.

1. Elsahy NI, Waters WR: The branchio-skeleto-genital syndrome. Plast Reconstr Surg 48:542-550, 1971
2. Gorlin RJ, Cohen MM Jr, Levin LS: Syndromes of the Head and Neck. 3rd ed. New York: Oxford University Press, 1990
3. Shafai J, et al: The branchioskeletogenital syndrome. Birth Defects 18:193-196, 1982

BRANHAM SIGN, compression of an arteriovenous malformation causing slowing of the heartbeat and disappearance of a murmur. Cross-reference: Nicoladoni sign. (Henry H. Branham, U.S. surgeon)

1. Casas EC: Diccionario Terminologico de Ciencias Medicas. 5th ed. Salvat Editores, SA, 1954

BRAQUEHAYE OPERATION, surgery for correction of a vesicovaginal fistula.

1. Maffei WE: Os Fundamentos da Medicina. 2nd ed. Livraria Editora Artes Medicas Ltd, 1978

BRASDOR OPERATION, peripheral ligature of an aneurysmal vessel. (Pierre Brasdor, 1721-1798, French surgeon)

1. Maffei WE: Os Fundamentos da Medicina. 2nd ed. Livraria Editora Artes Medicas Ltd, 1978

BRAUER OPERATION, cardiolysis.

1. Maffei WE: Os Fundamentos da Medicina. 2nd ed. Livraria Editora Artes Medicas Ltd, 1978

BRAUN-FERNWALD SIGN, an asymmetrical increase in the size of the uterus; an indication of pregnancy.

1. Casas EC: Diccionario Terminologico de Ciencias Medicas. 5th ed. Salvat Editores, SA, 1954

BRAUNWALD SIGN, the patient has a weak pulse immediately following a premature ventricular contraction. (Eugene Braunwald, U.S. cardiologist)

1. Dorland's Medical Dictionary. 28th ed. Philadelphia: WB Saunders, 1994

BRAXTON HICKS CONTRACTION, intermittent contractions of the uterus occurring after the first trimester of pregnancy. Cross-reference: Hicks sign. (John Braxton Hicks, 1823-1897, British obstetrician)

1. Casas EC: Diccionario Terminologico de Ciencias Medicas. 5th ed. Salvat Editores, SA, 1954

BREAK-OFF PHENOMENON, a state of disconnectedness or unreality often experienced during high-altitude flight.

1. Dorland's Medical Dictionary. 28th ed. Philadelphia: WB Saunders, 1994

BREDA DISEASE, see Charlouis disease. (Achille Breda, 1850-1933, Italian dermatologist)

BREISKY DISEASE, kraurosis vulvae. (August Breisky, 1832-1889, Czech gynecologist)

1. Breisky A: Hand Allgspec Chir 4:1-256, 1879

BRENNEMANN SYNDROME, mesenteric and retroperitoneal lymphadenitis (often noted following throat infections). (Joseph Brennemann, 1872-1944, U.S. pediatrician)

1. Brennemann J: JAMA 89:2183-2186, 1927

BRENNER OPERATION, a modification of the Bassini operation in which the abdominal muscles are sutured to the cremaster.

1. Maffei WE: Os Fundamentos da Medicina. 2nd ed. Livraria Editora Artes Medicas Ltd, 1978

BRENNER SIGN, a metallic sound heard behind the ribs in the case of stomach perforation with gas under the diaphragm.
1. Casas EC: Diccionario Terminologico de Ciencias Medicas. 5th ed. Salvat Editores, SA, 1954

BRETONNEAU DISEASE, diphtheria. (Pierre Bretonneau, 1778-1862, French)
1. Casas EC: Diccionario Terminologico de Ciencias Medicas. 5th ed. Salvat Editores, SA, 1954

BREWER OPERATION, occlusion of arterial wounds by applying a net embedded in a special glue.
1. Maffei WE: Os Fundamentos da Medicina. 2nd ed. Livraria Editora Artes Medicas Ltd, 1978

BRICKER OPERATION, surgical creation of an ileal conduit for the collection of urine. (Eugene Bricker, U.S. urologist)
1. Maffei WE: Os Fundamentos da Medicina. 2nd ed. Livraria Editora Artes Medicas Ltd, 1978

BRICKNER SIGN, slowness of ocular muscles and auricular motion in facial nerve paralysis. (Richard Brickner, 1896-1959, U.S. neurologist)
1. Casas EC: Diccionario Terminologico de Ciencias Medicas. 5th ed. Salvat Editores, SA, 1954

BRIGHT DISEASE, nephritis; a term once used for kidney disease with proteinuria, usually glomerulonephritis. (Richard Bright, 1789-1858, British internist-pathologist)
1. Bright R: Guys Hops Rep, 1836

BRIGHTON OPERATION, this technique uses Teflon-insulated K-wires with an exposed tip inserted percutaneously, under radiographic visualization, into a fracture so that the tip is located at the fracture site and connected to a battery power pack.
1. Schwartz SI: Principles of Surgery. 4th ed. New York: McGraw-Hill, 1983

BRILL DISEASE, BRILL-ZINSSER DISEASE, probably represents a recrudescence of epidemic typhus in patients in whom the infection is latent. First noted in New York City, it has also been encountered in other populous areas. In the majority of cases, not characterized by any cutaneous lesions, and its severity is less than that of the initial infection of epidemic typhus. (Nathan Brill, 1860-1925, U.S.; Hans Zinsser, 1878-1940, U.S. bacteriologist and immunologist)
1. Brill NE: Am J Med Sci 139:484-502, 1910
2. Hoeprich PD, Jordan MC: Infectious Diseases. 4th ed. Philadelphia: WB Saunders, 1989

BRILL-SYMMERS DISEASE, giant follicle lymphoma. (Nathan Brill; Douglas Symmers, 1879-1952, U.S. pathologist)
1. Casas EC: Diccionario Terminologico de Ciencias Medicas. 5th ed. Salvat Editores, SA, 1954

BRINTON DISEASE, linitis gastrica. (William Brinton, 1823-1867, British)
1. Casas EC: Diccionario Terminologico de Ciencias Medicas. 5th ed. Salvat Editores, SA, 1954

BRION-KAYSER DISEASE, see Schottmüller disease. (Albert Brion, German; Heinrich Kayser, 1876-1940, German)

BRIQUET SYNDROME, a somatization disorder; the patient has recurrent complaints of symptoms involving almost every bodily system. Described by Guzé initially. Cross-reference: Branchio-skeleton syndrome. (Paul Briquet, 1796-1881, French)
1. Bennett JC, Plum F (eds): Cecil Textbook of Medicine. 20th ed. Philadelphia: WB Saunders, 1996
2. Rowland LP (ed): Merritt's Textbook of Neurology. 9th ed. Baltimore: Williams & Wilkins, 1995

BRISSAUD SIGN, BRISSAUD-MARIE SIGN, the hysterical contraction of the tensor fasciae lata. (Edouard Brissaud, 1852-1909, French neurologist; Pierre Marie, 1853-1940, French neurologist)
1. Baker AB, Baker LH: Clinical Neurology. Revised ed. Philadelphia: Harper & Row, 1982
2. Bordas LB (ed): Neurologia Fundamental. 2nd ed. Barcelona: Ed. Toray, 1968

BRISSAUD-MARIE SYNDROME, hysterical glossolabial hemispasm with contralateral weakness. (Edouard Brissaud; Pierre Marie)
1. Brissaud E, Marie P: Prog Med 5:84, 1887

BRISSAUD-SICARD SYNDROME, facial hemispasm associated with contralateral paralysis of extremities due to lesions of the pons; either intrapontine or extrapontine and may cause facial spasm and paralysis of the contralateral limbs. (Edouard Brissaud; Jean A. Sicard, 1872-1929, French radiologist)
1. Brissaud EA, Sicard JA: Type special de syndrome alterne. Rev Neurol 16:86, 1908
2. Haymaker W: Bing's Local Diagnosis in Neurological Diseases. 15th ed. St Louis: CV Mosby, 1969

BRISTOWE SYNDROME, tumor of the corpus callosum. (John S. Bristowe, 1827-1895, British)

1. Bristowe JS: Brain 7:315-333, 1884

BRITTAIN SIGN, palpitation of the right iliac fossa causes retraction of the right testicle; seen in the patient with appendicitis.
1. Casas EC: Diccionario Terminologico de Ciencias Medicas. 5th ed. Salvat Editores, SA, 1954

BRITTLE BONES SYNDROME, osteogenesis imperfecta associated with multiple fractures.
1. Dorland's Medical Dictionary. 28th ed. Philadelphia: WB Saunders, 1994

BRITTLE CORNEA SYNDROME, an X-linked recessively inherited syndrome characterized by corneal abnormality, blue sclerae, and red hair. Reported in Tunisian Jewish families.
1. Dorland's Medical Dictionary. 28th ed. Philadelphia: WB Saunders, 1994

BROAD THUMBS SYNDROME, see Rubinstein-Taybi syndrome.

BROADBENT SIGN, systolic retraction of the intercostal spaces at the diaphragmatic attachment; an indication of adherent pericardium. (Sir Walter H. Broadbent, 1835-1907, British)
1. Fowler NO: Cardiac Diagnosis and Treatment. 3rd ed. Cambridge: Harper & Row, 1980

BROCA APHASIA, motor aphasia; aphasia in which the patient is able to speak only a few words and is unable to write, although the patient is aware of what to say. Results from a lesion in the Broca area (i.e., the portion of the frontal lobe just anterior to the face, lip, tongue, and mouth area of the motor cortex). (Pierre Paul Broca, 1824-1880, French surgeon-neurologist)
1. Bennett JC, Plum F (eds): Cecil Textbook of Medicine. 20th ed. Philadelphia: WB Saunders, 1996
2. Broca PP: Bull Soc Anat Paris 36:330-357, 1861

BROCK-BROCCA DISEASE, BROCK SYNDROME, see Middle lobe syndrome. (Russel C. Brock, 1903-1980, British thoracic surgeon)

BROCKENBROUGH SIGN, BROCKENBROUGH-BRAUNWALD-MORROW SIGN, diminished pulse pressure in the post-extrasystolic beat; an indication of hypertrophic cardiomyopathy. (E.C. Brockenbrough, U.S. surgeon)
1. Criley JM, et al: The Brockenbrough-Braunwald-Morrow sign. N Engl J Med 331:1589-1590, 1994 (Letter)
2. Pollock SG: Pressure tracings in obstructive cardiomyopathy. N Engl J Med 331:238, 1994

BROCQ DISEASE, parakeratosis in psoriasiformis. (A.J. Louis Brocq, 1856-1928, French dermatologist)
1. Casas EC: Diccionario Terminologico de Ciencias Medicas. 5th ed. Salvat Editores, SA, 1954

BROCQ-DUHRING DISEASE, see Duhring disease. (A. J. Louis Brocq; Louis A. Duhring, 1845-1913, U.S. dermatologist)

BRODERS CLASSIFICATION, a classification for carcinoma of the rectum. Simplified later by the Dukes grading system. Low-grade = well-differentiated tumors with an 11% good prognosis; average = 64% fair prognosis; high-grade = anaplastic tumors with 25% poor prognosis. (Albert Broders, 1885-1964, U.S. pathologist)
1. Bailey H, Love M: A Short Practice of Surgery. 12th ed. London: HK Lewis & Co, 1962

BRODIE ABSCESS, a localized form of infection of the metaphysis of a long bone, caused by a *Staphylococcus* of low or attenuated virulence. The most frequent sites are the lower and upper ends of the tibia, the lower end of the femur, and the upper end of the humerus. (Sir Benjamin Brodie, 1783-1862, British surgeon)
1. Lumley JS, Clain A: Hamilton Bailey's Demonstration of Physical Signs in Clinical Surgery. 18th ed. London: Butterworth-Heinemann, 1997

BRODIE DISEASE, serocystic sarcoma of the breast. (Sir Benjamin Brodie)
1. Lumley JS, Clain A: Hamilton Bailey's Demonstration of Physical Signs in Clinical Surgery. 18th ed. London: Butterworth-Heinemann, 1997

BRODIE SIGN, the presence of a black spot in the glans penis; an indication of urinary infiltration in corpus spongiosum. (Sir Benjamin Brodie)
1. Casas EC: Diccionario Terminologico de Ciencias Medicas. 5th ed. Salvat Editores, SA, 1954

BRODIE-TRENDELENBURG TEST, a measurement of the presence of varicose veins; while lying on a couch, the patient's limb is raised to allow the blood to drain from the veins. The fingers or thumb of the examiner are placed firmly over the saphenous vein opening. Keeping firm pressure over this point, the limb is lowered and the patient instructed to stand. The examiner's hand is removed suddenly. If the veins fill immediately, the valves in the saphenous vein are incompetent and the test is pos-

itive. (Sir Benjamin Brodie; Friedrich Trendelenburg, 1844-1924, surgeon)
1. Bailey H: Physical Signs in Clinical Surgery. 16th ed. Baltimore: Williams & Wilkins, 1983

BRONZE BABY SYNDROME, describes infants who develop a gray-brown discoloration of the skin, serum, and urine while undergoing phototherapy.
1. Kopelman AE, et al: J Pediatr 87:466-472, 1972
2. Moschella SL, Hurley HJ: Dermatology. 2nd ed. Philadelphia: WB Saunders, 1985

BROOKE DISEASE, coccidiosis. (Henry A.G. Brooke, 1854-1919, British dermatologist)
1. Casas EC: Diccionario Terminologico de Ciencias Medicas. 5th ed. Salvat Editores, SA, 1954

BROOKE TUMOR, a form of carcinoma in which the cell type is thought to be derived from the germinal epithelium of the hair follicles and/or sweat glands. The lesion is exceedingly rare but may involve either the auricle or the external auditory canal. (Henry A.G. Brooke)
1. Ballenger JJ: Diseases of the Nose, Throat, Ear, Head and Neck. 12th ed. Philadelphia: Lea & Febiger, 1977
2. Dillaha , Janset, Honeycutt, et al: Clinical Dermatology. Hagerstown: Harper & Row, 1979, Vol 4

BROPHY OPERATION, surgery for cleft palate. (Truman W. Brophy, 1848-1928, U.S. oral surgeon)
1. Maffei WE: Os Fundamentos da Medicina. 2nd ed. Livraria Editora Artes Medicas Ltd, 1978

BROWN SYNDROME, a superior oblique tendon sheath syndrome in the patient with rheumatoid arthritis. May be unilateral or bilateral and may be associated with orbital pain that is generalized or localized to the superior nasal region. Cross-reference: Tendon sheath syndrome. (Harold W. Brown, U.S. ophthalmologist)
1. Brown HW: Congenital structural motor anomalies, in Allen JH (ed): Strabismus. St Louis: CV Mosby, 1950

BROWN TEST, the application of pressure with a Siegle otoscope causes an increase in pulsation as the pressure is raised until sudden blanching occurs.
1. Ballenger JJ: Diseases of the Nose, Throat, Ear, Head and Neck. 12th ed. Philadelphia: Lea & Febiger, 1977

BROWN-SÉQUARD SYNDROME, spinal hemiparaplegia; cutaneous anesthesia found mostly on the side of a spinal cord injury and on the same side as the resulting paralysis and ipsilateral signs of posterior column dysfunction. (Charles E. Brown-Séquard, 1817-1894, French physiologist/neurologist)
1. Bennett JC, Plum F (eds): Cecil Textbook of Medicine. 20th ed. Philadelphia: WB Saunders, 1996
2. Brown-Séquard CE: Compt Rendu Soc Biol 2:33-34, 1850
3. Rowland LP (ed): Merritt's Textbook of Neurology. 9th ed. Baltimore: Williams & Wilkins, 1995

BROWN-SYMMERS DISEASE, acute serous encephalitis in infants. (Charles Brown, 1899-1959, U.S.; Douglas Symmers, 1879-1952, U.S. pathologist)
1. Brown C: Am J Dis Child 29:174-181, 1925

BROWNE OPERATION, urethroplasty using the "buried strip" principle for hypospadias repair; described in 1953. (Denis Browne, Australian surgeon)
1. Campbell MF, Walsh PC: Campbell's Urology. 5th ed. Philadelphia: WB Saunders, 1986

BRUCK DISEASE, characterized by bone deformity, multiple fractures, ankylosis, and muscular atrophy. (Alfred Bruck, German)
1. Bruck A: Dtsch Med Wochenschr 23:152-155, 1897

BRUCK-DE LANGE DISEASE, congenital muscular hypertrophy, mental deficiency, and extrapyramidal disturbances are features.
1. Casas EC: Diccionario Terminologico de Ciencias Medicas. 5th ed. Salvat Editores, SA, 1954

BRUDZINSKI CHEEK SIGN, pressure against the cheeks on or just below the zygoma is accompanied by a reflex flexion of the elbows with an upward jerking of the arms. (Jósef von Brudzinski, 1874-1917, Polish)
1. Baker AB, Baker LH: Clinical Neurology. Revised ed. Philadelphia: Harper & Row, 1982

BRUDZINSKI CONTRALATERAL LEG SIGN, passive flexion of one hip (especially if the hip is flexed while the knee is extended) is followed by flexion of the opposite hip and knee; a sign of meningeal irritation. (Jósef von Brudzinski)
1. Baker AB, Baker LH: Clinical Neurology. Revised ed. Philadelphia: Harper & Row, 1982

BRUDZINSKI NECK SIGN, passive flexion of the head on the chest is followed by flexion of both thighs and legs so that both lower extremities may be strongly flexed on the pelvis. (Jósef von Brudzinski)
1. Baker AB, Baker LH: Clinical Neurology. Revised ed. Philadelphia: Harper & Row, 1982

BRUEGHEL SYNDROME, see Meige syndrome. (Pieter Brueghel the Elder, 1525-1569, Flemish painter)

BRUGADA SYNDROME, characterized electrocardiographically by an ST-segment elevation in V1 through V3 and a rapid polymorphic ventricular tachycardia that can degenerate into ventricular fibrillation. Apparently related to a cardiac sodium channel mutation, of which the arrhythmogenicity is revealed only at temperatures approaching the physiological range. Some patients may be more at risk during febrile states. A major cause of sudden death, particularly among young men of Southeast Asian and Japanese origin.
  1. Dumaine R, Towbin JA, Brugada P, et al: Circ Res 85:803-809, 1999
  2. Makita N, Shirai N, Wang DW, et al: Circulation 101:54-60, 2000

BRUGSCH SYNDROME, acropachyderma with large fingers, hypertrophy of the long bones, and acromegaly are features. (K.L. Theodor Brugsch, German internist)
  1. Casas EC: Diccionario Terminologico de Ciencias Medicas. 5th ed. Salvat Editores, SA, 1954

BRUHL DISEASE, congestive splenomegaly and hyperthermia.
  1. Casas EC: Diccionario Terminologico de Ciencias Medicas. 5th ed. Salvat Editores, SA, 1954

BRUN SYNDROME, see Nothnagel syndrome. (Theodor Brun, 1878-1963, German)

BRUNATI SIGN, the cornea appears opaque in the patient with typhoid fever or pneumonia. (M. Brunati, Italian)
  1. Casas EC: Diccionario Terminologico de Ciencias Medicas. 5th ed. Salvat Editores, SA, 1954

BRUNN DISEASE, epidemic syphilis in Moravia; described in 1578.
  1. Casas EC: Diccionario Terminologico de Ciencias Medicas. 5th ed. Salvat Editores, SA, 1954

BRUNS SYNDROME, vertigo Bruns; headache, nystagmus, and ataxia are features. A cyst or tumor within or overlying the 4th ventricle may give rise to this syndrome. (Ludwig von Bruns, 1858-1916, German neurologist)
  1. Baker AB, Baker LH: Clinical Neurology. Revised ed. Philadelphia: Harper & Row, 1982
  2. Von Bruns L: Neurol Centralbl 21:561-567, 1902

BRUNS-GARLAND SYNDROME, diabetic amyotrophy; characterized by severe pain in the hip and thigh followed by asymmetric weakness and wasting affecting the leg muscles. This syndrome, originally described by Bruns and later by Garland and Taverner, who coined the term diabetic amyotrophy, continues to be a topic for debate and discussion 100 years after its original description.
  1. Barohn RJ, et al: The Bruns-Garland syndrome (diabetic amyotrophy) revisited 100 years later. Arch Neurol 48:1130-1135, 1991

BRUNSCHWIG OPERATION, pancreatoduodenectomy performed in two stages. (Alexander Brunschwig, 1901-1969, U.S. surgeon)
  1. Maffei WE: Os Fundamentos da Medicina. 2nd ed. Livraria Editora Artes Medicas Ltd, 1978

BRUNSTING SYNDROME, benign pemphigoid; recurrent eruptions of grouped vesicular lesions at the head and neck regions, affecting middle-aged men and resulting in scarring. (Louis A. Brunsting, U.S.)
  1. Dorland's Medical Dictionary. 28th ed. Philadelphia: WB Saunders, 1994

BRUSHFIELD SPOTS, pigmented spots on the iris seen in the patient with Down syndrome (chromosome 21 trisomy). (Thomas Brushfield, 1858-1937, British)
  1. Braunwald E: Heart Disease: A Textbook of Cardiovascular Medicine. 4th ed. Philadelphia: WB Saunders, 1992
  2. Smith DW, Jones KL: Recognizable Patterns of Human Malformation: Genetic, Embryologic, and Clinical Aspects. 3rd ed. Philadelphia: WB Saunders, 1982

BRUSHFIELD-WYATT SYNDROME, a congenital syndrome of extensive unilateral port-wine nevus flammeus, hemianopia affecting the right or left halves of the visual fields of both eyes, cerebral angioma, contralateral hemiplegia, and mental retardation; probably related to the Sturge-Weber syndrome. (Thomas Brushfield; W. Wyatt, British)
  1. Brushfield T, Wyatt W: Hemiplegia associated with extensive naevus and mental defect. Br J Child Dis 24:98-106, 1927

BRUTON DISEASE, X-linked agammaglobulinemia; T cells develop normally, but the patient lacks B cells and the formation of immunoglobulins and antibodies is impaired. One of the more common genetically determined immunodeficiencies. X-linked recessive trait inheritance. (Ogden C. Bruton,

U.S. pediatrician)
1. Bruton OC: Pediatrics 9:722-728, 1952

BRYANT OPERATION, lumbar colotomy through an incision between the lowest rib and the iliac crest.
1. Maffei WE: Os Fundamentos da Medicina. 2nd ed. Livraria Editora Artes Medicas Ltd, 1978

BRYANT SIGN, axillary fullness seen in the patient with shoulder dislocation. (Sir Thomas Bryant, 1828-1914, British surgeon)
1. Casas EC: Diccionario Terminologico de Ciencias Medicas. 5th ed. Salvat Editores, SA, 1954

BUCHANAN OPERATION, mediolateral lithotomy.
1. Maffei WE: Os Fundamentos da Medicina. 2nd ed. Livraria Editora Artes Medicas Ltd, 1978

BUCK OPERATION, cuneiform resection of the patella and the proximal portions of the fibula and tibia. (Gurdon Buck, 1807-1877, U.S. surgeon)
1. Maffei WE: Os Fundamentos da Medicina. 2nd ed. Livraria Editora Artes Medicas Ltd, 1978

BUCKLEY SYNDROME, see Job syndrome. (Rebecca H. Buckley, U.S.)

BUDD DISEASE, BUDD-CHIARI SYNDROME, acute parenchymatous jaundice; thrombosis of the hepatic veins, which may follow abdominal trauma or the use of birth control pills or may occur in the patient with diseases such as polycythemia rubra vera and paroxysmal nocturnal hemoglobinuria, which has an associated hypercoagulable state. Cross-references: Chiari-Budd syndrome; Rokitansky disease. (George Budd, 1808-1882, British; Hans Chiari, 1851-1916, Austrian pathologist)
1. Bennett JC, Plum F (eds): Cecil Textbook of Medicine. 20th ed. Philadelphia: WB Saunders, 1996
2. Budd G: On Diseases of the Liver. London: Churchill, 1945
3. Ritchie AC: Boyd's Textbook of Pathology. 9th ed. Philadelphia: Lea & Febiger, 1990

BUDIN SIGN, compression of the female breast elicits milk and pus; seen in the patient with mastitis. (Pierre-Constant Budin, 1846-1907, French gynecologist)
1. Casas EC: Diccionario Terminologico de Ciencias Medicas. 5th ed. Salvat Editores, SA, 1954

BÜDINGER-LUDLOFF-LAEWEN DISEASE, pathological fracture of the patellar cartilage.
1. Casas EC: Diccionario Terminologico de Ciencias Medicas. 5th ed. Salvat Editores, SA, 1954

BUERGER DISEASE, thromboangiitis obliterans; an inflammatory, segmental obliterative disease of medium and small arteries and less commonly of veins. There has been considerable controversy as to whether it is an entity distinct from arteriosclerosis (McKusick et al, 1962). Cross-references: Leo Buerger disease; Winiwarter disease. (Leo Buerger, 1879-1943, Austrian-U.S. urologist)
1. Buerger L: Am J Med 136:567-580, 1908

BUERGER POSTURAL TEST, the patient lies supine and lifts both legs high, keeping the knees straight. The examiner supports the legs while the patient flexes and extends the ankles and toes to the point of mild fatigue. The feet are lowered and the patient adopts a sitting position. In two to three minutes a ruddy, cyanotic hue spreads over the affected foot. This sequence signifies that a major lower limb artery is occluded. (Leo Buerger)
1. Bailey H: Physical Signs in Clinical Surgery. 16th ed. Baltimore: Williams & Wilkins, 1983

BUHL DISEASE, acute adipose degeneration in the newborn, associated with jaundice and intestinal hemorrhage. (Ludwig von Buhl, 1816-1880, German)
1. Casas EC: Diccionario Terminologico de Ciencias Medicas. 5th ed. Salvat Editores, SA, 1954

BULBAR SYNDROME, see Déjerine syndrome.

BULLDOG SYNDROME, see Simpson-Golabi-Behmel syndrome.

BUMKE PUPIL, dilatation of the pupils caused by emotional excitement. (Oswald C.E. Bumke, 1877-1950, German neurologist)
1. Casas EC: Diccionario Terminologico de Ciencias Medicas. 5th ed. Salvat Editores, SA, 1954

BURCKHARDT OPERATION, opening of a retropharyngeal abscess through a neck incision.
1. Maffei WE: Os Fundamentos da Medicina. 2nd ed. Livraria Editora Artes Medicas Ltd, 1978

BUREN OPERATION, treatment of prolapse of the rectum using a thermocautery.
1. Maffei WE: Os Fundamentos da Medicina. 2nd ed. Livraria Editora Artes Medicas Ltd, 1978

BURGER SIGN, see Heryng sign.

BÜRGER-GRÜTZ SYNDROME, see Chylomicronemia syndrome. (Max Bürger, German; Otto

Grütz, German)

BURKITT LYMPHOMA, lymphatic neoplasm; a malignant disease of lymphoreticular origin. (Denis Burkitt, British surgeon)
1. Burkitt D: Br J Surg 46:218-223, 1958
2. Campbell MF, Walsh PC: Campbell's Urology. 5th ed. Philadelphia: WB Saunders, 1986

BURNETT SYNDROME, see Milk-alkali syndrome. (Charles H. Burnett, 1913-1967)

BURNING FEET SYNDROME, see Gopalan syndrome.

BUROW OPERATION, plastic operation for extirpation of tumors leaving no scars. (Karl A. von Burow, 1809-1874, German surgeon)
1. Maffei WE: Os Fundamentos da Medicina. 2nd ed. Livraria Editora Artes Medicas Ltd, 1978

BURTON SYNDROME, consists of Kniest-like skeletal dysplasia, microstomia, pursed lips, and dislocated lenses.
1. Burton BK, Sumner T, Langer LO Jr, et al: A new skeletal dysplasia: clinical, radiologic, and pathologic findings. J Pediatr 109:642-648, 1986
2. Gorlin RJ, Cohen MM Jr, Levin LS: Syndromes of the Head and Neck. 3rd ed. New York, NY: Oxford University Press, 1990

BURY DISEASE, erythema elevatum diutinum; a variant of erythema multiforme. (Judson S. Bury, 1852-1944, British dermatologist)
1. Casas EC: Diccionario Terminologico de Ciencias Medicas. 5th ed. Salvat Editores, SA, 1954

BUSCHKE-LÖWENSTEIN TUMOR, verrucous carcinoma or giant condyloma acuminatum; a lesion occurring in the genital or anal areas, large in size and resembling a condyloma acuminatum. The characteristics were recognized by Buschke in 1925 and by Löwenstein in 1939. (Abraham Buschke, 1868-1943, German dermatologist; Ludwig W. Löwenstein, 1885-1959, German-born U.S.)
1. Löwenstein LW: Med Clin North Am 23:789-795, 1939

BUSCHKE-OLLENDORFF SYNDROME, generalized eruptive histiocytoma or dermatofibrosis lenticularis disseminata with osteopoikilosis. A rare autosomal-dominant syndrome. (Abraham Buschke; Helene Ollendorff, German dermatologist)
1. Buschke A, Ollendorff H: Dermatol Wochenschr 86:251-262, 1928
2. Moschella SL, Hurley HJ: Dermatology. 2nd ed. Philadelphia: WB Saunders, 1985

BUSQUET DISEASE, exostosis of the dorsum of the foot caused by metatarsal periostitis. (G. Paul Busquet, 1866-1930, French)
1. Casas EC: Diccionario Terminologico de Ciencias Medicas. 5th ed. Salvat Editores, SA, 1954

BUSSE-BUSCHKE DISEASE, cryptococcoses. (Otto Busse, 1867-1922, German; Abraham Buschke, 1868-1943, German dermatologist)
1. Buschke A: Dtsch Med Wochenschr 21, 1895

BUTCHER OPERATION, surgical correction of a double harelip.
1. Maffei WE: Os Fundamentos da Medicina. 2nd ed. Livraria Editora Artes Medicas Ltd, 1978

BUZZI OPERATION, creation of an artificial pupil by passing a needle through the cornea.
1. Maffei WE: Os Fundamentos da Medicina. 2nd ed. Livraria Editora Artes Medicas Ltd, 1978

BYARS OPERATION, two-stage method for urethroplasty; described in 1955.
1. Campbell MF, Walsh PC: Campbell's Urology. 5th ed. Philadelphia: WB Saunders, 1986

BYLER DISEASE, a rare, progressive, intrahepatic cholestasia; severe obstructive jaundice develops in infancy and persists. The defect seems to be in the excretion of bile from the hepatocytes. At first, liver biopsy is normal, but cholestasis soon develops around the terminal hepatic veins. Autosomal recessive transmission. (An Amish kindred in the U.S.)
1. Freese D: Intracellular cholestatic syndromes of infancy. Semin Liver Dis 2:255, 1982
2. Ritchie AC: Boyd's Textbook of Pathology. 9th ed. Philadelphia: Lea & Febiger, 1990

BYRD OPERATION, creation of an artificial anus in the perineal region prior to colotomy for an imperforate anus.
1. Maffei WE: Os Fundamentos da Medicina. 2nd ed. Livraria Editora Artes Medicas Ltd, 1978

BYRON-SMITH OPERATION, a classic procedure for involutional ectropion; a modification of the Kuhnt-Szymanowski procedure.
1. Spaeth GL: Ophthalmic Surgery, Principles and Practice. Philadelphia: WB Saunders, 1982

BYWATERS SYNDROME, see Compression syndrome. (Eric G.L. Bywaters, British)

C SYNDROME, trigonocephaly, unusual facial features, wide alveolar ridges, multiple frenula, limb defects, visceral anomalies, redundant skin, mental deficiency, and hypotonia are characteristics. Cross-reference: Opitz trigonocephaly syndrome.

1. Gorlin RJ, Cohen MM Jr, Levin LS: Syndromes of the Head and Neck. 3rd ed. New York: Oxford University Press, 1990
2. Opitz JM, et al: The C syndrome of multiple congenital anomalies. Birth Defects 5(2):161-166, 1969

CACCIAPUOTI SIGN, when the normal limb is pushed down from the elevated position, the paralyzed limb goes up.

1. Casas EC: Diccionario Terminologico de Ciencias Medicas. 5th ed. Salvat Editores, SA, 1954

CADET DE GASSICOURT DISEASE, acute pulmonary congestion in the newborn (abortive pneumonia).

1. Casas EC: Diccionario Terminologico de Ciencias Medicas. 5th ed. Salvat Editores, SA, 1954

CAFFEY SYNDROME, CAFFEY-SILVERMAN SYNDROME, infantile cortical hyperostosis; visualized in skull x-rays. (John Caffey, 1895-1966, U.S. radiologist; William A. Silverman)

1. Caffey J, Silverman WA: Am J Roentgenol 54:1-16, 1945

CAFFEY-PSEUDO-HURLER SYNDROME, gangliosidosis G_{M1} type I; a glycogen storage disorder with the characteristics of growth deficiency (short stature), coarse features with a low nasal bridge and broad nose, moderate joint limitation with thick wrists, contractures of elbows and knees, and the development of claw hand. A cherry-red macular spot is present in about one half of patients. Autosomal recessive inheritance. Cross-reference: Generalized gangliosidosis syndrome type I. (John Caffey)

1. Caffey J: Gargoylism (Hunter-Hurler disease, dysostosis multiplex, lipochondrodystrophy); prenatal and neonatal bone lesions and their early postnatal evolution. Bull Hosp Joint Dis 12:38, 1951
2. Smith DW, Jones KL: Recognizable Patterns of Human Malformation: Genetic, Embryologic, and Clinical Aspects. 3rd ed. Philadelphia: WB Saunders, 1982

CAISSON DISEASE, sickness induced by a too-rapid decrease in air pressure after a stay in a compressed atmosphere, caused by nitrogen bubbles forming in blood and tissues.

1. Campbell WC, Crenshaw AH: Campbell's Operative Orthopaedics. 7th ed. St Louis: CV Mosby, 1987

CALABRO SYNDROME, synostosis of the coronal and metopic sutures, unilateral ulnar aplasia and oligodactyly, down-slanting palpebral fissures, micrognathia, short neck, micropenis, cryptorchidism, and pulmonic stenosis are features.

1. Gorlin RJ, Cohen MM Jr, Levin LS: Syndromes of the Head and Neck. 3rd ed. New York: Oxford University Press, 1990

CALDWELL-LUC OPERATION, radical maxillary sinusotomy. Cross-reference: Luc operation. (George W. Caldwell, 1834-1918, U.S.; Henri Luc, 1855-1925, French laryngologist)

1. DeWeese DD, Saunders WH: Textbook of Otolaryngology. 6th ed. St Louis: CV Mosby, 1982
2. Maffei WE: Os Fundamentos da Medicina. 2nd ed. Livraria Editora Artes Medicas Ltd, 1978

CALIFORNIA ENCEPHALITIS, the true clinical spectrum is not known, but includes nonspecific febrile illness, aseptic meningitis, and meningoencephalitis. Occurs in California, New Mexico, Utah, and Texas. Death is extremely uncommon.

1. Bennett JC, Plum F (eds): Cecil Textbook of Medicine. 20th ed. Philadelphia: WB Saunders, 1996

CALL SYNDROME, characteristics include headache, seizures, and multifocal brain signs that are transient or sometimes persistent. Cerebral edema and increased intracranial pressure can also occur. Women are affected more often than men, and a history of migraine is frequent. The syndrome is most common during the puerperium but can occur at any time, even after menopause. Probably a vasospastic disorder and not arteritis.

1. Call GK, Fleming MC, Sealfon S, et al: Reversible cerebral segmental restriction. Stroke 19:1159-1170, 1988

CALLISEN OPERATION, lumbar colotomy through a vertical incision.

1. Maffei WE: Os Fundamentos da Medicina. 2nd ed. Livraria Editora Artes Medicas Ltd, 1978

CALOT OPERATION, surgery for correction of a tuberculous gibbosity.

1. Maffei WE: Os Fundamentos da Medicina. 2nd ed. Livraria Editora Artes Medicas Ltd, 1978

CALVÉ-PERTHES DISEASE, see Legg disease. (Jacques Calvé, 1875-1954, French orthopedic surgeon; Georg Perthes, 1869-1927, German surgeon)

CAMERON-HAIGHT OPERATION, surgery for primary repair of esophageal atresia and tracheo-esophageal fistula in pediatric surgery.
1. Schwartz SI: Principles of Surgery. 4th ed. New York: McGraw-Hill, 1983

CAMPTOMELIC SYNDROME, growth hormone deficiency, large brain with gross cellular disorganization, flat-appearing face, anterior bowing of the tibiae, short and somewhat flat vertebrae, and incomplete cartilaginous development with tracheobronchomalacia are features. Autosomal recessive inheritance.
1. Smith DW, Jones KL: Recognizable Patterns of Human Malformation: Genetic, Embryologic, and Clinical Aspects. 3rd ed. Philadelphia: WB Saunders, 1982
2. Spranger J, et al: Increasing frequency of a syndrome of multiple osseous defects? Lancet 2:716, 1970

CAMURATI-ENGELMANN DISEASE, diaphyseal dysplasia; a progressive developmental disorder characterized by hyperostosis of the long bones, osteosclerosis, and muscular dystrophy. The typical case begins in early childhood, with a peculiar waddling gait as the first symptom. (Mario Camurati, 1896-1948, Italian; Guido Engelmann, 1876-1959, Austrian orthopedic surgeon)
1. Camurati M: Di un raro caso di osteite Simmetrica ereditaria degli arti inferiori. Chir Organi Mov 6:662-665, 1922
2. Engelmann G: Fortschr Roentgenstr 39:1101-1106, 1929
3. Gorlin RJ, Cohen MM Jr, Levin LS: Syndromes of the Head and Neck. 3rd ed. New York: Oxford University Press, 1990

CANAVAN DISEASE, a disorder is grouped with the diffuse cerebral scleroses but is considered a separate entity. The process begins between the 3rd and 9th months of life and pursues a rapid course, with death occurring within 3 to 15 months. (Myrtelle M. Canavan, 1879-1953, U.S. pathologist)
1. Canavan MM: Arch Neurol 25:299-308, 1931
2. Ritchie AC: Boyd's Textbook of Pathology. 9th ed. Philadelphia: Lea & Febiger, 1990

CANTELLI SIGN, dissociation of movement between the head and eyes. Cross-reference: Doll's eye sign.
1. Casas EC: Diccionario Terminologico de Ciencias Medicas. 5th ed. Salvat Editores, SA, 1954

CANTON DISEASE, CANTON FEVER, a typhus-like disease described in persons in the Cantonese region of China.
1. Casas EC: Diccionario Terminologico de Ciencias Medicas. 5th ed. Salvat Editores, SA, 1954

CANTRELL SYNDROME, a congenital heart disease (left ventricular diverticulum) consisting of a defect of the pericardium, diaphragm, sternum, and anterior abdomen wall. Cross reference: Pentalogy of Cantrell.
1. Borges AJ, Hazebroek FW, Hess J: Eur J Cardiothorac Surg 7:334-335, 1993
2. Czarnecki L, Mikolajczak-Mejir U, Zinka E: Wiad Lek 46:301-304, 1993
3. Genberg L, et al: Circulation 101:109-110, 2000

CAPGRAS SYNDROME, delusional misidentification; the delusional negation of identity of a familiar person and the conviction that the person has been replaced by a physically identical double. A variant of the delusional misidentification syndrome, the other three subtypes being the syndromes of Frégoli, intermetamorphosis, and subjective doubles. There is evidence that organic factors play a major part in the pathogenesis of these syndromes, although all Capgras syndrome cases cannot be explained on this basis. (Jean M. Capgras, 1873-1950, French psychiatrist)
1. Capgras J, Reboul-Lachaux J: Illusion des sosies dans un délire systématisé chronique. Bull Soc Clin Med Ment 11: 6-16, 1923
2. Christodoulou GN: The Delusional Misidentification Syndromes. Basel: Karger, 1986
3. Enoch D, Trethowan W: Some Uncommon Psychiatric Syndromes. Bristol, Engl: John Wright and Son, 1991, pp 1-23

CAPLAN SYNDROME, rheumatoid pneumoconiosis; pulmonary involvement in rheumatoid arthritis, giving rise to pleuritis with or without effusion, diffuse interstitial pneumonitis, and rheumatoid nodules are features. Often associated with dust exposure or pneumoconiosis. A frequent and often unsuspected manifestation of arthritis. (Anthony Caplan, 1907-1976, British)
1. Bennett JC, Plum F (eds): Cecil Textbook of Medicine. 20th ed. Philadelphia: WB Saunders, 1996
2. Caplan A: Thorax 8:29-37, 1953

CAPSULAR THROMBOSIS SYNDROME, hemiplegia due to thrombotic stroke affecting the internal capsule.
1. Fisher CM: Capsular infarct. Arch Neurol 36:65-73, 1979

CAPSULOTHALAMIC SYNDROME, hemiplegia, hemianopia, and abnormal pain perception due to lesions of the thalamus and internal capsule.

CAR SYNDROME, *c*ancer-*a*ssociated *r*etinopathy (CAR); a paraneoplastic disorder that appears to be an autoimmune process (oat cell or small cell carcinomas). Subacutely progressive bilateral blindness.
1. Walsh FB, Hoyt EF, Miller NR: Clinical Neuro-Ophthalmology. 4th ed. Baltimore: Williams & Wilkins, 1982

CARCINOID SYNDROME, carcinoidosis; alludes to the various humoral manifestations (such as rash, precordial murmur, and flushing) that may occur in a patient with carcinoid tumors. Cross-references: Argentaffinoma syndrome; Malignant carcinoid syndrome; Metastatic carcinoid syndrome.
1. Ballenger JJ: Diseases of the Nose, Throat, Ear, Head and Neck. 14th ed. Philadelphia: Lea & Febiger, 1991
2. Moschella SL, Hurley HJ: Dermatology. 2nd ed. Philadelphia: WB Saunders, 1985
3. Obendorfer S: Z Pathol 1:416-429, 1901

CARDARELLI SIGN, deviation of the trachea seen in the patient with aortic aneurysm. (Antonio Cardarelli, 1831-1927, Italian)
1. Casas EC: Diccionario Terminologico de Ciencias Medicas. 5th ed. Salvat Editores, SA, 1954

CARDARELLI-JAKSCH DISEASE, bending of the trachea to one side; may be present with an aneurysm of the aorta. (Antonio Cardarelli)
1. Casas EC: Diccionario Terminologico de Ciencias Medicas. 5th ed. Salvat Editores, SA, 1954

CARDIOFACIAL SYNDROME, see Caylor syndrome.

CARDIO-FACIO-CUTANEOUS SYNDROME, features include a characteristic retarded-like facial appearance, ectodermal abnormalities, growth failure, and variable cardiac defects. Etiology unknown.
1. Baraitser M, Patton MA: A Noonan-like short stature syndrome with sparse hair. J Med Genet 23:161-164, 1986
2. Gorlin RJ, Cohen MM Jr, Levin LS: Syndromes of the Head and Neck. 3rd ed. New York: Oxford University Press, 1990

CARDIORESPIRATORY SIGN, a change in the normal pulse/respiration ratio from 4:1 to 2:1; seen in the patient with infantile scurvy.
1. Dorland's Medical Dictionary. 28th ed. Philadelphia: WB Saunders, 1994

CARDIOVOCAL SYNDROME, see Ortner syndrome.

CAREY COOMBS MURMUR, a short, early diastolic murmur of the aortic valve or a soft pansystolic murmur of mitral valve incompetence. (Carey Coombs, 1879-1932, British)
1. Cheitlin MD, Sokolow M: Clinical Cardiology. 5th ed. Norwalk, Conn: Appleton & Lange, 1993

CARNETT SIGN, pain of visceral origin on compression of relaxed abdominal muscles. (John B. Carnett, 1876-1934, U.S. surgeon)
1. Casas EC: Diccionario Terminologico de Ciencias Medicas. 5th ed. Salvat Editores, SA, 1954

CARNETT TEST, lying flat, the patient is asked to extend both legs; while keeping the knees stiff, to raise both feet from the bed. This renders the abdominal muscles tense. (John B. Carnett)
1. Bailey H: Physical Signs in Clinical Surgery. 16th ed. Baltimore: Williams & Wilkins, 1983

CARNEVALE SYNDROME, consists of down-slanting palpebral fissures, ptosis of the upper eyelids, convergent strabismus, limited extension of the forearms, and hip dysplasia. Also includes mental deficiency, cryptorchidism, and partial agenesis of the abdominal musculature with diastasis.
1. Carnevale F, Krajewska G, Fischetto R, et al: New syndrome: ptosis of eyelids, strabismus, diastasis recti, hip defect, cryptorchidism, and developmental delay in two sibs. Am J Med Genet 33:186-189, 1989
2. Gorlin RJ, Cohen MM Jr, Levin LS: Syndromes of the Head and Neck. 3rd ed. New York: Oxford University Press, 1990

CARNEY SYNDROME, see LAMB syndrome.

CARNEY TRIAD, a rare disorder affecting young females and characterized by the presence of at least two of three neoplasms: gastric epithelioid leiomyosarcoma, extra-adrenal paraganglioma, and pulmonary chondroma.
1. Carney JA: The triad of gastric epithelioid leiomyosarcoma, functioning extra-adrenal paraganglioma and pulmonary chondroma. Cancer 43:374-382, 1979
2. Margulies KB, Sheps SG: Carney's triad: guidelines for management. Mayo Clin Proc 63:496-502, 1988

CARNOCHAN OPERATION, arterial ligature; seen in elephantiasis.
1. Maffei WE: Os Fundamentos da Medicina. 2nd ed. Livraria Editora Artes Medicas Ltd, 1978

CAROLI DISEASE, saccular intrahepatic bile duct dilatations that most often become symptomatic in the patient between the ages of 20 and 50 years; due to intrahepatic stone formation and cholangitis. (Jacques Caroli, French)

1. Adair DC, et al: Caroli's disease complicating pregnancy. South Med J 88, 1995
2. Ritchie AC: Boyd's Textbook of Pathology. 9th ed. Philadelphia: Lea & Febiger, 1990

CAROTID SYNDROME, CAROTID SINUS SYNDROME, cardio-inhibitory carotid sinus; syncope when associated with convulsive seizures due to overactivity of the carotid sinus reflex when pressure is applied to one or both carotid sinuses. Cross-reference: Charcot-Weiss-Baker syndrome.

1. Baker AB, Baker LH: Clinical Neurology. Revised ed. Philadelphia: Harper & Row, 1982
2. Charcot JM: Leçons sur les Maladies du Système Nerveaux Faites à la Salpétrière. Paris, 1872-1873
3. Weiss S, Baker JP: Medicine 12:297-354, 1933

CARPAL LIFT SIGN, the patient's hand is fixed on the examination table; the examiner applies pressure to the dorsum of the digit being examined. The patient is asked to lift the finger off the table. A carpal fracture or sprain is present when there is pain at the dorsum of the wrist.

1. Evans RC: Illustrated Essentials in Orthopedic Physical Assessment. St Louis: Mosby Yearbook, 1994

CARPAL SIGN, abnormally shaped bones in the proximal carpal row; frequently present in gonadal dysgenesis.

1. Gold JJ, Josimovich JB: Gynecologic Endocrinology. 3rd ed. New York: Plenum Medical, 1980

CARPAL TUNNEL SYNDROME, acroparesthesia; a result of compression or constriction of the median nerve in the carpal tunnel due to thickening of the transverse carpal ligament secondary to wrist injury or a space-occupying lesion.

1. Grinker RR, Sahs AL: Neurology. 6th ed. Springfield: Charles C Thomas, 1966
2. Haymaker W: Bing's Local Diagnosis in Neurological Diseases. 15th ed. St Louis: CV Mosby, 1969

CARPENTER SYNDROME, acrocephalopolysyndactyly type II. Characterized by acrocephaly, syndactyly, and a characteristic facial appearance, and associated with polydactyly of the feet, obesity, mental retardation, and hypogonadism. (George Carpenter, 1859-1910, British)

1. Carpenter G: Two sisters showing malformation of the skull and other congenital abnormalities. Rep Soc Study Dis Child (Lond) 1:110-118, 1901
2. Gorlin RJ, Cohen MM Jr, Levin LS: Syndromes of the Head and Neck. 3rd ed. New York: Oxford University Press, 1990
3. Wilson JD, Foster DW, Kronenberg HM, et al (eds): Williams Textbook of Endocrinology. 9th ed. Philadelphia: WB Saunders, 1998

CARPUE OPERATION, surgical technique for rhinoplasty that originated in India. (Joseph Carpue, 1764-1846, British surgeon)

1. Maffei WE: Os Fundamentos da Medicina. 2nd ed. Livraria Editora Artes Medicas Ltd, 1978

CARRIÓN DISEASE, see Oroya fever. (Daniel A. Carrión, 1859-1885, Peruvian)

CARTER DISEASE, Persian recurrent fever. (Henry V. Carter, 1831-1897, Anglo-Indian)

1. Casas EC: Diccionario Terminologico de Ciencias Medicas. 5th ed. Salvat Editores, SA, 1954

CARTER OPERATION, osseous rhinoplasty using a flap from the rib.

1. Maffei WE: Os Fundamentos da Medicina. 2nd ed. Livraria Editora Artes Medicas Ltd, 1978

CARVALLO SIGN, the mid-diastolic rumble of tricuspid stenosis and the holosystolic murmur of tricuspid regurgitation are increased during inspiration; distinguishes tricuspid from mitral involvement. (J.M. Rivera Carvallo, Mexican cardiologist)

1. Fowler NO: Cardiac Diagnosis and Treatment. 3rd ed. Cambridge: Harper & Row, 1980

CASAL DISEASE, necklace-like erythema and pigmentation around the neck in pellagra. (Gasper Casal, 1691-1759, Spanish)

1. Casas EC: Diccionario Terminologico de Ciencias Medicas. 5th ed. Salvat Editores, SA, 1954

CASCADE SIGN, when flexing the fingers, if the axes converge toward the scaphoid tubercle, either rheumatoid arthritis or internal derangement of the wrist and hand is indicated.

1. Evans RC: Illustrated Essentials in Orthopedic Physical Assessment. St Louis: Mosby Yearbook, 1994

CASSAN SIGN, "cracked pot" noise seen in the patient with brain tumors.

1. Casas EC: Diccionario Terminologico de Ciencias Medicas. 5th ed. Salvat Editores, SA, 1954

CASSEL OPERATION, resection of a middle ear exostosis through the external auditory canal.

1. Maffei WE: Os Fundamentos da Medicina. 2nd ed. Livraria Editora Artes Medicas Ltd, 1978

CAST SYNDROME, vascular compression of the duodenum leading to acute duodenal obstruction and gastric dilatation. Cross-reference: Plaster cast syndrome.

1. Campbell WC, Crenshaw AH: Campbell's Operative Orthopaedics. 7th ed. St Louis: CV Mosby, 1987

2. Evarts CM: The cast syndrome: report of a case after spinal fusion for scoliosis. Clin Orthop 75:164, 1971

CASTELLANI DISEASE, hemorrhagic bronchitis caused by *Spirochaeta bronchialis*. (Sir Aldo Castellani, 1878-1971, Italian-born Britain)

1. Castellani A: Lancet 1:13-15, 1912

CAT EYE SYNDROME, mild mental deficiency, coloboma iris, and anal atresia are features. Occurs because of an extra segment derived from chromosome 22 in the karyotype; associated with partial trisomy or tetrasomy 22pter-q11.

1. Campbell MF, Walsh PC: Campbell's Urology. 5th ed. Philadelphia: WB Saunders, 1986
2. Gorlin RJ, Cohen MM Jr, Levin LS: Syndromes of the Head and Neck. 3rd ed. New York: Oxford University Press, 1990
3. Haab O: Graefes Arch Klin Ophthalmol 24:257-262, 1878

CATEL-MANZKE SYNDROME, includes cleft palate, micrognathia, and bilateral clinodactyly (radial angulation) of the index finger. Cross-reference: Palatodigital syndrome.

1. Brude E: Pierre Robin sequence and hyperphalangy—a genetic entity (Catel-Manzke syndrome). Eur J Pediatr 142:222-223, 1984
2. Catel W: Differential diagnose von Krankheitssymptomon bei Kindern und Jugendlichen. Stuttgart: Thieme, 1961
3. Gorlin RJ: Type A2 brachydactyly syndrome. Birth Defects 2(2):41-42, 1975
4. Manzke H: Fortschr Roentgenstr 105:425-427, 1996

CAT'S CRY SYNDROME, see Cri du chat syndrome.

CATTANEO SIGN, firm compression of the dorsal spinal process causes redness; an indication of tracheobronchial adenopathy.

1. Casas EC: Diccionario Terminologico de Ciencias Medicas. 5th ed. Salvat Editores, SA, 1954

CAUDA EQUINA SYNDROME, caused by tumors of the cauda equina, lumbar spine stenosis, ruptured lumbar disc, arachnoiditis, and spinal fracture and manifested by paralysis and neurogenic involvement of the urinary bladder.

1. Rowland LP (ed): Merritt's Textbook of Neurology. 9th ed. Baltimore: Williams & Wilkins, 1995

CAUDAL DYSPLASIA SYNDROME, CAUDAL REGRESSION SYNDROME, sacral agenesis; failure of development of part or all of the coccygeal, sacral, and occasionally lumbar vertebral units and the corresponding segments of the caudal spinal cord, with resulting neurogenic dysfunction of bowel and bladder.

1. Duhamel B: From the mermaid to anal imperforation: the syndrome of caudal regression. Arch Dis Child 36:152, 1961
2. Smith DW, Jones KL: Recognizable Patterns of Human Malformation: Genetic, Embryologic, and Clinical Aspects. 3rd ed. Philadelphia: WB Saunders, 1982

CAVARÉ-WESTPHAL DISEASE, familial hypokalemic paralysis and cramps; usually nocturnal. (C. Cavaré, Italian; Karl F.O. Westphal, 1833-1890, German neurologist)

1. Bordas LB: Neurologia Fundamental. 2nd ed. Barcelona: Ed. Toray, 1968
2. Cavaré C: Berl Klin Wochenschr 22:489-491, 1885

CAVERNOUS SINUS SYNDROME, ophthalmoplegia and paralysis of the 3rd-6th cranial nerves caused by infections or tumors (rarely pituitary), intracranial aneurysms, or thrombosis involving the cavernous and/or lateral sinuses. Cross-references: Foix syndrome; Godtfredsen syndrome; Hillemand syndrome.

1. Foix C: Rev Neurol (Par) 38:827-832, 1922
2. Godtfredsen E: Studies on the cavernous sinus syndrome. Acta Neurol Scand 40:69-75, 1964
3. Gorlin RJ, Cohen MM Jr, Levin LS: Syndromes of the Head and Neck. 3rd ed. New York: Oxford University Press, 1990

CAVITE DISEASE, endemic fever similar to dengue in which the patient complains of muscle pain, fever, and pain in the globi.

1. Casas EC: Diccionario Terminologico de Ciencias Medicas. 5th ed. Salvat Editores, SA, 1954

CAYLER SYNDROME, asymmetric crying facies, usually affecting the right side, associated with cardiac defects. Present from birth. Cross-reference: Cardiofacial syndrome.

1. Cayler GG: Cardiofacial syndrome. Congenital heart disease and facial weakness, a hitherto unrecognized association. Arch Dis Child 44:69-75, 1969

CAZENAVE DISEASE, lupus erythematosus. (Pierre L.A. Cazenave, 1795-1877, French)

1. Casas EC: Diccionario Terminologico de Ciencias Medicas. 5th ed. Salvat Editores, SA, 1954

CEELEN-GELLERSTEDT SYNDROME, see Goodpasture syndrome.

CEGKA SIGN, respiratory sounds do not change when the chest is percussed; an indication of pericardial effusion. (Josephus J. Cegka, 1812-1862, Czech)
1. Casas EC: Diccionario Terminologico de Ciencias Medicas. 5th ed. Salvat Editores, SA, 1954

CELIAC SYNDROME, see Gee syndrome.

CELSIO OPERATION, 1) circular amputation; 2) perineal lithotomy; 3) extirpation of a labial epithelioma using a V-shaped incision; 4) embryotomy by decapitation.
1. Maffei WE: Os Fundamentos da Medicina. 2nd ed. Livraria Editora Artes Medicas Ltd, 1978

CENTRAL ALVEOLAR HYPOVENTILATION SYNDROME, characterized by major changes in respiratory function during sleep, including central sleep apnea and hypopnea associated with recurrent hypoxemia, hypercapnia, and a decreased tidal and minute volume. Cross-reference: Ondine curse. (Named after Ondine, a water nymph who punished her husband for betraying her, by depriving him of automatic breathing.)
1. Rowland LP (ed): Merritt's Textbook of Neurology. 9th ed. Baltimore: Williams & Wilkins, 1995

CENTRAL CORD SYNDROME, represents the clinical correlate of the central part of the spinal cord damaged from injury just above the concussive blow. Disproportionately more involvement of the upper extremities than the lower. Usually a result of hyperextension injury in the patient with cervical spondylosis.
1. Bennett JC, Plum F (eds): Cecil Textbook of Medicine. 20th ed. Philadelphia: WB Saunders, 1996
2. Campbell WC, Crenshaw AH: Campbell's Operative Orthopaedics. 7th ed. St Louis: CV Mosby, 1987

CENTRAL CORE DISEASE, the central portion of the muscle fiber appears rather amorphous, in contrast to the fibrillar appearance of the surrounding normal portion.
1. Bennett JC, Plum F (eds): Cecil Textbook of Medicine. 20th ed. Philadelphia: WB Saunders, 1996

CENTRAL SLEEP APNEA SYNDROME, see Sleep apnea syndrome.

CENTROPOSTERIOR SYNDROME, a syndrome of syringomyelic dissociation of sensibility and vasomotor disorders, owing to lesions of the centroposterior portion of the gray matter of the spinal cord.
1. Dorland's Medical Dictionary. 28th ed. Philadelphia: WB Saunders, 1994

CEPHALIC ZOSTER SYNDROME, see Ramsay Hunt syndrome.

CEREBELLAR SYNDROME, hereditary cerebellar ataxia (particularly the Marie type) with hyperreflexia, optic atrophy, and possibly oculomotor palsy.
1. Dorland's Medical Dictionary. 28th ed. Philadelphia: WB Saunders, 1994

CEREBELLOPONTINE ANGLE SYNDROME, damage to the 8th cranial nerve in the region between the porus acusticus and the edge of the lowermost pons, giving rise to the variety of clinical disturbances known as this syndrome.
1. Baker AB, Baker LH: Clinical Neurology. Revised ed. Philadelphia: Harper & Row, 1982
2. Haymaker W: Bing's Local Diagnosis in Neurological Diseases. 15th ed. St Louis: CV Mosby, 1969
3. Henneberg, Koch: Ueber 'Central'-neurofibromatose und die Geschwülste des Kleinhirnbrückenwinkels. Arch Psychiatr Nervenkr 36:251-304, 1902

CEREBROCOSTOMANDIBULAR SYNDROME, a hereditary developmental disorder with features of mental deficiency, short stature, unusual cough, severe micrognathia with glossoptosis and cleft palate, and a bell-shaped small thorax. Autosomal recessive inheritance. Cross-reference: Rib-gap syndrome.
1. Burton EM, Oestreich AE: Cerebro-costo-mandibular syndrome with stippled epiphyses and cystic fibrosis. Pediatr Radiol 18:365-367, 1988
2. Gorlin RJ, Cohen MM Jr, Levin LS: Syndromes of the Head and Neck. 3rd ed. New York: Oxford University Press, 1990
3. Smith DW, Jones KL: Recognizable Patterns of Human Malformation: Genetic, Embryologic, and Clinical Aspects. 3rd ed. Philadelphia: WB Saunders, 1982

CEREBROHEPATORENAL SYNDROME, see Zellweger syndrome.

CEREBRO-OCULO-FACIAL-SKELETAL SYNDROME, see Pena-Shokeir syndrome type II.

CERVICAL RIB SYNDROME, a form of the thoracic outlet syndrome in which the thoracic inlet has moved cranially one vertebral segment. The rib articulating with the 7th cervical vertebra has all or most of the characteristic features and muscle attachments of what is regarded as a normal 1st thoracic rib, while the 7th cervical vertebra presents the features of the 1st thoracic vertebra. The vertebral series now shows six cervical and 13 thoracic vertebrae. Cross-reference: Thoracic outlet syndrome.

1. Sunderland S: Nerves and Nerve Injuries. Edinburgh: Churchill Livingstone, 1972

CERVICAL-FUSION SYNDROME, see Klippel-Feil syndrome.

CERVICO-BRACHIAL SYNDROME, compression of the subclavian vessels and/or the lower trunk of the brachial plexus causes tension and friction which impair circulation to the limb and alter function in the distribution of the 8th cervical and 1st thoracic nerve fibers. The syndrome is both neural and vascular in origin.

1. Sunderland S: Nerves and Nerve Injuries. Edinburgh: Churchill Livingstone, 1972

CERVICO-OCULO-ACOUSTIC SYNDROME, see Wildervanck syndrome.

CÉSTAN SIGN, see Dutemps-Céstan sign. (E.J.M. Raymond Céstan, 1872-1934, French neurologist)

CÉSTAN-CHENAIS SYNDROME, CÉSTAN PARALYSIS, includes the same features as Babinski-Nageotte syndrome plus paralysis of the ipsilateral vocal cord and soft palate with dysphagia. (E.J.M. Raymond Céstan; Louis J. Chenais, 1872-1950, French)

1. Baker AB, Baker LH: Clinical Neurology. Revised ed. Philadelphia: Harper & Row, 1982
2. Céstan EJ, Chenais J: Gaz Hop 76:1229-1233, 1903
3. Gorlin RJ, Cohen MM Jr, Levin LS: Syndromes of the Head and Neck. 3rd ed. New York: Oxford University Press, 1990

CÉSTAN-RAYMOND SYNDROME, see Raymond-Céstan syndrome. (E.J.M. Raymond Céstan)

CHABERT DISEASE, symptomatic anthrax.

1. Casas EC: Diccionario Terminologico de Ciencias Medicas. 5th ed. Salvat Editores, SA, 1954

CHADDOCK SIGN, elicited by stimulating the lateral aspect of the foot with a blunt point, producing the Babinski sign; seen in the patient with upper motor neuron lesions of the pyramidal tracts. Cross-reference: External malleolar sign. (Charles G. Chaddock, 1861-1936, U.S. neurologist)

1. Baker AB, Baker LH: Clinical Neurology. Revised ed. Philadelphia: Harper & Row, 1982

CHADWICK SIGN, purplish color of the cervix and vagina in the fourth week of pregnancy. (James R. Chadwick, 1844-1905, U.S.)

1. Casas EC: Diccionario Terminologico de Ciencias Medicas. 5th ed. Salvat Editores, SA, 1954

CHAGAS DISEASE, CHAGAS-CRUZ DISEASE, produced by a protozoan, *Trypanosoma cruzi*, which is harbored by hematophagous insects common in South and Central America. Cross-reference: Cruz-Chagas disease. (Carlos Chagas, 1879-1934, Brazilian; Oswaldo G. Cruz, 1872-1917, Brazilian)

1. Bennett JC, Plum F (eds): Cecil Textbook of Medicine. 20th ed. Philadelphia: WB Saunders, 1996
2. Chagas C: Mem Inst Oswaldo Cruz 1:159-218, 1909
3. Shafii A: Chagas' disease with cardiopathy and hemiplegia. NY State J Med 77:418-419, 1977

CHAGRES DISEASE, a severe type of malarial fever. Cross-reference: Panama disease.

1. Casas EC: Diccionario Terminologico de Ciencias Medicas. 5th ed. Salvat Editores, SA, 1954

CHALIER-LEVRAT DISEASE, tropical eosinophilia.

1. Casas EC: Diccionario Terminologico de Ciencias Medicas. 5th ed. Salvat Editores, SA, 1954

CHANCRIFORM SYNDROME, a characteristic chancre at the site of entry of the causative organism, accompanied by regional lymphadenopathy. These infections are usually self-limiting and seldom result in disseminated disease; often seen in laboratory or autopsy workers. May be a manifestation of extrapulmonary coccidioidomycosis.

1. Moschella SL, Hurley HJ: Dermatology. 2nd ed. Philadelphia: WB Saunders, 1985

CHANDRA-KHETARPAL SYNDROME, repeated fever with symptoms of bronchiectasis associated with levocardia.

1. Chandra RK, Khetarpal SK: Levocardia with bronchiectasis and paranasal sinus abnormalities. Indian J Pediatr 30:78-80, 1963

CHAPPLE SIGN, the examiner flexes the thigh of a newborn (under 3 months of age) to 90 degrees in an attempt to adduct it. The sign is present when no more than 45 degrees of adduction can be obtained and is found in congenital dislocation of the hip.

1. Casas EC: Diccionario Terminologico de Ciencias Medicas. 5th ed. Salvat Editores, SA, 1954

CHAPUT OPERATION, a technique for creation of an artificial anus followed by enteroanastomosis. (Henry Chaput, 1857-1919, French surgeon)

1. Maffei WE: Os Fundamentos da Medicina. 2nd ed. Livraria Editora Artes Medicas Ltd, 1978

CHARCOT DISEASE, CHARCOT JOINT DISEASE, neuroarthropathic arthritis; a progressive joint disease as a result of neurological disorders. Occurs secondary to syphilis, syringomyelia, and other lesions of the nervous system. An arthropathy that occurs 85% of the time in the lower limbs, the knee being the commonest joint affected. Two quite distinct types of neuropathic joint are distinguishable radiologically: hypertrophic and atrophic. (Jean M. Charcot, 1825-1893, French neurologist)

1. Charcot JM: Arch Physiol Paris 1:161-178, 1868

CHARCOT HYSTERICAL BLUE EDEMA, long-standing disuse of a limb due to hysteria; may present to the surgeon in two ways. First, the dependent limb becomes cyanosed and swollen from lack of use; this is usually seen in the lower limbs. In the upper limbs, muscle wasting consequent to disuse atrophy occurs and a radiograph shows bone decalcification similar to that seen in Sudeck posttraumatic bone atrophy. (Jean M. Charcot)

1. Guinon G: Prog Med Paris 12:259-264, 1890

CHARCOT SIGN, depression of the eyebrow on the paralyzed side when trying to contract the eyebrow.

1. Casas EC: Diccionario Terminologico de Ciencias Medicas. 5th ed. Salvat Editores, SA, 1954

CHARCOT SYNDROME, a progressive disease of the joints resulting from neural disorders including neuroarthropathy; amyotrophic lateral sclerosis, intermittent claudication, and intermittent fever due to cholangitis are features. The Charcot triad consists of intention tremor, scanning speech, and nystagmus. (Jean M. Charcot)

1. Bailey H, Love M: A Short Practice of Surgery. 12th ed. London: HK Lewis & Co, 1962
2. Charcot JM: Arch Physiol 1:161-178, 1868
3. Charcot JM: Compt Rendu Soc Biol 5:225-258, 1858

CHARCOT-MARIE SIGN, quick, short tremor in exophthalmic goiter. Cross-reference: Marie sign. (Jean M. Charcot; Pierre Marie, 1853-1940, French neurologist)

1. Casas EC: Diccionario Terminologico de Ciencias Medicas. 5th ed. Salvat Editores, SA, 1954

CHARCOT-MARIE-TOOTH DISEASE, spinocerebellar degeneration with onset in the first or second decade and slow progression. Reflexes are absent and there is moderate sensory loss and predominantly peroneal muscle atrophy. Nerves may be hypertrophic, with optic and acoustic nerve involvement. Usually autosomal dominant. (Jean M. Charcot; Pierre Marie; Howard Tooth, 1856-1925, British)

1. Bennett JC, Plum F (eds): Cecil Textbook of Medicine. 20th ed. Philadelphia: WB Saunders, 1996
2. Charcot JM, Marie P: Rev Med Paris 6:97-138, 1886
3. Tooth H: The Peroneal Type of Progressive Muscular Atrophy. London: Lewis, 1886

CHARCOT-VIGOUROUX SIGN, see Vigouroux sign. (Jean M. Charcot)

CHARCOT-WEISS-BAKER SYNDROME, see Carotid sinus syndrome. (Jean M. Charcot; Soma Weiss, 1898-1942, U.S.; James P. Baker, U.S.)

CHARCOT-WILBRAND SYNDROME, visual agnosia; the patient with this disease has difficulty picturing or describing familiar objects or people not in his/her immediate view. The pathological lesion is usually near dominant angular gyrus. (Jean M. Charcot; Hermann Wilbrand, 1851-1935, German neuro-ophthalmologist)

1. Charcot JM: Sur un Cas de Ceocite Verbales. Paris: Delahaye, 1887

CHARLEVOIX DISEASE, see Andermann syndrome.

CHARLIE M. SYNDROME, hypertelorism, absent or conically crowned incisors, cleft palate, and variable degrees of hypodactyly of the hands and feet are characteristics. Facial paralysis is present in some instances.

1. Gorlin RJ: Some facial syndromes. Birth Defects 5(2):65-76, 1969
2. Gorlin RJ, Cohen MM Jr, Levin LS: Syndromes of the Head and Neck. 3rd ed. New York: Oxford University Press, 1990
3. Kaplan P, et al: A "community" of face-limb malformation syndromes. J Pediatr 89:241-247, 1976

CHARLIN SYNDROME, ciliary neuralgia; an eye disturbance of nasal origin. Pain is associated with corneal and iris inflammation, rhinorrhea, and tenderness along the nose producing recurrent headaches. (Carlos Charlin, 1886-1945, Chilean ophthalmologist)

1. Charlin C: Dia Med 2:839, 1930

CHARLOUIS DISEASE, yaws; an infectious disease caused by *Treponema pertenue*. Cross-reference: Breda disease. (M. Charlouis, Dutch surgeon)
1. Charlouis M: Vjersch Derm Syph, 1881, pp 431-466

CHARRIN DISEASE, pyocyanic infection.
1. Casas EC: Diccionario Terminologico de Ciencias Medicas. 5th ed. Salvat Editores, SA, 1954

CHASE PHENOMENON, CHASE-SULZBERGER PHENOMENON, see Sulzberger-Chase phenomenon.

CHASE SIGN, compression of the descending colon with one hand and the transverse colon with the other hand results in pain near the cecum.
1. Casas EC: Diccionario Terminologico de Ciencias Medicas. 5th ed. Salvat Editores, SA, 1954

CHASSAIGNAC SIGN, pus is elicited when the nipple is squeezed; an indication of mastitis.
1. Casas EC: Diccionario Terminologico de Ciencias Medicas. 5th ed. Salvat Editores, SA, 1954

CHAUFFARD SYNDROME, CHAUFFARD-STILL SYNDROME, an inflammatory condition affecting multiple joints; consists of fever and enlargement of the spleen and lymph nodes in persons infected with nonhuman tuberculosis. (Anatole M.E. Chauffard; 1855-1932, French; George F. Still, 1868-1941, British)
1. Ramon F: Rev Med Par 16:345-359, 1896
2. Still GF: Med Chir Trans R Med Chir Soc Lond 80:47-59, 1897

CHAUSSIER SIGN, pain in the epigastric region preceding eclampsia. (François Chaussier, 1746-1828, French)
1. Casas EC: Diccionario Terminologico de Ciencias Medicas. 5th ed. Salvat Editores, SA, 1954

CHEADLE DISEASE, see Möller-Barlow disease.

CHEATLE DISEASE, see Bloodgood disease.

CHÉDIAK-HIGASHI SYNDROME, CHÉDIAK-STEINBRINCK-HIGASHI SYNDROME, an autosomally inherited defect in the production of lysosomes, the membrane-enclosed granular organelles that are found in almost every type of cell. Chronic polyneuropathy, diminished uveal or retinal pigmentation, mental deficiency, and hyperhidrosis are present. (Moises Chédiak, Cuban; Ototaku Higashi, Japanese pediatrician; W. Steinbrinck, West German)
1. Chédiak M: Rev Hematol 7:362-367, 1952
2. Farmer TW: Pediatric Neurology. 2nd ed. Hagerstown: Harper & Row, 1975
3. Higashi O: Tohoku J Exp Med 59:315-332, 1953/54
4. Steinbrinck W: Dtsch Arch Klin Med 193:577-581, 1948

CHÉDIAK-HIGASHI-LIKE SYNDROME, see Griscelli syndrome. (Moises Chédiak; Ototaku Higashi)

CHEEK PHENOMENON, following pressure on both cheeks just under the zygomas, there is a reflex upward jerk of both arms with bending of both elbows; seen in meningitis.
1. Dorland's Medical Dictionary. 28th ed. Philadelphia: WB Saunders, 1994

CHEEVER OPERATION, tonsillectomy through a neck incision.
1. Maffei WE: Os Fundamentos da Medicina. 2nd ed. Livraria Editora Artes Medicas Ltd, 1978

CHEMKE SYNDROME, see Walker-Warburg syndrome.

CHENEY SYNDROME, see Hajdu syndrome.

CHERCHEVSKY DISEASE, adynamic ileus of hysterical origin.
1. Casas EC: Diccionario Terminologico de Ciencias Medicas. 5th ed. Salvat Editores, SA, 1954

CHERRY-RED SPOT MYOCLONUS SYNDROME, sialidosis type 1; cherry-red spot in the macula presenting before 10 years of age and myoclonus precipitated by thought of movement but not by light due to deficiency of sialidase.
1. Rapin I, Goldfischer S, Katzman R, et al: The cherry red spot-myoclonus syndrome. Ann Neurol 3:234-242, 1978

CHEYNE OPERATION, surgical technique for crural hernia using a flap from the pectineal muscle.
1. Maffei WE: Os Fundamentos da Medicina. 2nd ed. Livraria Editora Artes Medicas Ltd, 1978

CHEYNE-STOKES RESPIRATION, a respiratory pattern of apnea and hyperpnea; some patients with severe heart failure display periodic breathing characterized by alternating periods of apnea and hyperventilation. (John Cheyne, 1777-1836, Scottish; William Stokes, 1804-1878, Irish)

1. Cheitlin MD, Sokolow M: Clinical Cardiology. 5th ed. Norwalk, Conn: Appleton & Lange, 1993
2. Cheyne J: Dublin Hosp Rep 2:216-223, 1818
3. Stokes W: The Diseases of the Heart and Aorta. Dublin: Hodges & Smith, 1854, pp 320-327

CHIARI SYNDROME, see Arnold-Chiari syndrome. (Johann B.V.L. Chiari, 1817-1854, Austrian gynecologist)

CHIARI-BUDD SYNDROME, see Budd syndrome. (Johann B.V.L. Chiari)

CHIARI-FROMMEL SYNDROME, galactorrhea and amenorrhea persisting, without evident pituitary involvement, for more than 6 months postpartum in the absence of nursing. A poorly understood syndrome. Cross-references: Amenorrhea-galactorrhea syndrome; Forbes-Albright syndrome; Frommel disease. (Johann B.V.L. Chiari; Richard J.E. Frommel, 1854-1912, German gynecologist)

1. Ahumada JC, Del Castille EB: Sobre un caso de galactorrhea y amenorrhea. Bull Soc Obstet Gen Buenos Aires 11:64-72, 1932
2. Chiari J: Klinik der Geburtschilke und Gynekologie. Erlagen: Enke, 1855
3. Frommel RJE: Zschr Geburtsh 7:305-313, 1882

CHIASMAL SYNDROME, CHIASMATIC SYNDROME, impairment of vision, field vision limitation, central scotoma, syncope, headache, and vertigo are characteristics. Virtually any lesion that in some way damages the optic chiasma produces this syndrome.

1. Cushing H: The chiasma syndrome of primary optic atrophy and bitemporal field defects in adults with a normal sella turcica. Arch Ophthalmol 3:505-551, 704-735, 1930

CHIAZZI OPERATION, omentopexy.

1. Maffei WE: Os Fundamentos da Medicina. 2nd ed. Livraria Editora Artes Medicas Ltd, 1978

CHICAGO DISEASE, North American blastomycosis.

1. Casas EC: Diccionario Terminologico de Ciencias Medicas. 5th ed. Salvat Editores, SA, 1954

CHIENNE OPERATION, 1) resection of a cuneiform portion of the medial condyle of the femur for treatment of genu valgus; 2) opening of the retropharyngeal space through a cervicolateral incision in the posterior border of the sternocleidomastoid muscle.

1. Maffei WE: Os Fundamentos da Medicina. 2nd ed. Livraria Editora Artes Medicas Ltd, 1978

CHIKUNGUNYA DISEASE, an arthropod-borne viral infection indigenous to Africa and Asia. Its native name is from its outstanding symptoms (i.e., a state of being "doubled up" owing to fulminating severe joint pain).

1. Baker AB, Baker LH: Clinical Neurology. Revised ed. Philadelphia: Harper & Row, 1982
2. Harrison VR, Marshall JD, Guilloud NB: The presence of antibody to chikungunya and other serologically related viruses in the sera of subhuman primate imports to the U.S. J Immunol 98:979-981, 1967

CHILAIDITI SYNDROME, migration of the colon between the liver and diaphragm; the condition is usually asymptomatic in adults, but symptoms are evident in children and include vomiting, abdominal pain, anorexia, constipation, and aerophagia. Signs include abdominal distention and absence of liver dullness. (Demetrius Chilaiditi, German radiologist)

1. Chilaiditi D: Fortschr Roentgenstr 16:173-208, 1910
2. Melester T, Burt ME: Chilaiditi syndrome: report of three cases. JAMA 254:944-945, 1985

CHILD SYNDROME, *c*ongenital *h*emidysplasia with *i*chthyosiform erythroderma and *l*imb *d*efects (CHILD); see Jadassohn syndrome.

CHIN-RETRACTION SIGN, the chin and larynx move downward during inspiration.

1. Casas EC: Diccionario Terminologico de Ciencias Medicas. 5th ed. Salvat Editores, SA, 1954

CHINESE RESTAURANT SYNDROME, ingestion of food containing large amounts of monosodium glutamate (MSG) followed by burning retrosternal distress resembling the pain of angina pectoris. Named after a type of restaurant where MSG is frequently used in cooking.

1. Fowler NO: Cardiac Diagnosis and Treatment. 3rd ed. Cambridge: Harper & Row, 1980
2. Haymaker W: Bing's Local Diagnosis in Neurological Diseases. 15th ed. St Louis: CV Mosby, 1969
3. Kwok RHM: The Chinese restaurant syndrome. N Engl J Med 278:796, 1968

CHIPAULT OPERATION, lengthening of the tibial nerves in the treatment of peripheral diabetic vasculopathy (diabetic foot).

1. Maffei WE: Os Fundamentos da Medicina. 2nd ed. Livraria Editora Artes Medicas Ltd, 1978

CHIPRE DISEASE, see Malta fever.

CHIRAY-FOIX-NICOLESCO SYNDROME, see Mari-Foix sign.

CHITRAL DISEASE, pappataci (phlebotomus) fever.
1. Casas EC: Diccionario Terminologico de Ciencias Medicas. 5th ed. Salvat Editores, SA, 1954

CHOLESTATIC HEPATITIS SYNDROME, a complication of acute viral hepatitis.
1. Bennett JC, Plum F (eds): Cecil Textbook of Medicine. 20th ed. Philadelphia: WB Saunders, 1996

CHOPART OPERATION, 1) a method of amputation; 2) plastic operation on the lip. (François Chopart, 1743-1795, French surgeon)
1. Maffei WE: Os Fundamentos da Medicina. 2nd ed. Livraria Editora Artes Medicas Ltd, 1978

CHORDA TYMPANI SYNDROME, reddening and sweating involving the whole of one side of the face, neck, upper back, and chest. A subjective feeling of warmth in the involved area is common. An objective sensory deficit and a decrease or loss of thermal sweating in the area may also be present.
1. Baker AB, Baker LH: Clinical Neurology. Revised ed. Philadelphia: Harper & Row, 1982
2. Haymaker W: Bing's Local Diagnosis in Neurological Diseases. 15th ed. St Louis: CV Mosby, 1969

CHOTZEN SYNDROME, see Saethre-Chotzen syndrome.

CHRIST-SIEMENS-TOURAINE SYNDROME, ectodermal dysplasia with diminished sweat; hypotrichosis and partial or total anodontia are characteristics. Cross-references: Anhidrotic ectodermal dysplasia syndrome; Rapp-Hodgkin syndrome. (Joseph Christ, 1871-1948, German; Hermann W. Siemens, 1891-1969, German dermatologist; Albert Touraine, 1883-1961, French dermatologist)
1. Christ J: Arch Dermatol Syph 116:685-703, 1913
2. Siemens HW: Arch Dermatol Syph 175:567-717, 1937
3. Touraine A: Presse Med 44:145-149, 1946

CHRISTIAN SYNDROME, consists of microcephaly, craniosynostosis, arthrogryposis, and cleft palate. An autosomal recessive disorder. Cross-reference: Adducted thumbs syndrome. (Joe C. Christian, U.S. geneticist)
1. Christian JC, Andrews PA, Conneally PM, et al: Clin Genet 2:95-103, 1971
2. Gorlin RJ, Cohen MM Jr, Levin LS: Syndromes of the Head and Neck. 3rd ed. New York: Oxford University Press, 1990

CHRISTIAN-WEBER DISEASE, see Weber disease. (Henry A. Christian, 1876-1951, U.S. internist)

CHRISTMAS DISEASE, hemophilia can be caused by a mutation at either of two distinct loci on the X chromosome, one leading to a deficiency of factor VIII (classic hemophilia) and one leading to a deficiency of factor IX (Christmas disease). (Christmas is the surname of a child with this disease.)
1. Bennett JC, Plum F (eds): Cecil Textbook of Medicine. 20th ed. Philadelphia: WB Saunders, 1996
2. Ritchie AC: Boyd's Textbook of Pathology. 9th ed. Philadelphia: Lea & Febiger, 1990

CHRONIC BRAIN SYNDROME, see Organic mental syndrome.

CHRONIC FATIGUE SYNDROME, fatigue dysphoria; a weariness or decreased motivation to engage in physical or mental effort is described. Work tolerance is diminished and there is a subjective feeling of tiredness along with dissatisfaction with his/her state of health. Dispute exists regarding the etiology of this condition.
1. Albrecht R, Oliver VL, Poskanzer DC: JAMA 187:904-907, 1964

CHRONIC HYPERVENTILATION SYNDROME, see Hyperventilation syndrome.

CHURG-STRAUSS SYNDROME, allergic granulomatous angiitis; a disease similar to classic polyarthritis nodosa, except for the divergent features of allergic angitis and granulomatosis. (Jacob Churg, U.S. pathologist; Lotte Strauss, 1913-1985, U.S. pathologist)
1. Bennett JC, Plum F (eds): Cecil Textbook of Medicine. 20th ed. Philadelphia: WB Saunders, 1996
2. Churg J, Strauss L: Am J Pathol 27:277-294, 1951

CHVOSTEK SIGN, CHVOSTEK-WEISS SIGN, in cases of tetany, gently tapping the 7th cranial nerve as it emerges in front of the external auditory meatus with a percussion hammer provokes a brisk muscular twitch on the same side of the face. Cross-references: Schultze-Chvostek sign; Weiss sign. (Franz Chvostek, 1834-1884, Austrian surgeon; Nathan Weiss, 1851-1883, Austrian)
1. Bailey H: Physical Signs in Clinical Surgery. 16th ed. Baltimore: Williams & Wilkins, 1983
2. Grinker RR, Sahs AL: Neurology. 6th ed. Springfield: Charles C Thomas, 1966

CHYLOMICRONEMIA SYNDROME, hyperlipoproteinemia type I of familial origin; marked chylomicronemia with plasma triglyceride levels in excess of 2000 mg/dl associated with a constellation of signs and symptoms such as colicky abdominal pain, malaise, anorexia, recurrent attacks of pancreatitis with hepatosplenomegaly, and paresthesias similar to carpal tunnel syndrome. Cross-reference: Bürger-Grütz syndrome.

1. Bennett JC, Plum F (eds): Cecil Textbook of Medicine. 20th ed. Philadelphia: WB Saunders, 1996

CIARROCCHI DISEASE, dermatitis of the third interdigital space.

1. Casas EC: Diccionario Terminologico de Ciencias Medicas. 5th ed. Salvat Editores, SA, 1954

CIRCLE OF WILLIS, connections between both internal carotid arteries via the anterior communicating artery and with the basilar artery via the posterior communicating arteries. Willis first noted the sweetness of diabetic urine and described myasthenia gravis. (Thomas Willis, 1621-1675, British)

1. Krayenbühl HA, Yasargil MG: Cerebral Angiography. 2nd ed. Philadelphia: JB Lippincott, 1968

CITELLI SYNDROME, loss of power of concentration and drowsiness, mental retardation, sleep disturbance, and sinusitis and adenoiditis are features. (Salvatore Citelli, 1875-1947, Italian laryngologist)

1. Citelli S: Vegetazioni adenoidi e sordomutismo. Boll Mal Orecchio Gola Naso 22:141-150, 1904

CIVATTE DISEASE, poikiloderma; reticulated, blotchy, reddish-brown hyperpigmentation and telangiectasia with interspersed atrophic pale puncta develop in a fairly symmetrical distribution on sun-exposed areas of the neck and face. Occurs predominantly in middle-aged women. A common, benign, mild cosmetic problem. (Achille Civatte, 1877-1956, French dermatologist)

1. Civatte A: Ann Derm Syph 4:605-620, 1923

CIVIALE OPERATION, lithotripsy.

1. Maffei WE: Os Fundamentos da Medicina. 2nd ed. Livraria Editora Artes Medicas Ltd, 1978

CLAIRMONT OPERATION, puncture of the right auricle for aspiration of an air embolism.

1. Maffei WE: Os Fundamentos da Medicina. 2nd ed. Livraria Editora Artes Medicas Ltd, 1978

CLARK GRADING SYSTEM, a grading system for malignant melanoma. I = intra-epidermal (in situ). II = in the papillary dermis. III = filling the papillary dermis and stopping at the interphase between the papillary and reticular dermis. IV = in the reticular dermis. V = in the subcutaneous fat.

1. Rosai J: Ackerman's Surgical Pathology. 7th ed. St Louis: CV Mosby, 1989

CLARK OPERATION, plastic surgery for repairing a urethral fistula.

1. Maffei WE: Os Fundamentos da Medicina. 2nd ed. Livraria Editora Artes Medicas Ltd, 1978

CLARK SIGN, liver percussion is not audible due to distention of the abdomen; seen in peritonitis. (Alonzo Clark, 1809-1887, U.S.)

1. Casas EC: Diccionario Terminologico de Ciencias Medicas. 5th ed. Salvat Editores, SA, 1954

CLARKE NUCLEUS, a prominent and discrete cell group situated at the base of the posterior horn medially (nucleus dorsalis). (Jacob Clarke, 1817-1880, British anatomist)

1. Haymaker W: Bing's Local Diagnosis in Neurological Diseases. 15th ed. St Louis: CV Mosby, 1969

CLARKE SIGN, assesses the presence of chondromalacia patellae; the patient is asked to contract the quadriceps muscle while the examiner pushes down on the patella. If the test causes retropatellar pain and the patient cannot hold the contraction without pain, the sign is positive.

1. Evans RC: Illustrated Essentials in Orthopedic Physical Assessment. St Louis: Mosby Yearbook, 1994

CLARKE-HADFIELD SYNDROME, cystic fibrosis; congenital pancreatic disease with characteristics of infantilism, obesity, hepatomegaly, and extensive atrophy of the pancreas in an undersized, underweight child. Cross-reference: Andersen triad. (Cecil Clarke, British; Geoffrey Hadfield, 1889-1968, British)

1. Clarke C, Hadfield G: Q J Med 17:358-364, 1924

CLAUDE BERNARD-HORNER SYNDROME, see Horner syndrome. (Claude Bernard, 1813-1878, French physiologist; Johann F. Horner, 1831-1886, Swiss ophthalmologist)

CLAUDE HYPERKINESIS SIGN, reflex movements of paretic muscles elicited by painful stimuli. Cross-reference: Hyperkinesis sign. (Henri C.J. Claude, 1869-1945, French neuropsychiatrist/neurologist)

1. Dorland's Medical Dictionary. 28th ed. Philadelphia: WB Saunders, 1994

CLAUDE SYNDROME, a neurological disorder that results from the involvement of the red nucleus and brachium conjunctivum producing ipsilateral 3rd nerve paralysis and contralateral asynergia, ataxia, and dysmetria. May also result from thrombosis of the medial interpeduncular branch of the posterior cerebral artery. Symptoms are similar to those of the Weber syndrome associated with unilateral cerebellar dysfunction. Cross-reference: Inferior nucleus ruber syndrome. (Henri C.J. Claude)

1. Claude HCJ: Syndrome pédonculaire de la région du noyau rouge. Rev Neurol 23:311-313, 1912

CLAUDE-NOTHNAGEL SYNDROME, see Nothnagel syndrome.

CLAUDE-SORDEL DISEASE, senilism caused by endocrine disturbances.
1. Casas EC: Diccionario Terminologico de Ciencias Medicas. 5th ed. Salvat Editores, SA, 1954

CLAVICULAR SIGN, see Higouménaki sign.

CLAYBROOK SIGN, auscultation of the abdomen allows the examiner to hear heart and lung sounds; an indication of abdominal rupture. Cross-reference: Federici sign. (Edwin B. Claybrook, 1871-1931, U.S. surgeon)
1. Casas EC: Diccionario Terminologico de Ciencias Medicas. 5th ed. Salvat Editores, SA, 1954

CLEIDOCRANIAL DYSOSTOSIS SYNDROME, characteristics include slight to moderate short-ness of stature, brachycephaly with bossing of frontal, parietal, and occipital bones, and late eruption of permanent teeth; hand anomalies include short, tapering 2nd and 5th distal phalanges with or without down-curving nails. Autosomal dominant inheritance.
1. Grieg DM: Neanderthal skull presenting features of cleidocranial dysostosis and other peculiarities. Edinb Med J 40:407, 1933
2. Smith DW, Jones KL: Recognizable Patterns of Human Malformation: Genetic, Embryologic, and Clinical Aspects. 3rd ed. Philadelphia: WB Saunders, 1982

CLELAND-ARNOLD-CHIARI MALFORMATION, the deformity responsible for the type of hydrocephalus in which there is herniation of the brain stem and cerebellar vermis through the fora-men magnum. (John Cleland, 1835-1925; Julius Arnold, 1835-1915, German; Hans Chiari, 1851-1916, German)
1. Campbell MF, Walsh PC: Campbell's Urology. 5th ed. Philadelphia: WB Saunders, 1986
2. Cleland J: J Anat Physiol 17:257-291, 1883

CLENCHED FIST SYNDROME, an entity in which the patient keeps one or both hands tightly clenched against the chest. Seen in all age groups; hand dominance or compensation is not a factor. Often a conversion phenomenon that follows a minor inciting incident and is associated with swelling, pain, and paradoxical stiffness.
1. Campbell WC, Crenshaw AH: Campbell's Operative Orthopaedics. 7th ed. St Louis: CV Mosby, 1987
2. Simmons BP, et al: The clenched fist syndrome. J Hand Surg 5:420-427, 1980

CLERC-LEVY CRISTECO SYNDROME, see Lown-Ganong-Levine syndrome.

CLICK SYNDROME, CLICK-MURMUR SYNDROME, see Mitral valve prolapse syndrome.

CLIMACTERIC SYNDROME, see Menopausal syndrome.

CLOSED HEAD SYNDROME, the complex of symptoms characteristic of nonpenetrative cerebral injury.
1. Dorland's Medical Dictionary. 28th ed. Philadelphia: WB Saunders, 1994

CLOQUET SIGN, if a needle is plunged into the biceps, it will be oxidized if the patient is not dead. Cross-reference: Laborde sign.
1. Casas EC: Diccionario Terminologico de Ciencias Medicas. 5th ed. Salvat Editores, SA, 1954

CLOUGH-RICHTER SYNDROME, see Cold hemagglutinin syndrome. (Mildred C. Clough, U.S. hematologist; Ina M. Richter, U.S. hematologist)

CLOUSTON SYNDROME, hidrotic ectodermal dysplasia with hyperkeratosis of the palms and soles. (H.R.C. Clouston, Canadian)
1. Clouston HR: A hereditary ectodermal dystrophy. Can Med Assoc J 21:18-31, 1929

CLOVÉ-ESCAT OPERATION, maxillary sinus trephination using a nasal approach.
1. Maffei WE: Os Fundamentos da Medicina. 2nd ed. Livraria Editora Artes Medicas Ltd, 1978

CLUTTON JOINT DISEASE, a congenital syphilitic joint disease appearing around puberty and characterized as the halt (Clutton), the deaf (because of otitis interna), the blind (following interstitial keratitis), and the impotent (secondary to orchitis). (Henry H. Clutton, 1850-1909, British surgeon)
1. Bailey H, Love M: A Short Practice of Surgery. 12th ed. London: HK Lewis & Co, 1962
2. Clutton HH: Lancet 1:391-393, 1886

COAKLEY OPERATION, opening of the maxillary sinus through the cheek with resection of the anterior wall and rasping of the mucosa.
1. Maffei WE: Os Fundamentos da Medicina. 2nd ed. Livraria Editora Artes Medicas Ltd, 1978

COATS DISEASE, telangiectatic retinal vessels associated with telangiectasis of the face, breasts, conjunctivae, and nailbeds; a port wine stain has been reported with retinal telangiectasis without central nervous system involvement. (George Coats, 1876-1915, British ophthalmologist)

1. Coats G: Ophthalmol Hosp Rep 17:440-525, 1908
2. Hurst JW, Schlant RC, Alexander RW: The Heart: Arteries and Veins. 8th ed. New York: McGraw-Hill, 1994
3. Moschella SL, Hurley HJ: Dermatology. 2nd ed. Philadelphia: WB Saunders, 1985

COBB SYNDROME, a rare entity exhibiting both cutaneous and meningospinal angiomas. Vascular nevi, including port wine stains, are present within two dermatomes of the site of spinal cord angiomatosis. (Stanley Cobb, U.S. neuropathologist)

1. Cobb S: Haemangioma of the spinal cord associated with skin naevi of these same metamers. Ann Surg 62:641-649, 1915
2. Moschella SL, Hurley HJ: Dermatology. 2nd ed. Philadelphia: WB Saunders, 1985

COCK OPERATION, urethrotomy through an incision in the perineal midline.

1. Maffei WE: Os Fundamentos da Medicina. 2nd ed. Livraria Editora Artes Medicas Ltd, 1978

COCKAYNE SYNDROME, familial microcephaly with calcification; follows the characteristic evolution of a degenerative rather than a developmental disease (i.e., affected children may be normal at birth but during infancy or early childhood begin to have seizures that recur frequently). Somatic features include dwarfism, a beaked nose, and dermatitis in a butterfly distribution. A rare disorder with autosomal recessive inheritance. (Edward A. Cockayne, 1880-1956, British)

1. Cockayne EA: Arch Dis Child 11:1-8, 1936
2. Farmer TW: Pediatric Neurology. 2nd ed. Hagerstown: Harper & Row, 1975
3. McKusick VA: Heritable Disorders of Connective Tissue. 4th ed. St Louis: CV Mosby, 1972

COCKAYNE-TOURAINE SYNDROME, dominant dystrophic epidermolysis bullosa. (Edward A. Cockayne; Albert Touraine, 1883-1961, French dermatologist)

1. Touraine A: L'Hérédité en Medicine. Paris: Masson, 1955

CODIVILLA OPERATION, surgery for pseudoarthrosis using osseous grafts from the tibia.

1. Maffei WE: Os Fundamentos da Medicina. 2nd ed. Livraria Editora Artes Medicas Ltd, 1978

CODMAN SIGN, the arm can be abducted with support; seen in the case of rupture of the supraspinatus tendon. (Ernest A. Codman, 1869-1940, U.S. surgeon)

1. Casas EC: Diccionario Terminologico de Ciencias Medicas. 5th ed. Salvat Editores, SA, 1954

COFARD SYNDROME, paranoia and suicidal tendencies.

1. Casas EC: Diccionario Terminologico de Ciencias Medicas. 5th ed. Salvat Editores, SA, 1954

COFFEY OPERATION, fixation of the greater omentum to the parietal peritoneum for treating gastroptosis. (Robert Coffey, 1869-1933, U.S. surgeon)

1. Maffei WE: Os Fundamentos da Medicina. 2nd ed. Livraria Editora Artes Medicas Ltd, 1978

COFFIN-LOWRY SYNDROME, COFFIN-SIRIS SYNDROME, females have mild mental retardation, short stature, short hyperextensible hands, and tufted distal phalanges. Males are much more severely affected, with severe mental deficiency, short stature, stiff joints, coarse facial features, pectus carinatum, and large soft hands. (George S. Coffin, U.S. pediatrician; R. Brian Lowry, Canadian; Evelyn Siris, U.S. radiologist)

1. Coffin GS, Siris E, Wegienka LC: Am J Dis Child 112:205-213, 1966
2. Haymaker W: Bing's Local Diagnosis in Neurological Diseases. 15th ed. St Louis: CV Mosby, 1969
3. Lowry RB, Miller JR, Fraser FC: Am J Dis Child 121:496-500, 1971

COGAN SYNDROME, nonsyphilitic interstitial keratitis; an uncommon vasculitis presenting in young adults, with vertigo, deafness, and interstitial keratitis as well as other systemic manifestations. Disease is usually nonsyphilitic. (David Cogan, U.S. neuro-ophthalmologist)

1. Bennett JC, Plum F (eds): Cecil Textbook of Medicine. 20th ed. Philadelphia: WB Saunders, 1996
2. Cogan D: Arch Ophthalmol 33:144-149, 1945

COGWHEEL PHENOMENON, see Negro phenomenon.

COGWHEEL SIGN, rigidity of joint muscles in which passive motion elicits movement that can be felt by the examiner.

1. Mazion JM: Illustrated Manual of Neurological Reflexes/Signs/Tests For Office Procedure. 2nd ed. Arizona City: Daniels Publishing, 1980

COH SYNDROME, cloverleaf skull, polymicrogyria, absent olfactory tracts and bulbs, proptosis, a low nasal bridge, short upturned nose, down-turned mouth, narrow palate, thumb duplication, small fifth fingers, micropenis, bifid scrotum, agenesis of the cervical thymic lobes, and bilobed lungs are characteristics. COH stands for *C*hildren's *O*rthopedic *H*ospital, where the first identified patient was seen as a newborn.

1. Gorlin RJ, Cohen MM Jr, Levin LS: Syndromes of the Head and Neck. 3rd ed. New York: Oxford University Press, 1990

COHEN SYNDROME, a genetic disease featuring microcephaly, severe mental retardation, short stature, facial abnormalities, and moderate obesity. (M. Michael Cohen, Jr., U.S. oral pathologist)

1. Cohen MM: J Pediatr 83:280-284, 1973
2. Wilson JD, Foster DW, Kronenberg HM, et al (eds): Williams Textbook of Endocrinology. 9th ed. Philadelphia: WB Saunders, 1998

COITAL CEPHALGIA SYNDROME, acute headache occurring during sexual intercourse. Patient has a history of migraine in almost one half of cases.

1. Pearce JMS: Headache. J Neurol Neurosurg Psychiatry 57:134-144, 1944

COLD HEMAGGLUTININ SYNDROME, caused by hemagglutinins that are 19s or α-M globulins and agglutinate erythrocytes of all groups at temperatures of 0° to 5°C. A rare, chronic primary type is seen in elderly persons, and a secondary type is associated with infections, connective tissue diseases, malignant tumors, and cirrhosis of the liver. Cross-references: Clough-Richter syndrome; Cryopathic hemolytic syndrome.

1. Clough MC, Richter IM: Bull John Hopkins Hosp 29:86-93, 1918
2. Moschella SL, Hurley HJ: Dermatology. 2nd ed. Philadelphia: WB Saunders, 1985

COLE SIGN, a radiological sign of deformity of the duodenal ulcer. (Lewis G. Cole, 1874-1954, U.S. roentgenologist)

1. Casas EC: Diccionario Terminologico de Ciencias Medicas. 5th ed. Salvat Editores, SA, 1954

COLLES FRACTURE, fracture of the distal radius. Named before the use of x-rays and has come to mean dorsally angulated fractures of the ulnar styloid bone. (Abraham Colles, 1773-1843, Irish surgeon)

1. Colles A: Edinb Med Surg J 10:182-186, 1814
2. Schwartz SI: Principles of Surgery. 4th ed. New York: McGraw-Hill, 1983

COLLET SYNDROME, COLLET-SICARD SYNDROME, manifests as unilateral involvement of the last four cranial nerves. May also occur as a result of tumor, inflammatory lesion, aneurysm of the internal or external carotid artery, or fibromuscular dysplasia of the carotid artery. A variant of the Villaret syndrome, without Horner syndrome. Cross-reference: Sicard syndrome. (Frédéric J. Collet, French otolaryngologist; Jean A. Sicard, 1872-1929, French neurologist)

1. Collet FJ: Sur un nouveau syndrome paralytique pharyngolaryné par blessure de guerre. Lyon Med 124:121-129, 1916
2. Gorlin RJ, Cohen MM Jr, Levin LS: Syndromes of the Head and Neck. 3rd ed. New York: Oxford University Press, 1990
3. Sicard JA: Marseilles Med 53:385-397, 1916/1917

COLLIE PHENOMENON, when enclosed and shaken in a glass tube with a globule of mercury, pure neon glows with a bright red-orange color.

1. Dorland's Medical Dictionary. 28th ed. Philadelphia: WB Saunders, 1994

COLLIER SIGN, pathological lid retraction; may be a sign of midbrain (posterior commissure) disease. Cross-references: Epstein sign; Setting-sun sign. (James S. Collier, 1870-1930, British)

1. Rowland LP (ed): Merritt's Textbook of Neurology. 9th ed. Baltimore: Williams & Wilkins, 1995
2. Smith JL: Neuro-Ophthalmology. Vol 6. St Louis: CV Mosby, 1972

COLLINS OPERATION, extraction of calculi from the ampulla of Vater prior to incision of the duodenum.

1. Maffei WE: Os Fundamentos da Medicina. 2nd ed. Livraria Editora Artes Medicas Ltd, 1978

COLORADO TICK FEVER, a tick-borne, nonexanthematous, febrile, viral disease occurring in the Rocky Mountain region of the U.S. Cross-reference: American mountain disease.

1. Bennett JC, Plum F (eds): Cecil Textbook of Medicine. 20th ed. Philadelphia: WB Saunders, 1996

COMA VIGILE SYNDROME, see Apallic syndrome.

COMBY SIGN, whitish patches in the oral mucosa; an early indication of measles. (Jules Comby, 1853-1947, French pediatrician)

1. Casas EC: Diccionario Terminologico de Ciencias Medicas. 5th ed. Salvat Editores, SA, 1954

COMÉL SYNDROME, see Netherton syndrome.

COMOLLI SIGN, a triangular bulge indicating fracture of the scapula. (Antonio Comolli, Italian pathologist)
1. Casas EC: Diccionario Terminologico de Ciencias Medicas. 5th ed. Salvat Editores, SA, 1954

COMPARTMENTAL SYNDROME, arises when increased tissue pressure in a confined anatomical space causes ischemia and subsequently dysfunction of contained myoneural elements; marked by pain, muscle weakness, sensory loss, and palpable tenseness in the involved compartment. Ischemia can lead to necrosis resulting in permanent impairment of function.
1. Dorland's Medical Dictionary. 28th ed. Philadelphia: WB Saunders, 1994

COMPLETE CORD SYNDROME, an acute disorder, occurring over minutes, usually associated with areflexia (spinal shock).

COMPRESSION SYNDROME, a shock-like state with hematuria and oliguria following long continuous pressure on a limb, as may occur in people caught in bombed buildings. Cross-references: Bywaters syndrome; Crush syndrome.
1. Bywaters EGL, Beall D: Br Med J 1:417-432, 1941

CONCATO DISEASE, a rare polyserositis of uncertain etiology that causes massive effusions into the serous cavities and may result in constrictive pericarditis or perihepatic or perisplenic fibrosis. (Luigi M. Concato, 1825-1882, Italian)
1. Concato LM: Giorg Ingerm Sci Med Napoli 3:1037-1053, 1881
2. Ritchie AC: Boyd's Textbook of Pathology. 9th ed. Philadelphia: Lea & Febiger, 1990

CONCUSSION SYNDROME, see Postconcussion syndrome.

CONDOMINE OPERATION, surgical method for treating an umbilical hernia.
1. Maffei WE: Os Fundamentos da Medicina. 2nd ed. Livraria Editora Artes Medicas Ltd, 1978

CONE SYNDROME, characterized by complaints of severely diminished color vision, decreased visual acuity, and decreased vision with bright illumination (day blindness, not photophobia). Cross-reference: Retinal cone dystrophy syndrome.
1. Goodman G, et al: Cone dysfunction syndromes. Arch Ophthalmol 70:214, 1963

CONGENITAL ANDROGEN INSENSITIVITY SYNDROME, see Testicular feminization syndrome.

CONGENITAL FLAT NOSE SYNDROME, see Binder syndrome.

CONGENITAL RUBELLA SYNDROME, a maternal infection with the rubella virus during the first trimester of pregnancy causing fetal abnormalities, including features seen in infants with chronic inflammatory disease, such as hepatosplenomegaly, jaundice, petechial and purpuric rashes, thrombocytopenia, microcephaly, and mental retardation. Cross-reference: Rubella syndrome.
1. Krugman S, Katz SL: Infectious Diseases of Children. 7th ed. Philadelphia: JB Lippincott, 1989

CONLEY OPERATION, an eversion endarterectomy that has made endarterectomy more satisfactory.
1. Schwartz SI: Principles of Surgery. 4th ed. New York: McGraw-Hill, 1983

CONN SYNDROME, primary hyperaldosteronism; the salient features are hypertension, episodic muscular weakness, polyuria, paresthesia, tetany, headache, and hypokalemic alkalosis. (Jerome W. Conn, U.S.)
1. Conn JW: J Lab Clin Med 45:3-17, 1955
2. Farmer TW: Pediatric Neurology. 2nd ed. Hagerstown: Harper & Row, 1975

CONOR-BRUCH DISEASE, a tick-borne boutonneuse ("pimply") fever or exanthematic fever. First described in 1910. Cross-references: Kenya tick typhus; Marseilles disease.
1. Casas EC: Diccionario Terminologico de Ciencias Medicas. 5th ed. Salvat Editores, SA, 1954

CONRADI SYNDROME, CONRADI-HÜNERMANN SYNDROME, chondrodystrophia congenita punctata. A rare bone disorder involving multisystem defects; the skeletal, cardiovascular, and central nervous systems as well as the skin and eyes are affected. Involvement appears within the first 9 months of life. Cross-references: Hünermann syndrome; Rhizomelic chondrodysplasia punctata syndrome. (Erich Conradi, German; Carl Hünermann, German)
1. Conradi E: Jahrb Kinderheilkd 80:86-97, 1914
2. Heselson NG, Cremin BJ, Beighton P: Lethal chondrodysplasia punctata. Clin Radiol 29:679, 1978

3. Hünermann C: Chondrodystrophia calcificans congenital als abortive Form der chondrodystrophie. Z Kinderheilkd 51:1-19, 1931

CONTIGUOUS GENE SYNDROME, naturally occurring deletions that result in the clinical disease state as a result of loss of multiple genes located in the same region; the patient with these deletions can develop multiple diseases and malformations that would normally be inherited separately and in a Mendelian fashion.

CONUS SYNDROME, infrequently encountered, and then only in certain lesions such as small intramedullary tumor metastases, hemorrhagic infarct, or gliotic foci cysts. In its pure form, offers no diagnostic difficulties.
1. Haymaker W: Bing's Local Diagnosis in Neurological Diseases. 15th ed. St Louis: CV Mosby, 1969

COOLEY ANEMIA, hereditary hemolytic anemia or severe ß-thalassemia usually in persons of Mediterranean extract. Occurs in the patient who is homozygous for mutations that lead to a decrease in ß-globin synthesis. Cross-reference: Mediterranean disease. (Thomas B. Cooley, 1871-1945, U.S. pediatrician)
1. Baker AB, Baker LH: Clinical Neurology. Revised ed. Philadelphia: Harper & Row, 1982
2. Cooley TB, Lee P: Trans Am Pediatr Soc 37:29, 1925

COOPER DISEASE, chronic cystic disease of the breast. (Sir Astley Cooper, 1768-1841, British surgeon)
1. Casas EC: Diccionario Terminologico de Ciencias Medicas. 5th ed. Salvat Editores, SA, 1954

COOPER OPERATION, 1) ligature of the external iliac artery through an incision parallel to the ligament of Poupart; 2) basal ganglia surgery for dystonia.
1. Maffei WE: Os Fundamentos da Medicina. Livraria Editora Artes Médicas Ltda, 1978

COOPERNAIL SIGN, ecchymosis of the perineum and scrotum; an indication of pelvic fracture. (George P. Coopernail, 1876-1962, U.S.)
1. Casas EC: Diccionario Terminologico de Ciencias Medicas. 5th ed. Salvat Editores, SA, 1954

COPE SIGN, extension of the leg causes stretching of the psoas muscle and results in pain; seen in appendicitis. Cross-reference: Psoas sign. (Sir Vincent Cope, 1881-1974, British surgeon)
1. Casas EC: Diccionario Terminologico de Ciencias Medicas. 5th ed. Salvat Editores, SA, 1954

CORBUS DISEASE, gangrenous balanitis. (Budd Corbus, 1876-1954, U.S. urologist)
1. Casas EC: Diccionario Terminologico de Ciencias Medicas. 5th ed. Salvat Editores, SA, 1954

CORD SIGN, a linear area of increased density indicating a clot in the veins or sinus; seen on computed tomography of the superior sagittal sinus.
1. Rowland LP (ed): Merritt's Textbook of Neurology. 9th ed. Baltimore: Williams & Wilkins, 1995

CORI DISEASE, CORI-FORBES DISEASE, see Forbes disease.

CORNELIA DE LANGE SYNDROME, see De Lange syndrome.

CORNELL SIGN, compression of the phrenic nerve causing pain; seen in cases of malaria.
1. Casas EC: Diccionario Terminologico de Ciencias Medicas. 5th ed. Salvat Editores, SA, 1954

CORRADI OPERATION, see Moore-Corradi operation.

CORRIGAN SIGN, chronic copper intoxication indicated by a purple color between the gums and teeth. (Sir Dominic J. Corrigan, 1802-1880, Irish)
1. Casas EC: Diccionario Terminologico de Ciencias Medicas. 5th ed. Salvat Editores, SA, 1954

CORVISART DISEASE, chronic hypertrophic myocarditis. (Jean N. Corvisart des Marets, 1755-1821, French)
1. Casas EC: Diccionario Terminologico de Ciencias Medicas. 5th ed. Salvat Editores, SA, 1954

COSTEN SYNDROME, see Temporomandibular joint syndrome. (James B. Costen, U.S. otorhinolaryngologist)

COSTOCLAVICULAR SYNDROME, costoclavicular compression; pain and dysesthesia in the arm and/or hand, apparently due to pressure, stretching, or friction on the nerves or vessels at the cervicobrachial outlet. Dispute exists regarding the exact mechanism of pain. Cross-reference: Thoracic outlet syndrome.
1. Dorland's Medical Dictionary. 28th ed. Philadelphia: WB Saunders, 1994

COTARD SYNDROME, paranoia with delusions of negation, a tendency toward self-inflicted injury, and sensory disturbances are features. (Jules Cotard, 1840-1887, French neurologist)

1. Cotard J: Arch Neurol 4:152-282, 1882

COTTE OPERATION, removal of the presacral nerve. (Gaston Cotte, 1879-1951, French surgeon)

1. Maffei WE: Os Fundamentos da Medicina. 2nd ed. Livraria Editora Artes Medicas Ltd, 1978

COTTING OPERATION, surgery for an ingrown nail using a lateral incision of the border of the toe or finger. (Benjamin Cotting, 1812-1898, U.S. surgeon)

1. Maffei WE: Os Fundamentos da Medicina. 2nd ed. Livraria Editora Artes Medicas Ltd, 1978

COTUGNO DISEASE, COTUNNIIS DISEASE, sciatica. (Domenico Cotugno, 1736-1822, Italian anatomist)

1. Cotugno D: De Ischiade Nervoso Commentarius. Napoli: Fratres Simonis, 1764

COUGH IMPULSE TEST, laying the fingers on the thigh just below the saphenous vein opening, the patient is asked to cough. A fluid thrill is imparted to the examiner's finger if the valve at the saphenofemoral junction is incompetent.

1. Bailey H: Physical Signs in Clinical Surgery. 16th ed. Baltimore: Williams & Wilkins, 1983

COUGH TEST, when asked to cough, a patient with inflammation of the pleura feels pain in the abdomen; when positive, suggests an inflammatory process at the site of pain.

1. Bailey H: Physical Signs in Clinical Surgery. 16th ed. Baltimore: Williams & Wilkins, 1983

COUGHING SIGN, see Huntington coughing sign.

COURTOIS SIGN, in coma due to a cerebral lesion, passive neck flexion causes automatic flexion of the limb on the same side as the lesion.

1. Casas EC: Diccionario Terminologico de Ciencias Medicas. 5th ed. Salvat Editores, SA, 1954

COURVOISIER LAW, COURVOISIER SIGN, distention of the gallbladder with jaundice; more indicative of a tumor than of gallstones. (Ludwig G. Courvoisier, 1843-1918, Swiss surgeon)

1. Bailey H: Physical Signs in Clinical Surgery. 16th ed. Baltimore: Williams & Wilkins, 1983

COURVOISIER-TERRIER SYNDROME, see Bard-Pic syndrome. (Ludwig G. Courvoisier; Felix Terrier, 1837-1908, French surgeon)

COUTON DISEASE, tuberculous spondylosis.

1. Casas EC: Diccionario Terminologico de Ciencias Medicas. 5th ed. Salvat Editores, SA, 1954

COWDEN DISEASE, multiple hamartomas and neoplasias. The diagnostic mucocutaneous lesions are facial papules, oral mucosal papillomatosis, and acral and palmoplantar keratoses. Early detection of an associated malignancy has a greater chance of cure. Autosomal dominant inheritance trait with incomplete penetrance and variable expressivity. (Cowden is the surname of family from which the condition is known.) Cross-reference: Multiple hamartoma syndrome.

1. Albecht S, Haber RM, Goodman JC, et al: Cowden syndrome and Lhermitte-Duclos disease. Cancer 70:869-876, 1992
2. Gorlin RJ, Cohen MM Jr, Levin LS: Syndromes of the Head and Neck. 3rd ed. New York: Oxford University Press, 1990
3. Moschella SL, Hurley HJ: Dermatology. 2nd ed. Philadelphia: WB Saunders, 1985

COWEN SIGN, light shined into one eye elicits jerky constriction of the contralateral pupil; an indication of Graves disease.

1. Dorland's Medical Dictionary. 28th ed. Philadelphia: WB Saunders, 1994

COX SIGN, occurs during straight leg raising when, instead of the hip flexing, the pelvis rises from the table; an indication of a prolapse of nuclear material into the neural foramen.

1. Evans RC: Illustrated Essentials in Orthopedic Physical Assessment. St Louis: Mosby Yearbook, 1994

COXSACKIE ENCEPHALITIS, brain inflammation seen mostly in infants caused by *Enterovirus* Coxsackie B. (Coxsackie, New York is where disease was first identified.)

1. Pedro-Pons A: Patologia-y-Clinica Medicus. Salvat Editores, SA, 1952

COZEN TEST, the patient is asked to clench a fist and keep it clenched while extending the arm. The examiner grasps the lower forearm and, while the patient attempts to keep the wrist extended, flexes the wrist firmly and steadily. This places considerable tension on the origin of the extensor tendons at the lateral epicondyle and causes pain.

1. Bailey H: Physical Signs in Clinical Surgery. 16th ed. Baltimore: Williams & Wilkins, 1983

CRANDALL SYNDROME, see Björnstad syndrome. (Barbara F. Crandall, U.S.)

CRANE-HEISE SYNDROME, involves cleft lip/palate, agenesis of the clavicles and cervical vertebrae, and talipes equinovarus.
1. Crane JP, Heise RL: New syndrome in three affected siblings. Pediatrics 68:235-237, 1981
2. Gorlin RJ, Cohen MM Jr, Levin LS: Syndromes of the Head and Neck. 3rd ed. New York: Oxford University Press, 1990

CRANIODIGITAL SYNDROME, see Scott syndrome.

CRANIOMETAPHYSEAL DYSPLASIA SYNDROME, a congenital disorder with a bony wedge over the bridge of the nose, mild splaying of the metaphyses, compression of the foramina with cranial nerve deficits, headache, and a narrow nasal passage with rhinitis. An autosomal dominant and a presumed autosomal recessive type exist.
1. Gorlin RJ, et al: Genetic craniotubular bone dysplasias and hyperostoses. A critical analysis. Birth Defects 5(4):79-95, 1969
2. Smith DW, Jones KL: Recognizable Patterns of Human Malformation: Genetic, Embryologic, and Clinical Aspects. 3rd ed. Philadelphia: WB Saunders, 1982

CREDÉ MANEUVER, manual pressure on the bladder to expel urine. Should be used in managing the spastic bladder associated with spinal cord injury in preference to continued catheter drainage. (Karl S.F. Credé, 1819-1892, German obstetrician and gynecologist)

CREDÉ OPERATION, resection of the pubis followed by hysterectomy. (Karl S.F. Credé)
1. Credé KSF: Zschr Ges Neuropsychiatr 57:1-18, 1920
2. Maffei WE: Os Fundamentos da Medicina. 2nd ed. Livraria Editora Artes Medicas Ltd, 1978

CRESCENT SIGN, implies tilt of the humerus either medially or laterally in supracondylar fracture. Cross-reference: Meniscus sign.
1. Campbell WC, Crenshaw AH: Campbell's Operative Orthopaedics. 7th ed. St Louis: CV Mosby, 1987

CREST SYNDROME, a type of scleroderma, consisting of *c*alcinosis cutis, *R*aynaud phenomenon, *e*sophageal dysfunction, *s*clerodactyly, and *t*elangiectasia (CREST).
1. Moschella SL, Hurley HJ: Dermatology. 2nd ed. Philadelphia: WB Saunders, 1985
2. Ritchie AC: Boyd's Textbook of Pathology. 9th ed. Philadelphia: Lea & Febiger, 1990

CREUTZFELDT-JAKOB DISEASE, a rare viral encephalopathy that causes progressive dementia. Cross-references: Jakob-Creutzfeldt disease; Nevin-Jones disease. (Hans G. Creutzfeldt, 1885-1964, German neuropsychiatrist; Alfons M. Jakob, 1884-1931, German neuropsychiatrist)
1. Creutzfeldt HG: Histologie und Histopathologie. Jena, 1921
2. Creutzfeldt HG: Zschr Ges Neuropsychiatr 57:1-18, 1920
3. Esmonde T, Lueck CJ, Symon L, et al: Creutzfeldt-Jakob disease and lyophilised dura mater grafts: report of two cases. J Neurol Neurosurg Psychiatry 56:999-1000, 1993
4. Jakob AM: Zschr Ges Neuropsychiatr 64:147-228, 1921
5. Traub RD: Recent data and hypotheses on Creutzfeldt-Jakob disease. Adv Neurol 38:149-164, 1983

CRI DU CHAT SYNDROME, "cat's cry"; an underlying chromosome aberration, with partial deletion of the short arm of chromosome 5. There is a cat-like cry in infancy, microcephaly, downward slant of palpebral fissures, low birth weight, mental deficiency, strabismus, and facial asymmetry. Cross-reference: Cat's cry syndrome.
1. Breg WR, et al: The cri-du-chat syndrome in adolescents and adults. J Pediatr 77:782, 1970
2. Smith DW, Jones KL: Recognizable Patterns of Human Malformation: Genetic, Embryologic, and Clinical Aspects. 3rd ed. Philadelphia: WB Saunders, 1982

CRICHTON-BROWNE SIGN, tremor of the lateral aspect of the eyelid and the labial commissure; a sign of syphilis. (Sir James Crichton-Browne, 1840-1938, British)
1. Casas EC: Diccionario Terminologico de Ciencias Medicas. 5th ed. Salvat Editores, SA, 1954

CRICOPHARYNGEAL ACHALASIA SYNDROME, see Asherson syndrome.

CRIGLER-NAJJAR SYNDROME, an exceedingly rare and almost uniformly lethal type of hyperbilirubinemia, with an impaired ability of the liver to transport or conjugate bilirubin, producing non-hemolytic jaundice. (John F. Crigler, Jr., U.S. pediatrician; Victor A. Najjar, Lebanese-born U.S. microbiologist)
1. Crigler JF, Najjar VA: Congenital familial non-hemolytic jaundice with kernicterus. Pediatrics 10:169-179, 1952
2. Farmer TW: Pediatric Neurology. 2nd ed. Hagerstown: Harper & Row, 1975

CRILE-MATAS OPERATION, local anesthesia by intraneural injection of the anesthetic agent.
1. Maffei WE: Os Fundamentos da Medicina. 2nd ed. Livraria Editora Artes Medicas Ltd, 1978

CRIMEAN HEMORRHAGIC FEVER, CRIMEAN-CONGO HEMORRHAGIC FEVER, an acute febrile disease often marked by severe hemorrhage, a high mortality rate, and nosocomial transmission, occurring in the Soviet Union, Bulgaria, the Middle East, and Pakistan.
1. Bennett JC, Plum F (eds): Cecil Textbook of Medicine. 20th ed. Philadelphia: WB Saunders, 1996

CRIPPS OPERATION, a method of colotomy via the iliac region.
1. Maffei WE: Os Fundamentos da Medicina. 2nd ed. Livraria Editora Artes Medicas Ltd, 1978

CRITCHETT OPERATION, excision of the anterior segment of the globe.
1. Maffei WE: Os Fundamentos da Medicina. 2nd ed. Livraria Editora Artes Medicas Ltd, 1978

CROCODILE TEARS SYNDROME, see Bogorad syndrome.

CROCQ-CASSIRER SYNDROME, acrocyanosis. (Jean B. Crocq, 1868-1925, Belgian; Richard Cassirer)
1. Casas EC: Diccionario Terminologico de Ciencias Medicas. 5th ed. 1954

CROHN DISEASE, segmental enteritis; a subacute and chronic inflammatory process of uncertain etiology that may involve any part of the intestinal tract, especially the distal ileum, colon, and anorectal region. (Burrill B. Crohn, 1884-1983, U.S. gastroenterologist)
1. Crohn BB, et al: JAMA 99:1323-1329, 1932
2. Kirsner JB, et al: N Engl J Med 306:837-848, 1982
3. Moschella SL, Hurley HJ: Dermatology. 2nd ed. Philadelphia: WB Saunders, 1985

CRONKHITE-CANADA SYNDROME, refers to the rare association of generalized intestinal polyposis, dystrophy of the fingernails, alopecia, and cutaneous hyperpigmentation. A familial association has not been clearly established. (Leonard W. Cronkhite, Jr., U.S.; Wilma J. Canada, U.S. radiologist)
1. Cronkhite LW, Canada WJ: Generalized gastrointestinal polyposis. N Engl J Med 252:1011-1015, 1955
2. Moschella SL, Hurley HJ: Dermatology. 2nd ed. Philadelphia: WB Saunders, 1985
3. Ritchie AC: Boyd's Textbook of Pathology. 9th ed. Philadelphia: Lea & Febiger, 1990

CROSBY-COONEY OPERATION, surgical creation of a subcutaneous pouch for collecting ascitic fluid to allow absorption by the lymphatic system.
1. Maffei WE: Os Fundamentos da Medicina. 2nd ed. Livraria Editora Artes Medicas Ltd, 1978

CROSS SYNDROME, CROSS-McKUSICK-BREEN SYNDROME, oculocutaneous albinism along with microphthalmia, small opaque corneas, and oligophrenia with spasticity. The hair bulbs show weakly positive tyrosinase reactions and a high-arched palate, gingival hypertrophy, and scoliosis are features. This rare syndrome has been described in one multiply-consanguineous Amish family. Melanocytes are scanty but there is no block in maturation. Cross-reference: Oculocerebral-hypopigmentation syndrome. (Harold E. Cross, U.S.; Victor A. McKusick, U.S. geneticist; William Breen, U.S.)
1. Bennett JC, Plum F (eds): Cecil Textbook of Medicine. 20th ed. Philadelphia: WB Saunders, 1996
2. Cross HE, McKusick VA, Breen W: A new oculocerebral syndrome with hypopigmentation. J Pediatr 70:398-406, 1967
3. Moschella SL, Hurley HJ: Dermatology. 2nd ed. Philadelphia: WB Saunders, 1985

CROSSED SCIATIC SIGN, see Fajersztajn sign.

CROUZON SYNDROME, craniofacial dysostosis; bilateral coronal suture synostoses are associated with hypertelorism and hypoplasia of the maxilla, resulting in a frog-like facial appearance. (Octave Crouzon, 1874-1938, French neurologist)
1. Crouzon MO: Presse Med 20:737-739, 1912
2. Rowland LP (ed): Merritt's Textbook of Neurology. 9th ed. Baltimore: Williams & Wilkins, 1995
3. Smith DW, Jones KL: Recognizable Patterns of Human Malformation: Genetic, Embryologic, and Clinical Aspects. 3rd ed. Philadelphia: WB Saunders, 1982

CROW-FUKASE SYNDROME, see POEMS syndrome. (R.S. Crow, British; Masaichi Fukase, Japanese)

CROWE SIGN, compression of the internal jugular vein on one side produces engorgement of the retinal veins; sometimes seen in lateral saphenous varicosity. (Samuel J. Crowe, 1883-1955, U.S. otolaryngologist)
1. Casas EC: Diccionario Terminologico de Ciencias Medicas. 5th ed. Salvat Editores, SA, 1954

CROWE SIGN OF NEUROFIBROMATOSIS, freckles in the axillae, especially when seen with irregular hyperpigmented mottling of the skin elsewhere.
1. Bennett JC, Plum F (eds): Cecil Textbook of Medicine. 20th ed. Philadelphia: WB Saunders, 1996

CRST SYNDROME, *c*alcification of the skin, *R*aynaud phenomenon, *s*clerodactyly, and *t*elangiectasia (CRST), but without evidence of visceral involvement. Similar to CREST syndrome, when esophageal dysfunction is prominent.
  1. Alarcon-Segovia D: Mixed connective tissue disease. Semin Arthritis Rheum 13:114, 1983
  2. Ritchie AC: Boyd's Textbook of Pathology. 9th ed. Philadelphia: Lea & Febiger, 1990

CRUCHET DISEASE, epidemic encephalomyelitis.
  1. Casas EC: Diccionario Terminologico de Ciencias Medicas. 5th ed. Salvat Editores, SA, 1954

CRUSH SYNDROME, see Compression syndrome.

CRUVEILHIER SIGN OF SAPHENA VARIX, when the patient coughs or blows his/her nose while in the erect position, a tremor is imparted to the palpating fingers as if a jet of water is entering and filling the pouch. (Jean Cruveilhier, 1791-1874, French pathologist)
  1. Bailey H: Physical Signs in Clinical Surgery. 16th ed. Baltimore: Williams & Wilkins, 1983

CRUVEILHIER-BAUMGARTEN SYNDROME, a loud venous hum audible over the path of the umbilical vein associated with cirrhosis of the liver and portal hypertension. (Jean Cruveilhier; Walter Baumgarten, 1873-1945, U.S.)
  1. Bennett JC, Plum F (eds): Cecil Textbook of Medicine. 20th ed. Philadelphia: WB Saunders, 1996
  2. Cruveilhier J: Anatomie Pathologique de Corps Humain, Vol 1. Paris: Baillière, 1829-1835

CRUZ-CHAGAS DISEASE, see Chagas disease.

CRYOPATHIC HEMOLYTIC SYNDROME, see Cold hemagglutinin syndrome.

CRYPTOPHTHALMOS SYNDROME, see Fraser syndrome.

CSILLAG DISEASE, chronic atrophic acrodermatitis.
  1. Casas EC: Diccionario Terminologico de Ciencias Medicas. 5th ed. Salvat Editores, SA, 1954

CUBITAL TUNNEL SYNDROME, see Kiloh-Nevin syndrome.

CULLEN SIGN, a bluish discoloration in the area of the umbilicus; a possible sign of acute hemorrhagic pancreatitis, a ruptured common bile duct, or a perforated duodenal ulcer. Cross-references: Hellendall sign; Hoffstatter-Cullen sign. (Thomas S. Cullen, 1869-1953, U.S. gynecologist)
  1. Bailey H: Physical Signs in Clinical Surgery. 16th ed. Baltimore: Williams & Wilkins, 1983
  2. Bennett JC, Plum F (eds): Cecil Textbook of Medicine. 20th ed. Philadelphia: WB Saunders, 1996

CULP PYELOPLASTY, CULP-DE WEERD OPERATION, pyeloplasty using a spiral type of flap (1951). (Ormond Culp, 1910-1977, U.S. urologist; James De Weerd, U.S. surgeon)
  1. Campbell MF, Walsh PC: Campbell's Urology. 5th ed. Philadelphia: WB Saunders, 1986

CULTURE-SPECIFIC SYNDROME, a form of behavior specific to certain cultural systems and that does not conform to Western nosological entities (examples are amok, koro, piblokto, and Windigo).
  1. Dorland's Medical Dictionary. 28th ed. Philadelphia: WB Saunders, 1994

CUNEO OPERATION, surgical method for treating exstrophy of the bladder by creating an artificial one from a portion of the small intestine, where the ureters are implanted.
  1. Maffei WE: Os Fundamentos da Medicina. 2nd ed. Livraria Editora Artes Medicas Ltd, 1978

CURRY-HALL SYNDROME, see Weyers syndrome. (Cynthia J.R. Curry, U.S.; Bryan D. Hall, U.S.)

CURRY-JONES SYNDROME, consists of unilateral coronal synostosis and plagiocephaly, unilateral microphthalmia, iris coloboma, broad thumbs, complete 1-4 syndactyly of one hand with partial 1-3 syndactyly of the other, bilateral preaxial polydactyly of the feet, and unusual skin lesions.
  1. Gorlin RJ, Cohen MM Jr, Levin LS: Syndromes of the Head and Neck. 3rd ed. New York: Oxford University Press, 1990

CURSCHMANN DISEASE, thickening of the hepatic peritoneum that gives the liver a frosted (frozen) appearance. (Heinrich Curschmann, 1846-1910, German)
  1. Casas EC: Diccionario Terminologico de Ciencias Medicas. 5th ed. Salvat Editores, SA, 1954

CURSCHMANN-STEINERT DISEASE, see Steinert disease. (Hans Curschmann, 1875-1950, German; Hans Steinert, German)

CURTIS DISEASE, pseudomyxoma of the skin containing *Saccharomyces*.
  1. Casas EC: Diccionario Terminologico de Ciencias Medicas. 5th ed. Salvat Editores, SA, 1954

CURTIUS SYNDROME, congenital hemihypertrophy; hypertrophy of a portion of one side of the body, as of the face. Cross-reference: Steiner syndrome (when schizophrenia is present). (Friedrich Curtius, 1896-1975, German internist)

1. Barwell R: Case of unilateral hypertrophy of the head and face involving bones and soft parts. Trans Pathol Soc Lond 32:282-284, 1881
2. Curtius F: Dtsch Arch Klin Med 147:310-319, 1925

CUSHING DISEASE, similar to Cushing syndrome except associated with an adrenocorticotrophic hormone-producing adenoma. (Harvey W. Cushing, 1869-1939, U.S. neurosurgeon)

1. Cushing HW: Bull Johns Hopkins Hosp 50:137-195, 1932

CUSHING OPERATION, subtemporal extradural approach for removal of the gasserian ganglion. (Harvey W. Cushing)

1. Maffei WE: Os Fundamentos da Medicina. 2nd ed. Livraria Editora Artes Medicas Ltd, 1978

CUSHING PHENOMENON, a rise in systemic blood pressure following an increase in intracranial pressure. (Harvey W. Cushing)

1. Dorland's Medical Dictionary. 28th ed. Philadelphia: WB Saunders, 1994

CUSHING SYNDROME, pituitary basophilism; results from increased adrenocortical secretion of cortisol. Plethora, moon face, acne, obesity, bruises, ecchymoses, hypertension, and osteoporosis are features. Back pain is very common and vertebral collapse may occur. (Harvey W. Cushing)

1. Bennett JC, Plum F (eds): Cecil Textbook of Medicine. 20th ed. Philadelphia: WB Saunders, 1996
2. Cushing H: The basophil adenomas of the pituitary body and their clinical manifestations (pituitary basophilism). Bull Johns Hopkins Hosp 50:137-195, 1932
3. Cushing H: Tumors of the Nervus Acusticus. Philadelphia: WB Saunders, 1917

CUTIS VERTICIS GYRATA SYNDROME, see Touraine-Solente-Golé syndrome.

CUTLER-BEARD OPERATION, a procedure used for reconstruction of very large upper eyelid defects.

1. Spaeth GL: Ophthalmic Surgery. Principles and Practice. Philadelphia: WB Saunders, 1982

CYRIAX SYNDROME, diagnosed when slipped rib cartilage compresses the nerves at the interchondral joint, resulting in pain in the region of the cartilage, radiation of pain to the shoulder and arm, or pain similar to that of angina pectoris. Cross-reference: Slipping rib syndrome. (Edward F. Cyriax, British orthopedic surgeon)

1. Cyriax EJ: On various conditions that may simulate referred pain of visceral disease. Practitioner 2:314-322, 1919

CYSTOURETHRAL SYNDROME, a vague denomination often used for the patient with the classic symptoms of "cystitis" but who lacks significant bacteriuria.

1. Campbell MF, Walsh PC: Campbell's Urology. 5th ed. Philadelphia: WB Saunders, 1986

CZERNY DISEASE, periodic hydrarthrosis of the patella.

1. Casas EC: Diccionario Terminologico de Ciencias Medicas. 5th ed. Salvat Editores, SA, 1954

CZERNY OPERATION, surgical method for treating an inguinal hernia.

1. Maffei WE: Os Fundamentos da Medicina. 2nd ed. Livraria Editora Artes Medicas Ltd, 1978

DAAE DISEASE, DAAE-FINSEN DISEASE, epidemic pleurodynia. (Anders Daae, 1838-1910, Norwegian)

1. Casas EC: Diccionario Terminologico de Ciencias Medicas. 5th ed. Salvat Editores, SA, 1954

DA COSTA SYNDROME, functional asthenia; a mitral valve prolapse anxiety-associated illness, with autonomic disturbance. Cross-reference: Egg white syndrome. (Jacob M. Da Costa, 1833-1900, U.S. surgeon)

1. Da Costa JM: Am J Med 61:17-52, 1871

DA COSTA SYNDROME, see Mendes Da Costa syndrome. (Samuel Mendes da Costa, Dutch)

DAGNINI EXTENSION-ADDUCTION REFLEX, percussion of the radial aspect of the dorsum of the hand elicits extension and slight adduction of the wrist; seen in hyperreflexia or pyramidal tract lesion. (Guido Dagnini, Italian)

1. Baker AB, Baker LH: Clinical Neurology. Revised ed. Philadelphia: Harper & Row, 1982

DAGNINI SIGN, DAGNINI-ASCHER SIGN, an oculocardiac reflex; if the eyes are compressed, the heart rate decreases. (Guido Dagnini)

1. Casas EC: Diccionario Terminologico de Ciencias Medicas. 5th ed. Salvat Editores, SA, 1954

DALLAS OPERATION, obliteration of the conduit of an inguinal or femoral hernia that has been caused by an inflammatory process provoked by mechanical irritation.
1. Maffei WE: Os Fundamentos da Medicina. 2nd ed. Livraria Editora Artes Medicas Ltd, 1978

DALRYMPLE SIGN, abnormal, widened palpebral fissures; seen in the patient with exophthalmic goiter. (John Dalrymple, 1804-1852, English ophthalmologist)
1. Casas EC: Diccionario Terminologico de Ciencias Medicas. 5th ed. Salvat Editores, SA, 1954

D'AMATO SIGN, in the patient with pleural effusion, the findings at the percussion zone change as the patient changes position. (Luigi D'Amato, Italian)
1. Casas EC: Diccionario Terminologico de Ciencias Medicas. 5th ed. Salvat Editores, SA, 1954

DANBOLT-CLOSS SYNDROME, acrodermatitis enteropathica; characterized by chronic and severe diarrhea and desquamation in the mouth and anus. (Niels C. Danbolt, Norwegian dermatologist; Karl Closs, Norwegian)
1. Nelson WE, Vaughan VC, McKay RJ: Tratado de Pediatria. 6th ed. Salvat Editories, SA, 1971, Volumes 1 and 2

DANCING EYE-DANCING FOOT SYNDROME, a unique form of encephalopathic myoclonus. The onset is usually within the first 3 years of life, often after a prodromal illness that may include gastrointestinal or upper respiratory tract symptoms or fever. Cross-reference: Kingsbourne syndrome.
1. Kingsbourne M: J Neurol Neurosurg Psychiatry 27:271-276, 1962

DANDY OPERATION, intracranial section of the glossopharyngeal nerve in cases of glossopharyngeal neuralgia; the first intracranial cure of a carotid artery aneurysm (1938). (Walter E. Dandy, 1886-1946, U.S. neurosurgeon)
1. Maffei WE: Os Fundamentos da Medicina. 2nd ed. Livraria Editora Artes Medicas Ltd, 1978

DANDY-WALKER SYNDROME, atresia of the foramen of Magendie. While this condition may result in progressive hydrocephalus in infancy, it commonly remains compensated for long periods, resulting in the development of symptoms in late childhood or young adulthood. (Walter E. Dandy; Arthur Earl Walker, 1907-1995, U.S. neurosurgeon)
1. Dandy WE: Surg Gynecol Obstet 32:112-124, 1921
2. Farmer TW: Pediatric Neurology. 2nd ed. Hagerstown: Harper & Row, 1975
3. Krayenbühl HA, Yasargil MG: Cerebral Angiography. 2nd ed. Philadelphia: JB Lippincott, 1968
4. Walker AE: J Neuropathol Exp Neurol 3:368-373, 1944

DANIELOPOLU OPERATION, resection of the sympathetic cervical roots (except for the inferior cervical ganglion) and section of the thoracic branch of the vagus nerve, vertebral nerve, and communicating branches for the treatment of angina pectoris.
1. Maffei WE: Os Fundamentos da Medicina. 2nd ed. Livraria Editora Artes Medicas Ltd, 1978

DARIER DISEASE, DARIER-WHITE DISEASE, keratosis follicularis; a papulosquamous disorder usually first noted in late childhood. Autosomal dominant inheritance, affecting both sexes equally. (Jean F. Darier, 1856-1938, French dermatologist; James White, 1833-1916, U.S. dermatologist)
1. Darier JF: Ann Derm Syph 10:597-612, 1889
2. Moschella SL, Hurley HJ: Dermatology. 2nd ed. Philadelphia: WB Saunders, 1985
3. White J: J Cutan Genitourin Dis 7:201-209, 1889

DARLING DISEASE, histoplasmosis. (Samuel T. Darling, 1872-1925, U.S.)
1. Darling ST: JAMA 46:1283-1285, 1906

DARRACH OPERATION, indicated as a solitary procedure because of the risk of late ulnar angulation and translocation of the carpus upon the distal radius for excision of the distal ulna.
1. Schwartz SI: Principles of Surgery. 4th ed. New York: McGraw-Hill, 1983

DARWINIAN TUBERCLE, DARWIN TUBERCLE, tuberculum auriculare; the prominent rim of the auricle is called the helix. Where the helix turns downward, a small projection known as a Darwin tubercle is frequently seen. (Charles R. Darwin, 1809-1882, British biologist and evolutionist)
1. Ballenger JJ: Diseases of the Nose, Throat, Ear, Head, and Neck. 12th ed. Philadelphia: Lea & Febiger, 1977

DAVAT OPERATION, a technique for compression of veins in treating varicocele.
1. Maffei WE: Os Fundamentos da Medicina. 2nd ed. Livraria Editora Artes Medicas Ltd, 1978

DAVID DISEASE, hemorrhage of the mucosa and gums caused by endocrine dysfunction and seen in women. (W. Walter David, German)
1. Casas EC: Diccionario Terminologico de Ciencias Medicas. 5th ed. Salvat Editores, SA, 1954

DAVID DISEASE, see Pott disease. (John-Pierre David, 1737-1784, French surgeon)

DAVIDENKOW SYNDROME, hereditary sensorimotor polyneuropathy. The distinction of this syndrome from scapuloperoneal humeroperoneal neuromuscular disease can be made by the clinical finding of distal glove and stocking-type sensory loss and the presence of abnormal sensory nerve conduction. The pelvic girdle and hands are never involved. (S. Davidenkow, Russian)
  1. Davidenkow S: Arch Neurol Psychiatr 41:694-701, 1939

DAVIEL OPERATION, extraction of a cataract through a corneal incision without cutting the iris. (Jacques Daviel, 1696-1762, French oculist)
  1. Maffei WE: Os Fundamentos da Medicina. 2nd ed. Livraria Editora Artes Medicas Ltd, 1978

DAVIES-COLLEY OPERATION, cuneiform resection of a portion of the tarsus in cases of pes abductus. (R. Colley, British)
  1. Colley R: Br Med J 1:432, 1922
  2. Maffei WE: Os Fundamentos da Medicina. 2nd ed. Livraria Editora Artes Medicas Ltd, 1978

DAWSON ENCEPHALITIS, subacute sclerosing panencephalitis. An uncommon disorder most often occurring in children and young adults between the ages of 4 and 20 years. Onset is usually insidious and characterized by deterioration in school work and behavioral disorders, followed in weeks or months by overt mental deterioration and neurological signs, the most characteristic of which is myoclonus. (James R. Dawson, U.S. pathologist)
  1. Bennett JC, Plum F (eds): Cecil Textbook of Medicine. 20th ed. Philadelphia: WB Saunders, 1996
  2. Dawson JR: Am J Pathol 9:7-15, 1933
  3. Rowland LP (ed): Merritt's Textbook of Neurology. 9th ed. Baltimore: Williams & Wilkins, 1995

DE BARSY SYNDROME, consists of intrauterine growth retardation, wrinkled atrophic skin, open fontanels and sutures, somatic and mental retardation, brisk deep tendon reflexes, athetoid posturing, hypermobility of small joints, and muscular hypotonia. Autosomal recessive inheritance. (A.M. De Barsy, Belgian)
  1. De Barsy AM, Moens E, Dierckx L: Dwarfism, oligophrenia, and degeneration of the elastic tissue in skin cornea. A new syndrome? Helv Paediatr Acta 23:305-313, 1968
  2. Gorlin RJ, Cohen MM Jr, Levin LS: Syndromes of the Head and Neck. 3rd ed. New York: Oxford University Press, 1990
  3. Kunze J, Majewski F, Montgomery P, et al: De Barsy syndrome: an autosomal recessive progeroid syndrome. Eur J Pediatr 144:348-354, 1985

DÉBOVE DISEASE, essential splenomegaly. (Georges M. Débove, 1845-1920, French)
  1. Cruhl I: Bull Soc Med Hop Paris 9:596-613, 1892

DEBRÉ-SÉMÉLAIGNE SYNDROME, cretinism-muscular hypertrophy; has been described as a combination of muscular hypertrophy of the "infant Hercules" type associated with pronounced hypertoxicity and cretinism. Enlargement and stiffness of the muscles are likely due to their being packed with mucopolysaccharide. Cross-reference: Kocher-Debré-Sémélaigne syndrome. (Robert Debré, 1882-1978, French pediatrician; Georges Sémélaigne, French pediatrician)
  1. Debré R, Sémélaigne G: Bull Soc Pediatr 32:699-706, 1934
  2. Kocher T: Dtsch Z Chir 34:556-626, 1892

DEFIBRINATION SYNDROME, see Disseminated intravascular coagulation syndrome.

DEGOS DISEASE, small bowel ischemia characterized by necrotic skin lesions and vasculitis of the small gut. May also cause malabsorption, although the far more serious and common clinical manifestation is infarction of the gut. (Robert Degos, French dermatologist)
  1. Delort J, Tricort R: Arch Derm Syph 2:148-150, 1942
  2. Hurst JW, Schlant RC, Alexander RW: The Heart: Arteries and Veins. 8th ed. New York: McGraw-Hill, 1994
  3. Moschella SL, Hurley HJ: Dermatology. 2nd ed. Philadelphia: WB Saunders, 1985

DEJARDIN OPERATION, section of the round ligaments at the point of entrance into the inguinal conduit and suturing to the superior border of the broad ligaments.
  1. Maffei WE: Os Fundamentos da Medicina. 2nd ed. Livraria Editora Artes Medicas Ltd, 1978

DÉJERINE SYNDROME, diphtheric neuritis; 1) a syndrome of cortical sensory disturbances characterized by impairments in sensory discrimination in half of the body. 2) bulbar lesions. Cross-reference: Bulbar syndrome. 3) symptoms of radiculitis resembling tabes dorsalis due to a lesion of the long nerve root fibers of the posterior column. (Joseph Jules Déjerine, 1849-1917, French neurologist/pathologist)
  1. Déjerine J: Semiologie des Affections du System Nerveux. Paris: Masson, 1914

2. Gorlin RJ, Cohen MM Jr, Levin LS: Syndromes of the Head and Neck. 3rd ed. New York: Oxford University Press, 1990

DÉJERINE-KLUMPKE SYNDROME, see Klumpke syndrome. (Augusta Déjerine-Klumpke, 1859-1927, French neurologist)

DÉJERINE-LICHTHEIM PHENOMENON, see Lichtheim sign. (J.J. Déjerine; Ludwig Lichtheim, 1845-1928, German)

DÉJERINE-MOUZON SYNDROME, dysfunction of cortical sensation and tactile discrimination owing to parietal lobe lesions. (J.J. Déjerine)

1. Bordas LB (ed): Neurologia Fundamental. Toray, 1968

DÉJERINE-ROUSSY SYNDROME, consists of mild, transient initial hemiparesis on the side contralateral to the causative thalamic lesion, persistent hemianesthesia involving tactile sensation and proprioception, and thermoanalgesia with a complaint of ineffable pain referred to the parts affected, but usually not specifiable as to site or locus of distress. Cross-references: Posterior-thalamic syndrome; Thalamic syndrome. (J.J. Déjerine; Gustave Roussy, 1874-1948, French neuropathologist)

1. Dejerine J, Roussy G: Le syndrome thalamique. Rev Neurol 14:521-532, 1906
2. Grinker RR, Sahs AL: Neurology. 6th ed. Springfield: Charles C Thomas, 1966

DÉJERINE-SOTTAS DISEASE, hypertrophic neuritis; spinocerebellar degeneration, with onset in the first or second decades and slow progression. Reflexes are absent and there is moderate sensory loss, dysarthria, nystagmus, tremor, hypertrophic nerves, scoliosis, and elevated cerebrospinal fluid protein. Autosomal dominant trait. (J.J. Déjerine; Jules Sottas, 1866-1943, French neurologist)

1. Bennett JC, Plum F (eds): Cecil Textbook of Medicine. 20th ed. Philadelphia: WB Saunders, 1996
2. Campbell WC, Crenshaw AH: Campbell's Operative Orthopaedics. 7th ed. St Louis: CV Mosby, 1987
3. Déjerine JJ: Compt Rendu Soc Biol 2:43-53, 1890

DÉJERINE-THOMAS ATAXIA, olivopontocerebellar atrophy; progressive degeneration that may occur sporadically or in a hereditary setting. (J.J. Déjerine; André A.H. Thomas, 1867-1943, French neurologist)

1. Baker AB, Baker LH: Clinical Neurology. Revised ed. Philadelphia: Harper & Row, 1982
2. Déjerine JJ, Thomas AAH: Nouv Icon Salpetriere 13:330-370, 1900

DE LANGE SYNDROME, a syndrome of growth deficiency, mental retardation, and anomalies of the extremities. The face is characterized by an upturned nose, midline fusion of the eyebrows, micrognathia, and a small midline beak on the upper eyelid; the head is microbrachycephalic. Cross-reference: Brachmann-de Lange syndrome. (Cornelia de Lange, 1871-1950, Dutch pediatrician)

1. Brachmann W: Jahrb Kinderheilkd 84:225-235, 1916
2. De Lange C: Arch Med Enf 36:713-719, 1933
3. Farmer TW: Pediatric Neurology. 2nd ed. Hagerstown: Harper & Row, 1975

DEL CASTILLO SYNDROME, see Sertoli-cell-only syndrome. (E.B. Del Castillo, Argentine endocrinologist)

DEL TORO OPERATION, thermal destruction of the vertex of a conical cornea.

1. Maffei WE: Os Fundamentos da Medicina. 2nd ed. Livraria Editora Artes Medicas Ltd, 1978

DEL(1q) SYNDROME, deletion of the long arm of chromosome 1; characteristics include somatic and mental retardation, seizures, hypotonia, a high-pitched cry, microbrachycephalic head, characteristic facies, hypospadias, cryptorchidism, cleft lip and/or palate, and missing or bifid uvula.

1. Gorlin RJ, Cohen MM Jr, Levin LS: Syndromes of the Head and Neck. 3rd ed. New York: Oxford University Press, 1990
2. Juberg RC, Haney NR, Stallard R: New deletion syndrome 1q4. Am J Hum Genet 33:455-463, 1981
3. Zabel BV, et al: 1q deletion syndrome. Clin Genet 19:544-545, 1981

DEL(2q) SYNDROME, two deletions are found. The first involves deletion of q21-q31 and characteristics of somatic and mental retardation, macrocephaly, small nose, cataracts, microphthalmia, ptosis, micrognathia, flexion deformity of the fingers, and congenital heart disease. The second involves deletion of 2q31-q33 and characteristics of mental and somatic retardation, eye anomalies, and finger deformities of the first type; cleft lip and/or palate is also noted.

1. Fryns JP, Van Bosstraeten B, Malbrain H, et al: Interstitial deletion of the long arm of chromosome 2 in polymalformed newborn—karyotype 46, XX,del(2)(q21;q24). Hum Genet 39:233-238, 1977
2. Gorlin RJ, Cohen MM Jr, Levin LS: Syndromes of the Head and Neck. 3rd ed. New York: Oxford University Press, 1990

3. McConnell TS, Kornfield M, McClellan G, et al: Partial deletion of chromosome 2 mimicking a phenotype of tri-somy 18: case report of autopsy. Hum Pathol 11:202-205, 1980

DEL(3p) SYNDROME, deletion of the short arm of chromosome 3; characteristics include low birth weight, severe postnatal growth retardation, severe mental retardation, microcephaly, brachycephaly, unusual facies, and developmental delay with severe psychomotor retardation.

1. Beneck D, Sutherland MJ, Dicker R, et al: Deletion of the short arm of chromosome 3: a case report with necropsy findings. J Med Genet 21:307-310, 1984
2. Garcia-Sagredo JM, Quintana Castilla A, Ludeña Carpio ML, et al: The phenotype of partial monosomy 3 (p25Æpter) observed in two unrelated patients. Clin Genet 20:387, 1981 (Abstract)
3. Gorlin RJ, Cohen MM Jr, Levin LS: Syndromes of the Head and Neck. 3rd ed. New York: Oxford University Press, 1990

DEL(4p) SYNDROME, see Wolf-Hirschhorn syndrome.

DEL(4q) SYNDROME, the critical deletion segment is 4q31→qter. Common features are mild post-natal growth retardation and mild to moderately severe mental retardation. Craniofacial anomalies, low-set posteriorly angulated pinnae and various skeletal anomalies are also found in some cases. Congenital heart disease and aspiration pneumonia are the leading causes of death within the first 2 years of life.

1. Davis JM, Clarren SK, Salk DJ, et al: The del(4)(q31) syndrome—a recognizable disorder with atypical Robin malfor-mation sequence. Am J Med Genet 9:113-117, 1981
2. Gorlin RJ, Cohen MM Jr, Levin LS: Syndromes of the Head and Neck. 3rd ed. New York: Oxford University Press, 1990

DEL(5q) SYNDROME, deletion of the long arm of chromosome 5; severe mental retardation and a characteristic facies of downward slanting, palpebral fissure, strabismus, frontal bossing, hypertelorism, epicanthal folds, and low-set malformed ears are features. There is no evidence of growth retardation.

1. Gorlin RJ, Cohen MM Jr, Levin LS: Syndromes of the Head and Neck. 3rd ed. New York: Oxford University Press, 1990
2. Harprecht-Beato W, Kaiser P, Steuber E, et al: Interstitial deletion in the long arm of chromosome no. 5. Clin Genet 23:167-171, 1983

DEL(6q) SYNDROME, deletion of the long arm of chromosome 6; mental retardation, microcephaly, facial asymmetry, up-slanting palpebral fissures, hypertelorism, microphthalmia, strabismus, epicanthal folds, a broad nasal bridge, prominent nose, long philtrum, large low-set dysmorphic pinnae, thin upper lip, micrognathia, cleft palate, and short neck are features.

1. Bartoshesky L, Lewis MB, Pashayan HM: Developmental abnormalities associated with long arm deletion of chro-mosome No. 6. Clin Genet 13:68-71, 1978
2. Gorlin RJ, Cohen MM Jr, Levin LS: Syndromes of the Head and Neck. 3rd ed. New York: Oxford University Press, 1990

DEL(7p) SYNDROME, deletion of the short arm of chromosome 6; variable craniosynostosis, micro-cephaly, flat occiput, prominent forehead, trigonocephaly, and cranial asymmetry are features. Intelligence varies from severe retardation to normal.

1. Gorlin RJ, Cohen MM Jr, Levin LS: Syndromes of the Head and Neck. 3rd ed. New York: Oxford University Press, 1990
2. Zackai EH, Breg WR: Ring chromosome 7 with variable phenotypic expression. Cytogenet Cell Genet 12:40-48, 1973

DEL(7q) SYNDROME, deletion of 7q32→7qter results in pre- and postnatal growth retardation, feeding problems, severe mental retardation, hypotonia, microcephaly with prominent forehead, a broad nasal bridge with bulbous tip, various eye anomalies, large dysplastic pinnae, a large mouth, micrognathia, and a short neck.

1. Gorlin RJ, Cohen MM Jr, Levin LS: Syndromes of the Head and Neck. 3rd ed. New York: Oxford University Press, 1990
2. Young RS, Weaver DD, Kukolich MK, et al: Terminal and interstitial deletions of the long arm of chromosome 7: a review of five new cases. Am J Med Genet 17:437-450, 1984

DEL(8p) SYNDROME, deletion of the short arm of chromosome 8; intrauterine growth retardation, abnormal facial appearance, congenital heart defects, and genital anomalies are found. As the child grows older, postnatal growth deficiency, mental retardation, developmental delay, microcephaly, and some lessening of facial changes become evident.

1. Gorlin RJ, Cohen MM Jr, Levin LS: Syndromes of the Head and Neck. 3rd ed. New York: Oxford University Press, 1990

2. Leisti J, Aula P: A case of deletion of short arm of chromosome 8. Birth Defects 13:187-194, 1977

DEL(9p) SYNDROME, deletion of the short arm of chromosome 9; characteristics include mental and somatic retardation, normal birth weight, characteristic facies, wide-set nipples, congenital heart disease, omphalocele or umbilical hernia, inguinal hernia, long fingers or toes because of dolichomesophalangy, relative shortness of the metacarpal bones, square hyperconvex nails, and an increased number of fingertip whorls.

1. Fryns JP, Pedersen JC, Duyck H, et al: Deletion of the short arm of chromosome 9. A clinically recognisable entity. Eur J Pediatr 134:201-204, 1980
2. Gorlin RJ, Cohen MM Jr, Levin LS: Syndromes of the Head and Neck. 3rd ed. New York: Oxford University Press, 1990

DEL(10p) SYNDROME, deletion of the short arm of chromosome 10. Severe mental retardation, frequent postnatal growth retardation, characteristic facies, and widely spaced nipples are features. Also frequently found are congenital heart anomalies, cryptorchidism, hernia, and renal abnormalities. Hypoplasia or aplasia of the olfactory bulb and tracts has been found with more proximal deletions.

1. Elstner CL, Carey JC, Livingston G, et al: Further delineation of the 10p deletion syndrome. Pediatrics 73:670-675, 1984
2. Gorlin RJ, Cohen MM Jr, Levin LS: Syndromes of the Head and Neck. 3rd ed. New York: Oxford University Press, 1990

DEL(10q) SYNDROME, deletion of the long arm of chromosome 10. Severe mental and growth retardation, microcephaly, a prominent beaked nose, apparent hypertelorism, strabismus, malformed pinnae, and a short neck are features. Cleft lip has also been noted.

1. Gorlin RJ, Cohen MM Jr, Levin LS: Syndromes of the Head and Neck. 3rd ed. New York: Oxford University Press, 1990
2. Mulcahy MT, Pemberton PJ, Thompson E, et al: Is there a monosomy 10qter syndrome? Clin Genet 21:33-35, 1982

DEL(11q) SYNDROME, deletion of the long arm of chromosome 11. Involves del(11)(q23→qter) or terminal deletion. Mental retardation, postnatal somatic retardation, frequent respiratory infections, characteristic facies, various heart anomalies, joint contractures and/or minor digital anomalies, single flexion creases, and thrombocytopenia are usually exhibited. About 25% of affected persons die before 2 years of age, usually from congenital heart disease.

1. Ferry AP, Marchevsky A, Strauss L: Ocular abnormalities in deletion of the long arm of chromosome 11. Ann Ophthalmol 13:1373-1377, 1981
2. Gorlin RJ, Cohen MM Jr, Levin LS: Syndromes of the Head and Neck. 3rd ed. New York: Oxford University Press, 1990

DEL(14q) SYNDROME, deletion of the long arm of chromosome 14; the patient with this syndrome usually has ring chromosomes. Features include microcephaly with a flat occiput, epicanthal folds, downward-slanting palpebral fissures, a narrow elongated face, short palpebral fissures, a flat nasal bridge, large low-set pinnae, micrognathia, and a short neck. Severe mental retardation, hypotonia, and seizures are also found. Recurrent respiratory infections are common.

1. Gorlin RJ, Cohen MM Jr, Levin LS: Syndromes of the Head and Neck. 3rd ed. New York: Oxford University Press, 1990
2. Schmidt R, Eviatar L, Nitowsky HM, et al: Ring chromosome 14: a distinct clinical entity. J Med Genet 18:304-307, 1981

DEL(15q) SYNDROME, deletion of the long arm of chromosome 15; in the young patient, the most characteristic findings are prenatal growth retardation, variable mental retardation, microcephaly, hypertelorism, a triangular face, and limb anomalies including delayed bone development, clinodactyly of the fifth fingers, and thumb hypoplasia. Congenital heart anomalies and café-au-lait spots are found in some patients. In the adult patient, severe mental and somatic retardation become evident and a bossed forehead, triangular face, anomalous pinnae, and broad high-bridged nose are found; the male is hypogonadal.

1. Gorlin RJ, Cohen MM Jr, Levin LS: Syndromes of the Head and Neck. 3rd ed. New York: Oxford University Press, 1990
2. Kousseff BG: Ring chromosome 15 and failure to thrive. Am J Dis Child 134:798-799, 1980

DEL(16q) SYNDROME, deletion of the long arm of chromosome 16; low birth weight, delayed growth and development, feeble suck response, hypotonia, distinct craniofacies such as a high forehead and prominent metopic suture, diverse skeletal anomalies, and cardiac, renal, and intestinal anomalies are features.

1. Gorlin RJ, Cohen MM Jr, Levin LS: Syndromes of the Head and Neck. 3rd ed. New York: Oxford University Press, 1990
2. Rivera H, Vargos-Moyeda E, Möller M, et al: Monosomy 16q: a distinct syndrome. Apropos of a de novo del(16)(q2100q 2300). Clin Genet 28:84-86, 1985

DEL(17p) SYNDROME, deletion of the short arm of chromosome 17; includes developmental delay, brachycephaly, mid-face hypoplasia with a broad nasal bridge, highly arched palate, malformed and/or malpositioned pinnae, hearing deficit, relative mandibular prognathism, and short broad thumbs.

1. Bridge J, Sanger W, Mosher G, et al: Partial deletion of distal 17q. Am J Med Genet 21:225-229, 1985
2. Gorlin RJ, Cohen MM Jr, Levin LS: Syndromes of the Head and Neck. 3rd ed. New York: Oxford University Press, 1990

DEL(22q) SYNDROME, deletion of the long arm of chromosome 22; in the young child, the face tends to be round. Also found are horizontal, wide almond-shaped palpebral fissures, epicanthal folds, ptosis, low-set eyebrows, large pinnae, severe mental retardation, hypotonia, and poor motor coordination; the nose has a bulbous tip in infancy. Decreased head circumference is found in 65% of patients.

1. Gorlin RJ, Cohen MM Jr, Levin LS: Syndromes of the Head and Neck. 3rd ed. New York: Oxford University Press, 1990
2. Hunter AGW, Ray M, Wang HS, et al: Phenotypic correlations in patients with ring chromosome 22. Clin Genet 12:239-249, 1977

DELAYED SLEEP-PHASE SYNDROME, a specific chronobiological sleep disorder; a chronic inability to sleep at a desired time to meet required work or study schedules is described.

1. Association of Sleep Centers: Diagnostic classification of sleep and arousal disorders. Sleep 2:1-154, 1979
2. Rowland LP (ed): Merritt's Textbook of Neurology. 9th ed. Baltimore: Williams & Wilkins, 1995

DELBET SIGN, in the patient with an aneurysm of the main artery of a limb, effective collateralization is suggested by the nutrition of the tissues even in the absence of a pulse. (Pierre Delbet, 1861-1957, French surgeon)

1. Casas EC: Diccionario Terminologico de Ciencias Medicas. 5th ed. Salvat Editores, SA, 1954

DELEAGE DISEASE, myotonia atrophica.

1. Casas EC: Diccionario Terminologico de Ciencias Medicas. 5th ed. Salvat Editores, SA, 1954

DELLEMAN SYNDROME, see Oculocerebrocutaneous syndrome.

DELMEGE SIGN, flatness of the deltoid muscle; seen in the patient with incipient tuberculosis. (Jean A. Delmege, French)

1. Casas EC: Diccionario Terminologico de Ciencias Medicas. 5th ed. Salvat Editores, SA, 1954

DELORME OPERATION, excision of a portion of the pleura.

1. Maffei WE: Os Fundamentos da Medicina. 2nd ed. Livraria Editora Artes Medicas Ltd, 1978

DELPECH OPERATION, ligature of the axillary artery between the pectoralis major and deltoid muscles.

1. Maffei WE: Os Fundamentos da Medicina. 2nd ed. Livraria Editora Artes Medicas Ltd, 1978

DEMARQUAY SIGN, fixation or lowering of the larynx during phonation and deglutition; an indication of syphilis of the trachea. (Jean N. Demarquay, 1814-1875, French surgeon)

1. Dorland's Medical Dictionary. 28th ed. Philadelphia: WB Saunders, 1994

DEMIANOFF SIGN, see Straight leg raising test. (G.S. Demianoff, French)

DEMONS-MEIGS SYNDROME, see Meigs syndrome.

DEMOURS DISEASE, exophthalmic goiter.

1. Casas EC: Diccionario Terminologico de Ciencias Medicas. 5th ed. Salvat Editores, SA, 1954

DE MUSSET SIGN, see Musset sign.

DENANS OPERATION, a technique for intestinal anastomosis using metallic cylinders.

1. Maffei WE: Os Fundamentos da Medicina. 2nd ed. Livraria Editora Artes Medicas Ltd, 1978

DENGUE SHOCK SYNDROME, hemorrhagic dengue.

1. Dorland's Medical Dictionary. 28th ed. Philadelphia: WB Saunders, 1994

DENNIE SIGN, see Morgan line. (Charles C. Dennie, 1883-1971, U.S. dermatologist)

DENNIE-MARFAN SYNDROME, spastic paralysis and mental deficiency in association with congenital syphilis. (Charles C. Dennie; Antoine B.J. Marfan, 1858-1942, French pediatrician)

1. Dennie C: Partial paralysis of the lower extremities in children accompanied by backward mental development. Am J Syph 13:157-163, 1929

DENONVILLIERS OPERATION, autoplasty of the ala nasi using a triangular flap adjacent to the nose. (Charles P. Denonvilliers, 1808-1872, French surgeon)
1. Maffei WE: Os Fundamentos da Medicina. 2nd ed. Livraria Editora Artes Medicas Ltd, 1978

DENT DISEASE, a mutation of the X-linked renal specific chloride channel (CLCN5) characterized by low-molecular weight proteinuria.
1. Igarashi T, Gunther W, Sekine T, et al: Kidney Int 54:1850-1856, 1998
2. Norden AG, Scheinman SJ, Deschodt-Lanckman MM, et al: Kidney Int 57:240-249, 2000

DENTAL PHENOMENON, thermal and tactile sensations in the gums with toothache, produced by repeated faradic stimulation of hyperesthetic lines on the body.
1. Dorland's Medical Dictionary. 28th ed. Philadelphia: WB Saunders, 1994

DENYS-LECLÉF PHENOMENON, enhanced phagocytosis occurring in a test tube following the mixing of leukocytes, bacteria, and immune serum specific for the bacteria. (Joseph Denys, 1857-1932, Belgian bacteriologist)
1. Dorland's Medical Dictionary. 28th ed. Philadelphia: WB Saunders, 1994

DE QUERVAIN DISEASE, tenosynovitis of the abductor pollicis longus and extensor pollicis brevis muscles. (Fritz de Quervain, 1868-1940, Swiss)
1. Ballenger JJ: Diseases of the Nose, Throat, Ear, Head, and Neck. 12th ed. Philadelphia: Lea & Febiger, 1977
2. De Quervain F: Arch Klin Chir Berl 67:706-714, 1902
3. Wilson JD, Foster DW, Kronenberg HM, et al (eds): Williams Textbook of Endocrinology. 9th ed. Philadelphia: WB Saunders, 1998

DERCUM DISEASE, a rare, progressive disease that usually affects menopausal, obese females, although has also been reported in males. The patient develops multiple, painful subcutaneous plaques and ecchymoses; lesions usually occur on the shoulders, arms, forearms, trunk, and legs, although any part of the body, with the exception of the face and hands, may be involved. The overlying skin may be normal or inflamed. Pain may be spontaneous or may follow minor pressure. (Francis X. Dercum, 1856-1931, U.S. neurologist)
1. Campbell MF, Walsh PC: Campbell's Urology. 5th ed. Philadelphia: WB Saunders, 1986
2. Dercum FX: Univ Med Gaz Phila 1:140-150, 1888/1889
3. Moschella SL, Hurley HJ: Dermatology. 2nd ed. Philadelphia: WB Saunders, 1985

DERRICK-BURNETT DISEASE, Q fever.
1. Casas EC: Diccionario Terminologico de Ciencias Medicas. 5th ed. Salvat Editores, SA, 1954

DE SANCTIS-CACCHIONE SYNDROME, xerodermic idiocy; xeroderma pigmentosa, microcephaly, and hypogonadism are features. Autosomal recessive inheritance. (Carlo De Sanctis, Italian psychiatrist; Aldo Cacchione, Italian psychiatrist)
1. De Sanctis C, Cacchione A: L'idiozia xerodermica. Riv Sper Freniatr 56:269-292, 1932
2. Smith DW, Jones KL: Recognizable Patterns of Human Malformations: Genetic, Embryologic, and Clinical Aspects. 3rd ed. Philadelphia: WB Saunders, 1982

DESAULT OPERATION, opening of the larynx through an incision in the thyroid cartilage. (Pierre J. Desault, 1744-1795, French surgeon)
1. Maffei WE: Os Fundamentos da Medicina. 2nd ed. Livraria Editora Artes Medicas Ltd, 1978

DESAULT SIGN, a deformity of the greater trochanteric arch caused by rotation; seen in cases of intrascapular fracture of the femur. (Pierre Desault)
1. Casas EC: Diccionario Terminologico de Ciencias Medicas. 5th ed. Salvat Editores, SA, 1954

DESNOS DISEASE, see Grancher disease.

D'ÉSPINE SIGN, see Espine sign.

DE TONI-DEBRÉ-FANCONI SYNDROME, cystinosis; represents a heterogeneous group of disorders and characterized by hypophosphatemia, glycosuria, and aminoaciduria. (Guido De Toni, 1892-1973, Swedish pediatrician; Robert Debré, 1882-1978, French pediatrician; Giovanni Fanconi, 1896-1973, Italian pediatrician)
1. Bennett JC, Plum F (eds): Cecil Textbook of Medicine. 20th ed. Philadelphia: WB Saunders, 1996
2. De Toni G: Acta Paediatr Uppsala 16:479-484, 1933
3. Debré R: Arch Med Enf 37:597-606, 1934

DEUTSCHLÄNDER DISEASE, fracture of the third metacarpal bone, resulting from excessive strain; discovered after formation of a corn. (Carl E.W. Deutschländer, 1872-1942, German surgeon)

1. Deutschländer CEW: Arch Klin Chir Berl 118:530-549, 1921

DEVERGIE DISEASE, pityriasis rubra pilaris. (Marie G. Devergie, 1798-1879, French)
1. Devergie MG: Gaz Hebd Med Paris 3:197-201, 1856

DEVIC DISEASE, neuromyelitis optica; characterized by the occurrence of partial or complete transverse myelopathy and optic neuritis. Loss of vision and paraplegia may occur, and days or weeks may elapse between the onsets of the two symptom complexes. (Eugène Devic, 1869-1930, French)
1. Devic E: Bull Med (Par) 8:1033-1034, 1894
2. Devic E: Cong Fr Med Lyon 1:434-439, 1894

DEVIL'S GRIP, see Bornholm disease.

DEW SIGN, with the patient in a sitting position and bent forward, percussion of the right upper quadrant produces resonance; seen in the patient with hydatidosis. (Sir Harold R. Dew, 1891-1962, Australian)
1. Casas EC: Diccionario Terminologico de Ciencias Medicas. 5th ed. Salvat Editores, SA, 1954

DEWEE SIGN, expectoration of mucus and whitish sputum in pregnant women.
1. Casas EC: Diccionario Terminologico de Ciencias Medicas. 5th ed. Salvat Editores, SA, 1954

DEYERLE SIGN, the affected leg is extended until pain is produced; the knee is then flexed and pressure is applied in the popliteal fossa. The test is positive if radiculitis symptoms are increased.
1. Evans RC: Illustrated Essentials in Orthopedic Physical Assessment. St Louis: Mosby Yearbook, 1994
2. Mazion JM: Illustrated Manual of Neurological Reflexes/Signs/Tests For Office Procedure. 2nd ed. Arizona City: Daniels Publishing, 1980

D'HERELLE PHENOMENON, see Twort-d'Herelle phenomenon.

DIABETIC FOOT SYNDROME, the consequence of coexisting vascular insufficiency and neuropathy; neuropathy is more important.
1. Wilson JD, Foster DW, Kronenberg HM, et al (eds): Williams Textbook of Endocrinology. 9th ed. Philadelphia: WB Saunders, 1998

DIALYSIS DYSEQUILIBRIUM SYNDROME, a well-known complication during hemodialysis. Characteristics are nausea, vomiting, headache, visual acuity disturbance, tremor, muscle twitching, disorientation, agitation, confusion, convulsion, loss of consciousness, electroencephalogram abnormalities, and elevation of intracranial pressure.
1. Lancet 1:410-411, 1962
2. Neurosurgery 20:716-721, 1987

DIAMOND-BLACKFAN SYNDROME, see Aase-Smith syndrome II. (Louis Diamond, U.S.; Kenneth Blackfan, 1883-1941, U.S.)

DIAPHRAGM PHENOMENON, see Litten sign.

DIARRHEOGENIC SYNDROME, see Verner-Morrison syndrome.

DIASTROPHIC DYSPLASIA SYNDROME, diastrophic dwarfism; short tubular bones, joint limitation with talipes, and hypertrophy of the auricular cartilage are features. Autosomal recessive inheritance. Cross-reference: Lamy-Maroteaux syndrome.
1. Smith DW, Jones KL: Recognizable Patterns of Human Malformations: Genetic, Embryologic, and Clinical Aspects. 3rd ed. Philadelphia: WB Saunders, 1982
2. Walker BA, Scott CI, Hall JG, et al: Diastrophic dwarfism. Medicine 51:41-59, 1972

DIDE-BOTCAZO SYNDROME, bilateral lesions of the posterior cerebral artery causing visual impairment (central), spatial sense impairment, agnosia, and amnesia.
1. Bordas LB (ed): Neurologia Fundamental. Toray, 1968

DIEFFENBACH OPERATION, disarticulation of the hip; autoplasty by sliding a quadrangular flap. (Johann F. Dieffenbach, 1792-1847, German surgeon)
1. Dieffenbach JF: Uges Kr Laegner 92:798-801, 1930
2. Maffei WE: Os Fundamentos da Medicina. 2nd ed. Livraria Editora Artes Medicas Ltd, 1978

DIENCEPHALIC SYNDROME, see Russell syndrome.

DIEULAFOY DISEASE, multiple and superficial ulcerations of the stomach. (Georges Dieulafoy, 1839-1911, French)
1. Dieulafoy G: Sem Med Paris, 1900, p 263

DI GEORGE SYNDROME, congenital absence of the thymus and parathyroid glands causing hypoparathyroidism, an aortic arch anomaly, hypertelorism, and a short philtrum. Cross-reference: Pharyngeal pouch syndrome. (Angelo M. DiGeorge, U.S. pediatrician)

1. Bennett JC, Plum F (eds): Cecil Textbook of Medicine. 20th ed. Philadelphia: WB Saunders, 1996
2. DiGeorge AM: J Pediatr 67:907-908, 1965
3. Krugman S, Katz SL: Infectious Diseases of Children. 7th ed. St Louis: CV Mosby, 1981

DI GUGLIELMO SYNDROME, a rare, acute myeloproliferative syndrome characterized by anemia, increased numbers of markedly abnormal erythroblasts in the peripheral circulation, and marked erythroblastic overgrowth of the bone marrow. (Giovanni Di Guglielmo, 1886-1962, Italian hematologist)

1. Di Guglielmo G: Folia Med 3:319, 1917

DIMAURO DISEASE, myoglobinuria. The missing enzyme is carnitine palmityl transferase, which plays a vital role in the oxidation of long-chain fatty acids.

1. Bennett JC, Plum F (eds): Cecil Textbook of Medicine. 20th ed. Philadelphia: WB Saunders, 1996

DIMITRI DISEASE, see Sturge-Kalischer-Weber syndrome

DIMPLE SIGN, dimpling occurring when a lesion is squeezed; habitual crossing of the legs may produce an oval area of pressure atrophy involving the tissues overlying the peroneal nerve at the head of the fibula.

1. Baker AB, Baker LH: Clinical Neurology. Revised ed. Philadelphia: Harper & Row, 1982

DIOGENES SYNDROME, a syndrome occurring in the elderly population characterized by gross self-neglect, social withdrawal, and squalid living conditions. This complex geriatric problem poses clinical, social, and ethical challenges. The condition is not clearly defined, and the reference to the Greek philosopher Diogenes is misleading.

1. Roberge RF: Can Fam Phys 44:812-817, 1998
2. Sikdar S: Hosp Med 60:679, 1999

DISAPPEARING SIGN, while still comparatively small, a cyst can disappear on acute flexion of the joint and reappear on extension, reaching its maximum dimensions when the joint is nearly, but not quite, fully extended. (Anthony J. Pisani, U.S. orthopedic surgeon)

1. Bailey H: Physical Signs in Clinical Surgery. 16th ed. Baltimore: Williams & Wilkins, 1983

DISCONJUGATE GAZE SIGN, the patient is unable to move the eyeball to the normal medial extreme, while the opposite eye exhibits nystagmus during the attempt. The sign may be reversed (i.e., the inability to move the eye to the normal lateral extreme while the opposite eye reveals nystagmus).

1. Mazion JM: Illustrated Manual of Neurological Reflexes/Signs/Tests For Office Procedure. 2nd ed. Arizona City: Daniels Publishing, 1980

DISEQUILIBRIUM SYNDROME, see Dialysis disequilibrium syndrome.

DISSEMINATED INTRAVASCULAR COAGULATION SYNDROME, thrombotic thrombocytopenic purpura; this syndrome encompasses a number of clinical situations in which excess thrombin gains access to the general circulation. Cross-reference: Defibrination syndrome.

1. Bennett JC, Plum F (eds): Cecil Textbook of Medicine. 20th ed. Philadelphia: WB Saunders, 1996

DISTAL ARTHROGRYPOSIS SYNDROME, distal congenital contractures; clenched hands with medial overlapping of the fingers and thumb adduction at birth are features. Autosomal dominant inheritance.

1. Lundblom A: On congenital ulnar deviation of the fingers of familial occurrence. Acta Orthop Scand 3:393-404, 1932
2. Smith DW, Jones KL: Recognizable Patterns of Human Malformations: Genetic, Embryologic, and Clinical Aspects. 3rd ed. Philadelphia: WB Saunders, 1982

DISTAL OPTIC NERVE SYNDROME, junctional scotoma; loss of vision in one eye and a superior temporal field defect in the contralateral, asymptomatic eye.

1. Walsh FB, Hoyt EF, Miller NR: Clinical Neuro-Ophthalmology. 4th ed. Baltimore: Williams & Wilkins, 1982

DISTICHIASIS-LYMPHEDEMA SYNDROME, features include an extra row of eyelashes, lymphedema (predominantly from the knees downward), epidural spinal cysts, and sometimes secondary vertebral anomalies. Autosomal dominant inheritance.

1. Robinow M, Johnson GF, Verhagen AD, et al: Distichiasis-lymphedema. A hereditary syndrome of multiple congenital defects. Am J Dis Child 119:343, 1970
2. Smith DW, Jones KL: Recognizable Patterns of Human Malformations: Genetic, Embryologic, and Clinical Aspects. 3rd ed. Philadelphia: WB Saunders, 1982

DITTEL OPERATION, enucleation of the lateral lobules of the hypertrophied prostate through an

external incision. (Leopold R. von Dittel, 1815-1898, Italian urologist)
1. Maffei WE: Os Fundamentos da Medicina. 2nd ed. Livraria Editora Artes Medicas Ltd, 1978

DIXON MANN SIGN, see Mann sign.

DÖHLE DISEASE, syphilitic aortitis. Cross-reference: Heller-Döhle disease. (Karl G. Döhle, 1855-1928, German pathologist)
1. Casas EC: Diccionario Terminologico de Ciencias Medicas. 5th ed. Salvat Editores, SA, 1954

DOLÉRIS OPERATION, shortening of the round ligaments and fixation of each one to the corresponding iliac spine through an opening into the rectus abdominis muscle.
1. Maffei WE: Os Fundamentos da Medicina. 2nd ed. Livraria Editora Artes Medicas Ltd, 1978

DOLL'S EYE SIGN, see Cantelli sign.

DOLL'S HEAD PHENOMENON, an abnormal muscle manifestation, with the eyes depressing as the head is bent backward.
1. Dorland's Medical Dictionary. 28th ed. Philadelphia: WB Saunders, 1994

DONNELLY SIGN, pain is present if the leg is adducted and extended and pressure is present at the McBurney point; seen in retrocecal appendicitis.
1. Casas EC: Diccionario Terminologico de Ciencias Medicas. 5th ed. Salvat Editores, SA, 1954

DONOHUE SYNDROME, leprechaunism; consists of failure to thrive, unusual facies, sexual precocity, retarded bone age, and insulin resistance with glucose intolerance and hyperinsulinemia. Autosomal recessive inheritance. Cross-reference: Leprechaunism syndrome. (William L. Donohue, Canadian pathologist)
1. Adams JM, Gordon LP, Dutton RV, et al: Leprechaunism (Donohue's syndrome) in a low birth weight infant. South Med J 70:998-1001, 1977
2. Ayraud N, Rovinski J, Lambert JC, et al: Délétion interstitielle du bras long d'un chromosome 7 chez une enfant lepréchaune. Ann Genet 19:265-268, 1976
3. Donohue WL: Dysendocrinism. J Pediatr 32:739-748, 1948
4. Donohue WL, Uchida I: Leprechaunism. A euphemism for a rare familial disorder. J Pediatr 45:505-519, 1954

DOPPLER OPERATION, injection of phenol into the tissues around the sympathetic nerve innervating the gonads in order to increase the production of hormones and obtain rejuvenescence.
1. Maffei WE: Os Fundamentos da Medicina. 2nd ed. Livraria Editora Artes Medicas Ltd, 1978

DORENDORF SIGN, bulging of the supraclavicular fossa in an aortic arch aneurysm. (Hans Dorendorf, 1866-1953, German)
1. Casas EC: Diccionario Terminologico de Ciencias Medicas. 5th ed. Salvat Editores, SA, 1954

DORSOCUBOIDAL SIGN, see Mendel reflex.

DORSOLATERAL MIDBRAIN SYNDROME, due largely to occlusion of the quadrigeminal artery and characterized by ipsilateral signs of cerebellar deficiency, Horner syndrome, and contralateral sensory deficit and hypacusis.
1. Haymaker W: Bing's Local Diagnosis in Neurological Diseases. 15th ed. St Louis: CV Mosby, 1969

DOUGLAS SIGN, acute verbal reaction by the patient during laparotomy when the surgeon manipulates the fundus of the uterus. (John C. Douglas, 1770-1850, Irish obstetrician)
1. Casas EC: Diccionario Terminologico de Ciencias Medicas. 5th ed. Salvat Editores, SA, 1954

DOWELL OPERATION, 1) surgery for an inguinal hernia; 2) hemicraniectomy; 3) abdominal hysterectomy for prolapse of the uterus; 4) resection of the gasserian ganglion through a vertical incision anterior to the acoustic meatus.
1. Maffei WE: Os Fundamentos da Medicina. 2nd ed. Livraria Editora Artes Medicas Ltd, 1978

DOWN SYNDROME, mongolism or trisomy 21; multiple congenital abnormalities including developmental defects of nervous, cutaneous, osseous, ligamentous, cardiac, and hematopoietic tissue. Features include hypotonia, mental deficiency, slanted palpebral fissures, and small ears. Cross-reference: Trisomy 21 syndrome. (John L.H. Down, 1828-1891, British)
1. Down JLH: Clin Lect Rep Lond Hosp 3:259-262, 1866
2. Grinker RR, Sahs AL: Neurology. 6th ed. Springfield: Charles C Thomas, 1966
3. Smith DW, Jones KL: Recognizable Patterns of Human Malformations: Genetic, Embryologic, and Clinical Aspects. 3rd ed. Philadelphia: WB Saunders, 1982

DOYEN OPERATION, 1) eversion of the tunica vaginalis in the treatment of hydrocele; 2) exposure of the heart through a U-shaped incision of the costal cartilage; 3) pericardial paracentesis; 4) panhysterectomy through the abdomen.

1. Maffei WE: Os Fundamentos da Medicina. 2nd ed. Livraria Editora Artes Medicas Ltd, 1978

DRAGSTEDT OPERATION, transthoracic supradiaphragmatic division of the vagus nerve for treatment of a peptic ulcer. (Lester R. Dragstedt, 1893-1975, U.S. surgeon)

1. Maffei WE: Os Fundamentos da Medicina. 2nd ed. Livraria Editora Artes Medicas Ltd, 1978

DRANGEDAD DISEASE, epidemic pleurodynia.

1. Casas EC: Diccionario Terminologico de Ciencias Medicas. 5th ed. Salvat Editores, SA, 1954

DREIFUSS SIGN, see Arnoss sign.

DRESBACH SYNDROME, hereditary elliptocytosis; a hematological disorder characterized by the presence of elliptical erythrocytes in the blood. (Melvin Dresbach, 1874-1946, U.S.)

1. Dresbach M: Science 19:469-470, 1904

DRESSLER SYNDROME, a postmyocardial infarction pericarditis; characterized by the onset of typical pericardial pain, particularly that precipitated by changes in position or cough, and may be accompanied by fever and significant pericardial effusion. Cross-reference: Postmyocardial infarction syndrome. (William Dressler, 1890-1969, U.S.)

1. Cheitlin MD, Sokolow M: Clinical Cardiology. 5th ed. Norwalk, Conn: Appleton & Lange, 1993
2. Dressler W: Arch Intern Med 163:28-42, 1959
3. Ritchie AC: Boyd's Textbook of Pathology. 9th ed. Philadelphia: Lea & Febiger, 1990

DREYER SIGN, while lying down with the knee extended, the patient is unable to raise the leg without help; seen in the patient with fracture of the patella.

1. Evans RC: Illustrated Essentials in Orthopedic Physical Assessment. St Louis: Mosby Yearbook, 1994
2. Mazion JM: Illustrated Manual of Orthopedic Signs/Tests/Maneuvers for Office Procedure. 2nd ed. Orlando: Daniels Publishing, 1980

DRUMMOND SIGN, bruit of an aortic aneurysm that can be heard by the examiner when the patient breathes with the mouth open. (Sir David Drummond, 1852-1932, British)

1. Casas EC: Diccionario Terminologico de Ciencias Medicas. 5th ed. Salvat Editores, SA, 1954

DRUMMOND-MORISON OPERATION, surgical technique for the treatment of ascites, consisting of opening the abdomen, friction of the hepatic and splenic peritoneum, and suturing the epiploon to the abdominal wall.

1. Maffei WE: Os Fundamentos da Medicina. 2nd ed. Livraria Editora Artes Medicas Ltd, 1978

DRY EYE SYNDROME, see Sjögren syndrome.

DTP SIGN, *d*istal *t*ingling on *p*ercussion (DTP); see Tinel sign.

DUANE SYNDROME, congenital retraction; a hereditary congenital disorder where the lateral rectus muscles are converted to fibrous cords. Characterized by a marked deficiency of abduction, a limitation of adduction, and retraction of the eye several millimeters into the orbit on turning medially. Cross-reference: Stilling-Türk-Duane syndrome. (Alexander Duane, 1858-1926, U.S. ophthalmologist)

1. Duane A: Congenital deficiency of adduction associated with impairment of abduction, retardation movements, contractions of the palpebral fissure and oblique movements of the eye. Arch Ophthalmol 34:133-159, 1905
2. Gorlin RJ, Cohen MM Jr, Levin LS: Syndromes of the Head and Neck. 3rd ed. New York: Oxford University Press, 1990
3. Stilling J: Untersuchungen ueber die Entstehung der Kurzsichtigkiet. Wiesbaden, 1887
4. Türk S: Dtsch Med Wochenschr 22:199, 1896

DUBARD SIGN, appendicitis pain referred to the right cervical region.

1. Casas EC: Diccionario Terminologico de Ciencias Medicas. 5th ed. Salvat Editores, SA, 1954

DUBIN-JOHNSON SYNDROME, DUBIN-SPRINZ SYNDROME, idiopathic jaundice which may mimic acquired hepatobiliary disease. Cross-references: Sprinz-Dubin syndrome; Sprinz-Nelson syndrome. (Isidore Dubin, 1913-1981, U.S. pathologist; Frank B. Johnson, U.S. pathologist)

1. Dubin IN, Johnson FB: Medicine 33:157-197, 1954
2. Ritchie AC: Boyd's Textbook of Pathology. 9th ed. Philadelphia: Lea & Febiger, 1990
3. Sprinz H, Nelson RS: Ann Intern Med 41:952-962, 1954

DUBINI DISEASE, see Bergeron disease. (Angelo Dubini, 1813-1902, Italian)

DUBOIS SIGN, abnormal shortness of the little finger; seen in the patient with congenital syphilis. (Paul DuBois, 1795-1871, French obstetrician)

1. Dorland's Medical Dictionary. 28th ed. Philadelphia: WB Saunders, 1994

DUBOWITZ SYNDROME, peculiar facies, infantile eczema, small stature, and mild microcephaly are features. Autosomal recessive inheritance. (Victor Dubowitz, British)

1. Dubowitz V: Familial low birth weight dwarfism with an unusual facies and a skin eruption. J Med Genet 2:12-17, 1969
2. Smith DW, Jones KL: Recognizable Patterns of Human Malformations: Genetic, Embryologic, and Clinical Aspects. 3rd ed. Philadelphia: WB Saunders, 1982

DUBREUIL-CHAMBARDEL SYNDROME, dental caries of the incisors (mostly only the upper ones), usually appearing during adolescence; within a few years, the teeth are irreparably damaged. (Louis Dubreuil-Chambardel, 1879-1927, French dentist)

1. Casas EC: Diccionario Terminologico de Ciencias Medicas. 5th ed. Salvat Editores, SA, 1954

DUCHENNE DISEASE, degeneration of the posterior roots and spinal cord column. (G.B.A. Duchenne, 1806-1875, French neurologist)

1. Duchenne GBA: Arch Gen Med 12:641-652, 1858

DUCHENNE MUSCULAR DYSTROPHY, infantile muscular atrophy with pseudohypertrophy. At onset, this disease affects the pelvic muscles; symptoms begin early (ages 2 to 6 years) and then cause pseudohypertrophy of the distal muscles. Occurs in males only. There are no symptoms in the first year of life, but walking may be somewhat delayed beyond 18 months. The child waddles when ambulating and is never able to run. (Guillaume B.A. Duchenne)

1. Duchenne GBA: Recherchés sur la paralysie musculaire pseudohypertrophique or paralsyie myo-sclérosique. Arch Gen Med 11:5-25, 1868

DUCHENNE SIGN, depression of the epigastric region during inspiration; seen in the patient with diaphragmatic paralysis. (Guillaume B.A. Duchenne)

1. Casas EC: Diccionario Terminologico de Ciencias Medicas. 5th ed. Salvat Editores, SA, 1954

DUCHENNE SYNDROME, DUCHENNE-ERB SYNDROME, upper radicular syndrome; lesions of the upper nerve roots (4th, 5th, and 6th cervical roots or upper primary trunk) are characterized by paralysis of the deltoid, biceps, brachialis anticus, brachioradialis, pectoralis major, supraspinatus, intraspinatous, subscapularis, and teres major muscles. (G.B.A. Duchenne; Wilhelm H. Erb, 1840-1921, German neurologist)

1. Duchenne GBA: De l'Electrisation Localisée et de son Application à la Pathologie et à la Therapeutique. Paris: Bailliere, 1855
2. Erb WH: Verh Naturhist Med Verein 2:130-137, 1874
3. Rowland LP (ed): Merritt's Textbook of Neurology. 9th ed. Baltimore: Williams & Wilkins, 1995

DUCKWORTH PHENOMENON, DUCKWORTH SIGN, apnea precedes cardiac asystole by a significant period of time in certain fatal conditions. (Sir Dyce Duckworth, 1840-1928, British)

1. Casas EC: Diccionario Terminologico de Ciencias Medicas. 5th ed. Salvat Editores, SA, 1954

DUDLEY OPERATION, 1) suturing the retroverted uterus to the anterior wall of the vagina by shortening the round ligaments through an abdominal incision; 2) posterior sagittal incision of the uterine neck for the treatment of dysmenorrhea and sterility.

1. Maffei WE: Os Fundamentos da Medicina. 2nd ed. Livraria Editora Artes Medicas Ltd, 1978

DUGAS SIGN, DUGAS TEST, adduction is not possible in the patient with subluxation of the shoulder. (Louis A. Dugas, 1806-1884, U.S.)

1. Casas EC: Diccionario Terminologico de Ciencias Medicas. 5th ed. Salvat Editores, SA, 1954

DUGUET SIGN, ulceration of the palate; seen in the patient with typhoid fever.

1. Casas EC: Diccionario Terminologico de Ciencias Medicas. 5th ed. Salvat Editores, SA, 1954

DUHRING DISEASE, dermatitis herpetiformis; a multisystem disease in which the clinical manifestations are primarily cutaneous. Cross-reference: Brocq-Duhring disease. (Louis A. Duhring, 1845-1913, U.S. dermatologist)

1. Duhring LA: JAMA 3:225-228, 1884

DÜHRSSEN OPERATION, vaginal fixation of the uterus. (Alfred Dührssen, 1862-1933, German obstetrician-gynecologist)

1. Maffei WE: Os Fundamentos da Medicina. 2nd ed. Livraria Editora Artes Medicas Ltd, 1978

DUKES DISEASE, DUKES-FILATOV DISEASE, scarlatinella; characteristics are headache, anorexia, drowsiness, chills, and occasionally backache, followed within several hours by a diffuse, bright rosy red, slightly raised eruption that quickly covers the body. Cross-references: Filatov disease;

76

Fourth disease. (Clement Dukes, 1845-1925, British; Nils Filatov, 1847-1902, Russian pediatrician)

1. Dukes C: Lancet 2:89-94, 1900
2. Moschella SL, Hurley HJ: Dermatology. 2nd ed. Philadelphia: WB Saunders, 1985

DUKES GRADING SYSTEM, a classification of carcinoma of the colon. Dukes stages A, B, and C depend on the involvement of the tumor, the lymph nodes involved, and the surrounding area invaded. (Cuthbert E. Dukes, 1890-1977, British pathologist)

1. Rosai J: Ackerman's Surgical Pathology. 7th ed. St Louis: CV Mosby, 1989

DUMPING SYNDROME, see Postprandial dumping syndrome.

DUNCAN DISEASE, an X-linked lymphoproliferative disease characterized by an impaired immune response to the Epstein-Barr virus. (Surname of boys afflicted with what is now known as this disease.)

1. Bennett JC, Plum F (eds): Cecil Textbook of Medicine. 20th ed. Philadelphia: WB Saunders, 1996
2. JAMA 235:2066, 1976

DUNCAN-BIRD SIGN, see Bird sign.

DUNNIGAN SYNDROME, acanthosis nigricans, decreased subcutaneous fat, an enlarged clitoris, insulin-resistant diabetes, thickened nails, pineal hyperplasia, premature eruption of teeth, open bite and macrodontia of the upper central incisors with palatal cusps arising from the cingulum, and enlargement of the filiform and fungiform papillae of the tongue are features. Autosomal recessive inheritance. (M.G. Dunnigan, British)

1. Gorlin RJ, Cohen MM Jr, Levin LS: Syndromes of the Head and Neck. 3rd ed. New York: Oxford University Press, 1990

DUP(1q) SYNDROME, somatic and mental retardation, low birth weight, abnormal facies, variable cardiac malformations, thymic hypoplasia or aplasia, and sometimes neonatal death are features.

1. Gorlin RJ, Cohen MM Jr, Levin LS: Syndromes of the Head and Neck. 3rd ed. New York: Oxford University Press, 1990
2. Rosenthal J, Abeliovich D, Carmi R: Clinical variability of partial duplication. 1q: a clinical report and literature review. Am J Med Genet 27:787-792, 1987

DUP(2p) SYNDROME, involves trisomy of the 2p21 or p23→pter region. Characteristics are severe mental retardation, pre- and postnatal growth retardation, microcephaly, characteristic facies, slender body build, hypotonia, skeletal anomalies, widely spaced toes, congenital hearing anomalies (35% incidence), micropenis (60%), hypospadias (15%), and cryptorchidism (10%).

1. Francke U, Jones KL: The 2p partial trisomy syndrome. Duplication of region 2p23Æ2pter in two members of a t(2;7) translocation kindred. Am J Dis Child 130:1244-1249, 1976
2. Gorlin RJ, Cohen MM Jr, Levin LS: Syndromes of the Head and Neck. 3rd ed. New York: Oxford University Press, 1990

DUP(2q) SYNDROME, deletion of q31→qter to q34→qter; findings include mental retardation, frontal bossing, microbrachycephaly with temporal retraction, hypertelorism, a short-beaked nose, elongated philtrum, abnormal pinnae and other eye findings, thoracic kyphosis, clinodactyly of the fifth finger, and cleft palate. Birth weight and length are normal.

1. Gorlin RJ, Cohen MM Jr, Levin LS: Syndromes of the Head and Neck. 3rd ed. New York: Oxford University Press, 1990
2. Yu CW, Chen H: De novo inverted tandem duplication of the long arm of chromosome 2 (q34 leads to q37). Birth Defects 18:311-320, 1982

DUP(3p) SYNDROME, psychomotor retardation delayed prenatal growth (15% incidence), and slowed postnatal growth (25%), are features as well as characteristic facies, congenital heart defects, and excessive fingertip whorls. In 75% of affected males, hypospadias, micropenis, or cryptorchidism is found. About 40% of patients die in the first 2 years of life.

1. Gorlin RJ, Cohen MM Jr, Levin LS: Syndromes of the Head and Neck. 3rd ed. New York: Oxford University Press, 1990
2. Reiss JA, Sheffield J, Sutherland GR: Partial trisomy 3p syndrome. Clin Genet 30:50-58, 1986

DUP(3q) SYNDROME, findings include severe mental retardation, underlying brain anomalies, craniofacial anomalies, hand anomalies, and omphalocele. Approximately one third of patients die before the end of the 1st year of life due to heart malformations and infections.

1. Falek A, Schmidt R, Jervis GA: Familial de Lange syndrome with chromosomal abnormalities. Pediatrics 37:92-101, 1966
2. Gorlin RJ, Cohen MM Jr, Levin LS: Syndromes of the Head and Neck. 3rd ed. New York: Oxford University Press, 1990

DUP(4p) SYNDROME, usual findings include psychomotor retardation, postnatal growth retardation, an increase in fingertip whorls, micropenis, and characteristic facies such as a depressed nasal bridge and a small pointed mandible. IQ ranges from 20-65. There are other less common findings.

1. Dallapiccola B, Mastroiacovo PP, Montali E, et al: Trisomy 4p: five new observations and overview. Clin Genet 12:344-356, 1977
2. Gorlin RJ, Cohen MM Jr, Levin LS: Syndromes of the Head and Neck. 3rd ed. New York: Oxford University Press, 1990

DUP(4q) SYNDROME, ranges from trisomy 4q21→qter to 4q32→qter. Marked psychomotor retardation, frequent cardiac and genitourinary anomalies, low birth weight (in approximately one half the cases), characteristic facies, umbilical or inguinal hernia, cardiovascular anomalies, genitourinary abnormalities, and unusual hands and rockerbottom feet are features. Cryptorchidism is frequent in males.

1. Andrle M, Erlach A, Rett A: Partial trisomy 4q in two unrelated cases. Hum Genet 49:179-183, 1979

DUP(5p) SYNDROME, severe psychomotor retardation, postnatal growth retardation, hypotonia, seizures, craniofacial changes, and slender extremities with long fingers, short first toes, and club feet are features.

1. Carnevale A, Hernández M, Limón-Toledo I, et al: A clinical syndrome associated with dup(5p). Am J Med Genet 13:277-283, 1982

DUP(5q) SYNDROME, for trisomy 5q31→5qter, severe psychomotor retardation, low birth weight, characteristic facies, musculoskeletal anomalies, and various congenital heart defects (50% incidence) are features. For trisomy 5q13→q22, a high forehead, bulbous nose, short philtrum, large protruding pinnae, and micrognathia are features. A small deletion of 5q34→qter results in failure to thrive and strabismus.

1. Gorlin RJ, Cohen MM Jr, Levin LS: Syndromes of the Head and Neck. 3rd ed. New York: Oxford University Press, 1990
2. Rodewald A, Zankl M, Gley EO, et al: Partial trisomy 5q: three different phenotypes depending on different duplication segments. Hum Genet 55:191-198, 1980

DUP(6p) SYNDROME, low birth weight, characteristic facies, congenital cardiac abnormalities, renal anomalies, and musculoskeletal abnormalities are features. Most patients die during infancy due to respiratory or feeding problems.

1. Gorlin RJ, Cohen MM Jr, Levin LS: Syndromes of the Head and Neck. 3rd ed. New York: Oxford University Press, 1990
2. Smith BS, Petterson JC: An anatomical study of a duplication 6p band on two sibs. Am J Med Genet 20:649-663, 1985

DUP(6q) SYNDROME, characteristic facies, somatic and mental retardation, contractures, flexed or deviated fingers and wrists, club feet, scoliosis, and genital anomalies are found.

1. Fitch N: Partial trisomy 6. Clin Genet 14:181-185, 1978
2. Gorlin RJ, Cohen MM Jr, Levin LS: Syndromes of the Head and Neck. 3rd ed. New York: Oxford University Press, 1990

DUP(7p) SYNDROME, severe retardation, dolichocephaly, wide fontanels, hypertelorism, full cheeks, short beaked nose, micrognathia, cleft palate, craniosynostosis, choanal atresia, arachnodactyly, and congenital hip dislocation are features. The patient rarely survives infancy.

1. Gorlin RJ, Cohen MM Jr, Levin LS: Syndromes of the Head and Neck. 3rd ed. New York: Oxford University Press, 1990
2. Moore CM, Pfeiffer RA, Craig-Holmes AP, et al: Partial trisomy 7p in two families resulting from different balanced translocations. Clin Genet 21:112-121, 1982

DUP(7q) SYNDROME, dup(7q31→7qter) involves large fontanels, a square prominent forehead, short down-slanting palpebral fissures, long eyelashes, a short nose, long philtrum, thin vermilion, down-curved upper lip, micrognathia, cleft palate, and early death. Dup(7q32→7qter) differs, with no cleft palate; additional features are hypotonia, epicanthal folds, scoliosis, congenital hip dislocation, and strabismus.

1. Gorlin RJ, Cohen MM Jr, Levin LS: Syndromes of the Head and Neck. 3rd ed. New York: Oxford University Press, 1990
2. Pflueger SMV, Scott CI Jr, Moore CM: Trisomy 7 and Potter syndrome. Clin Genet 25:543-548, 1984

DUP(8p) SYNDROME, severe mental retardation, characteristic facies, long trunk and extremities, contractures that may restrict movement, and absence of the corpus callosum are found. Micropenis and cryptorchidism are frequent in males.

1. Gorlin RJ, Cohen MM Jr, Levin LS: Syndromes of the Head and Neck. 3rd ed. New York: Oxford University Press, 1990
2. Mattei JF, Mattei MG, Ardissone JP, et al: Clinical, enzyme, and cytogenetic investigations in three new cases of trisomy 8p. Hum Genet 53:315-321, 1980

DUP(8q) SYNDROME, mental retardation (IQ 20-70), low birth weight, prominent forehead and flat occiput, hypertelorism, upward-slanting palpebral fissures, a short nose with a broad base, beaked nose, thin upper lip and drooping lower lip, low-set pinnae, cleft palate and skeletal anomalies, and variable congenital heart defects are features.

1. Gorlin RJ, Cohen MM Jr, Levin LS: Syndromes of the Head and Neck. 3rd ed. New York: Oxford University Press, 1990
2. Townes PL, White MR: Inherited partial trisomy 8q (22Æqter) Am J Dis Child 132:498-501, 1978

DUP(9q) SYNDROME, severe mental retardation, microdolichocephaly, deep-set eyes, prominent beaked nose, relatively large pinnae, and microretropathia are features.

1. Aftimos SF, Hoo JJ, Parslow MI: Partial trisomy 9q due to maternal 9/17 translocation. Am J Dis Child 134:848-850, 1980
2. Gorlin RJ, Cohen MM Jr, Levin LS: Syndromes of the Head and Neck. 3rd ed. New York: Oxford University Press, 1990

DUP(10p) SYNDROME, severe mental and motor retardation with little or no speech. Characteristic facies, elbows, wrists, and fingers are often hyperextensible; common findings include flexion deformities of fingers and toes, club feet, and cystic kidneys.

1. Gorlin RJ, Cohen MM Jr, Levin LS: Syndromes of the Head and Neck. 3rd ed. New York: Oxford University Press, 1990
2. Yunis E, Silva R, Gerald A: Trisomy 10p. Ann Genet 19:57-60, 1976

DUP(10q) SYNDROME, severe mental retardation, pre- and postnatal growth retardation, characteristic facies, anomalies of the hands and feet, and kidney abnormalities are clinical features. Prognosis is poor; death usually occurs prior to the age of 4 years.

1. Gorlin RJ, Cohen MM Jr, Levin LS: Syndromes of the Head and Neck. 3rd ed. New York: Oxford University Press, 1990
2. Taysi K, Yang V, Monaghan N, et al: Partial trisomy 10q in three unrelated patients. Ann Genet 26:79-85, 1983

DUP(11q) SYNDROME, mental retardation, reduced birth weight and postnatal growth, hypertonia, craniofacial asymmetry and microcephaly and other facial findings, genitourinary anomalies, musculoskeletal anomalies, and congenital heart anomalies are common features.

1. Gorlin RJ, Cohen MM Jr, Levin LS: Syndromes of the Head and Neck. 3rd ed. New York: Oxford University Press, 1990
2. Iselius L, Lindsen J, Aurias A, et al: The 11q;22q translocation: a collaborative study of 20 new cases and analysis of 110 families. Hum Genet 64:343-355, 1983

DUP(14q) SYNDROME, mental retardation, pre- and postnatal growth retardation, a large face, chubby cheeks, facial asymmetry, hypertelorism, broad nose, short prominent philtrum, carp mouth, posteriorly rotated pinnae with prominent antitragus, cleft palate, and micrognathia are features. Brain, lung, and congenital heart defects are also common.

1. Cottrall K, Magrath I, Bootes JAH, et al: A case of proximal 14 trisomy with pathological findings. J Ment Defic Res 25:1-6, 1981
2. Gorlin RJ, Cohen MM Jr, Levin LS: Syndromes of the Head and Neck. 3rd ed. New York: Oxford University Press, 1990

DUP(15q) SYNDROME, trisomy for the long arm of chromosome exhibits characteristic facies, postnatal growth deficiency, scoliosis, pectus excavatum, cryptorchidism, arachnodactyly, hyperextensible thumbs, and cardiovascular anomalies. Mental retardation is severe and hypotonia frequent.

1. Gorlin RJ, Cohen MM Jr, Levin LS: Syndromes of the Head and Neck. 3rd ed. New York: Oxford University Press, 1990
2. Lacro RV, Jones KL, Mascarello JT, et al: Duplication of distal 15q: report of five new cases from two different translocation kindreds. Am J Med Genet 26:719-728, 1987

DUP(16q) SYNDROME, the most common trisomy found in spontaneous abortions during the first trimester. There have been only a few live-birth examples, with features including low birth weight, severe psychomotor and mental retardation, characteristic facies, flexion contractures, cryptorchidism, a ventricular septal defect, and foot deformities.

1. Balestrazzi P, Giovanneli G, Landucci Rubini L, et al: Partial trisomy 16q resulting from maternal translocation. Hum Genet 49:229-235, 1979

2. Gorlin RJ, Cohen MM Jr, Levin LS: Syndromes of the Head and Neck. 3rd ed. New York: Oxford University Press, 1990

DUP(17p) SYNDROME, severe mental and somatic retardation, microcephaly, narrow palpebral fissures, hypertelorism, a broad nasal bridge, dysplastic low-set ears, chronic open mouth, micrognathia, short webbed neck, flexion abnormalities of the first four digits with extension of the fifth finger, long and tapered fingers, inguinal hernia, a transverse palmar crease, and hypoplastic genitalia in males are features.

1. Feldman GM, Baumer JG, Sparkes RS, et al: The dup(17p) syndrome. Am J Med Genet 11:299-304, 1982
2. Gorlin RJ, Cohen MM Jr, Levin LS: Syndromes of the Head and Neck. 3rd ed. New York: Oxford University Press, 1990

DUP(17q) SYNDROME, usually involves bands q21, q22, or q23→qter. Profound psychomotor retardation, short stature, characteristic facies, serious congenital heart anomalies, central nervous system abnormalities, renal anomalies, and cryptorchidism are features. Quite rare.

1. Fryns J, Parloir C, Van den Berghe H: Partial trisomy 17q. Karyotype: 46, XYder(21), t(17;21)(q22;p13) Hum Genet 49:361-364, 1979
2. Gorlin RJ, Cohen MM Jr, Levin LS: Syndromes of the Head and Neck. 3rd ed. New York: Oxford University Press, 1990

DUP(19q) SYNDROME, mental retardation, marked postnatal growth retardation, low birth weight and short length, characteristic facies, barrel-shaped thorax, and musculoskeletal disorders are features.

1. Chen H, Yu CW, Wood MJ, et al: Mosaic trisomy 19 syndrome. Ann Genet 24:32-33, 1981
2. Gorlin RJ, Cohen MM Jr, Levin LS: Syndromes of the Head and Neck. 3rd ed. New York: Oxford University Press, 1990

DUP(20p) SYNDROME, mild to severe (but usually moderate) psychomotor retardation, poor motor coordination, delayed poor speech, and characteristic facies are features. Cardiac anomalies are found in one third of patients.

1. Chen H, Hoffman WH, Tyrkus M, et al: Partial trisomy 20p syndrome and maternal mosaicism. Ann Genet 26:21-25, 1983
2. Gorlin RJ, Cohen MM Jr, Levin LS: Syndromes of the Head and Neck. 3rd ed. New York: Oxford University Press, 1990

DUPLAY DISEASE, adhesive bursitis; inflammation of the acromial or subdeltoid bursa. (Simon Emmanuel Duplay, 1836-1924, French surgeon)

1. Duplay ES: Arch Gen Med Paris 20:513-542, 1872

DUPLAY OPERATION, designates various autoplastic methods for treating congenital anomalies of the penis. (Simon Emmanuel Duplay)

1. Maffei WE: Os Fundamentos da Medicina. 2nd ed. Livraria Editora Artes Medicas Ltd, 1978

DUPRÉ SYNDROME, pseudomeningitis; meningeal infection that sometimes follows an extracerebral infection. (Ernest Dupré, 1862-1921, French)

1. Capdevilla Cases F: Diccionario Terminologico de Ciencias Medicas. 5th ed. 1954
2. Dupré E: Cong Fr Med 1:411-423, 1895

DUPUYS-DUTEMPS OPERATION, 1) blepharoplasty of the lower eyelid with tissue from the upper lid; 2) dacryorhinostomy for draining the lacrimal sac. (Louis Dupuys-Dutemps, French ophthalmologist)

1. Maffei WE: Os Fundamentos da Medicina. 2nd ed. Livraria Editora Artes Medicas Ltd, 1978

DUPUYTREN OPERATION, 1) Dupuytren amputation; tenotomy of the sternocleidomastoid muscle; 2) section of the retracted aponeurosis palmar. (Guillaume Dupuytren, 1777-1835, French surgeon and surgical pathologist)

1. Maffei WE: Os Fundamentos da Medicina. 2nd ed. Livraria Editora Artes Medicas Ltd, 1978

DUPUYTREN SIGN, 1) a cracking sensation when sarcomatous bone is compressed; 2) upward and downward movements of the head of the femur, seen in congenital dislocation. (Guillaume Dupuytren)

1. Casas EC: Diccionario Terminologico de Ciencias Medicas. 5th ed. Salvat Editores, SA, 1954

DURAND-NICOLAS-FAVRE DISEASE, lymphogranuloma venereum. Cross-references: Favre-Durand-Nicolas disease; Frei disease; Nicolas-Favre disease. (J. Durand, French; Joseph Nicolas, 1868-1960, French; Maurice J. Favre, 1876-1954, French)

1. Durand J, Favre MJ: Bull Soc Med Hop Paris35:274-288, 1913
2. Frei W: Klin Wochenschr 4:2148-2149, 1925

DURANTE DISEASE, bone fragility. (Gustave Durante, 1865-1934, French)
1. Casas EC: Diccionario Terminologico de Ciencias Medicas. 5th ed. Salvat Editores, SA, 1954

DURET OPERATION, gastropexy by fixation of the pylorus and lesser curvature of the stomach to the abdominal wall.
1. Maffei WE: Os Fundamentos da Medicina. 2nd ed. Livraria Editora Artes Medicas Ltd, 1978

DUROZIEZ MURMUR, a "pistol shot" sound heard over the femoral artery; common in the patient with severe aortic insufficiency. May also be heard in the patient with other high-output states such as hyperthyroidism or severe anemia. (Paul L. Duroziez, 1826-1897, French)
1. Fowler NO: Cardiac Diagnosis and Treatment. 3rd ed. Cambridge: Harper & Row, 1980

DUROZIEZ SIGN, a double bruit heard in the femoral artery; seen in the patient with aortic insufficiency. (Paul L. Duroziez)
1. Casas EC: Diccionario Terminologico de Ciencias Medicas. 5th ed. Salvat Editores, SA, 1954

DUTEMPS-CÉSTAN SIGN, see Levator sign (Raymond E.J.M. Céstan, 1872-1934, French neurologist)
1. Casas EC: Diccionario Terminologico de Ciencias Medicas. 5th ed. Salvat Editores, SA, 1954

DUTTON DISEASE, trypanosomiasis. (Joseph E. Dutton, 1877-1905, British)
1. Casas EC: Diccionario Terminologico de Ciencias Medicas. 5th ed. Salvat Editores, SA, 1954

DWARFISM KNIEST SYNDROME, see Kniest syndrome.

DWYER-PATERSON OPERATION, the direct implantation of a direct-current bone-growth stimulator (the Osteo-Stim).
1. Schwartz SI: Principles of Surgery. 4th ed. New York: McGraw-Hill, 1983

DYGGVE-MELCHIOR-CLAUSEN SYNDROME, a disorder of short trunk dwarfism and mental retardation. Often mistaken for Morquio syndrome. (H.V. Dyggve, Danish)
1. Bonafede RP, Beighton P: The Dyggve-Melchior-Clausen syndrome in adult siblings. Clin Genet 14:24-30, 1978
2. Dyggve HV, Melchior JC, Clausen J: Morquio-Ullrich's disease. An inborn error of metabolism? Arch Dis Child 37:525-534, 1962
3. Gorlin RJ, Cohen MM Jr, Levin LS: Syndromes of the Head and Neck. 3rd ed. New York: Oxford University Press, 1990

DYKE-DAVIDOFF-MASSON SYNDROME, cerebral hemiatrophy; possibly due to injury or severe disease affecting one side of the brain during the neonatal period. Characterized by mental retardation, asymmetry of the face, and varying degrees of hemiplegia, neurological impairment, and atrophy of the side of the body contralateral to the lesion.
1. Dyke CG, Davidoff LM, Masson CB: Surg Gynecol Obstet 57:588-600, 1933

DYSKERATOSIS CONGENITA SYNDROME, see Zinsser-Engman-Cole syndrome.

EAGLE SYNDROME, facial pain due to the elongated styloid process; the second branchial arch (the Reichert cartilage) gives rise to the styloid process, the ligament, and the upper half of the body of the hyoid bone. In adults, the styloid process is about 2.5 cm in length and lies between the internal and external carotid arteries. Because of this anatomic proximity it may impinge on either artery, particularly if the tip of the process is deviated. The styloid process lies just lateral to the tonsillar fossa, and impingement here may also cause symptoms. (Watt W. Eagle, U.S. otolaryngologist)
1. Ballenger JJ: Diseases of the Nose, Throat, Ear, Head and Neck. 12th ed. Philadelphia: Lea & Febiger, 1977
2. Eagle WW: Elongated styloid process. Arch Otolaryngol 25:584-587, 1937

EAGLE-BARRETT SYNDROME, see Prune belly syndrome.

EALES DISEASE, recurrent retinal hemorrhage in young adults. Etiology uncertain. (Henry Eales, 1852-1913, British ophthalmologist)
1. Branwood AW: The enigma of vasculitis. Prog Surg Pathol 3:279, 1981
2. Eales H: Birmingham Med Rev 9:262-273, 1880
3. Resnick H, Esterly NB: Vasculitis in children. Int J Dermatol 24:139, 1985

EATON-LAMBERT SYNDROME, see Lambert syndrome.

EBEBOHL OPERATION, removal of the renal capsule; seen in Bright disease.
1. Maffei WE: Os Fundamentos da Medicina. 2nd ed. Livraria Editora Artes Medicas Ltd, 1978

EBSTEIN SIGN, obtuseness of the wide cardiohepatic angle on percussion; due to pericardial effusion. (Wilhelm Ebstein, 1836-1912, German)

1. Casas EC: Diccionario Terminologico de Ciencias Medicas. 5th ed. Salvat Editores, SA, 1954

EBSTEIN-PEL DISEASE, see Pel-Ebstein disease. (Wilhelm Ebstein)

ECHO SIGN, 1) an echo-like percussion sound heard over a hydatid cyst; 2) repetition of the last word or clause in a sentence; seen in several brain disorders.

1. Dorland's Medical Dictionary. 28th ed. Philadelphia: WB Saunders, 1994

ECTOPIC ACTH SYNDROME, a condition in which tumors arising from non-endocrine tissue produce adrenocorticotropic hormone (ACTH). Depending on its duration, the syndrome may be subtle, resembling true Cushing disease, but hypokalemic alkalosis and weakness are often the dominant manifestations.

1. Dorland's Medical Dictionary. 28th ed. Philadelphia: WB Saunders, 1994

ECTOPIC HYPERCALCEMIA SYNDROME, hypercalcemia resulting from ectopic production by a pancreatic islet-cell or other (lung or kidney) tumor of parathyroid polypeptide; a polypeptide with activity similar to that of parathyroid hormone.

1. Dorland's Medical Dictionary. 28th ed. Philadelphia: WB Saunders, 1994

ECTRODACTYLY-ECTODERMAL DYSPLASIA-CLEFTING SYNDROME, see Rüdiger syndrome.

EDDOWES SYNDROME, see Osteogenesis imperfecta type I. (Alfred Eddowes, 1850-1946, British dermatologist)

EDSALL DISEASE, cramps caused by heat. (David Edsall, 1869-1945, U.S.)

1. Casas EC: Diccionario Terminologico de Ciencias Medicas. 5th ed. Salvat Editores, SA, 1954

EDWARDS OPERATION, closure of a long arteriotomy with a vein roof patch; used for semi-closed endarterectomy.

1. Schwartz SI: Principles of Surgery. 4th ed. New York, NY: McGraw-Hill, 1983

EDWARDS SYNDROME, see Trisomy 18 syndrome. (Jack H. Edwards, British geneticist)

EFFORT SYNDROME, see Da Costa syndrome.

EGAS MONIZ OPERATION, frontal leukotomy. A pioneer in the development of neurosurgery, Egas Moniz developed angiography in 1927 and Pantopaque myelography in 1942. (Antonio Egas Moniz, 1874-1955, Portuguese neurosurgeon)

1. Maffei WE: Os Fundamentos da Medicina. 2nd ed. Livraria Editora Artes Medicas Ltd, 1978

EGAWA SIGN, with the palm flat on the table, the patient is asked to raise the extended middle finger and abduct it from the ulnar side to the radial side.

1. Campbell WC, Crenshaw AH: Campbell's Operative Orthopaedics. 7th ed. St Louis: CV Mosby, 1987

EGG WHITE SYNDROME, see Da Costa syndrome.

EHLERS-DANLOS SYNDROME, cutis laxa; a group of inherited disorders of the connective tissue sharing phenotypic expressions, including hyperextensible skin and joints, easy bruisability, and friability of tissues with poor wound healing. Eleven forms of the condition are recognized. (Edward L. Ehlers, 1863-1937, Danish dermatologist; Henri A. Danlos, 1844-1912, French dermatologist)

1. Danlos H: Bull Soc Fr Dermatol Syph 19:70-72, 1908
2. Ehlers E: Derm Zschr 8:173-174, 1901
3. Gorlin RJ, Cohen MM Jr, Levin LS: Syndromes of the Head and Neck. 3rd ed. New York: Oxford University Press, 1990
4. Krayenbühl HA, Yasargil MG: Cerebral Angiography. 2nd ed. Philadelphia: JB Lippincott, 1968

EHLERS-DANLOS SYNDROME TYPE IX, see Occipital horn syndrome.

EHRET DISEASE, paralysis of the peroneal muscles caused by contraction of their antagonists. (Heinrich Ehret, German)

1. Ehret H: Arch Unfallheilkd 3:32-56, 1898

EICHHORST SIGN, differences in percussion sounds found in cavitary lung diseases according to the fullness of the cavities.

1. Casas EC: Diccionario Terminologico de Ciencias Medicas. 5th ed. Salvat Editores, SA, 1954

EICHSTEDT DISEASE, tinea versicolor.

1. Casas EC: Diccionario Terminologico de Ciencias Medicas. 5th ed. Salvat Editores, SA, 1954

EINHORN DISEASE, hemorrhagic ulcers of the stomach with dyspepsia.

1. Casas EC: Diccionario Terminologico de Ciencias Medicas. 5th ed. Salvat Editores, SA, 1954

EISENMENGER SYNDROME, a congenital heart disease with marked elevation of pulmonary vascular resistance with reversed or bidirectional shunt, which is intracardiac or between the aorta and pulmonary arteries. Syncopal crises occur. (Victor Eisenmenger, 1864-1932, German)

1. Cheitlin MD, Sokolow M: Clinical Cardiology. 5th ed. Norwalk, Conn: Appleton & Lange, 1993
2. Eisenmenger V: Zschr Klin Med 32 (Suppl):1-28, 1897

EKBOM SYNDROME, see Restless legs syndrome. (Karl-Axel Ekbom, Swedish neurologist)

ELEJALDE SYNDROME, a disorder of spectacular overgrowth; consists of complete fusion of all cranial sutures, closure of fontanels, epicanthic folds, down-slanting palpebral fissures, a hypoplastic nose, craniosynostosis, rudimentary auricles, and redundant neck skin.

1. Elejalde BR, Giraldo C, Jemenez R, et al: Birth Defects 13:53-56, 1977
2. Gorlin RJ, Cohen MM Jr, Levin LS: Syndromes of the Head and Neck. 3rd ed. New York: Oxford University Press, 1990

ELFIN FACIES SYNDROME, see Williams syndrome.

ELLIOT LINE, ELLIOT SIGN, hardness of syphilitic cutaneous lesions.

1. Casas EC: Diccionario Terminologico de Ciencias Medicas. 5th ed. Salvat Editores, SA, 1954

ELLIOT OPERATION, sclerectomy by trephine for relief of increased tension in glaucoma. (Robert H. Elliot, 1864-1936, British ophthalmologist)

1. Maffei WE: Os Fundamentos da Medicina. 2nd ed. Livraria Editora Artes Medicas Ltd, 1978

ELLIS SIGN, the line of dullness discovered during resorption of pleuritic effusion. Cross-reference: Damoiseau sign. (Calvin Ellis, 1826-1883, U.S.)

1. Casas EC: Diccionario Terminologico de Ciencias Medicas. 5th ed. Salvat Editores, SA, 1954

ELLIS-VAN CREVELD SYNDROME, chondroectodermal dysplasia; characterized by polydactyly of the hands and rarely of the feet, dwarfism, and dysplasia of the fingernails. Autosomal recessive inheritance. (Richard W.B. Ellis, 1902-1966, British; Simon van Creveld, 1894-1971, Dutch pediatrician)

1. Bennett JC, Plum F (eds): Cecil Textbook of Medicine. 20th ed. Philadelphia: WB Saunders, 1996
2. Ellis RWB, van Creveld S: Arch Dis Child 15:65-84, 1940
3. Fowler NO: Cardiac Diagnosis and Treatment. 3rd ed. Cambridge: Harper & Row, 1980

ELSAHY-WATERS SYNDROME, see Branchio-skeleto-genital syndrome.

ELY OPERATION, the use of a cutaneous graft on the granulation surface of suppurative chronic otitis media.

1. Maffei WE: Os Fundamentos da Medicina. 2nd ed. Livraria Editora Artes Medicas Ltd, 1978

ELY SIGN, ELY TEST, probable indication of contracture of the fascia lata. Elicited with the patient lying prone on the examination table; the examiner flexes the patient's leg on the thigh, bringing the heel toward the buttock. In a positive test, the pelvis rises from the table during such flexion and the thigh is abducted. (Leonard W. Ely, 1868-1944, U.S. orthopedic surgeon)

1. Baker AB, Baker LH: Clinical Neurology. Revised ed. Philadelphia: Harper & Row, 1982

EMBRYONIC TESTICULAR REGRESSION SYNDROME, see Vanishing testis syndrome.

EMERY-DREIFUSS MUSCULAR DYSTROPHY, an X-linked recessive form of muscular dystrophy, which differs from Duchenne and Becker muscular dystrophies in that pseudohypertrophy is not found and enzymes are normal or only minimally increased. (Alan E.H. Emery, British geneticist; F.E. Dreifuss, British)

1. Bennett JC, Plum F (eds): Cecil Textbook of Medicine. 20th ed. Philadelphia: WB Saunders, 1996
2. Emery A, Dreifuss FE: J Neurol Neurosurg Psychiatry 29:338-342, 1966

EMERY-NELSON SYNDROME, a syndrome of short stature, mild mental and somatic retardation, increased upper strength/lower strength ratio, deformities of the first three metacarpophalangeal joints of both thumbs, clawed toes, and an unusual facies. (Alan E.H. Emery; Matilda M. Nelson, British)

1. Emery AEH, Nelson MM: A familial syndrome of short stature, deformities of the hands and feet and an unusual facies. J Med Genet 7:379-382, 1970
2. Gorlin RJ, Cohen MM Jr, Levin LS: Syndromes of the Head and Neck. 3rd ed. New York: Oxford University Press, 1990

EMG SYNDROME, *e*xomphalos, *m*acroglossia, and *g*igantism (EMG); see Beckwith syndrome.

EMMET OPERATION, 1) trachelorrhaphy; suture of the uterine cervix; 2) creation of an artificial vesicovaginal fistula for vesical drainage in cystitis. (Thomas A. Emmet, 1828-1919, U.S. gynecologist)
1. Maffei WE: Os Fundamentos da Medicina. 2nd ed. Livraria Editora Artes Medicas Ltd, 1978

EMPTY DELTA SIGN, a radiological sign that appears after injection of contrast material, which outlines the periphery of the sinus where blood still flows, leaving the central area of the clot dark. Enhancement of the gyri or tentorium may also be present.
1. Rowland LP (ed): Merritt's Textbook of Neurology. 9th ed. Baltimore: Williams & Wilkins, 1995

EMPTY SELLA SYNDROME, syndrome in which the pituitary is displaced and the sella turcica enlarged and filled with spinal fluid; the optic chiasm herniates into the sella turcica and may cause visual field defects.
1. Bennett JC, Plum F (eds): Cecil Textbook of Medicine. 20th ed. Philadelphia: WB Saunders, 1996
2. Busch W: Arch Pathol Anat 320:437-440, 1951

ENCEPHALOTRIGEMINAL VASCULAR SYNDROME, see Sturge-Weber syndrome.

ENDOCRINE CANDIDOSIS SYNDROME, a variable combination of superficial mucocutaneous candidosis, hypoparathyroidism, hypoadrenocorticism, ovarian atrophy, keratoconjunctivitis, alopecia, intestinal malabsorption, pernicious anemia, diabetes mellitus, hepatitis, and thyroiditis.
1. Ahonen P: Autoimmune polyendocrinopathy-candidosis-ectodermal dystrophy (APECED): autosomal recessive inheritance. Clin Genet 27:535-542,1985
2. Arulanantham K, Dwyer JM, Genel M: Evidence for defective immunoregulation in the syndrome of familial candidiasis endocrinopathy. N Engl J Med 300:164-168, 1979
3. Gorlin RJ, Cohen MM Jr, Levin LS: Syndromes of the Head and Neck. 3rd ed. New York: Oxford University Press, 1990

ENGEL-VON RECKLINGHAUSEN DISEASE, osteitis fibrosa cystica; a bone disorder seen in advanced hyperparathyroidism. (Gerhard Engel, German; Friedrich von Recklinghausen, 1833-1910, German pathologist)
1. Engel G: Ueber einen Fall cystoider Entartung des Gesamten Skeletts. Giessen, 1864
2. Von Recklinghausen F: Untersuchungen ueber Rachitis und Osteomalacie. Jena: G Fisher, 1910

ENGMAN DISEASE, infectious eczematoid dermatitis. (Martin F. Engman, U.S.)
1. Engman MF: Am Med 4:769-773, 1902

ENROTH SIGN, unusual fullness of the eyelids; seen in the patient with Graves disease. (Emil E. Enroth, 1879-1953, Finnish)
1. Dorland's Medical Dictionary. 28th ed. Philadelphia: WB Saunders, 1994

ENVIRONMENTAL DEPENDENCY SYNDROME, associated with lesions of the inferior half of the anterior portion of one or both frontal lobes and believed to represent a release of parietal lobe activities that results from impairment of frontal lobe inhibition.
1. Walsh FB, Hoyt EF, Miller NR: Clinical Neuro-Ophthalmology. 4th ed. Baltimore: Williams & Wilkins, 1982

EPICONUS SYNDROME, an uncommon disorder characterized by considerable motor disability. External rotation and extension (dorsal flexion) of the thigh are most affected; also usually involved are abduction at the hip, flexion at the knee, and flexion and extension at the ankle. The "Achilles jerk" is lost.
1. Haymaker W: Bing's Local Diagnosis in Neurological Diseases. 15th ed. St Louis: CV Mosby, 1969

EPIDERMAL NEVUS SYNDROME, characterized by the association of epidermal nevi with abnormalities of the central nervous system, eyes, and bones, as well as other cutaneous alterations and malignancies. Cross-references: Feuerstein-Mims syndrome; Linear nevus sebaceous syndrome; Schimmelpenning-Feuerstein syndrome; Solomon syndrome.
1. Feuerstein RC, Mims LC: Am J Dis Child 104:675-679, 1962
2. Gorlin RJ, Cohen MM Jr, Levin LS: Syndromes of the Head and Neck. 3rd ed. New York: Oxford University Press, 1990
3. Schimmelpenning GW: Fortschr Roentgenol 87:716-720, 1957
4. Solomon LL, et al: Arch Dermatol 97:273-285, 1968

EPIDERMOLYSIS BULLOSA SYNDROME, a hereditary skin disease; characteristics include bullous and vesicular eruptions brought about by minor trauma or heat. Cross-references: Fox disease; Goldston syndrome; Köbner disease.
1. Köbner H: Dtsch Med Wochenschr 2:21-22, 1886

EPIPHYSEAL SYNDROME, precocious development of external genitalia and sexual function, and precocious abnormal growth of the long bones. Signs of internal hydrocephalus, in the absence of all other motor and sensory symptoms, indicate a lesion of the pineal body. Cross-references: Pellizzi syndrome; Pineal syndrome.

1. Pellizzi GB: La sindrome episfario "macrogenitosomia precoce." Rev Ital Neuropatol 3:193-207, 1907

EPSTEIN SIGN, see Collier sign.

EPSTEIN-BARR VIRUS, a herpes-like virus found in cell cultures of the Burkitt lymphoma; also associated with infectious mononucleosis. The usual symptoms and signs are headache, sore throat, malaise, fever, enlargement of the cervical lymph nodes, occasionally enlargement of the spleen, and hematological changes. Occurs sporadically and in small epidemics; is most common in children and young adults. (M. Anthony Epstein, British virologist; Yvonne M. Barr, British virologist)

1. Hurst JW, Schlant RC, Alexander RW: The Heart: Arteries and Veins. 8th ed. New York: McGraw-Hill, 1994
2. Rosair J: "Lymphoepithelioma-like" thymic carcinoma: another tumor related to Epstein-Barr virus? N Engl J Med 312:1320-1322, 1985 (Letter)

ERB DISEASE, progressive muscular dystrophy. Cross-reference: Myasthenia gravis syndrome. (Wilhelm H. Erb, 1840-1921, German neurologist)

1. Erb WH: Arch Klin Med 34:467-519, 1884
2. Erb WH: Arch Psychiatr 9:369-388, 1879
3. Rowland LP (ed): Merritt's Textbook of Neurology. 9th ed. Baltimore: Williams & Wilkins, 1995

ERB SIGN, electric irritability of the motor nerves is increased; seen in the patient with tetany. (Wilhelm H. Erb)

1. Baker AB, Baker LH: Clinical Neurology. Revised ed. Philadelphia: Harper & Row, 1982
2. Farmer TW: Pediatric Neurology. 2nd ed. Hagerstown: Harper & Row, 1975

ERB-CHARCOT SYNDROME, locomotor ataxia (tabes dorsalis). Cross-reference: Spiller syndrome. (Wilhelm H. Erb; Jean M. Charcot, 1825-1893, French neurologist)

1. Erb WH: Arch Pathol Anat Berl 70:241-267, 1877

ERB-GOLDFLAM DISEASE, ERB-GOLDFLAM-OPPENHEIM DISEASE, see Goldflam disease. (Wilhelm H. Erb; Samuel Goldflam, 1852-1932, Polish neurologist)

ERB-LANDOUZY DISEASE, progressive muscular dystrophy. (Wilhelm H. Erb; Louis T.J. Landouzy, 1845-1917, French neurologist)

1. Erb WH: Dtsch Zschr Nervenheilkd 1:173, 1892
2. Landouzy LTJ, Déjerine J: Compt Rendu Acad Sci Paris 98:53-55, 1884

ERB-WESTPHAL SIGN, see Westphal sign. (Wilhelm H. Erb; Karl F.O. Westphal, 1833-1890, German neurologist)

ERDHEIM-CHESTER DISEASE, lipogranulomatosis; characterized by infiltration of the viscera and bones by foamy, lipid-containing histiocytes that are associated with fibrosis. Involves the long bones, lungs, retroperitoneum, and central nervous system. A rare disorder of uncertain etiology. (Jakob Erdheim, 1874-1937, Austrian; William Chester)

1. Athanasou NA, Barbatis C: Erdheim-Chester disease with epiphyseal and systemic disease. J Clin Pathol 46:481-482, 1993
2. Babu, RP, Lansen TA, Chadburn A, et al: Erdheim-Chester disease of the central nervous system. J Neurosurg 86:888-892, 1997
3. Chester W: Virch Arch Anat Physiol 279:561-602, 1930
4. Dee P, Westgaard T, Langholm R: Erdheim-Chester disease: case with chronic discharging sinus from bone. AJR 134:837-839, 1980
5. Miller RL, Sheeler LR, Bauer TW, et al: Erdheim-Chester disease. Case report and review of the literature. Am J Med 80:1230-1236, 1986

ERICHSEN DISEASE, accident neurosis.

1. Casas EC: Diccionario Terminologico de Ciencias Medicas. 5th ed. Salvat Editores, SA, 1954

ERICHSEN SIGN, pain is felt when the iliac bones are sharply pressed toward each other; seen in the patient with sacroiliac disease. (Sir John E. Erichsen, 1818-1896, British)

1. Mazion JM: Illustrated Manual of Orthopedic Signs/Tests/Maneuvers for Office Procedure. 2nd ed. Orlando: Daniels Publishing, 1980

ERNI SIGN, percussion of the apex of the lung stimulates coughing in the patient with tuberculosis. (H. Erni, 1859-1937, Swiss)

1. Casas EC: Diccionario Terminologico de Ciencias Medicas. 5th ed. Salvat Editores, SA, 1954

ESCHERICH SIGN, contraction of the lips, masseter muscle, and tongue following percussion of the inner surface of the lips or of the tongue; seen in hypoparathyroidism. (Theodor Escherich, 1857-1911, German)

1. Baker AB, Baker LH: Clinical Neurology. Revised ed. Philadelphia: Harper & Row, 1982

ESCOBAR SYNDROME, multiple pterygia, camptodactyly, and syndactyly are features. Autosomal recessive inheritance. (Victor Escobar, U.S.)

1. Escobar V, Bixler D, Gleiser S, et al: Multiple pterygium syndrome. Am J Dis Child 132:609-611, 1978
2. Smith DW, Jones KL: Recognizable Patterns of Human Malformations: Genetic, Embryologic, and Clinical Aspects. 3rd ed. Philadelphia: WB Saunders, 1982

ESCOMEL DISEASE, paracoccidioidomycosis.

1. Casas EC: Diccionario Terminologico de Ciencias Medicas. 5th ed. Salvat Editores, SA, 1954

ESCUDERO DISEASE, erythrocytosis caused by syphilis.

1. Casas EC: Diccionario Terminologico de Ciencias Medicas. 5th ed. Salvat Editores, SA, 1954

ESMARCH OPERATION, cuneiform resection of the horizontal portion of the mandibula in mandibular ankylosis.

1. Maffei WE: Os Fundamentos da Medicina. 2nd ed. Livraria Editora Artes Medicas Ltd, 1978

ESPINE SIGN, hypertrophy at the hilum of the lymph nodes; checked by auscultation. Cross-reference: D'Espine sign. (Jean H.A. d'Espine, 1846-1930, Swiss pediatrician)

1. Casas EC: Diccionario Terminologico de Ciencias Medicas. 5th ed. Salvat Editores, SA, 1954

ESTES OPERATION, implantation of an ovary into the uterus for treating infertility. (William L. Estes, Jr., 1885-1940, U.S. surgeon)

1. Maffei WE: Os Fundamentos da Medicina. 2nd ed. Livraria Editora Artes Medicas Ltd, 1978

ESTLANDER OPERATION, partial subperiosteal resection of one or more ribs in order to obtain contact between the thoracic wall and the retracted lung in cases of empyema. (Jakob A. Estlander, 1831-1881, Finnish surgeon)

1. Maffei WE: Os Fundamentos da Medicina. 2nd ed. Livraria Editora Artes Medicas Ltd, 1978

EULENBURG SYNDROME, paramyotonia; a form of myotonia clinically most evident in a cold environment. (Albert Eulenburg, 1840-1917, German)

1. Eulenburg A: Zbl Neurol 5:265, 1886
2. Hudson AJ: Progressive neurological disorder and myotonia congenita associated with paramyotonia. Brain 86:811-826, 1963
3. Rowland LP (ed): Merritt's Textbook of Neurology. 9th ed. Baltimore: Williams & Wilkins, 1995

EUSTACE SMITH SIGN, see Smith sign.

EUTHYROID SICK SYNDROME, see Silvestrini-Corda syndrome.

EVANS SYNDROME, immune thrombocytopenia occurring in conjunction with immune hemolysis. (Robert S. Evans, U.S.)

1. Bennett JC, Plum F (eds): Cecil Textbook of Medicine. 20th ed. Philadelphia: WB Saunders, 1996
2. Evans RS, Takahashi K, Duane RT, et al: Arch Intern Med 87:48-65, 1951

EVERBUSCH OPERATION, surgery for eyelid ptosis by shortening the levator muscle of the upper eyelid. (Oskar Everbusch, 1853-1912, German ophthalmologist)

1. Maffei WE: Os Fundamentos da Medicina. 2nd ed. Livraria Editora Artes Medicas Ltd, 1978

EWART SIGN, an area of dullness and bronchial breathing beneath the angle of the left scapula; demonstrated in the patient with acute pericarditis with effusion. Cross-reference: Pins sign. (William Ewart, 1848-1929, British)

1. Fowler NO: Cardiac Diagnosis and Treatment. 3rd ed. Cambridge: Harper & Row, 1980

EWING SIGN, pain in the superior angle of the orbit; seen in the patient with obstruction of the frontal sinus. (James H. Ewing, 1798-1827)

1. Casas EC: Diccionario Terminologico de Ciencias Medicas. 5th ed. Salvat Editores, SA, 1954

EXOMPHALOS-MACROGLOSSIA-GIGANTISM SYNDROME, see Beckwith syndrome.

EXTERNAL MALLEOLAR SIGN, see Chaddock sign.

EXTRAPYRAMIDAL SYNDROME, any of a group of clinical disorders characterized by abnormal involuntary movements, including parkinsonism, athetosis, and chorea.

1. Dorland's Medical Dictionary. 28th ed. Philadelphia: WB Saunders, 1994

EYE SIGN, apparent exophthalmos is produced by lid retraction with staring and without true forward movement of the eyeball; the most frequent neurological syndrome is exophthalmos. Occurs as a result of the action of the sympathetically innervated Müller muscle.

1. Baker AB, Baker LH: Clinical Neurology. Revised ed. Philadelphia: Harper & Row, 1982

FABER SYNDROME, chronic hypochromic anemia. (Knud H. Faber, 1862-1956, Danish)

1. Faber KH: Med Klin 5:1310-1312, 1909

FABRY DISEASE, glycosphingolipidosis or diffuse angiokeratoma; a congenital defect of glycosphingolipid metabolism, characterized by telangiectatic skin lesions, hypohidrosis, corneal opacities, acral pain and paresthesias, intermittent fever, renal failure, and cardiovascular, gastrointestinal, and central nervous system disturbances. Symptoms and signs include intense burning in the hands and feet, a reddish-purple rash of the umbilicus, scrotum, and inguinal and gluteal areas, albuminuria, and subsequent uremia. (Johannes Fabry, 1860-1930, German dermatologist)

1. Bennett JC, Plum F (eds): Cecil Textbook of Medicine. 20th ed. Philadelphia: WB Saunders, 1996
2. Dyck PJ: Peripheral Neuropathy. 3rd ed. Philadelphia: WB Saunders, 1993
3. Fabry J: Arch Derm Syph 43:187-200, 1898

FACES SYNDROME, unique *f*acies, *a*norexia, *c*achexia, and *e*ye *s*kin lesions (FACES).

1. Friedman E, Goodman RM: The "FACES" syndrome: a new syndrome with unique facies, anorexia, cachexia, and eye and skin lesions. J Craniofac Genet Dev Biol 4:227-231, 1984
2. Gorlin RJ, Cohen MM Jr, Levin LS: Syndromes of the Head and Neck. 3rd ed. New York: Oxford University Press, 1990

FACIAL-DIGITAL-GENITAL SYNDROME, see Aarskog syndrome.

FACIO-AUDIO-SYMPHALANGISM SYNDROME, features include a characteristic facies, progressive conductive hearing loss, proximal symphalangism of fingers and toes, and various other skeletal abnormalities. Autosomal dominant inheritance. Cross-reference: Symphalangism-brachydactyly syndrome.

1. Gorlin RJ, Cohen MM Jr, Levin LS: Syndromes of the Head and Neck. 3rd ed. New York: Oxford University Press, 1990
2. Hurvitz SA, Goodman RM, Hertz M, et al: The facio-audio-symphalangism syndrome: report of a case and review of the literature. Clin Genet 28:61-68, 1985

FACIO-CARDIO-RENAL SYNDROME, severe mental retardation, congenital heart anomalies, characteristic facies, and horseshoe-shaped kidneys are features.

1. Eastman JR, Bixler D: Facio-cardio-renal syndrome: a newly delineated recessive disorder. Clin Genet 11:424-430, 1977
2. Gorlin RJ, Cohen MM Jr, Levin LS: Syndromes of the Head and Neck. 3rd ed. New York: Oxford University Press, 1990

FACIO-GENITO-POPLITEAL SYNDROME, see Popliteal pterygium syndrome.

FADEN OPERATION, a posterior fixation suture of the medial rectus muscle. ("Faden" is German for twine.)

1. Spaeth GL: Ophthalmic Surgery, Principles and Practice. Philadelphia: WB Saunders, 1982

FAGET SIGN, the classic sign of marked temperature-pulse dissociation; seen in the patient with yellow fever. (Jean C. Faget, 1818-1884, French)

1. Baker AB, Baker LH: Clinical Neurology. Revised ed. Philadelphia: Harper & Row, 1982

FAHR-VOLHARD DISEASE, the malignant form of arteriolar nephrosclerosis.

1. Casas EC: Diccionario Terminologico de Ciencias Medicas. 5th ed. Salvat Editores, SA, 1954

FAJERSZTAJN CROSSED SCIATIC SIGN, the hip can be flexed when the leg is flexed, but not when the leg is held straight; seen in cases of sciatica. Cross-reference: Crossed sciatic sign. (Jean Fajersztajn, French neurologist)

1. Baker AB, Baker LH: Clinical Neurology. Revised ed. Philadelphia: Harper & Row, 1982

FALL-AND-RISE PHENOMENON, at the beginning of drug treatment, the number of bacteria drops; a gradual rise follows while treatment continues.

1. Dorland's Medical Dictionary. 28th ed. Philadelphia: WB Saunders, 1994

FALLOT TETRALOGY, blue baby or tetralogy of Fallot; a congenital heart deficiency. (Etienne-Louis A. Fallot, 1850-1911, French)

1. Fallot A: Marseille Med 25:77-93, 1888

FAN SIGN, upon stroking the sole of the foot, the toes spread apart; seen in Babinski sign.

1. Dorland's Medical Dictionary. 28th ed. Philadelphia: WB Saunders, 1994

FANCONI ANEMIA, FANCONI SYNDROME, FANCONI PANCYTOPENIA SYNDROME, congenital pancytopenia; characterized by a constellation of disturbances due to proximal tubular dysfunction, including aminoaciduria, glycosuria, phosphaturia, bicarbonaturia, kaliuresis, and uricaciduria. The presenting conditions could be rickets (children) or osteomalacia (adults). Autosomal recessive inheritance. Cross-references: Lignac syndrome; Pancytopenia-dysmelia syndrome. (Guido Fanconi, 1882-1979, Swiss pediatrician)

1. Bennett JC, Plum F (eds): Cecil Textbook of Medicine. 20th ed. Philadelphia: WB Saunders, 1996
2. Fanconi G: Jahrb Kinderheilkd 117:257-280, 1927
3. Garriga S, Crosby WH: The incidence of leukemia in families of patients with hypoplasia of the marrow. Blood 14:1008, 1959
4. Lignac G: Dtsch Arch Klin Med 145:139-150, 1924

FARABEUF OPERATION, ischiopubiotomy.

1. Maffei WE: Os Fundamentos da Medicina. 2nd ed. Livraria Editora Artes Medicas Ltd, 1978

FARBER DISEASE, disseminated lipogranulomatosis; characterized by joint enlargement and contracture, hoarseness, pulmonary consolidation, mental retardation, hypotonia, and loss of tendon reflexes. Caused by a deficiency of acid ceramidase that degrades ceramide to sphingosine and fatty acids. Autosomal recessive disorder with onset in infancy. (Sidney Farber, 1903-1973, U.S. pediatrician-pathologist)

1. Braunwald E: Heart Disease: A Textbook of Cardiovascular Medicine. 4th ed. Philadelphia: WB Saunders, 1992
2. Dyck PJ: Peripheral Neuropathy. 3rd ed. Philadelphia: WB Saunders, 1993
3. Farber S: Am J Dis Child 84:499-500, 1952

FASENELLA-SERVAT OPERATION, frontalis muscle sling for severe ptosis.

1. Spaeth GL: Ophthalmic Surgery, Principles and Practice. Philadelphia: WB Saunders, 1982

FAT EMBOLISM SYNDROME, posttraumatic fat embolism; a lung disorder that results from the impaction of particulate fat globules in the pulmonary circulation. After long bone fractures, most patients develop fat embolism but most do not develop the fat embolism syndrome, which includes the presence of at least one of three major symptoms: respiratory insufficiency, cerebral symptoms, and petechiae.

1. Bennett JC, Plum F (eds): Cecil Textbook of Medicine. 20th ed. Philadelphia: WB Saunders, 1996

FAUCHARD DISEASE, periodontitis of the dental alveoli. Cross-reference: Riggs disease. (Pierre Fauchard, 1678-1761, French dentist)

1. Fauchard P: Le Chirurgien, ou Traite des Dents. Paris: Mariette, 1746
2. Riggs JM: Penn J Dent Sci 3:99-104, 1876

FAVRE-DURAND-NICOLAS DISEASE, see Durand-Nicolas-Favre disease. (Maurice Favre, 1876-1954, French)

FAVRE-RACOUCHOT SYNDROME, nodular elastoidosis of Favre and Racouchot. (Maurice Favre; Jean Racouchot, French)

1. Favre M, Racouchot J: Ann Dermatol Syph 78:681-702, 1951

FAZIO-LONDE DISEASE, progressive bulbar palsy; degeneration of motor nuclei in the brain stem results in the onset of motor symptoms during childhood. A rare disorder of uncertain etiology. (M. Fazio, 1849-1902, Italian; P.F.L. Londe, 1864-1944, French neurologist)

1. Farmer TW: Pediatric Neurology. 2nd ed. Hagerstown: Harper & Row, 1975, p 420
2. Fazio M: Rif Med 8:327, 1892
3. Gomez MR, Clermont V, Bernstein J: Progressive bulbar palsy in childhood (Fazio-Londe's disease). Arch Neurol 6:317, 1962
4. Londe PFL: Rev Med Paris 14:212-254, 1894

FEDE DISEASE, sublingual fibroma. (Francesco Fede, 1832-1913, Italian)

1. Fede F: Cong Pediatr Ital, 1891, pp 251-260

FEDERICI SIGN, see Claybrook sign. (Cesare Federici, 1838-1892, Italian)

FEER DISEASE, see Swift disease. (Emil Feer, 1864-1955, Swiss pediatrician)

FEER SIGN, as the fingernail grows, the line on the nail also disappears; seen in scarlet fever. (Emil Feer)

88

1. Casas EC: Diccionario Terminologico de Ciencias Medicas. 5th ed. Salvat Editores, SA, 1954

FEGAN METHOD, varicosities of the leg are marked with a skin pen while the patient is standing. The patient is asked to lie down, raise the affected leg, and rest the heel against the examiner's upper chest. The examiner palpates the line of the marked varicosities for gaps in the deep fascia through which the perforating veins pass; they are felt as circular openings with sharp edges and may be marked with an X. To confirm filling of the superficial varicosities from the perforating veins, the Brodie-Trendelenburg test can be applied. (George Fegan, Irish surgeon)

1. Bailey H: Physical Signs in Clinical Surgery. 16th ed. Baltimore: Williams & Wilkins, 1983

FEHLING OPERATION, suture of the anterior vaginal wall to treat a prolapsed uterus.

1. Maffei WE: Os Fundamentos da Medicina. 2nd ed. Livraria Editora Artes Medicas Ltd, 1978

FELTON PHENOMENON, immunological nonresponse or tolerance to pneumococcal polysaccharide; given to mice via large doses of the antigen. (Lloyd D. Felton, 1885-1953, U.S.)

1. Dorland's Medical Dictionary. 28th ed. Philadelphia: WB Saunders, 1994

FELTY SYNDROME, the triad of rheumatoid arthritis, splenomegaly, and neutropenia and/or thrombocytopenia. Appears between the 5th and 7th decades of life, and 60% to 70% of patients are women. Rare in Blacks. (Augustus R. Felty, 1895-1964, U.S.)

1. Felty AR: Bull Johns Hopkins Hosp 35:16-20, 1924
2. Moschella SL, Hurley HJ: Dermatology. 2nd ed. Philadelphia: WB Saunders, 1985
3. Ritchie AC: Boyd's Textbook of Pathology. 9th ed. Philadelphia: Lea & Febiger, 1990

FEMALE URETHRAL SYNDROME, see Urethral syndrome.

FEMINIZING SYNDROME, in males, caused by malignant adrenal tumors that occur in patients between the ages of 25 and 50 years. Gynecomastia is the most frequent finding and is usually bilateral. Testicular atrophy and diminished libido or potency occur in one half of patients.

1. Campbell MF, Walsh PC: Campbell's Urology. 5th ed. Philadelphia: WB Saunders, 1986

FEMORAL HYPOPLASIA-UNUSUAL FACIES SYNDROME, features include small stature, short nose, cleft palate, hypoplastic to absent femora and fibulae, and abnormalities of the lower spine. Etiology unknown.

1. Daentl DL, Smith DW, Scott CI, et al: Femoral hypoplasia-unusual facies syndrome. J Pediatr 86:107-111, 1975
2. De Palma L, Duray PH, Popeo VR: Femoral hypoplasia-unusual facies syndrome. Pediatr Pathol 5:1-8, 1986

FENWICK DISEASE, atrophy of the stomach in a patient with pernicious anemia. (Samuel Fenwick, 1821-1902, British)

1. Fenwick S: On Atrophy of the Stomach and on the Nervous Affections of the Digestive Organs. London: Churchill, 1880

FÉRÉOL-GRAUX DISEASE, paralysis of the medial rectus of one eye and lateral rectus of the other eye. (Louis H.F. Féréol, 1825-1891, French)

1. Casas EC: Diccionario Terminologico de Ciencias Medicas. 5th ed. Salvat Editores, SA, 1954

FERGUSON OPERATION, for hernia repair; the spermatic cord is placed deep to the reconstructed floor of the inguinal canal.

1. Schwartz SI: Principles of Surgery. 4th ed. New York: McGraw-Hill, 1983

FERGUSSON INCISION, FERGUSSON OPERATION, surgical method for resection of the maxilla. (William Fergusson, 1808-1877, British surgeon)

1. Maffei WE: Os Fundamentos da Medicina. 2nd ed. Livraria Editora Artes Medicas Ltd, 1978

FERRÉOL-BESNIER DISEASE, associated with recurrent meningitis. Extensive reddening and desquamation of skin in the palmar and plantar areas; fever, headache, and throat pain subside in 4 days. Neurological abnormalities other than meningism have not been found. Etiology uncertain; no infectious or viral agents have been found.

1. Meyer-Lindenberg A, Hotz M: Ferréol-Besnier disease with associated recurrent meningitis. J Neurol Neurosurg Psychiatry 62:297, 1997 (Letter)
2. Swithinbank IM, Rake MO: A case of Mollaret's meningitis associated with a lymphoma. Postgrad Med J 54:682-685, 1978

FERTILE EUNUCH SYNDROME, very rarely, a male presents with signs of eunuchoidism and variable secondary sexual development but with large testes. Testicular biopsy shows maturation of the terminal epithelium, but Leydig cells are absent. The ejaculate may even contain sperm. Cross-reference: Pasqualini syndrome.

1. Campbell MF, Walsh PC: Campbell's Urology. 5th ed. Philadelphia: WB Saunders, 1986
2. Gold JJ, Josimovich JB: Gynecologic Endocrinology. 3rd ed. New York: Plenum Medical, 1980

FETAL ALCOHOL SYNDROME, alcoholic embryopathy; a syndrome in infants whose mother received ethanol or its byproducts during gestation. Prenatal onset of growth deficiency, microcephaly, short palpebral fissures, and low IQ with fine motor dysfunction, joint anomalies, and heart murmur are features.

1. Jones KL, Smith DW, Ulleland CN, et al: Pattern of malformation in offspring of chronic alcoholic mothers. Lancet 1:1267-1271, 1973
2. Smith DW, Jones KL: Recognizable Patterns of Human Malformations: Genetic, Embryologic, and Clinical Aspects. 3rd ed. Philadelphia: WB Saunders, 1982
3. Sullivan WC: J Ment Sci 45:489-503, 1899

FETAL FACE SYNDROME, see Robinow syndrome.

FETAL HYDANTOIN SYNDROME, a syndrome in infants whose mother received anticonvulsant hydantoin during gestation. A two- to three-fold increase in the frequency of major fetal malformations is seen.

1. Meadow SR: Lancet 2:1296, 1968
2. Rowland LP (ed): Merritt's Textbook of Neurology. 9th ed. Baltimore: Williams & Wilkins, 1995

FETAL RUBELLA SYNDROME, maternal contraction of the rubella virus in the first trimester of gestation may cause infant deafness, cataracts, patent ductus arteriosis, mental deficiency, glaucoma, septal defects, and possibly death.

1. Hardy JB: Clinical and developmental aspects of congenital rubella. Arch Otolaryngol 98:230, 1973
2. Smith DW, Jones KL: Recognizable Patterns of Human Malformations: Genetic, Embryologic, and Clinical Aspects. 3rd ed. Philadelphia: WB Saunders, 1982

FETAL TRIMETHADIONE SYNDROME, a syndrome in infants whose mother received trimethadione during gestation. Mental deficiency, mild brachycephaly, septal defects, ambiguous genitalia, and a simian crease in the limbs are features. Cross-reference: Paramethadione syndrome.

1. Smith DW, Jones KL: Recognizable Patterns of Human Malformation: Genetic, Embryologic, and Clinical Aspects. 3rd ed. Philadelphia: WB Saunders, 1982
2. Zackai E, Mellman WJ, Neiderer B, et al: The fetal trimethadione syndrome. J Pediatr 87:280-290, 1975

FETAL WARFARIN SYNDROME, a syndrome in infants whose mother received coumarin derivatives during gestation, especially at 6-9 weeks. May cause nasal hypoplasia, mild hypoplasia of the nails, significant retardation (30% incidence), and sometimes death of the fetus.

1. Hall JG, Pauli RM, Wilson KM, et al: Maternal and fetal sequelae of anticoagulation during pregnancy. Am J Med 68:122-140, 1980
2. Smith DW, Jones KL: Recognizable Patterns of Human Malformations: Genetic, Embryologic, and Clinical Aspects. 3rd ed. Philadelphia: WB Saunders, 1982

FEUERSTEIN-MIMS SYNDROME, see Epidermal nevus syndrome.

FÈVRE-LANGUEPIN SYNDROME, see Popliteal pterygium syndrome. (Marcel Fèvre, French orthopedic surgeon; Anne Languepin, pediatrician)

FG SYNDROME, multiple congenital anomaly consisting of mental retardation, an imperforate anus, unusual facies, and other anomalies. X-linked inheritance. ("FG" indicates the surname of persons in whom the syndrome was first reported.)

1. Gorlin RJ, Cohen MM Jr, Levin LS: Syndromes of the Head and Neck. 3rd ed. New York: Oxford University Press, 1990

FIBRILLARIS SYNDROME, see Morvan chorea.

FIBROSIS SYNDROME, characterized by fibrosis of all extraocular muscles and of the Tenon capsule. Adhesions between muscles, the Tenon capsule and the globe, and inelasticity and fragility of the conjunctiva.

1. Walsh FB, Hoyt EF, Miller NR: Clinical Neuro-Ophthalmology. 4th ed. Baltimore: Williams & Wilkins, 1982

FICK PHENOMENON, a fogging of vision, including the appearance of halos around light sources; most often reported by individuals wearing contact lenses.

1. Dorland's Medical Dictionary. 28th ed. Philadelphia: WB Saunders, 1994

FIEDLER MYOCARDITIS, a form of myocarditis not accompanied by pericarditis or endocarditis; characterized by the sudden onset of dyspnea, pallor, cyanosis, vomiting, and marked tachycardia, with the rapid development of heart failure, collapse, and death. (Carl L.A. Fiedler, 1835-1921, German)

1. Fiedler CLA: Zentralbl Inn Med 21:212-213, 1900
2. Krugman S, Katz SL: Infectious Diseases of Children. 7th ed. St Louis: CV Mosby, 1981

FIESSINGER-LEROY-REITER SYNDROME, see Reiter syndrome.

FIESSINGER-RENDU SYNDROME, FIESSINGER-RENDU-STEVENS-JOHNSON DISEASE, see Stevens-Johnson syndrome.

FIFTH DISEASE, erythema infectiosum; a typical "slapped cheek" rash caused by *Parvovirus* B-19 infection. Disease is usually self-limiting. (After scarlatina, morbilli, rubella, and fourth disease.)
1. Sticker G: Zschr Prakt Arzte 8:353-358, 1899

FILATOV DISEASE, FILATOV-DUKES DISEASE, see Dukes disease. (Nils Filatov, 1847-1902, Russian pediatrician; Clement Dukes, 1845-1925, British)

FILATOV OPERATION, corneal transplantation using a graft from the conjunctiva.
1. Maffei WE: Os Fundamentos da Medicina. 2nd ed. Livraria Editora Artes Medicas Ltd, 1978

FILIPOVITCH [FILIPOWICZ] SIGN, yellowish discoloration of the palms and feet seen in typhoid fever. Cross-reference: Palmoplantar sign. (Casimir Filipovitch [Filipowicz], Polish)
1. Casas EC: Diccionario Terminologico de Ciencias Medicas. 5th ed. Salvat Editores, SA, 1954

FILUM TERMINALE SYNDROME, see Tethered cord syndrome.

FINDLAY DISEASE, lymphogranuloma inguinale (venereum).
1. Casas EC: Diccionario Terminologico de Ciencias Medicas. 5th ed. Salvat Editores, SA, 1954

FINGER PHENOMENON, FINGER SIGN, active elevation and extension of a paretic arm is followed by involuntary hyperextension and abduction of the fingers. Cross-references: Gordon sign; Interossei sign; Souques phenomenon.
1. Baker AB, Baker LH: Clinical Neurology. Revised ed. Philadelphia: Harper & Row, 1982

FINNEY OPERATION, pyloroplasty; reconstruction of the pyloric channel via a longitudinal incision through the pylorus and adjacent walls of the stomach and duodenum. (John M.T. Finney, 1863-1942, U.S. surgeon)
1. Maffei WE: Os Fundamentos da Medicina. 2nd ed. Livraria Editora Artes Medicas Ltd, 1978
2. Schwartz SI: Principles of Surgery. 4th ed. New York, NY: McGraw-Hill, 1983

FINSTERER SIGN, occurs when grasping or making a fist fails to show the normal prominence of the third metacarpal bone.
1. Evans RC: Illustrated Essentials in Orthopedic Physical Assessment. St Louis: Mosby Yearbook, 1994
2. Mazion JM: Illustrated Manual of Orthopedic Signs/Tests/Maneuvers for Office Procedure. 2nd ed. Orlando: Daniels Publishing, 1980

FIRST BRANCHIAL ARCH SYNDROME, malformation including macrostomia, hemignathia, and deformities of the external ear, resulting from an inhibitory process occurring around the 7th week of embryonic life.
1. McKenzie J: The first arch syndrome. Arch Dis Child 33:477-486, 1958

FIRST-SET PHENOMENON, the immunological reaction of a patient's body against an organ or tissue in a host not previously sensitized against the graft of antigens.
1. Dorland's Medical Dictionary. 28th ed. Philadelphia: WB Saunders, 1994

FISCHER SIGN, when the patient extends the neck, there is an audible bruit on the sternum caused by enlarged lymph nodes compressing the veins; seen in cases of tuberculosis of the mediastinal or peribronchial glands. (Louis Fischer, 1864-1944, U.S. pediatrician)
1. Casas EC: Diccionario Terminologico de Ciencias Medicas. 5th ed. Salvat Editores, SA, 1954

FISHER SIGN, presystolic bruit in the case of pericardial effusion.
1. Casas EC: Diccionario Terminologico de Ciencias Medicas. 5th ed. Salvat Editores, SA, 1954

FISHER SYNDROME, see One-and-a-half syndrome. (Miller Fisher, U.S. neurologist)

FISH-ODOR SYNDROME, a fishy odor due to the body's inability to break down trimethylamine, a fetid chemical derived from carnitine and choline, substances found in many foods. People with this condition emit a strong odor of rotting fish in their breath, sweat, urine, and other secretions, apparently caused by a recessive gene that a person must inherit from both parents.
1. Humbert JR, et al: Lancet 2:770-771, 1970

FITZ SYNDROME, acute hemorrhagic pancreatitis. (Reginald H. Fitz, 1843-1913, U.S.)
1. Fitz RH: Bost Med S J, 1889, pp 181-187

FITZ-HUGH AND CURTIS SYNDROME, gonococcal perihepatitis in women; caused by intra-abdominal spread of the infection to the right upper quadrant. May be mistaken for acute cholecystitis, but adnexal tenderness is usually present on pelvic examination. (Thomas Fitz-Hugh, Jr., 1894-1963, U.S.; Arthur H. Curtis, 1881-1955, U.S. gynecologist)
1. Curtis AH: JAMA 94:1221-1222, 1930
2. Fitz-Hugh T Jr: JAMA 102:2094-2096, 1934
3. Krugman S, Katz SL: Infectious Diseases of Children. 7th ed. St Louis: CV Mosby, 1981

FLAG SIGN, dyspigmentation of the hair; seen in the child recovering from kwashiorkor syndrome.
1. Dorland's Medical Dictionary. 28th ed. Philadelphia: WB Saunders, 1994

FLAJANI DISEASE, see Graves disease. (Giuseppe Flajani, 1741-1808, Italian surgeon)

FLAJANI OPERATION, iridodialysis using a needle introduced through the cornea.
1. Maffei WE: Os Fundamentos da Medicina. 2nd ed. Livraria Editora Artes Medicas Ltd, 1978

FLATAU-SCHILDER DISEASE, progressive subcortical encephalopathy. (Edward Flatau, 1869-1932, Polish neurologist; Paul Schilder, 1886-1940, German-U.S. psychiatrist)
1. Casas EC: Diccionario Terminologico de Ciencias Medicas. 5th ed. Salvat Editores, SA, 1954

FLEISCHNER DISEASE, osteochondritis of the second phalanges of the fingers. (Felix Fleischner, 1893-1969, U.S. radiologist)
1. Casas EC: Diccionario Terminologico de Ciencias Medicas. 5th ed. Salvat Editores, SA, 1954

FLES SIGN, an indication of undigested meat in the feces.
1. Casas EC: Diccionario Terminologico de Ciencias Medicas. 5th ed. Salvat Editores, SA, 1954

FLIP SIGN, with the patient lying supine, the examiner raises the affected leg, keeping the knee straight. If this movement is limited by pain or resistance, the patient is instructed to sit up with the legs flat on the table. If the patient is able to sit in this manner without pain, the test is positive.
1. Evans RC: Illustrated Essentials in Orthopedic Physical Assessment. St Louis: Mosby Yearbook, 1994

FLOATING HARBOR SYNDROME, see Pelletier-Leisti syndrome.

FLOPPY BABY SYNDROME, FLOPPY HEAD SYNDROME, FLOPPY INFANT SYN-DROME, limp child; paralytic muscular atrophies and congenital myopathies are characteristics.
1. Bennett JC, Plum F (eds): Cecil Textbook of Medicine. 20th ed. Philadelphia: WB Saunders, 1996
2. Rowland LP (ed): Merritt's Textbook of Neurology. 9th ed. Baltimore: Williams & Wilkins, 1995
3. Walton JN: The limp child. J Neurol Neurosurg Psychiatry 201:144-154, 1957

FLOPPY MITRAL VALVE SYNDROME, a valvular defect with a late systolic murmur, abnormal T-waves, and late systolic dysfunction of the mitral valve. Cross-references: Hypotonia syndrome; Mitral click syndrome.
1. McKusick VA: Heritable Disorders of Connective Tissue. 4th ed. St Louis: CV Mosby, 1972

FLORA SIGN, neurasthenia, lack of contraction after faradic stimulation of muscles.
1. Casas EC: Diccionario Terminologico de Ciencias Medicas. 5th ed. Salvat Editores, SA, 1954

FLUSH-TANK SIGN, a large amount of urine passes coincident with the temporary disappearance of lumbar swelling; seen in hydronephrosis.
1. Dorland's Medical Dictionary. 28th ed. Philadelphia: WB Saunders, 1994

FOCAL DERMAL HYPOPLASIA SYNDROME, see Goltz syndrome.

FODERE SIGN, edema of the lower eyelids in nephritic syndrome.
1. Casas EC: Diccionario Terminologico de Ciencias Medicas. 5th ed. Salvat Editores, SA, 1954

FOERSTER OPERATION, intradural bilateral section of the 7th, 8th, and 9th cranial nerve roots. Cross-reference: Mingazzini-Foerster operation.
1. Maffei WE: Os Fundamentos da Medicina. 2nd ed. Livraria Editora Artes Medicas Ltd, 1978

FOIX SYNDROME, see Cavernous sinus syndrome. (Charles Foix, 1882-1927, French neurologist)

FOIX-ALAJOUANINE DISEASE, progressive necrotic myelitis. Generally agreed that necrosis of the spinal cord is of ischemic origin, from narrowing or occlusion of arteries or veins. (Charles Foix; Théophile Alajouanine, 1890-1980, French neurologist)
1. Brion S, Netsky MG, Zimmerman HM: Vascular malformations of the spinal cord. Arch Neurol Psychiatr 68: 339, 1952
2. Foix C, Alajouanine T: Rev Neurol Paris 2:1-42, 1926
3. Vinken PJ, Bruyn GW (eds): Handbook of Clinical Neurology, Vol 9. Disorders of the Spinal Cord. New York: Elsevier-North Holland, 1970, p 620

FOIX-CHAVANY-MARIE SYNDROME, bilateral voluntary facial palsy with preserved emotional expression; may result from a pontine lesion and seems to prove that the fiber tracts subserving voluntary and emotional facial innervation are still anatomically distinct in the upper pons (i.e., just above the level of the motor facial nucleus). (Charles Foix; Jean A.E. Chavany, 1892-1959, French neurologist; Pierre Marie, 1853-1940, French neurologist)

1. Foix C, Chavany JAE, Marie P: Rev Neurol 33:214-219, 1926
2. Trepel M, Weller M, Dichgans J, et al: Voluntary facial palsy with a pontine lesion. J Neurol Neurosurg Psychiatry 61:531-532, 1996 (Letter)
3. Weller M: Anterior opercular cortex lesions cause dissociated lower cranial nerve palsies and anarthria but no aphasia: Foix-Chavany-Marie syndrome and "automatic voluntary dissociation" revisited. J Neurol 240:199-208, 1993

FØLLING DISEASE, phenylketonuria; a dysfunction in the enzymatic oxidation of phenylalanine. Recessive trait inheritance. (Ivar A. Følling, 1888-1973, Norwegian physiologist)

1. Baker AB, Baker LH: Clinical Neurology. Revised ed. Philadelphia: Harper & Row, 1982

FONTAINE SYNDROME, a disorder characterized by micrognathia, dysplastic ears, ectrodactyly and syndactyly of the feet, and, in some instances, submucous cleft palate and mental deficiency. Autosomal dominant inheritance.

1. Fontaine G, Farriaux JP, Delattre P, et al: Une observation familiale du syndrome ectrodactylie et dysostose mandibulo-faciale. J Genet Hum 22:289-307, 1974
2. Gorlin RJ, Cohen MM Jr, Levin LS: Syndromes of the Head and Neck. 3rd ed. New York: Oxford University Press, 1990

FONTAINE-FARRIAUX SYNDROME, consists of craniosynostosis, phalangeal hypoplasia with anonychia of the third, fourth, and fifth fingers, patches of lipodystrophy at the antecubital and popliteal fossae, aplasia of the abdominal muscles, genital hypoplasia, hypospadias, and cryptorchidism.

1. Gorlin RJ, Cohen MM Jr, Levin LS: Syndromes of the Head and Neck. 3rd ed. New York: Oxford University Press, 1990

FONTAN OPERATION, transposition of the great vessels; a corrective procedure usually performed in older children with a diagnosis of Fallot tetralogy. (François Fontan, French thoracic surgeon)

1. Schwartz SI: Principles of Surgery. 4th ed. New York, NY: McGraw-Hill, 1983

FORAMEN OF LUSCHKA, see Luschka foramen.

FORBES DISEASE, glycogen storage disease type III; cirrhosis of the liver with storage of abnormal glycogen. Cross-reference: Cori disease. (Gilbert B. Forbes, U.S. pediatrician)

1. Cori GT: Bibl Paediatr Basel 66:344-358, 1958
2. Forbes GB: J Pediatr 42:645-653, 1953
3. Grinker RR, Sahs AL: Neurology. 6th ed. Springfield: Charles C Thomas, 1966
4. Sidbury JB: The Genetics of the Glycogenosis Affecting Muscles.

FORBES OPERATION, division of the accessory tendons of the finger extensor muscles in order to gain more mobility of the ring finger.

1. Maffei WE: Os Fundamentos da Medicina. 2nd ed. Livraria Editora Artes Medicas Ltd, 1978

FORBES-ALBRIGHT SYNDROME, see Chiari-Frommel syndrome. (Anne P. Forbes, U.S.; Fuller Albright, 1900-1969, U.S. endocrinologist)

FORD-DUTTON DISEASE, trypanosomiasis; an infection with a member of the genus *Trypanosoma*.

1. Casas EC: Diccionario Terminologico de Ciencias Medicas. 5th ed. Salvat Editores, SA, 1954

FORDYCE DISEASE, see Fox-Fordyce disease. (John A. Fordyce, 1858-1925, U.S. dermatologist)

FOREARM SIGN, see Léri sign.

FORESTIER BOWSTRING SIGN, while standing, the patient performs side bending and reveals ipsilateral tightening and contracture of the paraspinal musculature; an indication of ankylosing spondylitis. (Jacques Forestier, French neurologist)

1. Evans RC: Illustrated Essentials in Orthopedic Physical Assessment. St Louis: Mosby Yearbook, 1994
2. Mazion JM: Illustrated Manual of Orthopedic Signs/Tests/Maneuvers for Office Procedure. 2nd ed. Orlando: Daniels Publishing, 1980

FORREST DISEASE, fever observed in the region of Rangpur, India. Cross-reference: Rangpur disease.

1. Casas EC: Diccionario Terminologico de Ciencias Medicas. 5th ed. Salvat Editores, SA, 1954

FORSIUS-ERIKSSON SYNDROME, ocular albinism, OA2, and Åland eye disease. An X-linked ocular albinism with males showing hypoplastic foveas, axial myopia, and protanomaly and females showing slightly defective color discrimination and latent nystagmus, but no mosaic pigment pattern in the fundus. (Henrik Forsius, Finnish; Aldur W. Eriksson, Finnish geneticist)

1. Forsius H, Eriksson W: Klin Monatsbl Augenheilkd 114:447-457, 1964

FÖRSTER DISEASE, cerebellar hypoplasia and atrophy of the frontal lobe with intellectual defects and incontinence; occurs in tertiary syphilis. (Carl F.R. Förster, 1825-1902, German ophthalmologist)

1. Pedro-Pons A: Patologia-y-Clinica Medicus. Salvat Editores, SA, 1952

FORT BRAGG DISEASE, pretibial fever; a *Leptospira autumnalis* infection, marked by a rash on the pretibial region, lumbar and postorbital pain, malaise, coryza, and fever.

1. Casas EC: Diccionario Terminologico de Ciencias Medicas. 5th ed. Salvat Editores, SA, 1954

FOSTER-KENNEDY SYNDROME, papilledema limited to one eye, while the other shows primary optic atrophy with a marked reduction in visual acuity. A result of a tumor on the inferior surface of the frontal lobe. Cross-references: Gowers syndrome; Paton syndrome. (Robert Foster-Kennedy, 1884-1952, Irish)

1. Foster-Kennedy R: Am J Med Sci 142:355-368, 1911
2. Gowers WR: Br Med J 2:89-92, 1902
3. Rowland LP (ed): Merritt's Textbook of Neurology. 9th ed. Baltimore: Williams & Wilkins, 1995

FOTHERGILL OPERATION, see Manchester-Fothergill operation. (William Fothergill, 1865-1926, British gynecologist)

FOTHERGILL SYNDROME, trigeminal neuralgia. (Samuel A. Fothergill, 1712-1780, British)

1. Fothergill SA: A Concise and Systematic Account of a Painful Affection of the Nerves of the Face, Commonly Called Tic Douloureux. London, 1804

FOUCHET SIGN, with the patient's knee in full extension, the examiner presses the patella against the femur, producing point tenderness and pain at the patellar margin; an indication of chondromalacia patellae.

1. Mazion JM: Illustrated Manual of Orthopedic Signs/Tests/Maneuvers for Office Procedure. 2nd ed. Orlando: Daniels Publishing, 1980

FOUNTAIN SYNDROME, a familial syndrome characterized by mental retardation, hearing loss, spina bifida, seizures, and facial edema with massive swelling of the upper and lower lips. (R.B. Fountain, British)

1. Fountain RB: Proc R Soc Med 67:878-879, 1974
2. Gorlin RJ, Cohen MM Jr, Levin LS: Syndromes of the Head and Neck. 3rd ed. New York: Oxford University Press, 1990

FOUR-DAY SYNDROME, respiratory distress syndrome of the newborn; so-called because the infant usually either recovers or dies within 4 days.

1. Dorland's Medical Dictionary. 28th ed. Philadelphia: WB Saunders, 1994

FOURNIER GANGRENE, idiopathic gangrene of the scrotum; localized in the scrotum and associated with local trauma, underlying urinary tract disease, and distant acute inflammatory processes. (Jean A. Fournier, 1832-1914, French syphilographer)

1. Campbell MF, Walsh PC: Campbell Urology. 5th ed. Philadelphia: WB Saunders, 1986
2. Moschella SL, Hurley HJ: Dermatology. 2nd ed. Philadelphia: WB Saunders, 1980

FOURNIER SIGN, a trophic ulcer of the foot; seen in syphilis. (Jean A. Fournier)

1. Bodechtel G: Diagnostico Diferencial de las Enfermedades Neurologicas. Madrid, 1967

FOURTH DISEASE, see Dukes disease.

FOVILLE SYNDROME, see Millard-Gubler syndrome. (Achille L.F. Foville, 1799-1878, French neurologist)

FOWLER OPERATION, decortication of the lung in empyema in order to achieve lung expansion.

1. Maffei WE: Os Fundamentos da Medicina. 2nd ed. Livraria Editora Artes Medicas Ltd, 1978

FOX DISEASE, see Epidermolysis bullosa syndrome. (William T. Fox, 1836-1879)

FOX-BACKER-ROSENBACH DISEASE, see Rosenbach syndrome.

FOX-FORDYCE DISEASE, a chronic, itchy, papular eruption of the apocrine gland areas, notably the axillae and pubes. Cross-reference: Fordyce disease. (George H. Fox, 1846-1937, U.S. dermatologist; John A. Fordyce, 1858-1925, U.S. dermatologist)

1. Fordyce JA: Trans Am Dermatol Assoc, 1896, pp 5-11
2. Fox GH, Fordyce JA: J Cutan Dis 20:1-5, 1902
3. Ritchie AC: Boyd's Textbook of Pathology. 9th ed. Philadelphia: Lea & Febiger, 1990

FRACK SIGN, hepatic pseudohemophilia.

1. Casas EC: Diccionario Terminologico de Ciencias Medicas. 5th ed. Salvat Editores, SA, 1954

FRACKE SIGN, pain in the posterior and deep part of the lung apex; seen in tuberculosis.

1. Casas EC: Diccionario Terminologico de Ciencias Medicas. 5th ed. Salvat Editores, SA, 1954

FRAENKEL SIGN, locomotor ataxia indicating decreased muscle tone; seen in tabes dorsalis. (Albert Fraenkel, 1884-1916, German)

1. Casas EC: Diccionario Terminologico de Ciencias Medicas. 5th ed. Salvat Editores, SA, 1954

FRAGILE X SYNDROME, a common cause of mental retardation, with mild facial abnormalities, and sometimes macro-orchidism in males. Cross-references: Macro-orchidism marker X syndrome; Martin-Bell syndrome.

1. Bennett JC, Plum F (eds): Cecil Textbook of Medicine. 20th ed. Philadelphia: WB Saunders, 1996

FRANCESCHETTI-JADASSOHN SYNDROME, a type of incontinentia pigmenti with an entirely different familial syndrome. Begins after infancy without preceding inflammation, appears on the trunk, and is slate-gray to brown in color. Reported in only one Swiss family pedigree as an autosomal dominant trait. Cross-reference: Naegeli syndrome. (Adolphe Franceschetti, Swiss ophthalmologist)

1. Bennett JC, Plum F (eds): Cecil Textbook of Medicine. 20th ed. Philadelphia: WB Saunders, 1996
2. Franceschetti A, Jadassohn W: Dermatologica 108:1-28, 1954
3. Naegli O: Schweiz Med Wochenschr 57:48, 1927

FRANCESCHETTI-KLEIN SYNDROME, see Treacher Collins syndrome. (Adolphe Franceschetti; David Klein, Swiss)

FRANCIS DISEASE, tularemia. (Edward Francis, 1872-1957, U.S. bacteriologist)

1. Casas EC: Diccionario Terminologico de Ciencias Medicas. 5th ed. Salvat Editores, SA, 1954

FRANCO OPERATION, suprapubic cystostomy. (Pierre Franco, 1500-1561, French surgeon)

1. Maffei WE: Os Fundamentos da Medicina. 2nd ed. Livraria Editora Artes Medicas Ltd, 1978

FRANÇOIS SYNDROME, chondrodermal corneal dystrophy; characterized by skeletal deformity of the hands and feet as well as "xanthomatous" nodules on the pinnae, the dorsal surface of the metacarpophalangeal and interphalangeal joints, the posterior surface of the elbows, or nose, and by corneal dystrophy. (Jules François, Belgian ophthalmologist)

1. François J: Ann Ocul 182:409-422, 1949
2. McKusick VA: Heritable Disorders of Connective Tissue. 4th ed. St Louis: CV Mosby, 1972

FRANK OPERATION, subcutaneous symphysiotomy. (Rudolf Frank, 1862-1913, Austrian surgeon)

1. Maffei WE: Os Fundamentos da Medicina. 2nd ed. Livraria Editora Artes Medicas Ltd, 1978

FRANKE OPERATION, extirpation of the intercostal nerves for relief of visceral crisis in tabes.

1. Maffei WE: Os Fundamentos da Medicina. 2nd ed. Livraria Editora Artes Medicas Ltd, 1978

FRANKE-HOCHWART DISEASE, infectious polyneuritis.

1. Casas EC: Diccionario Terminologico de Ciencias Medicas. 5th ed. Salvat Editores, SA, 1954

FRANKFORT-MARBURG SYNDROME, see Marburg virus disease

FRANTZEL SIGN, bruit in mitral stenosis.

1. Casas EC: Diccionario Terminologico de Ciencias Medicas. 5th ed. Salvat Editores, SA, 1954

FRASER SYNDROME, cryptophthalmos, usually with partial cutaneous syndactyly and incomplete development of genitalia. Autosomal recessive inheritance. Cross-reference: Cryptophthalmos syndrome. (G.R. Fraser, British geneticist)

1. Fraser GR: Ann Hum Genet 25:387-415, 1962
2. Gorlin RJ, Cohen MM Jr, Levin LS: Syndromes of the Head and Neck. 3rd ed. New York: Oxford University Press, 1990
3. Smith DW, Jones KL: Recognizable Patterns of Human Malformations: Genetic, Embryologic, and Clinical Aspects. 3rd ed. Philadelphia: WB Saunders, 1982

FRAZIER-SPILLER OPERATION, division of the sensory root of the gasserian ganglion for relief of trigeminal neuralgia. (Charles H. Frazier, 1870-1936, U.S. surgeon; William G. Spiller, 1864-1940, U.S. neurologist)

1. Maffei WE: Os Fundamentos da Medicina. 2nd ed. Livraria Editora Artes Medicas Ltd, 1978

FREDERICQ SIGN, a purple line in the gums and teeth; seen in the patient with tuberculosis.

1. Casas EC: Diccionario Terminologico de Ciencias Medicas. 5th ed. Salvat Editores, SA, 1954

FREDET-RAMSTEDT OPERATION, pyloromyotomy for gastroesophageal reflux in infants and small children. (Pierre Fredet, 1820-1946, French surgeon; Conrad Ramstedt, 1867-1936, German surgeon)

1. Maffei WE: Os Fundamentos da Medicina. 2nd ed. Livraria Editora Artes Medicas Ltd, 1978
2. Schwartz SI: Principles of Surgery. 4th ed. New York, NY: McGraw-Hill, 1983

FREEMAN OPERATION, frontal lobotomy, first performed in the U.S. by Freeman and Watts. Most operations were done using the transorbital technique. Cross-reference: Watts operation. (Walter Freeman, 1895-1972, U.S.)

FREEMAN-SHELDON SYNDROME, craniocarpotarsal dystrophy or mask-like "whistling" facies; hypoplastic alae nasi, talipes equinovarus, and ulnar deviation of hands are features. Autosomal dominant inheritance. Cross-reference: Whistling face syndrome. (E.A. Freeman, British orthopedic surgeon; Joseph H. Sheldon, 1920-1964, British)

1. Freeman EA, Sheldon JH: Cranio-carpo-tarsal dystrophy. An undescribed congenital malformation. Arch Dis Child 13:277-283, 1938
2. O'Connell DJ, Hall CM: Cranio-carpo-tarsal dysplasia. A report of seven cases. Radiology 123:719-722, 1977.
3. Smith DW, Jones KL: Recognizable Patterns of Human Malformations: Genetic, Embryologic, and Clinical Aspects. 3rd ed. Philadelphia: WB Saunders, 1982

FREI DISEASE, see Durand-Nicolas-Favre disease. (Wilhelm S. Frei, 1885-1943, German dermatologist)

FREIBERG DISEASE, osteochondrosis of the head of the second metatarsal bone. (Albert H. Freiberg, 1869-1940, U.S. surgeon)

1. Freiberg AH: Munch Med Wochenschr 67:1289-1290, 1920

FREUND OPERATION, thoracic chondrotomy; resection of cartilages of the chest wall to improve mechanics of restoration and restore elasticity. (Wilhelm A. Freund, 1833-1918, German gynecologist)

1. Maffei WE: Os Fundamentos da Medicina. 2nd ed. Livraria Editora Artes Medicas Ltd, 1978

FREY SYNDROME, the classic form of hyperemia and sweating in the distribution of the auriculotemporal nerve. Cross-references: Auriculotemporal nerve syndrome; Baillarger syndrome; Gustatory sweating syndrome. (Lucie Frey, 1889-1944, Polish)

1. Balfour HH Jr, Bloom JE: The auriculotemporal syndrome beginning in infancy. J Pediatr 77:872-874, 1970
2. Frey L: Rev Neurol 2:97-104, 1923
3. Gorlin RJ, Cohen MM Jr, Levin LS: Syndromes of the Head and Neck. 3rd ed. New York: Oxford University Press, 1990

FREYER OPERATION, suprapubic enucleation of the hypertrophied prostate. (Peter Freyer, 1851-1921, British surgeon)

1. Maffei WE: Os Fundamentos da Medicina. 2nd ed. Livraria Editora Artes Medicas Ltd, 1978

FRICK OPERATION, blepharoplasty for correction of the entropion using a tongue-like graft from the cheek.

1. Maffei WE: Os Fundamentos da Medicina. 2nd ed. Livraria Editora Artes Medicas Ltd, 1978

FRIED SYNDROME, congenitally absent or conically shaped deciduous teeth, fine slow-growing scalp hair, scanty eyebrows, thin fingernails, small thin concave toenails, and normal sweating are features.

1. Fried K: J Med Genet 14:137-139, 1977
2. Gorlin RJ, Cohen MM Jr, Levin LS: Syndromes of the Head and Neck. 3rd ed. New York: Oxford University Press, 1990

FRIEDERICHSEN SYNDROME, see Waterhouse-Friederichsen syndrome.

FRIEDLÄNDER DISEASE, endarteritis obliterans. (Karl Friedländer, 1847-1887, German pathologist)

1. Friedländer K: Zentralbl Med Wiss 14:65-70, 1876

FRIEDMANN SYNDROME, a vasomotor disorder seen following head injury with symptoms of subacute brain swelling. A train or cycle of symptoms due to a progressive subacute encephalitis of traumatic origin; includes a sense of fullness in the head, headache, vertigo, irritability, insomnia, easy fatigability, and defects of memory. (Max Friedmann, 1858-1925, German)

1. Friedmann M: Zur Pathologischen Anatomie der Multiplen Chronischen Enzephalitis. Wien, 1883

FRIEDREICH ATAXIA, spinal hereditary ataxia; ataxia and loss of deep sensibility are characteristics. Posterior column degeneration affects the spinocerebellar tracts and sometimes the pyramidal tracts. (Nikolaus Friedreich, 1825-1882, German neurologist)

1. Friedreich N: Virchows Arch 36:391-419, 1863; 68:145-245, 1876
2. Haymaker W: Bing's Local Diagnosis in Neurological Diseases. 15th ed. St Louis: CV Mosby, 1969
3. Rowland LP (ed): Merritt's Textbook of Neurology. 9th ed. Baltimore: Williams & Wilkins, 1995

FRIEDREICH PHENOMENON, the tympanic percussion sound in pleuritis with effusion; varies in pitch during inspiration and expiration. (Nikolaus Friedreich)

1. Dorland's Medical Dictionary. 28th ed. Philadelphia: WB Saunders, 1994

FRIEDREICH SIGN, diastolic collapse of the cervical veins in pericardial effusion. (Nikolaus Friedreich)

1. Casas EC: Diccionario Terminologico de Ciencias Medicas. 5th ed. Salvat Editores, SA, 1954

FRÖHLICH SYNDROME, adiposogenital dystrophy; a clinical syndrome frequently associated with parasellar tumors that involve both the hypophysis and the hypothalamus. Cross-references: Adiposogenital syndrome; Babinski-Fröhlich syndrome. (Alfred Fröhlich, 1871-1953, Austrian-born U.S. neurologist)

1. Babinski J: Rev Neurol Par 8:531-535, 1900
2. Fröhlich A: Wien Klin Rundshan 15:833-836, 906-908, 1901
3. Grinker RR, Sahs AL: Neurology. 6th ed. Springfield: Charles C Thomas, 1966

FROIN SYNDROME, increased coagulation of cerebrospinal fluid (CSF) due to increased levels of albumin. Seen in certain organic nervous diseases in which the lumbar CSF is cut off from communication with the CSF in the ventricles. Cross-reference: Spinal block syndrome. (Georges Froin, French)

1. Froin G: Gaz Hop 76:1005-1006, 1903
2. Pedro-Pons A: Patologia-y-Clinica Medicus. Salvat Editores, SA, 1952

FROMENT PAPER SIGN, FROMENT TEST, FROMENT THUMB SIGN, when a sheet of paper is firmly grasped between the patient's thumb and index finger and is pulled, the proximal phalanx of the thumb is extended and the distal phalanx is flexed in ulnar nerve paralysis; the proximal phalanx is flexed and the distal phalanx extended in median nerve paralysis. (Jules Froment, 1878-1946, French)

1. Baker AB, Baker LH: Clinical Neurology. Revised ed. Philadelphia: Harper & Row, 1982
2. Sutherland S: Nerve and Nerve Injuries. Edinburgh: Churchill Livingstone, 1972

FRUGONI-RUMPEL-LEEDE SIGN, see Rumpel-Leede sign.

FROMMEL DISEASE, see Chiari-Frommel syndrome. (Richard J.E. Frommel, 1842-1912, German gynecologist)

FROMMEL OPERATION, shortening of the uterosacral ligaments to correct a malpositioned uterus. (Richard J.E. Frommel)

1. Maffei WE: Os Fundamentos da Medicina. 2nd ed. Livraria Editora Artes Medicas Ltd, 1978

FRONTAL POLAR SYNDROME, a personality change after frontal lobe injury was probably one of the very first neuropathological behavioral syndromes discovered in humans. Despite over 100 years of study, including clinical observations with postmortem correlation, stimulation during surgery and excisions, psychological investigations, and the detailed study in animals of anatomy, physiology, and the effect of tissue removal, remain perplexing the fundamental mechanisms of behavioral change after frontal lobe damage.

1. Bennett JC, Plum F (eds): Cecil Textbook of Medicine. 20th ed. Philadelphia: WB Saunders, 1996

FRONTODIGITAL SYNDROME, see Greig cephalopolysyndactyly syndrome.

FROST-LANG OPERATION, insertion of a gold ball in place of an enucleated eyeball. (William A. Frost, 1853-1935, British ophthalmologist; Basil T. Lang, 1880-1928, British ophthalmologist)

1. Maffei WE: Os Fundamentos da Medicina. 2nd ed. Livraria Editora Artes Medicas Ltd, 1978

FRYDMAN TRIGONOCEPHALY SYNDROME, trigonocephaly, premature metopic synostosis, ridging of the metopic suture, mild synophrys, hypotelorism, S-curved lower eyelids, preauricular tag, omphalocele, a large phallus, and a hemivertebra at L5 are features. Mental development is normal. Autosomal dominant inheritance.

1. Gorlin RJ, Cohen MM Jr, Levin LS: Syndromes of the Head and Neck. 3rd ed. New York: Oxford University Press, 1990

FRYNS SYNDROME, a lethal syndrome of diaphragmatic hernia; coarse facies, acral hypoplasia, and cleft palate are features. (J.P. Fryns, Belgian)
1. Aymé S, Julian C, Gambarelli D, et al: Fryns syndrome: report on 8 new cases. Clin Genet 35:191-201, 1989
2. Fryns JP, Moerman F, Goddeeris P, et al: A new lethal syndrome with cloudy corneae, diaphragmatic defects, and distal limb deformities. Hum Genet 50:65-70, 1979

FUCHS SYNDROME, unilateral heterochromia, fine keratic precipitates, and secondary cataract are features. (Ernst Fuchs, 1851-1930, Austrian ophthalmologist)
1. Fuchs E: Zschr Augenheilkd 15:191, 1906

FUERSTNER DISEASE, spastic paralysis with trembling. (Carl Fuerstner, 1848-1906, German psychiatrist)
1. Casas EC: Diccionario Terminologico de Ciencias Medicas. 5th ed. Salvat Editores, SA, 1954

FUKALA OPERATION, extraction of the crystalline lens in cases of myopia. (Vincent Fukala, 1847-1911, Austrian ophthalmologist)
1. Maffei WE: Os Fundamentos da Medicina. 2nd ed. Livraria Editora Artes Medicas Ltd, 1978

FUKUHARA SYNDROME, see MERRF syndrome.

FUKUYAMA SYNDROME, congenital muscular dystrophy; less severe than Walker-Warburg syndrome and with no retinal changes. Autosomal recessive inheritance. (Yukio Fukuyama, Japanese)
1. Fukuyama Y, Kawazuza M, Haruna H: Paediatr Univ Tokyo 4:5-8, 1960
2. Volpe J: Neurology of the Newborn. 3rd ed. Philadelphia: WB Saunders, 1995

FULL VALVE BLADDER SYNDROME, the progression of upper tract dilatation despite adequate valvular ablation in some patients. May result from elevated intravesical pressures at relatively low bladder volumes. The lack of bladder compliance may lead to functional obstruction of the ureter at the level of the bladder. The sensation of a full bladder seems to be diminished in this patient, further compounding the problem.
1. Campbell MF, Walsh PC: Campbell's Urology. 5th ed. Philadelphia: WB Saunders, 1986

FULLER OPERATION, 1) incision of the seminal vesicles; 2) prostatectomy by hypogastric section of the bladder. (Eugene Fuller, 1858-1930, U.S. urologist)
1. Maffei WE: Os Fundamentos da Medicina. 2nd ed. Livraria Editora Artes Medicas Ltd, 1978

FUNCTIONAL HYPOGLYCEMIC SYNDROME, see Harris syndrome.

FÜRBRINGER SIGN, in the patient with a subphrenic abscess, the needle transmits the respiratory movement. (Paul W. Fürbringer, 1849-1936, German)
1. Casas EC: Diccionario Terminologico de Ciencias Medicas. 5th ed. Salvat Editores, SA, 1954

G SYNDROME, see Hypertelorism-hypospadias syndrome. ("G" is the first letter of the surname of the affected person reported.)

GAENSLEN SIGN, with the patient lying supine and holding one knee and hip in a flexed position, the examiner presses the other leg over the edge of the table to produce hyperextension of the hip. In lumbosacral disease, there is pain on the affected side. (Frederick J. Gaenslen, 187-1937, U.S. surgeon)
1. Dorland's Medical Dictionary. 28th ed. Philadelphia: WB Saunders, 1994

GAILLIARD SYNDROME, migration of the heart to the right from retraction of the lungs and pleura to the right.
1. Casas EC: Diccionario Terminologico de Ciencias Medicas. 5th ed. 1954

GAILLARD-ARLT SUTURE, subcutaneous sutures on the eyelid for treatment of entropion. (François Gaillard, 1805-1869, French; Carl F. von Arlt, 1812-1887, Austrian ophthalmologist)
1. Maffei WE: Os Fundamentos da Medicina. 2nd ed. Livraria Editora Artes Medicas Ltd, 1978

GAISBÖCK SYNDROME, pseudopolycythemia and stress erythrocytosis; the patient has mild, persistent polycythemia, but no other evidence of disease. (Felix Gaisböck, 1868-1955, Austrian)
1. Black VD: Neonatal hyperviscosity syndromes. Curr Probl Pediatr 17:73-130, 1987
2. Gaisböck F: Dtsch Arch Klin Med 83:363-409, 1905
3. Ritchie AC: Boyd's Textbook of Pathology. 9th ed. Philadelphia: Lea & Febiger, 1990

GALASSI PUPILLARY PHENOMENON, eye-closure pupil reaction.
1. Dorland's Medical Dictionary. 28th ed. Philadelphia: WB Saunders, 1994

GALBIATI OPERATION, double ischiopubiotomy and forceps utilization when childbirth is complicated by a narrow pelvis.

1. Maffei WE: Os Fundamentos da Medicina. 2nd ed. Livraria Editora Artes Medicas Ltd, 1978

GALEAZZI SIGN, congenital dislocation of the pelvis causing scoliosis; seen in children 6-18 months of age. (Riccardo Galeazzi, 1866-1952, Italian orthopedic surgeon)

1. Campbell WC, Crenshaw AH: Campbell's Operative Orthopaedics. 7th ed. St Louis: CV Mosby, 1987

GALIPPE DISEASE, infectious gingivitis of the dental alveoli.

1. Casas EC: Diccionario Terminologico de Ciencias Medicas. 5th ed. Salvat Editores, SA, 1954

GALLOP SYNDROME, see Hare eye syndrome.

GALVAGNI DISEASE, peritoneal effusion in young women during puberty, with spontaneous resolution.

1. Casas EC: Diccionario Terminologico de Ciencias Medicas. 5th ed. Salvat Editores, SA, 1954

GAMBIA DISEASE, trypanosomiasis. (Gambia, West Africa)

1. Casas EC: Diccionario Terminologico de Ciencias Medicas. 5th ed. Salvat Editores, SA, 1954

GAMNA DISEASE, splenomegaly with thickening of the splenic capsule and the presence of small brownish areas (Gamna nodules) caused by ferruginous pigment being deposited in the splenic pulp. (Carlos Gamna, 1886-1950, Italian)

1. Casas EC: Diccionario Terminologico de Ciencias Medicas. 5th ed. Salvat Editores, SA, 1954

GAMSTORP SYNDROME, hyperkalemic periodic paralysis; recurrent attacks of muscular weakness, hereditary episodic adynamia, or hyperkalemic periodic paralysis are features. Clinically similar to familial periodic paralysis. (Ingrid Gamstorp, Swedish pediatrician)

1. Farmer TW: Pediatric Neurology. 2nd ed. Hagerstown: Harper & Row, 1975
2. Gamstorp I: Acta Pediatr Uppsala Suppl 108:1-126, 1956

GANGOLPHE SIGN, strangulated hernia with serosanguinous effusion in the abdomen.

1. Casas EC: Diccionario Terminologico de Ciencias Medicas. 5th ed. Salvat Editores, SA, 1954

GANSER SYNDROME, hysterical pseudodementia; the giving of incomplete answers to questions, often associated with amnesia, disorientation, perceptual disturbances, fugue, and conversion symptoms sometimes recognized among persons on the death row. (Sigbert J.M. Ganser, 1853-1931, German psychiatrist)

1. Ganser SJ: Arch Psychiatr Nervenkr 30:633-640, 1898
2. Peszke MA, et al: The Ganser syndrome: a diagnostic and etiological enigma. Conn Med 51:79-83, 1987

GANT OPERATION, division of the diaphysis of the femur just below the lesser trochanter in ankylosis of the hip.

1. Maffei WE: Os Fundamentos da Medicina. 2nd ed. Livraria Editora Artes Medicas Ltd, 1978

GAPO SYNDROME, *g*rowth retardation, *a*lopecia, *p*seudoanodontia, and *o*ptic atrophy (GAPO).

1. Gorlin RJ, Cohen MM Jr: Syndromes of the Head and Neck. 3rd ed. New York: Oxford University Press, 1990
2. Shapira Y, et al: Case report 85: Growth retardation, alopecia, pseudoanodontia and optic atrophy. Syndrome Ident 8:14-16, 1982
3. Tipton RE, Gorlin RJ: Am J Med Genet 19:209-216, 1984

GARCIN SYNDROME, unilateral involvement of all cranial nerves in malignant tumors invading the base of the skull, although meningiomas, basal meningitis, and trauma have been implicated. Typical progression may be to complete ophthalmoplegia and unilateral paralysis of all cranial nerves. Cross-reference: Half-base syndrome. (Raymond Garcin, 1897-1971, French)

1. Gorlin RJ, Cohen MM Jr: Syndromes of the Head and Neck. 3rd ed. New York: Oxford University Press, 1990
2. Schoenberg BS, Massey EW: Tapia's syndrome. The erratic evolution of an eponym. Arch Neurol 36:257-260, 1979

GARDNER SYNDROME, hereditary adenomatosis; a disorder inherited as a dominant trait and characterized by the triad of adenomas of the colon, bone tumors (osteomas), and soft tissue tumors (lipomas, sebaceous cysts, fibromas, fibrosarcomas). Hamartomas become evident by 10-20 years of age. A high risk of colonic carcinoma. (Eldon J. Gardner, U.S. geneticist)

1. Bennett JC, Plum F (eds): Cecil Textbook of Medicine. 20th ed. Philadelphia: WB Saunders, 1996
2. Gardner EJ: Am J Human Genet 3:167-176, 1951
3. Smith DW, Jones KL: Recognizable Patterns of Human Malformations: Genetic, Embryologic, and Clinical Aspects. 3rd ed. Philadelphia: WB Saunders, 1982

GARDNER-DIAMOND SYNDROME, autoerythrocyte sensitization; produces recurrent, painful erythematous, and purpuric lesions. Psychiatric disturbances may also be present. Affects only women, often at various times after operations related to reproductive organs. Cross-references: Autoerythrocyte sensitization syndrome; Painful bruising syndrome. (Frank H. Gardner, U.S.; Louis K. Diamond, U.S.)

1. Bennett JC, Plum F (eds): Cecil Textbook of Medicine. 20th ed. Philadelphia: WB Saunders, 1996
2. Gardner RH, Diamond LK: Autoerythrocyte sensitization: a form of purpura producing painful bruising following autosensitization to red cells in certain women. Blood 10:675-690, 1955
3. Moschella SL, Hurley HJ: Dermatology. 2nd ed. Philadelphia: WB Saunders, 1985

GARDNER-SILENGO-WACHTEL SYNDROME, cleft palate, male pseudohermaphroditism (46,XY gonadal digenesis), and conotruncal anomalies are feat. Most infants die during the neonatal period. Cross-reference: Genito-palato-cardiac syndrome. (L.I. Gardner U.S., Margherita Silengo, Italian)

1. Gardner LI: Lancet 2:667-668, 1970
2. Haymaker W: Bing's Local Diagnosis in Neurological Diseases. 15th ed. St Louis: CV Mosby, 1969
3. Silengo M, Kaufman RL, Kissane JA: Humangenetik 25:65-68, 1974
4. Wachtel SS: X-Y Antigen and Biology of Sex Determination. New York: Grune & Stratton, 1983

GAREL SIGN, see Heryng sign. (Jean Garel, 1852-1931, French)

GARLAND TRIANGLE, a triangular area of relative resonance near the vertebral column, on the same side as pleural effusion. (George M. Garland, 1848-1926, U.S.)

1. Casas EC: Diccionario Terminologico de Ciencias Medicas. 5th ed. Salvat Editores, SA, 1954

GARRÉ DISEASE, nonsuppurative sclerosing osteomyelitis. (Carl Garré, 1857-1928, Swiss surgeon)

1. Garré C: Beitr Klin Chir 10:241-298, 1893

GARRICK DISEASE, name given a contagious fever occurring in Dublin in 1742.

1. Casas EC: Diccionario Terminologico de Ciencias Medicas. 5th ed. Salvat Editores, SA, 1954

GÄRTNER VEIN PHENOMENON, fullness of the veins of the arm as it is raised to varying heights; indicates the degree of pressure in the right atrium. (Gustav Gärtner, 1855-1937, Austrian pathologist)

1. Dorland's Medical Dictionary. 28th ed. Philadelphia: WB Saunders, 1994

GAS DISEASE, see Gerstmann-Sträussler syndrome.

GASPERINI SYNDROME, dysfunction in the region of the 5th through the 8th cranial nerves ipsi-lateral to the lesion in association with sensory disturbances in the contralateral limbs and paralysis of conjugate ocular movement to the side of the affected cranial nerves.

1. Haymaker W: Bing's Local Diagnosis in Neurological Diseases. 15th ed. St Louis: CV Mosby, 1969

GASSER SYNDROME, characterized by microangiopathic hemolytic anemia, thrombocytopenia, and acute renal failure; most frequently in infants and young children. Cross-reference: Hemolytic-ure-mic syndrome. (Conrad J. Gasser, Swiss pediatrician)

1. Bennett JC, Plum F (eds): Cecil Textbook of Medicine. 20th ed. Philadelphia: WB Saunders, 1996
2. Gasser C, Gantier E, Steck A, et al: Schweiz Med Wochenschr 85:905-909, 1955
3. Neild G: The haemolytic uremic syndrome: a review. Am J Med 63:367-378, 1987

GASTON SYNDROME, alcoholic pruritus.

1. Casas EC: Diccionario Terminologico de Ciencias Medicas. 5th ed. 1954

GASTROCARDIAC SYNDROME, intestinal gas with chest pain. Cross-reference: Roemheld syn-drome.

1. Roemheld L: Z Phys Diat Ther 16:339-349, 1912

GAUCHER DISEASE, familial splenic anemia; a familial condition in which an intracellular defect of lipid metabolism occurs. The lymph glands, spleen, liver, and bones are involved, but the nervous system is seldom affected. Autosomal recessive trait affecting homozygosity. (Phillippe C.E. Gaucher, 1854-1918, French)

1. Grinker RR, Sahs AL: Neurology. 6th ed. Springfield: Charles C Thomas, 1966
2. Winkelman MD, Banker BQ, Victor M, et al: Non-infantile neuropathic Gaucher's disease: a clinicopathologic study. Neurology 33:994-1008, 1983

GAUR SIGN, pressure by a hernial sac on the superficial epigastric and/or circumflex iliac veins caus-ing distention of one or both veins on the side of the hernia. (Durga D. Gaur, Indian surgeon)

1. Bailey H: Physical Signs in Clinical Surgery. 16th ed. Baltimore: Williams & Wilkins, 1983

GAUSS SIGN, abnormal mobility of the uterus in the 1st month of pregnancy. (Karl J. Gauss, 1875-1957, German gynecologist)

1. Casas EC: Diccionario Terminologico de Ciencias Medicas. 5th ed. Salvat Editores, SA, 1954

GAUVAIN SIGN, the femur is rotated, provoking a peculiar type of reflex spasm of the abdominal muscles; seen in the patient with tuberculosis of the hip.

1. Evans RC: Illustrated Essentials in Orthopedic Physical Assessment. St Louis: Mosby Yearbook, 1994
2. Mazion JM: Illustrated Manual of Orthopedic Signs/Tests/Maneuvers for Office Procedure. 2nd ed. Orlando: Daniels Publishing, 1980

GAY BOWEL SYNDROME, transmission of enteric pathogens by variant sexual practices such as cunnilingus or anal eroticism. The protozoa as well as bacterial and viral pathogens are known to cause this disease.

1. Campbell MF, Walsh PC: Campbell's Urology. 5th ed. Philadelphia: WB Saunders, 1986

GAYET DISEASE, GAYET-WERNICKE SYNDROME, see Wernicke syndrome. (Charles J.A. Gayet, 1833-1904, French)

GAZA OPERATION, section of the rami communicantes for treating gastric crises.

1. Maffei WE: Os Fundamentos da Medicina. 2nd ed. Livraria Editora Artes Medicas Ltd, 1978

GEE DISEASE, GEE-HERTER DISEASE, GEE-HERTER-HEUBNER DISEASE, GEE-THAYSEN DISEASE, nontropical sprue in children; characterized by the passage of offensive fatty stools and changes in the bones similar to osteomalacia. Recommended treatment is a diet low in fat and high in calcium. Cross-references: Celiac syndrome; Herter-Heubner disease. (Samuel J. Gee, 1839-1911, British; Christian A. Herter, 1865-1910, U.S.; Otto Johann L. Heubner, 1843-1926, German pediatrician; Thorwald Thaysen, 1883-1936, Danish)

1. Bailey H, Love M: A Short Practice of Surgery. 12th ed. London: HK Lewis & Co, 1962
2. Gee S: St Bartholomews Hosp Rep 24:17-20, 1888
3. Herter CA: On Infantilism from Chronic Intestinal Infection. New York: Macmillan, 1908
4. Heuber OJ: Jahrb Kinderheilkd 70:667, 1909
5. Thaysen ET: Lancet 1:1086-1089, 1880

GÉLINEAU SYNDROME, narcolepsy and catatonia. (Jean B.E. Gélineau, 1859-1906, French neurologist)

1. Gélineau JBE: De la narcolepsie. Gaz Hop (Par) 53:626-628, 635-637, 1880

GELLÉ SYNDROME, crossed paralysis of limbs and hypoacusia, with facial paralysis of same side.

1. Gellé M: Compt Rendu Soc Biol 53:997-1000, 1901
2. Pedro-Pons A: Patologia-y-Clinica Medicus. Salvat Editores, SA, 1952

GENDER DYSPHORIA SYNDROME, psychological problems associated with a discrepancy between the physical sex assignment and the psychological gender identity.

1. Dorland's Medical Dictionary. 28th ed. Philadelphia: WB Saunders, 1994

GENDRIN SIGN, the patient perceives a shock-like feeling near the apex; seen in pericardial effusion.

1. Casas EC: Diccionario Terminologico de Ciencias Medicas. 5th ed. Salvat Editores, SA, 1954

GENÉE-WIEDEMANN SYNDROME, see Miller syndrome.

GENERAL ADAPTATION SYNDROME, the aggregate of all nonspecific systemic reactions of the body to long-continued exposure to systemic stress. Cross-reference: Selye syndrome.

1. Dorland's Medical Dictionary. 28th ed. Philadelphia: WB Saunders, 1994

GENERALIZED ANAPHYLACTIC SYNDROME, signs and symptoms may be varied, as the chemical mediators producing this disorder may start with a localized manifestation and progress to a potentially life-threatening systemic reaction within minutes. Usually the clinical patterns involve the skin, respiratory, or cardiovascular system; however, combinations of these may also occur.

1. Moschella SL, Hurley HJ: Dermatology. 2nd ed. Philadelphia: WB Saunders, 1985

GENERALIZED GANGLIOSIDOSIS SYNDROME TYPE I, see Caffey-pseudo-Hurler syndrome.

GENICULATE GANGLION SYNDROME, see Ramsay Hunt syndrome.

GENITAL ULCER SYNDROME, may be either ulcerative or nonulcerative. A disease that causes genitalial ulceration. The most common sexually transmitted nonulcerative genital lesions are due to scabies, genital warts, molluscum contagiosum, or *Candida* species, but the differential diagnosis includes a long list of dermatological conditions.

1. Bennett JC, Plum F (eds): Cecil Textbook of Medicine. 20th ed. Philadelphia: WB Saunders, 1996

GENITO-PALATO-CARDIAC SYNDROME, see Gardner-Silengo-Wachtel syndrome.

GENSOUD OPERATION, technique for resection of the maxilla.
1. Maffei WE: Os Fundamentos da Medicina. 2nd ed. Livraria Editora Artes Medicas Ltd, 1978

GENSOUL DISEASE, purulent inflammation around the submaxillary gland, caused by *Streptococcus*. Cross-reference: Ludovici disease.
1. Casas EC: Diccionario Terminologico de Ciencias Medicas. 5th ed. Salvat Editores, SA, 1954

GÉRARD-MARCHAND OPERATION, fixation of the rectum to the fibrous tissue around the coccyx in prolapse of the rectum.
1. Maffei WE: Os Fundamentos da Medicina. 2nd ed. Livraria Editora Artes Medicas Ltd, 1978

GERARDINI OPERATION, denudation followed by suture of the anterior and posterior walls of the vagina in prolapse of the uterus.
1. Maffei WE: Os Fundamentos da Medicina. 2nd ed. Livraria Editora Artes Medicas Ltd, 1978

GERBASI SYNDROME, familial hypoparathyroidism with pernicious anemia, steatorrhea, mental deficiency, and adrenocortical insufficiency are features. Been reported to resemble pernicious anemia in Sicilian infants. (Michele Gerbasi, Italian)
1. Farmer TW: Pediatric Neurology. 2nd ed. Hagerstown: Harper & Row, 1975
2. Gerbasi M: Pediatria Napoli 48:505-526, 1940

GERHARDT SIGN, see Biermer-Gerhardt sign. (Carl A.C.J. Gerhardt, 1833-1902, German; Anton Biermer, 1827-1892, German)

GERHARDT SYNDROME, bilateral paralysis of the abductor muscle of the vocal cords causing inspiratory dyspnea. (Carl A.C.J. Gerhardt)
1. Bordas LB: Neurologia Fundamental. 2nd ed. Toray, 1968
2. Gerhardt C: Arch Path Anat Berl 27:309, 1863

GERLIER SYNDROME, paralytic vertigo. (E. Felix Gerlier, 1840-1914, Swiss)
1. Gerlier EF: Rev Med Suisse Rom 7:5-29, 1887

GERSTMANN SYNDROME, the inability to recognize and use the fingers, to differentiate right from left, to write, and to calculate, most commonly resulting from lesions involving the angular and supramarginal gyri and the contiguous part of the occipital lobe. (Josef Gerstmann, 1887-1969, Austrian neuropsychiatrist)
1. Gerstmann J: Wien Klin Wochenschr 37:1010-1012, 1924
2. Grinker RR, Sahs AL: Neurology. 6th ed. Springfield: Charles C Thomas, 1966

GERSTMANN-STRÄUSSLER SYNDROME, GERSTMANN-STRÄUSSLER-SCHEINKER SYNDROME, a rare transmissible dementia, an uncommon variant of Creutzfeldt-Jakob disease characterized by a typical familial pattern, a high incidence of ataxia, and somewhat slower progression. Hyporeflexia or areflexia of lower extremities with a positive Babinski sign. Cross-reference: Prion syndrome. (Josef Gerstmann; E. Sträussler, Austrian)
1. Dohura K, et al: Creutzfeldt-Jakob disease patients with congophilic kuru plaques have the missense variant prion protein common to Gerstmann-Sträussler syndrome. Ann Neurol 27:121-126, 1990
2. Gerstmann J: Some notes on the Gerstmann syndrome. Neurology 7:866-869, 1957
3. Gerstmann J, Sträussler E, Scheinker I: Z Gesamte Neurol Psychiatr 154:736-762, 1936

GIANELLI SIGN, see Tournay sign. (Giuseppe Gianelli, 1799-1871, Italian)

GIANNOTTI-CROSTI SYNDROME, infantile papular acrodermatitis or papular acrodermatitis of childhood; a benign disease of young children with a presumably viral origin. (Ferdinando Giannotti, Italian dermatologist; Agostini Crosti, Italian dermatologist)
1. Crosti A: Gior Ital Dermatol Sif 71:305-340, 1930
2. Crosti A, Giannotti F: Dermatologica (Basel) 115:671-677, 1957
3. Krugman S, Katz SL: Infectious Diseases of Children. 7th ed. St Louis: CV Mosby, 1981

GIANT PLATELET SYNDROME, see Bernard-Soulier syndrome.

GIBNEY DISEASE, perispondylitis. (Virgil Gibney, 1847-1927, U.S. surgeon)
1. Casas EC: Diccionario Terminologico de Ciencias Medicas. 5th ed. Salvat Editores, SA, 1954

GIBRALTAR DISEASE, GIBRALTAR FEVER, brucellosis.
1. Dorland's Pocket Medical Dictionary. 22nd ed. Philadelphia: WB Saunders, 1977

GIERKE DISEASE, see Von Gierke disease.

GIFFORD OPERATION, destruction of the lacrimal sac through instillation of trichloroacetic acid.

(Harold Gifford, 1858-1929, U.S. ophthalmologist and otologist)
1. Maffei WE: Os Fundamentos da Medicina. 2nd ed. Livraria Editora Artes Medicas Ltd, 1978

GIFFORD SIGN, difficulty in everting the eyelid; seen in the patient with exophthalmic goiter. (Harold Gifford)
1. Casas EC: Diccionario Terminologico de Ciencias Medicas. 5th ed. Salvat Editores, SA, 1954

GIGLI OPERATION, pubiotomy; lateral section of the os pubis via a Gigli saw when childbirth is complicated by a narrow pelvis. Cross-reference: Siebold operation. (Leonardo Gigli, 1863-1908, Italian gynecologist)
1. Maffei WE: Os Fundamentos da Medicina. 2nd ed. Livraria Editora Artes Medicas Ltd, 1978

GILBERT SIGN, increased urination in the patient with cirrhosis. (Nicholas A. Gilbert, 1858-1927, French)
1. Casas EC: Diccionario Terminologico de Ciencias Medicas. 5th ed. Salvat Editores, SA, 1954

GILBERT SYNDROME, familial nonhemolytic jaundice; mild unconjugated hyperbilirubinemia is recognized most commonly during the 2nd and 3rd decades of life, due to the presence of scleral icterus. Follows a benign course. (Nicholas A. Gilbert)
1. Bennett JC, Plum F (eds): Cecil Textbook of Medicine. 20th ed. Philadelphia: WB Saunders, 1996
2. Ritchie AC: Boyd's Textbook of Pathology. 9th ed. Philadelphia: Lea & Febiger, 1990

GILCHRIST DISEASE, dermatitis blastomycetica; may be entirely cutaneous with chronic or sub-acute ulcerating lesions or may be a highly lethal systemic disease. The usual gross picture is that of a single large abscess or multiple small abscesses in the cerebrum, brain stem, or cerebellum. (Thomas C. Gilchrist, 1862-1927, U.S.)
1. Baker AB, Baker LH: Clinical Neurology. Revised ed. Philadelphia: Harper & Row, 1982
2. Gilchrist TC: Johns Hopkins Hosp Rep 1:169-190, 1896

GILFORD-BURNIER SYNDROME, see Septo-optic dysplasia syndrome.

GILL-WYLIE OPERATION, see Wylie operation.

GILLES DE LA TOURETTE SYNDROME, a tic disorder in which vocalizations occur as various involuntary and compulsive sounds (barking, sniffing, throat clearing, yelping noises) and words or fragments of words, often obscene (coprolalia). Motor tics may also include obscene gestures (copro-praxia). The age of onset is usually between 2 and 15 years. No anatomic abnormalities have been observed in the brain, but the consistency of the clinical syndrome gives evidence that it is an organic disorder. Cross-references: Guinon disease; Tourette syndrome. (Georges Gilles de la Tourette, 1857-1904, French neurologist)
1. Bennett JC, Plum F (eds): Cecil Textbook of Medicine. 20th ed. Philadelphia: WB Saunders, 1996
2. Gilles de la Tourette G: Arch Neurol 9:19-42, 158-200, 1885

GILLESPIE OPERATION, carpal resection through a dorsal, vertical incision between the extensor digitorum and extensor carpi ulnaris muscles.
1. Maffei WE: Os Fundamentos da Medicina. 2nd ed. Livraria Editora Artes Medicas Ltd, 1978

GILLESPIE SYNDROME, chronic ataxia with absence of the iris. (Frank D. Gillespie, U.S. ophthal-mologist)
1. Gillespie F: Aniridia, cerebellar ataxia and oligophrenia in siblings. Arch Ophthalmol 73:338-341, 1965
2. Rosenberg S: Neuropediatria. Sarvier, 1992

GILLIAM OPERATION, surgery to correct uterine retroversion; consists of fixation of each round ligament to the abdominal aponeurosis. (David T. Gilliam, 1844-1923, U.S. gynecologist)
1. Maffei WE: Os Fundamentos da Medicina. 2nd ed. Livraria Editora Artes Medicas Ltd, 1978

GILLIAN TURNER-TYPE X-LINKED MENTAL DEFICIENCY SYNDROME, mental defi-ciency in the male, unusual facies, and macro-orchidism are features. X-linked recessive inheritance.
1. Cantu JM, Scaglia HE, Medina M, et al: Inherited congenital normofunctional testicular hyperplasia and mental defi-ciency. Hum Genet 33:23-33, 1976
2. Smith DW, Jones KL: Recognizable Patterns of Human Malformations: Genetic, Embryologic, and Clinical Aspects. 3rd ed. Philadelphia: WB Saunders, 1982

GIOVANNINI DISEASE, a rare hair disease caused by a fungus and producing nodules. (Sebastiano Giovannini, 1851-1920, Italian)
1. Giovannini S: Vjschr Derm Syph 14:1097-2075, 1887

GIRDLESTONE OPERATION, drainage of coxofemoral tuberculosis after resection of the major

and the head of the femur. (Gathorne R. Girdlestone, 1851-1950, British orthopedist)
1. Maffei WE: Os Fundamentos da Medicina. 2nd ed. Livraria Editora Artes Medicas Ltd, 1978

GITELMAN SYNDROME, an autosomal recessive disorder characterized by metabolic alkalosis, hypomagnesemia, hypokalemia, and hypocalciuria. Reported to be linked to thiazide-sensitive Na-Cl cotransporter (TSC) gene mutation.
1. Monkawa T, Kurihara I, Kobayashi K, et al: J Am Soc Nephrol 11:65-70, 2000
2. Takeuchi K, et al: J Clin Endocrinol Metab 81:4496-4499, 1996

GITTES AND MCLAUGHLIN OPERATION, technique to obtain an artificial erection; described in 1974.
1. Campbell MF, Walsh PC: Campbell Urology. 5th ed. Philadelphia: WB Saunders, 1986

GLANZMANN DISEASE, hemorrhagic thrombasthenia; a moderately severe platelet disorder. Autosomal recessive inheritance. (Eduard Glanzmann, 1887-1959, Swiss clinician)
1. Glanzmann E: Jahrb Kinderheilkd 88:1-42, 1918
2. Moschella SL, Hurley HJ: Dermatology. 2nd ed. Philadelphia: WB Saunders, 1980
3. Ritchie AC: Boyd's Textbook of Pathology. 9th ed. Philadelphia: Lea & Febiger, 1990

GLASGOW SIGN, a systolic sound over the brachial artery; seen in cases of aortic aneurysm. (William C. Glasgow, 1845-1907, U.S.)
1. Casas EC: Diccionario Terminologico de Ciencias Medicas. 5th ed. Salvat Editores, SA, 1954

GLEASON GRADING TABLE, GLEASON SCORE, a classification for cancer of the prostate by evaluating glandular differentiation. Grades 1, 2, 3a, 3b, 3c, 4a, 4b, 5a, and 5b and stages A, B, C, and D depend on the clinical stage/involvement of the lesion. (Donald Gleason, U.S. pathologist)
1. Rosai J: Ackerman Surgical Pathology. 7th ed. St Louis: CV Mosby, 1989

GLÉNARD DISEASE, splanchnoptosis; prolapse or downward displacement of the viscera. (Franz Glénard, 1848-1920, French)
1. Glénard F: Sem Med Paris 6:211-212, 1886

GLINSKI-SIMMONDS SYNDROME, see Sheehan syndrome (Leon K. Glinski, 1870-1918, Polish)

GLIOMA-POLYPOSIS SYNDROME, see Turcot syndrome.

GLISSON DISEASE, rickets; a metabolic disease of childhood and infancy. (Francis Glisson, 1597-1677, British)
1. Casas EC: Diccionario Terminologico de Ciencias Medicas. 5th ed. Salvat Editores, SA, 1954

GLOMERULONEPHRITIS SYNDROME, glomerular involvement in an immune-mediated response to an exogenous toxin; may present with the clinical features of glomerulonephritis, with insidious proteinuria, hematuria, and nitrogen retention. Cross-references: Klebs disease; Renal parenchymal syndrome.
1. Klebs TAE: Handbuch der Pathologische Anatomie. Berlin: Hirschwald, 1870

GLUCAGONOMA SYNDROME, a glucagon-secreting tumor of the alpha cells of the pancreas associated with increased serum levels of glucagon, mild diabetes mellitus, weight loss, anemia, glossitis, stomatitis, angular cheilitis, blepharitis, necrolytic migrating erythema, and increased susceptibility to deep vein thrombosis.
1. Bloom SR, Polak JM: Glucagonoma syndrome. Am J Med 82 (Suppl 5B):25-35, 1987
2. MacGavran MH, et al: A glucagon-secreting alpha cell carcinoma of the pancreas. N Engl J Med 274:1408-1413, 1966

GLUCORONIDASE DEFICIENCY MUCOPOLYSACCHARIDOSIS, mucopolysaccharidosis type VII; Most patients present by age 3 with a Hurler syndrome-like illness manifested by frequent upper respiratory infections, chest deformities, cardiac murmurs, hepatosplenomegaly, hernias, dysostosis multiplex, and mild to moderate mental retardation. Corneal clouding may also develop. Results from a ß-glucuronidase deficiency. Cross-reference: Sly syndrome.
1. Gorlin RJ, Cohen MM Jr, Levin LS: Syndromes of the Head and Neck. 3rd ed. New York: Oxford University Press, 1990
2. Sly WS, Quinton BA, McAlister WN, et al: Beta-glucuronidase deficiency. Report of clinical, radiological, and biochemical features of a new mucopolysaccharidosis. J Pediatr 82:249-257, 1973

GLUK OPERATION, total laryngectomy.
1. Maffei WE: Os Fundamentos da Medicina. 2nd ed. Livraria Editora Artes Medicas Ltd, 1978

GODTFREDSEN SYNDROME, see Cavernous sinus syndrome. (Erik Godtfredsen, Danish radiologist)

GOEMINNE SYNDROME, congenitally progressive muscular torticollis with facial asymmetry, multiple spontaneous keloids, cryptorchidism, chronic progressive pyelonephritis with hypertension, varicose veins of the legs, and multiple pigmented cutaneous nevi. The gene has been mapped at Xq28, distal to the G6PD locus. (Luc Goeminne, Belgian)
> 1. Goeminne L: Acta Genet Med Gemellol (Roma) 17:439-467, 1968
> 2. Gorlin RJ, Cohen MM Jr: Syndromes of the Head and Neck. 3rd ed. New York: Oxford University Press, 1990

GOFFE OPERATION, surgery for vaginal cystocele.
> 1. Maffei WE: Os Fundamentos da Medicina. 2nd ed. Livraria Editora Artes Medicas Ltd, 1978

GOGGIA SIGN, pinching does not produce muscle contraction of the biceps; seen in the patient with typhoid fever. (Carlo P. Goggia, 1871-1948, Italian)
> 1. Casas EC: Diccionario Terminologico de Ciencias Medicas. 5th ed. Salvat Editores, SA, 1954

GOLABI-ROSEN SYNDROME, see Simpson-Golabi-Behmel syndrome.

GOLDBERG SYNDROME, sialidase and ß-galactosidase deficiency. Resembles mucolipidosis type I, but is milder and seen more often in the patient of Japanese origin. (Morton Goldberg, U.S.)
> 1. Goldberg M: Arch Intern Med 128:387-398, 1971

GOLDBERG-MAXWELL SYNDROME, see Testicular feminization syndrome. (Minni B. Goldberg, U.S.)

GOLDBLATT PHENOMENON, ischemic tubular atrophy; a characteristic of renovascular hypertension. (Harry Goldblatt, 1891-1977, U.S. pathologist)
> 1. Dorland's Medical Dictionary. 28th ed. Philadelphia: WB Saunders, 1994

GOLDEN SIGN, a pale uterus indicating the possibility of a tubal pregnancy.
> 1. Casas EC: Diccionario Terminologico de Ciencias Medicas. 5th ed. Salvat Editores, SA, 1954

GOLDENHAR SYNDROME, oculoauriculovertebral dysplasia; features include defects in the 1st and 2nd branchial arches, oculoauriculovertebral dysplasia, hemifacial microsomia, hypoplasia of the facial musculature, malfunction of the soft palate, microtia, and hemivertebrae or hypoplasia of the vertebrae. Etiology unknown. Cross-reference: OAV syndrome. (Maurice Goldenhar, Swiss)
> 1. Converse JM, Coccaro PJ, Becker M, et al: On hemifacial microsomia. The first and second branchial arch syndrome. Plast Reconstr Surg 51:268-279, 1973
> 2. Goldenhar M: J Genet Hum 1:243-282, 1952
> 3. Smith DW, Jones KL: Recognizable Patterns of Human Malformations: Genetic, Embryologic, and Clinical Aspects. 3rd ed. Philadelphia: WB Saunders, 1982

GOLDFLAM DISEASE, myasthenia gravis; asthenic bulbar palsy without an anatomical basis. A chronic disorder characterized by variable weakness of the skeletal muscles following continued use. Cardiac and smooth muscles are not involved. Cross-references: Erb-Goldflam disease; Hoppe-Goldflam syndrome. (Samuel V. Goldflam, 1852-1932, Polish neurologist)
> 1. Erb W: Arch Psychiatr 9:336-350, 1879
> 2. Farmer TW: Pediatric Neurology. 2nd ed. Hagerstown: Harper & Row, 1975
> 3. Goldflam SV: Dtsch Z Nervenheilkd 4:312-352, 1893

GOLDSCHEIDER SYNDROME, see Weber-Cockayne syndrome (Johann K.A. E. Goldscheider, 1858-1935, German)

GOLDSPOHN OPERATION, destruction of uterine adherents using the surgeon's finger introduced through the abdomen.
> 1. Maffei WE: Os Fundamentos da Medicina. 2nd ed. Livraria Editora Artes Medicas Ltd, 1978

GOLDSTEIN DISEASE, hereditary hemorrhagic telangiectasia. (Hyman I. Goldstein, 1887-1954, U.S.)
> 1. Casas EC: Diccionario Terminologico de Ciencias Medicas. 5th ed. Salvat Editores, SA, 1954

GOLDSTEIN SIGN, the gap between the 1st and 2nd toes is larger than normal; seen in mongolism and in cretinism. (Hyman I. Goldstein)
> 1. Casas EC: Diccionario Terminologico de Ciencias Medicas. 5th ed. Salvat Editores, SA, 1954

GOLDSTON SYNDROME, see Epidermolysis bullosa syndrome. (Johann K. Goldston, 1858-1935, German)

GOLDTHWAIT OPERATION, surgery for recurrent luxation of the patella, consisting of a longitudinal incision in the patellar tendon and transplantation and suture of its lateral half to the periosteum of the anteromedial surface of the tibia. (Joel E. Goldthwait, 1866-1961, U.S. orthopedic surgeon)

1. Maffei WE: Os Fundamentos da Medicina. 2nd ed. Livraria Editora Artes Medicas Ltd, 1978

GOLDTHWAIT SIGN, a test for a sprain of the sacroiliac joint; with the patient lying supine, there is pain before the motion of the vertebral column begins when the leg is elevated. (Joel E. Goldthwait)

1. Casas EC: Diccionario Terminologico de Ciencias Medicas. 5th ed. Salvat Editores, SA, 1954

GOLONBOV SIGN, pain on percussion of the tibia; seen in the patient with idiopathic hypochromic anemia.

1. Casas EC: Diccionario Terminologico de Ciencias Medicas. 5th ed. Salvat Editores, SA, 1954

GOLTZ SYNDROME, poikiloderma with focal dermal hypoplasia, syndactyly, and dental anomalies are features. Cross-reference: Focal dermal hypoplasia syndrome. (Robert W. Goltz, U.S. dermatologist)

1. Goltz RW, Peterson WC, Gorlin RJ, et al: Focal dermal hypoplasia. Arch Dermatol 86:708-717, 1962
2. Smith DW, Jones KL: Recognizable Patterns of Human Malformations: Genetic, Embryologic, and Clinical Aspects. 3rd ed. Philadelphia: WB Saunders, 1982

GOMBO SYNDROME, *g*rowth retardation, *o*cular abnormalities, *m*icrocephaly, *b*rachydactyly, and *o*ligophrenia (GOMBO). Autosomal recessive inheritance.

1. Verloes A, et al: GOMBO syndrome of growth retardation, ocular abnormalities, microcephaly, brachydactyly and oligophrenia: a possible "new" recessively inherited MCA/MR syndrome. Am J Med Genet 32:15-18, 1989

GONDA SIGN, see Allen sign.

GONIN OPERATION, thermocautery of the fissure in the retina for retinal detachment. (Jules Gonin, 1870-1935, Swiss ophthalmic surgeon)

1. Maffei WE: Os Fundamentos da Medicina. 2nd ed. Livraria Editora Artes Medicas Ltd, 1978

GOOD SYNDROME, thymoma with chronic mucocutaneous candidiasis. Characteristically, this patient is healthy until the 3rd or 4th decade of life, at which time he/she develops signs of immunodeficiency including chronic mucocutaneous candidiasis, diarrhea, failure to thrive, recurrent bacterial and viral infections, and autoimmune disease. (Robert A. Good, U.S.)

1. Good RA: Bull Univ Minn Hosp 26:1-19, 1954
2. Mayo Clin Proc 68:1110-1123, 1993
3. Southern Med J 90:444, 1997

GOODELL SIGN, softening of the uterus; an indication of pregnancy. (William Goodell, 1829-1894, U.S. gynecologist)

1. Casas EC: Diccionario Terminologico de Ciencias Medicas. 5th ed. Salvat Editores, SA, 1954

GOODMAN SYNDROME, acrocephalopolysyndactyly type IV; clinodactyly, ulnar deviation, and congenital heart disease are features. (Richard M. Goodman)

1. Goodman RM, Steinberg M, Shem-Toy Y, et al: Acrocephalopolysyndactyly type IV: a new genetic syndrome in three siblings. Clin Genet 15:209-214, 1979

GOODPASTURE SYNDROME, characterized by diffuse pulmonary hemorrhage, interstitial lung disease, glomerulonephritis, and circulating antiglomerular basement membrane and antialveolar basement membrane antibodies. Can be mimicked by systemic lupus erythematosus, Wegener granulomatosis, or the systemic necrotizing vasculitides. Cross-reference: Ceelen-Gellerstedt syndrome. (Ernest W. Goodpasture, 1886-1960, U.S. pathologist)

1. Goodpasture EW: The significance of certain pulmonary lesions in relation to the etiology of influenza. Am J Med Sci 158:863-870, 1919
2. Ritchie AC: Boyd's Textbook of Pathology. 9th ed. Philadelphia: Lea & Febiger, 1990

GOPALAN SYNDROME, a constellation of symptoms resulting from malnutrition, with signs suggestive of riboflavin deficiency, a burning sensation in the extremities, a feeling of "pins and needles" in the distal limbs, and hyperhidrosis. Cross-reference: Burning feet syndrome. (C. Gopalan, Indian biochemist)

1. Gopalan C: Indian Med Gaz 81:22-26, 1946

GORDON SIGN, *See* Finger phenomenon. (Alfred Gordon, 1874-1953, U.S. neurologist/psychiatrist)

1. Dorland's Medical Dictionary. 28th ed. Philadelphia: WB Saunders, 1994

GORDON SYNDROME, distal arthrogryposis type IIa; camptodactyly, talipes, and cleft palate are features. Nevus flammeus, stenosis of the spinal canal, narrowed intervertebral spaces, and cryptorchism are sometimes associated. (Hymie Gordon, South African)

1. Gordon H, Davies D, Berman M: Camptodactyly, cleft palate and club foot. A syndrome showing the autosomal dominant pattern of inheritance. J Med Genet 6:266-274, 1969
2. Gorlin RJ, Cohen MM Jr: Syndromes of the Head and Neck. 3rd ed. New York: Oxford University Press, 1990
3. Hall JG, Reed SD, Greene G: The distal arthrogryposes: delineation of new entities. Review and nosologic discussion. Am J Med Genet 11:185-239, 1982

GORLIN SYNDROME, see Basal cell nevus syndrome. (Robert J. Gorlin, U.S. dental pathologist)

GOSSELIN SIGN, ether sprayed on a lesion becomes hard if it is a tumor, but exhibits no change if an abscess.

1. Casas EC: Diccionario Terminologico de Ciencias Medicas. 5th ed. Salvat Editores, SA, 1954

GOTTINGA DISEASE, typhoid fever.

1. Casas EC: Diccionario Terminologico de Ciencias Medicas. 5th ed. Salvat Editores, SA, 1954

GOTTRON SIGN, symmetrical macular violaceous erythema overlying the dorsal aspect of the interphalangeal joints of the hands; present in dermatomyositis. (Heinrich Gottron, 1890-1974, German dermatologist)

1. Dorland's Medical Dictionary. 28th ed. Philadelphia: WB Saunders, 1994

GOTTSCHALK OPERATION, shortening of the uterosacral ligaments through the vagina.

1. Maffei WE: Os Fundamentos da Medicina. 2nd ed. Livraria Editora Artes Medicas Ltd, 1978

GOUGEROT-CARTEAUD SYNDROME, acanthosis nigricans or confluent and reticulate papillomatosis. The primary lesion is a slightly keratotic papule up to 5 mm in diameter. The centrally located papules tend to become confluent and the peripherally located papules tend to become reticulate. This disorder is probably a genodermatosis; it favors girls, especially those at or near puberty. (Henri Gougerot, 1881-1955, French; Alexander Carteaud, French)

1. Gougerot H, Carteaud A: Bull Soc Fr Derm Syph 34:719-721, 1927
2. Moschella SL, Hurley HJ: Dermatology. 2nd ed. Philadelphia: WB Saunders, 1985

GOUGEROT-HOUWER-SJÖGREN SYNDROME, see Sjögren syndrome. (Henri Gougerot)

GOULD SIGN, in a peripheral lesion of the retina, the patient must bend forward and elevate the head while walking up an incline.

1. Casas EC: Diccionario Terminologico de Ciencias Medicas. 5th ed. Salvat Editores, SA, 1954

GOULEY OPERATION, total amputation of the penis and fixation of the urethra to the perineum. (John W.S. Gouley, 1832-1920, U.S. urologist)

1. Maffei WE: Os Fundamentos da Medicina. 2nd ed. Livraria Editora Artes Medicas Ltd, 1978

GOULEY SYNDROME, see Stiff heart syndrome.

GOULIAN OPERATION, dermal mastopexy.

1. Schwartz SI: Principles of Surgery. 4th ed. New York, NY: McGraw-Hill, 1983

GOURAND DISEASE, inguinal hernia.

1. Casas EC: Diccionario Terminologico de Ciencias Medicas. 5th ed. Salvat Editores, SA, 1954

GOWERS SIGN, GOWERS PHENOMENON, the inability of a patient to stand from a sitting position with the arms outstretched; present in Duchenne disease. (Sir William R. Gowers, 1845-1915, British neurologist))

1. Campbell WC, Crenshaw AH: Campbell's Operative Orthopaedics. 7th ed. St Louis: CV Mosby, 1987
2. Rowland LP (ed): Merritt's Textbook of Neurology. 9th ed. Baltimore: Williams & Wilkins, 1995

GOWERS SYNDROME, see Foster-Kennedy syndrome. (Sir William R. Gowers)

GRABER-DUVERNAY OPERATION, surgery for chronic arthritis of the hip, consisting of making small canals in the head of the femur in order to modify the blood circulation in the area.

1. Maffei WE: Os Fundamentos da Medicina. 2nd ed. Livraria Editora Artes Medicas Ltd, 1978

GRADENIGO SYNDROME, GRADENIGO-LANNOIS SYNDROME, disease in the petrous apex producing irritation and dysfunction of the 5th and 6th cranial nerves; lateral rectus paralysis is a feature. Cross-reference: Lannois-Gradenigo syndrome. (Giuseppe Gradenigo, 1859-1926, Italian otolaryngologist; Maurice Lannois, French)

1. Ballenger JJ: Diseases of the Nose, Throat, Ear, Head and Neck. 12th ed. Philadelphia: Lea & Febiger, 1977

2. Gradenigo G: Sulla leptomeninge circonscritta e sulla paralisi dell'abducente di origine otitica. Gior Accad Med Torino 10:59-84, 1904

GRADENIGO TRIAD, triad consists of otitis, abducens paralysis, and deep pain. (Giuseppe Gradenigo)
   1. Rimbaud L: Compendio de Neurologia. Livraria Editora Freitas Bastos, 1940

GRAEFE DISEASE, see Von Graefe syndrome. (Albrecht F.W.E.A. von Graefe, 1828-1870, German ophthalmologist)

GRAEFE OPERATION, 1) cataract surgery through an incision in the sclera, with laceration of the capsule, and iridectomy; 2) resection of the cornea and adjacent sclera prior to evisceration of the globe. (Albrecht F.W.E.A. von Graefe)
   1. Maffei WE: Os Fundamentos da Medicina. 2nd ed. Livraria Editora Artes Medicas Ltd, 1978

GRAEFE SIGN, see Von Graefe sign. (Albrecht F.W.E.A. von Graefe)

GRAHAM LITTLE SYNDROME, lichen planopilaris; characterized by the presence of cicatricial patches of alopecia of the scalp, with prominent follicular plugging and follicular keratoses involving the trunk and extremities and sometimes associated with noncicatricial alopecia of the axillae, pubes, trunk, and extremities. (Ernest G. Graham Little, 1867-1950, British)
   1. Dorland's Medical Dictionary. 28th ed. Philadelphia: WB Saunders, 1994

GRAHAM STEELL MURMUR, a diastolic murmur associated with pulmonary hypertension. (Graham Steell, 1851-1942, British)
   1. Fowler NO: Cardiac Diagnosis and Treatment. 3rd ed. Cambridge: Harper & Row, 1980

GRANCHER DISEASE, splenopneumonia. Cross-reference: Desnos disease. (Jacques J. Grancher, 1843-1907, French)
   1. Grancher JJ: Union Med Paris 36:1078-1081, 1883

GRANCHER SIGN, when the inspiratory and expiratory sounds are equal, there is obstruction of the airway.
   1. Casas EC: Diccionario Terminologico de Ciencias Medicas. 5th ed. Salvat Editores, SA, 1954

GRANDDAD SYNDROME, *g*rowth *r*etardation, *a*ged facies, *n*ormal *d*evelopment, *d*ecreased subcutaneous fat, *a*utosomal *d*ominant (GRANDDAD).
   1. Marion RW, et al: The GRANDDAD syndrome: a disorder combining aged facies, normal development and deficiency of subcutaneous fat. Am J Hum Genet 45 (Suppl 4):53, 1989

GRANDMONT OPERATION, surgery for eyelid ptosis.
   1. Maffei WE: Os Fundamentos da Medicina. 2nd ed. Livraria Editora Artes Medicas Ltd, 1978

GRANGER SIGN, on a skull x-ray of a child, poor visibility of the anterior wall of the lateral sinus indicates destruction of the mastoid process. (Amedee Granger, 1879-1939, U.S. radiologist)
   1. Casas EC: Diccionario Terminologico de Ciencias Medicas. 5th ed. Salvat Editores, SA, 1954

GRANT OPERATION, ablation of a lip tumor using a square en bloc resection. Triangular patches are obtained from each angle of the square and sutured to the center of the defect.
   1. Maffei WE: Os Fundamentos da Medicina. 2nd ed. Livraria Editora Artes Medicas Ltd, 1978

GRASSET SYNDROME, syringomyelia with vasomotor disturbance.
   1. Casas EC: Diccionario Terminologico de Ciencias Medicas. 5th ed. 1954

GRASSET-GAUSSEL PHENOMENON, see Phenomenon of Grasset and Gaussel. (Joseph Grasset; Amans Gaussel)

GRASSET-GAUSSEL-HOOVER SIGN, see Hoover sign. (Joseph Grasset; Amans Gaussel; Charles F. Hoover, 1865-1927, U.S.)

GRAVES DISEASE, a triad of hyperthyroidism, goiter, and exophthalmos. Hyperthyroidism has been stimulated by higher centers via the hypothalamus; imitates disorders of excessive sympathetic stimulation. Signs and symptoms include loss of strength, tachycardia, weight loss, and irritability. Cross-references: Basedow disease; Begbie disease; Flajani disease; Jod-Basedow syndrome; Parry disease; Von Basedow disease. (Robert J. Graves, 1796-1853, Irish)
   1. Flajani G: Sopra un Tumore Freddo nell'Anteriore parte del Collo. Rome, 1802
   2. Graves RJ: Lond Med Surg J, 1835, pp 516-517
   3. Grinker RR, Sahs AL: Neurology. 6th ed. Springfield: Charles C Thomas, 1966
   4. Von Basedow CA: Wochenschr Ges Heilkd, 1840, pp 197-204

GRAWITZ DISEASE, basophilia. (Paul A. Grawitz, 1850-1932, German pathologist)

1. Grawitz PA: Arch Pathol Berl 93:39-63, 1883

GRAY BABY SYNDROME, a potentially fatal condition seen in neonates, particularly premature infants, due to a reaction to chloramphenicol and characterized by an ashen gray cyanosis, listlessness, weakness, hypotension, and occasionally jaundice.

1. Dorland's Medical Dictionary. 28th ed. Philadelphia: WB Saunders, 1994

GRAY SIGN, pain caused by pressure applied 5 cm below and to the left of the umbilicus; seen in appendicitis.

1. Casas EC: Diccionario Terminologico de Ciencias Medicas. 5th ed. Salvat Editores, SA, 1954

GRAY SPINAL SYNDROME, muscular atrophy, syringomyelic disturbances of sensation, and vaso-motor dysfunction due to lesions of the gray matter of the spinal cord.

1. Dorland's Medical Dictionary. 28th ed. Philadelphia: WB Saunders, 1994

GREBE SYNDROME, achondrogenesis; marked distal limb reduction, polydactyly, and normal facies are features. Autosomal recessive inheritance. (Hans Grebe, German)

1. Grebe H: Erb Folia Hered Pathol 2:23-28, 1952
2. Scott CI: Skeletal dysplasias. Birth Defects 5(3):14, 1969
3. Smith DW, Jones KL: Recognizable Patterns of Human Malformations: Genetic, Embryologic, and Clinical Aspects. 3rd ed. Philadelphia: WB Saunders, 1982

GREEN MONKEY DISEASE, see Marburg virus disease.

GREENE SIGN, lateral displacement of the free cardiac edge in pleural effusion, determined by percussion. (Charles L. Greene, 1862-1929, U.S.)

1. Casas EC: Diccionario Terminologico de Ciencias Medicas. 5th ed. Salvat Editores, SA, 1954

GREENFIELD SYNDROME, late infantile form of metachromatic leukodystrophy. Autosomal recessive inheritance. (J. Godwin Greenfield, 1884-1958, British neuropathologist)

1. Greenfield JG: Brain 73:291-316, 1950
2. Greenfield JG: J Neuro Psychopathol 13:289-302, 1933
3. Greenfield JG: Proc R Soc Med Lond 26:690-697, 1932/1933
4. Haberg B: Neurometabolische Krankheiten in Padiatrische Neurologic. Berlin: Springer-Verlag, 1971

GREENHOW DISEASE, discoloration of the skin in persons subjected to louse bites over long periods. Cross-reference: Vagabond disease. (Edward H. Greenhow, 1814-1888, British)

1. Greenhow EH: Trans Clin Soc Lond 6:44-47, 1846

GREIG CEPHALOPOLYSYNDACTYLY SYNDROME, cephalopolysyndactyly, frontonasal dysplasia, or acrofacial dysostosis. The combination of frontal bossing, scaphocephaly, hypertelorism, broad thumbs and halluces, pre- and postaxial polydactyly of the hands and feet, and variable syndactyly of the fingers and toes. Cross-references: Frontodigital syndrome; Hootnick-Holmes syndrome. (David M. Greig, 1864-1936, Scottish)

1. Gorlin RJ, Cohen MM Jr: Syndromes of the Head and Neck. 3rd ed. New York: Oxford University Press, 1990
2. Greig DM: Oxicephaly. Edinb Med J 33:189-218, 1926
3. Volpe J: Neurology of the Newborn. 3rd ed. Philadelphia: WB Saunders, 1995

GREIG DISEASE, ocular hypertelorism as an isolated anomaly. (David M. Greig)

1. Baker AB, Baker LH: Clinical Neurology. Revised ed. Philadelphia: Harper & Row, 1982
2. Greig DM: Hypertelorism: a hitherto undifferentiated congenital craniofacial deformity. Edinb Med J 31:560-593, 1924

GREY BABY SYNDROME, see Gray baby syndrome.

GREY TURNER SIGN, a bruise-like discoloration of the skin of the left flank; seen in the patient with pancreatitis or other abdominal hemorrhage. Cross-reference: Turner sign. (George Grey Turner, 1877-1951, British surgeon)

1. Bennett JC, Plum F (eds): Cecil Textbook of Medicine. 20th ed. Philadelphia: WB Saunders, 1996

GRIESINGER SIGN, edematous bulging over the mastoid process due to thrombosis of the transverse sinus. (Wilhelm Griesinger, 1817-1868, German neurologist)

1. Casas EC: Diccionario Terminologico de Ciencias Medicas. 5th ed. Salvat Editores, SA, 1954

GRIESINGER-KUSSMAUL SIGN, a paradoxical pulse in pericardial effusion.

1. Casas EC: Diccionario Terminologico de Ciencias Medicas. 5th ed. Salvat Editores, SA, 1954

GRIFFITH SIGN, the lower eyelid is slow on upward gaze; seen in the patient with Graves disease. (J. Griffith, British ophthalmologist)

1. Dorland's Medical Dictionary. 28th ed. Philadelphia: WB Saunders, 1994

GRIP SIGN, with the examiner's fingers inserted into the contracted hand of the patient, the patient's grip is relaxed when the hand is passively flexed at the forearm but is increased as the hand is extended.
1. Baker AB, Baker LH: Clinical Neurology. Revised ed. Philadelphia: Harper & Row, 1982

GRIPPE-LIKE SYNDROME, rickettsialpox; within 1 week after the initial lesion develops, there is a sudden onset of fever, chills, headache, malaise, and backache.
1. Krugman S, Katz SL: Infectious Diseases of Children. 7th ed. St Louis: CV Mosby, 1981

GRISCELLI SYNDROME, characterized by hypomelanosis, frequent pyogenic infections, hepato-splenomegaly, neutro- and thrombopenia, and possible immunodeficiency. An autosomal recessive form of albinoidism. Cross-references: Chédiak-Higashi-like syndrome; Hypopigmentation-immunodeficiency disease. (Claude Griscelli, French)
1. Griscelli C, Durandy A, Guy-Grand D, et al: A syndrome associating partial albinism and immunodeficiency. Am J Med 65:691-702, 1978

GRISEL SYNDROME, "nasopharyngeal" torticollis; torticollis of the prevertebral muscles caused by acute inflammation of the nasopharynx. (P. Grisel, French)
1. Grisel P: Presse Med 38:50-53, 1930

GRISOLLE SIGN, the skin next to a bump is pulled. If the bump flattens, measles is indicated; if not, variola is indicated. (Augustin Grisolle, 1811-1869, French)
1. Casas EC: Diccionario Terminologico de Ciencias Medicas. 5th ed. Salvat Editores, SA, 1954

GROCCO SIGN, myocardial hypertrophy caused by exophthalmic goiter. (Pietro Grocco, 1856-1916, Italian)
1. Casas EC: Diccionario Terminologico de Ciencias Medicas. 5th ed. Salvat Editores, SA, 1954

GRÖNBLAD-STRANDBERG SYNDROME, GRÖNBLAD-STRANDBERG-TOURAINE SYNDROME, pseudoxanthoma elasticum; a generalized progressive connective tissue disorder primarily affecting the elastic fibers. Clinically, it manifests as characteristic cutaneous lesions, ocular changes, and widespread vascular abnormalities. (Ester E. Grönblad, 1898-1942, Swedish ophthalmologist; James Strandberg, 1883-1942, Swedish dermatologist)
1. Bennett JC, Plum F (eds): Cecil Textbook of Medicine. 20th ed. Philadelphia: WB Saunders, 1996
2. McKusick VA: Heritable Disorders of Connective Tissue. 4th ed. St Louis: CV Mosby, 1972

GROSS DISEASE, encysted rectum; formation of pouches on the mucous membrane of the rectum. (Samuel D. Gross, 1805-1884, U.S. surgeon)
1. Casas EC: Diccionario Terminologico de Ciencias Medicas. 5th ed. Salvat Editores, SA, 1954

GROSS-GROH-WEPPL SYNDROME, see Rosselli-Gulienetti syndrome.

GROSS-VOGT OPERATION, pediatric surgery for an esophageal fistula.
1. Schwartz SI: Principles of Surgery. 4th ed. New York: McGraw-Hill, 1983

GROSSMAN SIGN, myocardial hypertrophy; seen in pulmonary tuberculosis. (Morris Grossman, 1881-1955, U.S. neurologist)
1. Casas EC: Diccionario Terminologico de Ciencias Medicas. 5th ed. Salvat Editores, SA, 1954

GROSSMANN OPERATION, surgery for retinal detachment, consisting of aspiration of the subretinal fluid and slow injection of warm saline into the vitreous humor.
1. Maffei WE: Os Fundamentos da Medicina. 2nd ed. Livraria Editora Artes Medicas

GRUBER SYNDROME, see Meckel syndrome. (Georg Gruber, 1884-1977, German pathologist)

GRUBY DISEASE, a form of tinea capitis in children caused by *Trichophyton microsporon*. (David Gruby, 1810-1898, French)
1. Gruby D: Compt Rendu Acad Sci Paris 17:301-303, 1843

GRÜNTZIG OPERATION, a balloon angioplasty procedure. (Andreas Grüntzig, 1939-1985, German radiologist)
1. Schwartz SI: Principles of Surgery. 4th ed. New York: McGraw-Hill, 1983

GUBLER SIGN, a tumor on the back of the wrist caused by lead poisoning. (Adolphe M. Gubler, 1821-1879, French)
1. Casas EC: Diccionario Terminologico de Ciencias Medicas. 5th ed. Salvat Editores, SA, 1954

GUBLER SYNDROME, see Millard-Gubler syndrome. (Adolphe M. Gubler)

GUÉRIN OPERATION, 1) partial resection of the maxilla; 2) cruciform iridotomy through the cornea.
1. Maffei WE: Os Fundamentos da Medicina. 2nd ed. Livraria Editora Artes Medicas Ltd, 1978

GUGLIELMO SYNDROME, see Di Guglielmo syndrome.

GUILLAIM-THAOM SYNDROME, neurosyphilis with tabes dorsalis.
1. Casas EC: Diccionario Terminologico de Ciencias Medicas. 5th ed. 1954

GUILLAIN-BARRÉ SIGN, plantar flexion with fanning of the toes when the medioplantar region of the foot or the base of the heel is tapped. Cross-references: Heel reflex of Weingrow; Medioplantar reflex. (Georges Guillain, 1876-1961, French neurologist; Jean A. Barré, 1880-1967, French neurologist)
1. Baker AB, Baker LH: Clinical Neurology. Revised ed. Philadelphia: Harper & Row, 1982

GUILLAIN-BARRÉ SYNDROME, GUILLAIN-BARRÉ-STROHL SYNDROME, acute polyradiculoneuritis; characterized by the acute or subacute development of symmetrical paresis or paralysis of the limbs, at times of the trunk, or of muscles innervated by the cranial nerves. A variable degree of sensory disturbance accompanies the syndrome, and in severe cases sphincter disturbances are also present. In Zimbabwe, the condition is often associated with positive results of human immunodeficiency virus testing. Etiology uncertain. Cross-reference: Landry-Guillain-Barré syndrome. (Georges Guillain; Jean A. Barré)
1. Gorlin RJ, Cohen MM Jr, Levin LS: Syndromes of the Head and Neck. 3rd ed. New York: Oxford University Press, 1990
2. Guillain G, Barré J, Strohl A: Bull Soc Med Hop Paris 40:1462-1470, 1916
3. Landry O: Gaz Hebd Med 6:472-474, 1859

GUILLAND SIGN, pinching the skin over the quadriceps femoris muscle or squeezing the muscle on one side is followed by flexion of the contralateral hip and knee; an indication of meningeal irritation.
1. Baker AB, Baker LH: Clinical Neurology. Revised ed. Philadelphia: Harper & Row, 1982

GUINEA WORM DISEASE, dracontiasis; infection usually presents as a skin ulceration at the site of emergence of the female adult worm. Humans are probably the only reservoir. Disease is widespread in the tropics and occurs on ingesting flea-infested water from shallow wells or ponds.
1. Bennett JC, Plum F (eds): Cecil Textbook of Medicine. 20th ed. Philadelphia: WB Saunders, 1996

GUINON DISEASE, see Gilles de la Tourette syndrome. (Georges Guinon, 1859-1929, French)

GUIST OPERATION, surgical treatment for retinal detachment, consisting of multiple corneal trephinations and chemical cauterization of the choroid.
1. Maffei WE: Os Fundamentos da Medicina. 2nd ed. Livraria Editora Artes Medicas Ltd, 1978

GUITERAS DISEASE, a morbid condition similar to that of blastomycosis.
1. Casas EC: Diccionario Terminologico de Ciencias Medicas. 5th ed. Salvat Editores, SA, 1954

GULF WAR SYNDROME, a global term for various health problems, including fatigue, musculoskeletal pain, headache, memory loss, and diarrhea, occurring in U.S. military personnel after serving in the Persian Gulf conflict of 1991.

GULL DISEASE, adult cretinism or hypothyroidism; inadequate secretion of thyroid hormone for a prolonged period. Also called adult myxedema, from the Latin for slime or mucus. (Sir William Gull, 1816-1890, British)
1. Gull W: Trans Clin Soc Lond 7:180-185, 1874
2. Ritchie AC: Boyd's Textbook of Pathology. 9th ed. Philadelphia: Lea & Febiger, 1990

GULL-SUTTON DISEASE, arteriosclerotic fibrosis of the kidney. Cross-reference: Sutton-Gull disease. (Sir William W. Gull; Henry G. Sutton, 1837-1891, British)
1. Sutton HG: Med Chir Trans Lond 37:273-326, 1872

GUNN SIGN, see Marcus Gunn pupillary sign. (Robert Marcus Gunn, 1850-1909, Scottish ophthalmologist)

GUNN SYNDROME, see Marin-Amat syndrome. (Robert Marcus Gunn)

GÜNTHER DISEASE, congenital erythropoietic porphyria. (Hans Günther, 1884-1956, German)
1. Günther H: Dtsch Arch Klin Med 105:89-146, 1912

GÜNZBERG SIGN, tympanism between the gallbladder and the duodenum; seen in the patient with an ulcer. (Alfred Günzberg, 1861-1937, German)
1. Casas EC: Diccionario Terminologico de Ciencias Medicas. 5th ed. Salvat Editores, SA, 1954

GUSTATORY SWEATING SYNDROME, see Frey syndrome.

GUTTMAN SIGN, a bruit heard over the thyroid gland in the patient with goiter. (Paul Guttman, 1834-1893, German)
1. Casas EC: Diccionario Terminologico de Ciencias Medicas. 5th ed. Salvat Editores, SA, 1954

GUYE SIGN, deficiency of attention in the patient with adenoid hypertrophy.
1. Casas EC: Diccionario Terminologico de Ciencias Medicas. 5th ed. Salvat Editores, SA, 1954

GUYON OPERATION, amputation of the foot through an elliptical incision above the malleoli. (Felix J.C. Guyon, 1831-1920, French surgeon)
1. Maffei WE: Os Fundamentos da Medicina. 2nd ed. Livraria Editora Artes Medicas Ltd, 1978

GUYON SIGN, bulging on the side; seen in the patient with nephroptotic kidney. (Felix J.C. Guyon)
1. Casas EC: Diccionario Terminologico de Ciencias Medicas. 5th ed. Salvat Editores, SA, 1954

HAAB-BIBER-DIMMER DISEASE, reticular degeneration of the cornea. (Otto Haab, 1851-1931, Swiss ophthalmologist; Friedrich Dimmer, 1855-1926, Austrian ophthalmologist)
1. Dimmer F: Zschr Augenheilkd 2:354-399, 1899
2. Haab O: Zschr Augenheilkd 2:235-246, 1899

HABER SYNDROME, a persistent rosacea-like eruption seen on the face; a familial condition and rosacea-like eruption associated with follicular papules, scaly nodules, and depressed scars on the trunk and limbs. (Henry Haber, British)
1. Moschella SL, Hurley HJ: Dermatology. 2nd ed. Philadelphia: WB Saunders, 1985

HACKER OPERATION, surgery for hypospadias; posterior gastroenterostomy through an opening of the mesocolon in cases of pylorus stricture.
1. Maffei WE: Os Fundamentos da Medicina. 2nd ed. Livraria Editora Artes Medicas Ltd, 1978

HAENEL SIGN, analgesia of the eyeball; seen in the patient with tabes. (Hans G. Haenel, 1874-1942, German neurologist)
1. Casas EC: Diccionario Terminologico de Ciencias Medicas. 5th ed. Salvat Editores, SA, 1954

HAFF DISEASE, myoglobinuria; caused by eating fish and eels contaminated with poisonous resinous acids, the by-products of cellulose factories. Described among fishermen in Koenigsberg. (Haff is an arm of the Baltic Sea in East Prussia.)
1. Baker AB, Baker LH: Clinical Neurology. Revised ed. Philadelphia: Harper & Row, 1982
2. Pedro-Pons A: Patologia-y-Clinica Medicus. Salvat Editores, SA, 1952

HAGAR OPERATION, right lateral colotomy.
1. Maffei WE: Os Fundamentos da Medicina. 2nd ed. Livraria Editora Artes Medicas Ltd, 1978

HAGBERG SYNDROME, floppy baby, ataxia chronic but nonprogressive, does not put feet on the ground when held up by the arm ("sits in the air").
1. Rosenberg S: Neuropediatria. Sarvier, 1992

HAGNER OPERATION, drainage of blennorrhea though an incision in the epididymis.
1. Maffei WE: Os Fundamentos da Medicina. 2nd ed. Livraria Editora Artes Medicas Ltd, 1978

HAHN OPERATION, see Loreta operation.

HAHN SIGN, persistent rotation of the head; seen in the child with cerebellar disease. (Eugene H. Hahn, 1841-1902, German)
1. Casas EC: Diccionario Terminologico de Ciencias Medicas. 5th ed. Salvat Editores, SA, 1954

HAIDINGER BRUSHES, nerve bundles made visible by macular edema. (Wilhelm von Haidinger, 1795-1871, Austrian mineralogist)
1. Maffei WE: Os Fundamentos da Medicina. 2nd ed. Livraria Editora Artes Medicas Ltd, 1978

HAILEY-HAILEY DISEASE, a benign suprabasilar acantholytic disease; small flaccid vesicles are noted around the neck and in body folds, aggravated by heat and humidity. Incomplete penetrance of autosomal dominant genodermatosis. (Hugh Hailey, U.S. dermatologist; William Howard Hailey, 1898-1967, U.S. dermatologist)
1. Bennett JC, Plum F (eds): Cecil Textbook of Medicine. 20th ed. Philadelphia: WB Saunders, 1996
2. Hailey H, Hailey H: Arch Dermatol 39:679-685, 1939

HAIM-MUNK SYNDROME, see Papillon-Lefèvre syndrome.

HAIR-AN SYNDROME, in some cases, the patient with stromal hyperthecosis has *h*yperandrogenism (HA), *i*nsulin *r*esistance (IR), and *a*canthosis *n*igricans (AN). Less often, the syndrome develops in the patient with polycystic ovarian disease.

1. Coney P: Polycystic ovarian disease. Fertil Steril 42:667, 1984
2. Ritchie AC: Boyd's Textbook of Pathology. 9th ed. Philadelphia: Lea & Febiger, 1990

HAJDU SYNDROME, HAJDU-CHENEY SYNDROME, characterized by dissolution of the terminal phalanges of the hands and feet, malformation of the skull, generalized skeletal demineralization affecting in particular the vertebra, fractures, premature loss of teeth, scoliosis, and coarse hair. Cross-references: Acro-osteolysis syndrome; Cheney syndrome. (Nicholas Hajdu, Czech; William D. Cheney, U.S. radiologist)

1. Chaney WD: Am J Roentgenol 94:595-607, 1965
2. Hajdu N, Kauntze R: Cranio-skeletal dysplasia. Br J Radiol 21:42-48, 1948
3. Van den Houten BR, Ten-Kate LP, Gerding JC: The Hajdu-Cheney syndrome: a review of literature and report of three cases. Int J Oral Surg 14:113-125, 1985

HAKIM SYNDROME, HAKIM-ADAMS SYNDROME, constellation of symptoms producing normal-pressure hydrocephalus. (S. Hakim, U.S. neurologist; R.D. Adams, U.S.)

1. Hakim S, Adams RD: J Neurol Sci 2:307-327, 1965
2. Hill ME, Lougheed WM, Barnett HJM: A treatable form of dementia due to normal-pressure communicating hydrocephalus. Can Med Assoc J 97:1309-1320, 1967
3. Smith JL: Neuro-Ophthalmology. Vol 6. St Louis: CV Mosby, 1972

HALBAN SIGN, an increase in facial hair in a woman during pregnancy.

1. Casas EC: Diccionario Terminologico de Ciencias Medicas. 5th ed. Salvat Editores, SA, 1954

HALF-BASE SYNDROME, see Garcin syndrome.

HALISTERESIS PHENOMENON, withdrawal of bone salt selectively from previously already calcified tissue.

1. Dorland's Medical Dictionary. 28th ed. Philadelphia: WB Saunders, 1994

HALL SIGN, a tracheal diastolic pulsation; seen in the patient with aortic aneurysm. (Josiah N. Hall, 1859-1939, U.S.)

1. Casas EC: Diccionario Terminologico de Ciencias Medicas. 5th ed. Salvat Editores, SA, 1954

HALL SYNDROME, HALL-PALLISTER SYNDROME, hypothalamic hamartoblastoma, craniofacial anomalies, postaxial polydactyly, cardiac and renal defects, and renal dysfunction are features. Rapid growth and development with both height and weight are present. Cross-references: Hypothalamic hamartoblastoma syndrome; Pallister-Hall syndrome. (Josiah N. Hall.)

1. Gorlin RJ, Cohen MM Jr: Syndromes of the Head and Neck. 3rd ed. New York: Oxford University Press, 1990
2. Hall JG, Pallister PD, Clarren SK, et al: Congenital hypothalamic hamartoblastoma, hypopituitarism, imperforate anus, and postaxial polydactyly. Am J Med Genet 7:47-74, 1980

HALLERMANN-STREIFF SYNDROME, HALLERMANN-STREIFF-FRANÇOIS SYNDROME, dyscephalia mandibulo-oculofacialis; principally characterized by dyscephaly (usually brachycephaly), parrot nose, mandibular hypoplasia, proportionate nanism, hypotrichosis, bilateral congenital cataracts, and microphthalmia. Cross-reference: Oculomandibulofacial syndrome. (Wilhelm Hallermann, German ophthalmologist; Enrico B. Streiff, Swiss ophthalmologist; Jules François, Belgian ophthalmologist)

1. Cohen MM Jr: Hallermann-Streiff syndrome: a review. Am J Med Genet 41:488-499, 1991
2. François J: A new syndrome. Dyscephalia with bird face and dental anomalies, nanism, hypotrichosis, cutaneous atrophy, microphthalmia and congenital cataract. Arch Ophthalmol 60:842-862, 1958
3. François J: François' dyscephalic syndrome. Birth Defects 18(6):595-619, 1982
4. Hallermann W: Klin Monatsbl Augenheilkd 113:315-318, 1948
5. Streiff EB: Ophthalmologica 120:79-83, 1950

HALLERVORDEN SYNDROME, HALLERVORDEN-SPATZ DISEASE, progressive pallidal degeneration; established as a discrete entity through findings of abnormal iron deposits in the pallidum and the substantia nigra (pars reticulata). (Julian Hallervorden, 1882-1965, German neurologist; Hugo Spatz, 1888-1969, German neurologist/psychiatrist)

1. Farmer TW: Pediatric Neurology. 2nd ed. Hagerstown: Harper & Row, 1975
2. Grinker RR, Sahs AL: Neurology. 6th ed. Springfield: Charles C Thomas, 1966
3. Hallervorden J, Spatz H: Zschr Neurol 79:254-302, 1922

HALO SIGN, a radiological halo effect of the fetal head between the subcutaneous fat and the cranium; an indication of fetal death.

1. Dorland's Medical Dictionary. 28th ed. Philadelphia: WB Saunders, 1994

HALPIN OPERATION, extirpation of the lacrimal gland through a curved incision in the eyebrow.
1. Maffei WE: Os Fundamentos da Medicina. 2nd ed. Livraria Editora Artes Medicas Ltd, 1978

HALSTED OPERATION, 1) modification of the Bassini operation; 2) radical extirpation of the breast and axillary lymph nodes. (William S. Halsted, 1852-1922, U.S. surgeon)
1. Maffei WE: Os Fundamentos da Medicina. 2nd ed. Livraria Editora Artes Medicas Ltd, 1978

HALTIA-SANTAVUORI SYNDROME, a congenital amaurotic idiocy form of lipofuscinosis. (M. Haltia, Finnish; P. Santavuori)
1. Santavuori P, Haltia M: J Neurol Sci 18:257-267, 1973

HAMBURGER SIGN, a "glu glu" sound heard in the paravertebral region in the patient with mediastinal mass causing compression of the esophagus.
1. Casas EC: Diccionario Terminologico de Ciencias Medicas. 5th ed. Salvat Editores, SA, 1954

HAMMAN DISEASE, subcutaneous emphysema; pneumomediastinum causing severe pain, like that of a myocardial infarction, and a crackling, crunching noise as respiration and the heartbeat move the air. Rarely, interstitial emphysema causes cardiac tamponade. (Louis V. Hamman, 1877-1946, U.S.)
1. Hamman L: Mediastinal emphysema. JAMA 128:1-6, 1945
2. Hamman L: Spontaneous mediastinal emphysema. Bull Johns Hopkins Hosp 64:1-21, 1939

HAMMAN SIGN, a bubbling sound in the pericordial region; found in the patient with spontaneous emphysema of the mediastinum. (Louis V. Hamman)
1. Casas EC: Diccionario Terminologico de Ciencias Medicas. 5th ed. Salvat Editores, SA, 1954

HAMMAN-RICH SYNDROME, diffuse idiopathic interstitial pulmonary fibrosis; the acute, rapidly fatal form of diffuse interstitial pulmonary fibrosis. (Louis V. Hamman; Arnold R. Rich, 1893-1968, U.S. pathologist)
1. Hamman L, Rich AR: Trans Am Clin Climatol Assoc 51:154-163, 1935
2. Rich AR: Bull Johns Hopkins Hosp 74:177-212, 1944

HAMMERSCHLAG PHENOMENON, unusual fatigability when confronted with continuous sounds of gradually decreasing intensity. (Albert Hammerschlag, 1863-1935, Austrian)
1. Dorland's Medical Dictionary. 28th ed. Philadelphia: WB Saunders, 1994

HAND-FOOT-AND-MOUTH SYNDROME, a viral disease seen in children; Coxsackie A16 is the virus responsible for one of the clearest symptom complexes resulting from enterovirus infections. Vesicular rash is restricted to hands and feet; ovoid ulcers in mouth and cervical lymphadenopathy are present. First described in 1950, it is believed to occur much more commonly recently.
1. Cherry JD, John CL: Hand, foot, and mouth syndrome. Report of six cases due to Coxsackie virus, Group A type 16. Pediatrics 37:637-643, 1966
2. Krugman S, Katz SL: Infectious Diseases of Children. 7th ed. St Louis: CV Mosby, 1981

HAND-FOOT-UTERUS SYNDROME, features consist of small feet with unusually short great toes, and abnormal thumbs; in females, there is duplication of the genital tract, and in males, hypospadias. Autosomal dominant inheritance.
1. Stern AM, Gall JC, Perry BI, et al: The hand-foot-uterus syndrome. J Pediatr 77:109-116, 1970

HAND-SCHÜLLER-CHRISTIAN DISEASE, a chronic form of histiocytosis X; characterized by exophthalmos, and diabetes insipidus, and osteolytic bone lesions. Cross-references: Rowland disease; Schüller-Christian disease. (Alfred Hand, Jr., 1869-1949, U.S. pediatrician; Artur Schüller, 1874-1958, Austrian neurologist; Henry A. Christian, 1876-1951, U.S. internist)
1. Christian HA: Med Clin North Am 3:349-371, 1920
2. Grinker RR, Sahs AL: Neurology. 6th ed. Springfield: Charles C Thomas, 1966
3. Hand A Jr: Arch Pediatr 10:673-675, 1893
4. Rowland RS: Arch Intern Med 42:611-674, 1928
5. Schüller A: Fortschr Geb Roentgenstr 23:12-18, 1915

HAND-SHOULDER SYNDROME, see Shoulder-hand syndrome.

HANDLEY OPERATION, 1) method for mastectomy in case of breast cancer; 2) angioplasty for elephantiasis lymphedema.
1. Maffei WE: Os Fundamentos da Medicina. 2nd ed. Livraria Editora Artes Medicas Ltd, 1978

HANDYSIDE OPERATION, ovariotomy.
1. Maffei WE: Os Fundamentos da Medicina. 2nd ed. Livraria Editora Artes Medicas Ltd, 1978

HANHART SYNDROME, micrognathia with peromelia; microglossia, glossopalatine, and oromandibular-limb hypogenesis are characteristics. Cross-references: Hypoglossal-hypodactyly syndrome; Oromandibular syndrome. (Ernst Hanhart, 1891-1973, Swiss)

1. Bersu ET, Pettersen JC, Charboneau WJ, et al: Studies of malformation syndromes of man XXXXIA: anatomical studies in the Hanhart syndrome—a pathogenetic hypothesis. Eur J Pediatr 122:1-17, 1976
2. Gorlin RJ, Cohen MM Jr: Syndromes of the Head and Neck. 3rd ed. New York: Oxford University Press, 1990
3. Hanhart E: Arch Julius Klaus Stift 25:531-544, 1925
4. Hermann J, Pallister PD, Gilbert EF, et al: Studies of malformation syndromes of the man XXXXI B: nosologic studies in the Hanhart and the Möbius syndrome. Eur J Pediatr 122:19-55, 1976

HANKOW DISEASE, see Katayama disease.

HANOT SYNDROME, primary or secondary biliary cirrhosis producing palmar erythema, jaundice, skin pigmentation, and hepatosplenomegaly. (Victor C. Hanot, 1844-1896, French)

1. Dorland's Medical Dictionary. 28th ed. Philadelphia: WB Saunders, 1994

HANOT-CHAUFFARD SYNDROME, hypertrophic cirrhosis with diabetes and pigmentation. Cross-reference: Troisier syndrome. (Victor C. Hanot; Anatole M.E. Chauffard, 1855-1932, French)

1. Troisier CE: Bull Soc Anat Par 16:231, 1871

HANSEN DISEASE, leprosy; a communicable malady usually acquired by prolonged intimate contact between susceptible individuals and patients suffering from this affliction. Caused by *Mycobacterium leprae*. (Gerhard A. Hansen, 1841-1912, Norwegian)

1. Ballenger JJ: Diseases of the Nose, Throat, Ear, Head and Neck. 12th ed. Philadelphia: Lea & Febiger, 1977
2. Rowland LP (ed): Merritt's Textbook of Neurology. 9th ed. Baltimore: Williams & Wilkins, 1995

HANTAVIRUS PULMONARY SYNDROME, a respiratory distress syndrome with fever, chills, headache, myalgia, nausea, vomiting, diarrhea, hypotension, and shortness of breath. X-rays indicate bilateral diffuse infiltrates. (Named after the Hantaan River, Korea.)

1. Brackett LE, Rotenberg J, Sherman CB: Hantavirus pulmonary syndrome in New England and Europe. N Engl J Med 331:545, 1994 (Letter)
2. Centers for Disease Control and Prevention: Hantavirus pulmonary syndrome—Virginia, 1993. JAMA 272:1893, 1994

HAPPY PUPPET SYNDROME, see Angelman syndrome.

HARADA SYNDROME, a form of uveomeningitis encephalitis. Bilateral diffuse exudative choroiditis and retinal detachment when occurring in association with headache, vomiting, an increase of lymphocytes in the cerebrospinal fluid, and temporary or permanent deafness; loss of hair, vitiligo, and poliosis may be transient features. Cross-reference: Uveomeningitis syndrome. (Einosuke Harada, 1892-1947, Japanese ophthalmologist)

1. Harada E: Acta Soc Ophthalmol Jpn 30:356, 1926

HARD+E SYNDROME, *h*ydrocephalus-*r*etinal *d*ysplasia-*e*ncephalocele syndrome; see Walker-Warburg syndrome.

HARDY OPERATION, transsphenoidal hypophysectomy. (Jules Hardy, Canadian neurosurgeon)

1. Smith RR: Essentials of Neurosurgery. Philadelphia: JB Lippincott

HARE EYE SYNDROME, severe midface hypoplasia, brachycephaly, and an inability to close the eyes completely (Hare eye) are feat. Cross-references: Gallop syndrome; Hydrocephalus-retinal dysplasia-encephalocele syndrome.

1. Gallop TR: Fronto-facio-nasal dysostosis: a new autosomal recessive syndrome. Am J Med Genet 10:409-412, 1981 (Letter)

HARE SYNDROME, see Pancoast syndrome. (Edward Hare, British surgeon)

HARKAVY SYNDROME, a variant of autoimmune arteritis with pulmonary symptoms. Begins with asthma attacks, whereas the Wegner disease has oral lesions. Diffuse erythema, urticaria, and Raynaud phenomenon are frequent features. (Joseph Harkavy, U.S.)

1. Harkavy J: Arch Intern Med 67:709-734, 1941
2. Vannotti A: Clinique et Physiopathologie Médicales. Introduction a la Médecine Clinique. Libraire Maloine, SA, 1973

HARLEQUIN SIGN, reddening of the lower half of the body and blanching of the upper half; seen in temporary vasomotor disturbance in newborns.

1. Dorland's Medical Dictionary. 28th ed. Philadelphia: WB Saunders, 1994

HARRIS SYNDROME, hyperinsulinism due to organic endogenous factors, such as insulinoma, when presenting with symptoms of hypoglycemia, weakness, perspiration, jitteriness, tachycardia, mental confusion, and disturbances of vision. Cross-references: Functional hypoglycemic syndrome; McQuarrie syndrome. (Seale Harris, 1870-1957, British)

1. Harris S: Hyperinsulism and dysinsulism. JAMA 83:729-733, 1924

HARRISON OPERATION, puncture of the urinary bladder through the prostate.

1. Maffei WE: Os Fundamentos da Medicina. 2nd ed. Livraria Editora Artes Medicas Ltd, 1978

HARTLEY-KRAUSE OPERATION, excision of the gasserian ganglion and its roots in trigeminal neuralgia. Cross-reference: Krause operation. (Frank Hartley, 1857-1913, U.S. surgeon; Fedor V. Krause, 1857-1937, German surgeon)

1. Maffei WE: Os Fundamentos da Medicina. 2nd ed. Livraria Editora Artes Medicas Ltd, 1978

HARTNUP DISEASE, pellagra-cerebellar ataxia-renal aminoaciduria; characterized by gross aminoaciduria due to a defect in renal tubular absorption of neutral amino acids. An autosomal recessive disorder of childhood.

1. Farmer TW: Pediatric Neurology. 2nd ed. Hagerstown: Harper & Row, 1975
2. Grinker RR, Sahs AL: Neurology. 6th ed. Springfield: Charles C Thomas, 1966

HASAMIYAMI DISEASE, a mild fever caused by *Leptospira autumnalis* found in Japan.

1. Dorland's Pocket Medical Dictionary. 22nd ed. Philadelphia: WB Saunders, 1977

HASHIMOTO DISEASE, progressive painless enlargement of the thyroid gland with goiter; a goitrous form of autoimmune thyroiditis. (Hakaru Hashimoto, 1881-1934, Japanese surgeon)

1. Gold JJ, Josimovich JB: Gynecologic Endocrinology. 3rd ed. Hagerstown: Harper & Row, 1980
2. Hashimoto H: Arch Klin Chir Berl 97:219-248, 1912
3. Wilson JD, Foster DW, Kronenberg HM, et al (eds): Williams Textbook of Endocrinology. 9th ed. Philadelphia: WB Saunders, 1998

HASSIN SIGN, protrusion and posterior deviation of the ear; seen in the patient with cervical sympathetic lesion.

1. Casas EC: Diccionario Terminologico de Ciencias Medicas. 5th ed. Salvat Editores, SA, 1954

HASSIN SYNDROME, Horner syndrome with auricle protrusion.

1. Casas EC: Diccionario Terminologico de Ciencias Medicas. 5th ed. 1954

HATA PHENOMENON, an increase in severity of an infectious disease following the administration of a small dose of a chemotherapeutic remedy. (Sahachiro Hata, 1872-1938, Japanese bacteriologist)

1. Dorland's Medical Dictionary. 28th ed. Philadelphia: WB Saunders, 1994

HATCHCOCK SIGN, pain on touching the mandibular angle; seen in the patient with parotitis.

1. Casas EC: Diccionario Terminologico de Ciencias Medicas. 5th ed. Salvat Editores, SA, 1954

HAUDEK SIGN, a radiographic shadow in a patient with perforated ulcer of the stomach; seen with bismuth use. Cross-reference: Niche sign. (Martin Haudek, 1880-1931, Austrian radiologist)

1. Casas EC: Diccionario Terminologico de Ciencias Medicas. 5th ed. Salvat Editores, SA, 1954

HAVERHILL DISEASE, HAVERHILL FEVER, an acute form of a rat bite fever due to *Streptobacillus moniliformis*, with an erythematous eruption, severe generalized arthritis, adenitis, headache, and vomiting. (Named for Haverhill, Massachusetts, where an epidemic occurred in 1926.)

1. Casas EC: Diccionario Terminologico de Ciencias Medicas. 5th ed. Salvat Editores, SA, 1954

HAWAII DISEASE, a disease endemic to the Hawaiian islands, characterized by remittent fever, splenomegaly, jaundice, and headache.

1. Casas EC: Diccionario Terminologico de Ciencias Medicas. 5th ed. Salvat Editores, SA, 1954

HAWKINS SIGN, a thin line of subchondral atrophy along the dome of the talus, indicating the presence of vascularity and excluding the diagnosis of vascular necrosis.

1. Campbell WC, Crenshaw AH: Campbell's Operative Orthopaedics. 7th ed. St Louis: CV Mosby, 1987

HAY OPERATION, technique for subarachnoid blocks; described in 1959.

1. Smith RR: Essentials of Neurosurgery. Philadelphia: JB Lippincott

HAY-WELLS SYNDROME, ankyloblepharon-ectodermal dysplasia-cleft lip/palate; palmar and plantar keratoderma and absent or dystrophic nails are features. Autosomal dominant inheritance. Cross-references: AEC syndrome; Ankyloblepharon-ectodermal syndrome. (R.J. Hay, British dermatologist; Robert S. Wells, British dermatologist)

1. Gorlin RJ, Cohen MM Jr: Syndromes of the Head and Neck. 3rd ed. New York: Oxford University Press, 1990
2. Hay RJ, Wells RS: Br J Dermatol 94:277-284, 1976

3. Smith DW, Jones KL: Recognizable Patterns of Human Malformations: Genetic, Embryologic, and Clinical Aspects. 3rd ed. Philadelphia: WB Saunders, 1982

HAYEM-WIDAL SYNDROME, acquired hemolytic anemia and jaundice. Cross-reference: Widal syndrome. (George S. Hayem, 1841-1933, French hematologist; Georges F.I. Widal; 1862-1929, French)
1. Hayem GS: Presse Med 6:121-126, 1898
2. Widal GFI, Abrami P: Presse Med 15:749, 1907

HAYNES OPERATION, drainage of the cisterna magna in cases of suppurative meningitis.
1. Maffei WE: Os Fundamentos da Medicina. 2nd ed. Livraria Editora Artes Medicas Ltd, 1978

HEART-HAND SYNDROME, see Holt-Oram syndrome.

HEAT STRESS SYNDROME, thermal stress with sources either metabolic, ambient, or both; exercise and physical work may be important pathogenetically. Also caused by circulatory instability, water and electrolyte imbalance, and skin changes.
1. Moschella SL, Hurley HJ: Dermatology. 2nd ed. Philadelphia: WB Saunders, 1985

HEATH OPERATION, 1) resection of the posterior wall of the mastoid process, leaving a portion of bone between the epitympanum and the antrum. (Christopher J. Heath); 2) transoral division of the mandibular ramus in ankylosis of the temporomandibular joint. (Christopher H. Heath, 1835-1905, British surgeon)
1. Maffei WE: Os Fundamentos da Medicina. 2nd ed. Livraria Editora Artes Medicas Ltd, 1978

HEATON OPERATION, method for treating inguinal hernia through subcutaneous injection of astringent solutions in order to contract the hernia ring.
1. Maffei WE: Os Fundamentos da Medicina. 2nd ed. Livraria Editora Artes Medicas Ltd, 1978

HEBERDEN NODES, arthritic nodes; bony protuberance at the dorsal margins of the distal interphalangeal joints (osteoarthritis). Cross-references: Bouchard nodes; Rosenbach disease. (William Heberden, 1710-1801, British)
1. Bennett JC, Plum F (eds): Cecil Textbook of Medicine. 20th ed. Philadelphia: WB Saunders, 1996

HECHT SYNDROME, HECHT-BEALS SYNDROME, see Trismus-pseudocampylodactyly syndrome. (Frederick Hecht, U.S.; Rodney Beals, U.S. orthopedic surgeon)

HEEL REFLEX OF WEINGROW, see Guillain-Barré sign.

HEERFORDT SYNDROME, uveoparotid fever; the combination of uveal tract and lacrimal and salivary gland involvement with facial paralysis. Cross-reference: Waldenström uveoparotitis syndrome. (Christian F. Heerfordt, 1871-1953, Danish ophthalmologist)
1. Ballenger JJ: Diseases of the Nose, Throat, Ear, Head and Neck. 12th ed. Philadelphia: Lea & Fibiger, 1977
2. Heerfordt CF: Graefes Arch Ophthalmol 70:254-273, 1909
3. Ritchie AC: Boyd's Textbook of Pathology. 9th ed. Philadelphia: Lea & Febiger, 1990

HEFKE-TURNER SIGN, a radiographic sign involving the obturator muscle; seen in the patient with pathological conditions of the pelvis. Cross-reference: Obturator sign. (Hans W. Hefke, U.S. surgeon; Vernon C. Turner, U.S. orthopedic surgeon)
1. Casas EC: Diccionario Terminologico de Ciencias Medicas. 5th ed. Salvat Editores, SA, 1954

HEGAR OPERATION, perineorrhaphy through denudation of a triangular area of the posterior wall of the vagina. (Alfred Hegar, 1830-1914, German gynecologist)
1. Maffei WE: Os Fundamentos da Medicina. 2nd ed. Livraria Editora Artes Medicas Ltd, 1978

HEGAR SIGN, edema in the inferior segment of the uterus; an indication of pregnancy. (Alfred Hegar)
1. Casas EC: Diccionario Terminologico de Ciencias Medicas. 5th ed. Salvat Editores, SA, 1954

HEIDENHAIN SYNDROME, a rapidly progressive degenerative disease characterized by cortical blindness, presenile dementia, dysarthria, ataxia, athetoid movements, and generalized rigidity. (Adolf Heidenhain, German neurologist)
1. Grinker RR, Sahs AL: Neurology. 6th ed. Springfield: Charles C Thomas, 1966
2. Heidenhain A: Zschr Ges Neurol Psychiatr 118:49-114, 1929

HEILBRONNER SIGN, a lack of muscle tone with muscle atrophy; seen in organic paralysis. (Karl Heilbronner, 1869-1914, Dutch)
1. Casas EC: Diccionario Terminologico de Ciencias Medicas. 5th ed. Salvat Editores, SA, 1954

HEIM-KREYSIG SIGN, a depression in the left intercostal space during cardiac systole. Cross-reference: Kreysig sign. (Ernst L. Heim, 1747-1834, German; Friedrich L. Kreysig, 1770-1839, German)
  1. Casas EC: Diccionario Terminologico de Ciencias Medicas. 5th ed. Salvat Editores, SA, 1954

HEINE OPERATION, cyclodialysis in cases of glaucoma. (Leopold Heine, 1870-1940, German ophthalmologist)
  1. Maffei WE: Os Fundamentos da Medicina. 2nd ed. Livraria Editora Artes Medicas Ltd, 1978

HEINE-MEDIN DISEASE, poliomyelitis; at one time a common, occult viral infection that caused muscle weakness or paralysis as a result of concentrated damage to many motor cells in the spinal cord. (Jacob von Heine, 1800-1879, German; Karl Medin, 1847-1927, Swedish)
  1. Krugman S, Katz SL: Infectious Diseases of Children. 7th ed. St Louis: CV Mosby, 1981
  2. Pedro-Pons A: Patologia-y-Clinica Medicus. Salvat Editores, SA, 1952

HEINEKE OPERATION, a T-shaped surgical incision for rectal cancer.
  1. Maffei WE: Os Fundamentos da Medicina. 2nd ed. Livraria Editora Artes Medicas Ltd, 1978

HEINEKE-MIKULICZ OPERATION, pyloroplasty; enlargement of the pyloric sphincter by incising the pylorus longitudinally and suturing the incision transversely. (Walter Heineke, 1834-1901, German surgeon; Johann von Mikulicz-Radecki, 1850-1905, German surgeon)
  1. Maffei WE: Os Fundamentos da Medicina. 2nd ed. Livraria Editora Artes Medicas Ltd, 1978
  2. Schwartz SI: Principles of Surgery. 4th ed. New York: McGraw-Hill, 1983

HEINZ BODIES DISEASE, masses of denatured hemoglobin (Howell-Jolly bodies, Pappenheimer bodies) that may form in certain types of hemolytic anemia. (Robert Heinz, 1865-1924, German pathologist)
  1. Bennett JC, Plum F (eds): Cecil Textbook of Medicine. 20th ed. Philadelphia: WB Saunders, 1996

HEISRATH OPERATION, excision of the tarsal folds in trachoma.
  1. Maffei WE: Os Fundamentos da Medicina. 2nd ed. Livraria Editora Artes Medicas Ltd, 1978

HEITZ-BOYER-HOVELACQUE OPERATION, creation of an artificial urinary bladder and anus from the distal part of the rectum.
  1. Maffei WE: Os Fundamentos da Medicina. 2nd ed. Livraria Editora Artes Medicas Ltd, 1978

HEKTOEN PHENOMENON, antigens introduced into an animal body in the allergic state may stimulate antibody production that includes antibodies related to previous infections and immunizations. (Ludvig Hektoen, 1863-1951, U.S. pathologist)
  1. Dorland's Medical Dictionary. 28th ed. Philadelphia: WB Saunders, 1994

HELBING SIGN, the inward curve of the Achilles tendon associated with flat foot. (Carl E. Helbing, 1842-1914, German)
  1. Casas EC: Diccionario Terminologico de Ciencias Medicas. 5th ed. Salvat Editores, SA, 1954

HELLAT SIGN, a tuning fork is heard for a shorter time over the diseased area in mastoiditis.
  1. Casas EC: Diccionario Terminologico de Ciencias Medicas. 5th ed. Salvat Editores, SA, 1954

HELLENDALL SIGN, see Cullen sign.

HELLER-DÖHLE DISEASE, see Döhle disease. (Arnold L.G. Heller, 1840-1913, German pathologist)

HEMANGIOMA-THROMBOCYTOPENIA SYNDROME, see Kasabach-Merritt syndrome.

HEMOGLOBIN C DISEASE, a moderately severe anemia caused by an abnormality in hemoglobin formation. Occurs in 2%-3% of Black Americans. The spleen is usually enlarged, and abdominal pain and jaundice occasionally occurs.
  1. Kase NG, Weingold AB: Principles and Practice of Clinical Gynecology. New York: John Wiley & Sons, 1983

HEMOHISTIOBLASTIC SYNDROME, reticuloendotheliosis with a constellation of symptoms.
  1. Dorland's Medical Dictionary. 28th ed. Philadelphia: WB Saunders, 1994

HEMOLYTIC-UREMIC SYNDROME, see Gasser syndrome.

HEMOPLEUROPNEUMONIC SYNDROME, dyspnea, hemoptysis, tachycardia, and fever when associated with dullness at the base of the chest and tubular respiration over the middle zone of the chest; indicates pneumonia and hydrothorax when there is a puncture wound of the chest.
  1. Dorland's Medical Dictionary. 28th ed. Philadelphia: WB Saunders, 1994

HENCH-ROSENBERG SYNDROME, palindromic rheumatism; characterized by sudden attacks and pain and swelling of joints, often in late afternoons. (Philip S. Hench, 1896-1965, U.S., Edward F. Rosenberg, U.S.)

1. Hench PS, Rosenberg EF: Palindromic rheumatism; "new" often recurring disease of joints (arthritis, periarthritis, para-arthritis) apparently producing articular residues—report of 34 cases; its relation to "angioneural arthrosis," "allergic rheumatism" and rheumatoid arthritis. Arch Intern Med 73:293-321, 1944

HENLE LOOP, see Loop of Henle.

HENNEBERT SIGN, rotational nystagmus toward the affected ear; found in syphilitic labyrinthitis.

1. Casas EC: Diccionario Terminologico de Ciencias Medicas. 5th ed. Salvat Editores, SA, 1954

HENNEKAM SYNDROME, mental retardation, lymphedematous facies, marked edema of the lower extremities, and gastrointestinal lymphangiectasia are features.

1. Gorlin RJ, Cohen MM Jr: Syndromes of the Head and Neck. 3rd ed. New York: Oxford University Press, 1990
2. Hennekam RCM, Geerdink RA, Hamel BCJ, et al: Autosomal recessive intestinal lymphangiectasia and lymphedema, with facial anomalies and mental retardation. Am J Med Genet 34:593-600, 1989
3. Mücke J, Hoepffner W, Scheerschmidt G, et al: Early onset lymphoedema, recessive form—a new form of genetic lymphoedema syndrome. Eur J Pediatr 145:195-198, 1986

HENNEQUIN SIGN, after lower limb trauma, a sign of fracture of the neck of the femur if digital compression below the inguinal ligament elicits pain, tenderness, and crepitation.

1. Mazion JM: Illustrated Manual of Orthopedic Signs/Tests/Maneuvers for Office Procedure. 2nd ed. Orlando: Daniels Publishing, 1980

HENNINGS SIGN, a Gothic-arch shape of the angulus of the stomach seen in chronic gastric ulcer. (Wilhelm Hennings, 1716-1794, German)

1. Dorland's Medical Dictionary. 28th ed. Philadelphia: WB Saunders, 1994

HENOCH DISEASE, chronic progressive electric chorea. (Eduard H. Henoch, 1820-1910, German pediatrician)

1. Henoch EH: Beitr Kinderheilkd, 1868, p 113

HENOCH-SCHÖNLEIN PURPURA, see Schönlein-Henoch purpura. (Eduard H. Henoch)

HEPATONEPHORIC SYNDROME, HEPATORENAL SYNDROME, the combination of severe liver disease and renal failure. The patient with advanced cirrhosis of the liver or other severe liver disease (usually but not always with ascites) sometimes develops renal failure, which may be precipitated by minor complications, even as slight a thing as an abdominal paracentesis.

1. Haymaker W: Bing's Local Diagnosis in Neurological Diseases. 15th ed. St Louis: CV Mosby, 1969
2. Hoef JC: Hepatorenal syndrome, in Haubrich WS, Schaffner F, Berk JE (eds): Bockus Gastroenterology. 5th ed. Philadelphia: WB Saunders, 1995, pp 2023-2034
3. Ritchie AC: Boyd's Textbook of Pathology. 9th ed. Philadelphia: Lea & Febiger, 1990

HERBERT OPERATION, treatment of glaucoma using a cuneiform patch from the sclera. (Herbert Herbert, 1865-1942, British ophthalmologist)

1. Maffei WE: Os Fundamentos da Medicina. 2nd ed. Livraria Editora Artes Medicas Ltd, 1978

HEREDITARY BASAL NEVUS SYNDROME, multiple calcified fibromas in both ovaries are common. Basal cell carcinomas of the skin are developed at an early age and cysts in the jaws and mesentery, calcification of the dura, and other abnormalities are frequent.

1. Ritchie AC: Boyd's Textbook of Pathology. 9th ed. Philadelphia: Lea & Febiger, 1990

HEREDITARY BENIGN INTRAEPITHELIAL DYSKERATOSIS SYNDROME, consists of plaques of the conjunctiva and oral mucosal thickening clinically similar to white-folded hypertrophy (white sponge nevus of Cannon). Autosomal dominant trait inheritance, with a high degree of penetrance. Cross-reference: Witkop-Von Sallmann syndrome.

1. Gorlin RJ, Cohen MM Jr, Levin LS: Syndromes of the Head and Neck. 3rd ed. New York: Oxford University Press, 1990
2. Witkop CJ Jr, et al: Clinical, histologic, cytologic and ultrastructural characteristics of the oral lesions from hereditary mucoepithelial dysplasia: disease of gap junction and desmosomal formation. Oral Surg 46:645-657, 1978

HERING PHENOMENON, a faint murmur heard with a stethoscope over the lower end of the sternum; occurs for a short time after death. (Heinrich E. Hering, 1866-1948, German physiologist)

1. Dorland's Medical Dictionary. 28th ed. Philadelphia: WB Saunders, 1994

HERING-BREUER REFLEX, stretch receptors situated in the visceral pleura and/or the tracheobronchial tree initiate impulses that pass via the vagus nerve to the nucleus solitarius, hence to the reticular substance. Inhibition of respiration, preventing overdistention of the lungs, thus occurs. During expiration, the reflex operates in reverse. (Heinrich E. Hering; Josef R. Breuer, 1842-1925, Austrian)

1. Baker AB, Baker LH: Clinical Neurology. Revised ed. Philadelphia: Harper & Row, 1982

HERLITZ SYNDROME, epidermolysis bullosa lethalis.

1. Herlitz LG: Acta Paediatr 17:31-371, 1937

HERMANSKI [HERMANSKY]-PUDLAK SYNDROME, albinism with hemorrhagic diathesis; consists of the triad of tyrosinase-positive oculocutaneous albinism, hemorrhagic diathesis caused by storage pool-deficient platelets, and the accumulation of a ceroid-like material in the reticuloendothelial system, oral mucosa, and urine. A very rare syndrome of autosomal recessive inheritance. (F. Hermanski [Hermansky], Czech internist; P. Pudlak, Czech internist)

1. Bennett JC, Plum F (eds): Cecil Textbook of Medicine. 20th ed. Philadelphia: WB Saunders, 1996
2. Hermanski F, Pudlak P: Blood 14:162-169, 1959
3. Moschella SL, Hurley HJ: Dermatology. 2nd ed. Philadelphia: WB Saunders, 1985

HERNIG-LOMMEL SIGN, respiratory arrhythmia.

1. Casas EC: Diccionario Terminologico de Ciencias Medicas. 5th ed. Salvat Editores, SA, 1954

HERRMANN SYNDROME, a unique pattern syndrome consisting of craniosynostosis, severe symmetrical malformed limbs, and cleft lip/palate. (Christian Herrmann, Jr., U.S.)

1. Gorlin RJ, Cohen MM Jr: Syndromes of the Head and Neck. 3rd ed. New York: Oxford University Press, 1990
2. Herrmann C Jr: Birth Defects 10(5):23-53, 1974
3. Herrmann C Jr: Hereditary photomyoclonus associated with diabetes mellitus, deafness, nephropathy and cerebral dysfunction. Neurology 14:212-221, 1964

HERS DISEASE, glycogen storage disease type VI; an inborn glycogen metabolism disorder due to a deficiency of hepatophosphorylase. (G.H. Hers, French biochemist)

1. Grinker RR, Sahs AL: Neurology. 6th ed. Springfield: Charles C Thomas, 1966
2. Hers GH: Rev Int Hepatol 9:35-55, 1959

HERSH SYNDROME, a sensorineural hearing deficit; hypertelorism, a flat nasal bridge and broad nasal tip, micrognathia, and sparse curly hair are features. Coronal synostosis or dolichocephaly may be found.

1. Gorlin RJ, Cohen MM Jr: Syndromes of the Head and Neck. 3rd ed. New York: Oxford University Press, 1990
2. Hersh JA: Proc Greenwood Genet Ctr 5:186, 1986

HERTER-HEUBNER DISEASE, see Gee disease. (Christian A. Herter, 1865-1910, U.S.; Otto Johann L. Heubner, 1843-1926, German pediatrician)

HERTOGLIE SYNDROME, benign chronic hyperthyroidism.

1. Casas EC: Diccionario Terminologico de Ciencias Medicas. 5th ed. Salvat Editores, SA, 1954

HERTWIG-MAGENDIE SIGN, see Magendie sign. (Richard C.W.T. von Hertwig, 1850-1937, German zoologist; François Magendie, 1783-1855, French physiologist)

HERTZEL SIGN, when one arm and both legs are compressed, a 5-mm rise in the sphygmomanometer mercury on the opposite arm is usually noted; in the patient with atherosclerosis, this rise is 60 mm.

1. Casas EC: Diccionario Terminologico de Ciencias Medicas. 5th ed. Salvat Editores, SA, 1954

HERVA SYNDROME, see Hydrolethalus syndrome.

HERYNG SIGN, an infraorbital shadow produced by fluid or by a hypertrophied, hyperplastic, or neoplastic membrane in the maxillary antrum; seen in diseases of the maxillary sinus. Cross-references: Burger sign; Garel sign; Voltolini sign. (Théodor Heryng, 1847-1925, Polish otolaryngologist)

1. Casas EC: Diccionario Terminologico de Ciencias Medicas. 5th ed. Salvat Editores, SA, 1954

HESS OPERATION, modification of Pagenstecher operation for palpebral ptosis.

1. Maffei WE: Os Fundamentos da Medicina. 2nd ed. Livraria Editora Artes Medicas Ltd, 1978

HESS TOURNIQUET TEST, a measurement of capillary fragility. The examiner applies the cuff of a sphygmomanometer to a patient's arm and, after taking the blood pressure, inflates the cuff to register a pressure midway between that of the systolic and diastolic pressures. This is held for 5 minutes. The cubital fossa is then examined for petechiae. (Alfred F. Hess, 1875-1933, U.S. pediatrician)

1. Bailey H: Physical Signs in Clinical Surgery. 16th ed. Baltimore: Williams & Wilkins, 1983

HEUBNER ARTERITIS, HEUBNER ARTERY, in part, supplies the olfactory bulb and in very few cases the cerebral cortex; however, it mainly supplies the anterior limb of the internal capsule, the rostral and medial aspects of the putamen, the pallidum, and the head of the caudate nucleus. (Otto Johann L. Heubner, 1843-1926, German pediatrician)

1. Krayenbühl HA, Yasargil MG: Cerebral Angiography. 2nd ed. Philadelphia: JB Lippincott, 1968

HEUBNER SIGN, see Sicar sign.

HEUBNER-SCHILDER DISEASE, see Schilder disease. (Otto Johann L. Heubner)

HEY OPERATION, tarsometatarsal disarticulation with separation of a part of the cuneiform bone. (William Hey, 1736-1819, British surgeon)

1. Maffei WE: Os Fundamentos da Medicina. 2nd ed. Livraria Editora Artes Medicas Ltd, 1978

HEYD SYNDROME, postoperative hepatorenal syndrome. (Charles G. Heyd, 1884-1970, U.S. surgeon)

1. Heyd CG: Ann Surg 79:55-77, 1924

HIBBS OPERATION, surgery for vertebral column tuberculosis. (Russell Hibbs, 1869-1932, U.S. surgeon)

1. Maffei WE: Os Fundamentos da Medicina. 2nd ed. Livraria Editora Artes Medicas Ltd, 1978

HICKS SIGN, see Braxton Hicks contraction.

HIGOUMÉNAKI SIGN, an irregular thickening or enlargement of the sternoclavicular portion of the clavicle; usually unilateral rather than bilateral. The result of periostitis. Cross-reference: Clavicular sign. (G. Higouménaki, Polish)

1. Moschella SL, Hurley HJ: Dermatology. 2nd ed. Philadelphia: WB Saunders, 1985

HILL OPERATION, a posterior gastropexy performed transabdominally, but incorporating plicating sutures to narrow the esophagogastric junction. (Lucius Hill, U.S. thoracic surgeon)

1. Schwartz SI: Principles of Surgery. 4th ed. New York: McGraw-Hill, 1983

HILL SIGN, indirect measurements of blood pressure tend to show a systolic pressure considerably higher in the lower extremities than in the upper extremities; seen in severe aortic insufficiency. (Archibald V. Hill, 1886-1977, British biochemist)

1. Fowler NO: Cardiac Diagnosis and Treatment. 3rd ed. Cambridge: Harper & Row, 1980

HILLEMAND SYNDROME, see Cavernous sinus syndrome.

HINES-BANNICK SYNDROME, intermittent attacks of hypothermia and disabling sweating. (Edgar A. Hines, U.S.; Edwin Bannick, U.S.)

1. Dorland's Medical Dictionary. 28th ed. Philadelphia: WB Saunders, 1994

HIP-FLEXION PHENOMENON, when a hemiplegic person attempts to arise from a lying down posture, the hip on the paralyzed side is flexed first.

1. Dorland's Medical Dictionary. 28th ed. Philadelphia: WB Saunders, 1994

HIPO SYNDROME, *h*emihyperplasia, *i*ntestinal web, *p*reauricular skin tags, and *o*phthalmopathy (HIPO) consisting of a cloudy cornea.

1. Hanley TB, Simon JW: Ann Ophthalmol 16:342-344, 1984

HIPPEL SYNDROME, HIPPEL-LINDAU SYNDROME, HIPPEL-CZERMAK SYNDROME, see Von Hippel-Lindau syndrome.

HIRSCHBERG SIGN, internal rotation and adduction of the foot; seen in the patient with hemiplegia. (Leonard K. Hirschberg, U.S. neurologist)

1. Casas EC: Diccionario Terminologico de Ciencias Medicas. 5th ed. Salvat Editores, SA, 1954

HIRSCHFELD DISEASE, acute diabetes mellitus. (Felix V.B. Hirschfeld, German)

1. Hirschfeld FVB: Zbl Med Wiss 18:164-166, 1890

HIRSCHSPRUNG DISEASE, congenital megacolon. Occurs more commonly in males than females, but the affected female has a much greater risk of having affected children. (Harald Hirschsprung, 1830-1916, Danish pediatrician)

1. Baker AB, Baker LH: Clinical Neurology. Revised ed. Philadelphia: Harper & Row, 1982
2. Hirschsprung H: Jahrb Kinderheilkd 27:1-7, 1888

HIRST OPERATION, surgical correction of vaginismus; widening of the vagina through deep longitudinal incisions on each side of the vulva.

1. Maffei WE: Os Fundamentos da Medicina. 2nd ed. Livraria Editora Artes Medicas Ltd, 1978

HIS-WERNER DISEASE, see Trench fever. (Wilhelm His, Jr., 1863-1934, German; Heinrich Werner, 1874-1946, German)

HISTIOCYTOSIS SYNDROME, see Letterer-Siwe syndrome.

HOCHENEGG OPERATION, surgical method for treating rectal cancer. (Julius von Hochenegg, 1859-1940, Viennese surgeon)
1. Maffei WE: Os Fundamentos da Medicina. 2nd ed. Livraria Editora Artes Medicas Ltd, 1978

HOCHSINGER HAND SIGN, HOCHSINGER PHENOMENON, pressure on the inner aspect of the biceps muscle causes spasm and contraction of the hand. In carrying out this maneuver, it is possible to compress the brachial artery and thus may be a variation of the Trousseau sign; seen in hypocalcemia. (Karl Hochsinger, Austrian pediatrician)

HOCHSINGER SIGN, swelling of the inner third of the clavicle; seen in the patient with congenital syphilis. (Karl Hochsinger)
1. Casas EC: Diccionario Terminologico de Ciencias Medicas. 5th ed. Salvat Editores, SA, 1954

HODARA DISEASE, trichorrhexis nodosa; observed in women from ancient Constantinople. (Maneheim Hodara, Turkish)
1. Hodara M: Mschr Prakt Dermatol 19:173-188, 1894

HODGKIN DISEASE, HODGKIN-PALTAULF-STERNBERG DISEASE, malignant lymphogranulomatosis; a unique, malignant disorder, usually arising in the lymph nodes, with a characteristic histopathological appearance. First recognized as a distinct clinicopathological entity in 1832. Cross-references: Bonfils disease; Paltaulf-Sternberg disease; Reed-Hodgkin disease. (Thomas Hodgkin, 1798-1866, British; Richard Paltaulf, 1858-1924, British, C. Sternberg)
1. Bennett JC, Plum F (eds): Cecil Textbook of Medicine. 20th ed. Philadelphia: WB Saunders, 1996
2. Hodgkin T: On some morbid appearances of the absorbent glands and spleen. Med Chir Trans Lond 17:68-114, 1832

HODGSON DISEASE, aneurysmal dilatation of the proximal part of the aorta. (Joseph Hodgson, 1788-1869, British)
1. Casas EC: Diccionario Terminologico de Ciencias Medicas. 5th ed. Salvat Editores, SA, 1954

HODGSON OPERATION, femoral artery ligature in the vertex of Scarpa triangle (trigonum femoral).
1. Maffei WE: Os Fundamentos da Medicina. 2nd ed. Livraria Editora Artes Medicas Ltd, 1978

HOEHNE SIGN, the cessation of uterine contractions during childbirth; a sign of rupture of the uterus. (Ottomar Hoehne, 1871-1932, German gynecologist)
1. Casas EC: Diccionario Terminologico de Ciencias Medicas. 5th ed. Salvat Editores, SA, 1954

HOFFA DISEASE, solitary lipoma or hygroma of the patella caused by trauma. (Albert Hoffa, 1859-1907, German surgeon)
1. Casas EC: Diccionario Terminologico de Ciencias Medicas. 5th ed. Salvat Editores, SA, 1954

HOFFA SIGN, with the ankles in a symmetrical position, if the Achilles tendon on the injured side is less taut than on the contralateral side, there also may be increased dorsiflexion in the relaxed position on the affected side, an indication of a possible avulsion fracture of the calcaneus.
1. Mazion JM: Illustrated Manual of Orthopedic Signs/Tests/Maneuvers for Office Procedure. 2nd ed. Orlando: Daniels Publishing, 1980

HOFFA-LORENZ OPERATION, see Lorenz operation. (Albert Hoffa; Adolf Lorenz, 1854-1946, Austrian surgeon)

HOFFMAN-TINEL SIGN, refers to the radiating, tingling sensation felt in the cutaneous distribution of an injured nerve when the nerve trunk is lightly percussed.
1. Evans RC: Illustrated Essentials in Orthopedic Physical Assessment. St Louis: Mosby Yearbook, 1994
2. Sunderland S: Nerves and Nerve Injuries. Edinburgh: Churchill Livingstone, 1972

HOFFMANN SIGN, to elicit the finger flexor reflex, the examiner holds the middle phalanx of the patient's middle finger between the examiner's second and third fingers and, with a rapid flick of the examiner's thumb, nips the nail of the patient finger, thus suddenly flexing the finger. The examiner then manually flexes the finger again. The reflex consists of flexion of the other fingers, including the thumb. Cross-reference: Trömner sign. (Johann Hoffmann, 1857-1919, German neurologist)
1. Haymaker W: Bing's Local Diagnosis in Neurological Diseases. 15th ed. St Louis: CV Mosby, 1969

HOFFMANN SYNDROME, typical muscular abnormalities often observed in full-blown myxedema in adults. (Johann Hoffmann)
1. Farmer TW: Pediatric Neurology. 2nd ed. Hagerstown: Harper & Row, 1975

2. Hoffmann J: Dtsch Z Nervenkr 9:278-290, 1897

3. Wilson JD, Foster DW, Kronenberg HM, et al (eds): Williams Textbook of Endocrinology. 9th ed. Philadelphia: WB Saunders, 199

HOFFSTATTER-CULLEN SIGN, see Cullen sign.

HOLIDAY HEART SYNDROME, describes a condition associated with healthy persons who develop a variety of cardiac arrhythmias after brief drinking sprees. This particular alcohol-induced event occurs more frequently during holidays and weekends.

HOLLA DISEASE, epidemic hemolytic jaundice; observed in Holla, Norway.
1. Casas EC: Diccionario Terminologico de Ciencias Medicas. 5th ed. Salvat Editores, SA, 1954

HOLMAN-MILLER SIGN, a characteristic anterior bowing of the posterior wall of the maxillary sinus; seen when tumors expand to the pterygomaxillary space.
1. Ballenger JJ: Diseases of the Nose, Throat, Ear, Head and Neck. 12th ed. Philadelphia: Lea & Febiger, 1977

HOLMES OPERATION, resection of the calcaneus through an incision parallel to its superior edge and another incision in the plantar region to section the peroneal tendons.
1. Maffei WE: Os Fundamentos da Medicina. 2nd ed. Livraria Editora Artes Medicas Ltd, 1978

HOLMES SIGN, the patient attempts to flex the forearm against the examiner's resistance and the resistance is suddenly released. The patient is unable to quickly stop the further flexion of the arm and the hand may fly into the face. Cross-reference: Stewart-Holmes sign. (Sir Gordon M. Holmes, 1876-1965, British neurologist)
1. Grinker RR, Sahs AL: Neurology. 6th ed. Springfield: Charles C Thomas, 1966

HOLMES-ADIE SYNDROME, see Adie syndrome. (Sir Gordon M. Holmes; William J. Adie, 1886-1935, British neurologist)

HOLT OPERATION, HOLT-ANAGNOSTAKIS OPERATION, see Anagnostakis operation. (Andrei A. Holt, Cretan ophthalmologist; Andrei Anagnostakis, Cretan ophthalmologist)

HOLT-ORAM SYNDROME, HOLT-ORAM-ROBERT SYNDROME, a distinctive malformation concomitant with an ostium secundum atrial septal defect. The thumb is hypoplastic, with an accessory phalanx that gives it a crooked appearance. Opposition of the thumb with other digits is difficult and in some cases the thumb is rudimentary or absent. Cross-reference: Heart-hand syndrome. (Mary C. Holt, British cardiologist; Samuel Oram, British cardiologist)
1. Bennett JC, Plum F (eds): Cecil Textbook of Medicine. 20th ed. Philadelphia: WB Saunders, 1996

2. Holt M, Oram S: Familial heart disease with skeletal malformations. Br Heart J 22:236-242, 1960

HOLZINGER SIGN, a hypothenar reflex elicited by compression of the pisiform bone.
1. Casas EC: Diccionario Terminologico de Ciencias Medicas. 5th ed. Salvat Editores, SA, 1954

HOMANS SIGN, dorsiflexion of the foot results in calf tenderness and pain, suggesting venous thrombosis. (John Homans, 1877-1954, U.S. surgeon)
1. Campbell WC, Crenshaw AH: Campbell's Operative Orthopaedics. 7th ed. St Louis: CV Mosby, 1987

HOMÉN SYNDROME, a congenital, genetic lesion of the lenticular nucleus, marked by vertigo, ataxia, dysarthria, and gradually increasing dementia, with rigidity of the body, especially the legs. (Ernst A. Homén, 1851-1926, Finnish)
1. Homén EA: Neurol Zbl 9:514-518, 1890

HOMOCYSTINURIA SYNDROME, subluxation of the lens, malar flush, osteoporosis, mental defects, and medial degeneration of the aorta and elastic arteries with intimal hyperplasia and fibrosis leading to pads and ridges within the vessels. Autosomal recessive inheritance.
1. Finkelstein JD, Mudd SH, Irreverre F, et al: Homocystinuria due to cystathionine synthetase deficiency: the mode of inheritance. Science 146:785-787, 1964

2. Smith DW, Jones KL: Recognizable Patterns of Human Malformations: Genetic, Embryologic, and Clinical Aspects. 3rd ed. Philadelphia: WB Saunders, 1982

HONE DISEASE, endemic typhus.
1. Casas EC: Diccionario Terminologico de Ciencias Medicas. 5th ed. Salvat Editores, SA, 1954

HONG KONG EAR, otitis externa; seen more frequently in hot, damp conditions. Cross-reference: Singapore ear.
1. Bailey H: Physical Signs in Clinical Surgery. 16th ed. Baltimore: Williams & Wilkins, 1983

HOOK OPERATION, ureteroureterostomy.

1. Maffei WE: Os Fundamentos da Medicina. 2nd ed. Livraria Editora Artes Medicas Ltd, 1978

HOOKWORM DISEASE, caused by *Ancylostoma duodenale*; occurs in tropical and subtropical countries where the soil is contaminated by human feces.
1. Banwell JG, Schad GA: Hookworm. Clin Gastroenterol 7:129-156, 1978
2. Ritchie AC: Boyd's Textbook of Pathology. 9th ed. Philadelphia: Lea & Febiger, 1990

HOOTNICK-HOLMES SYNDROME, see Greig cephalopolysyndactyly syndrome.

HOOVER SIGN, a test for the presence of hysterical paralysis of one leg. The patient lies supine; when one leg is elevated, the other is pressed down, suggesting that it is not paralyzed. Cross-reference: Grasset-Gaussel-Hoover sign. (Charles F. Hoover, 1865-1927, U.S.)
1. Rowland LP (ed): Merritt's Textbook of Neurology. 9th ed. Baltimore: Williams & Wilkins, 1995

HOPE SIGN, double cardiac beat; seen in aortic aneurysm. (James Hope, 1801-1841, British)
1. Casas EC: Diccionario Terminologico de Ciencias Medicas. 5th ed. Salvat Editores, SA, 1954

HOPPE-GOLDFLAM SYNDROME, see Goldflam disease. (Herman H. Hoppe, 1867-1919, U.S. neurologist; Samuel V. Goldflam, 1852-1923, Polish neurologist)

HORN SIGN, traction on the right spermatic cord causes pain; seen in the patient with appendicitis. (C. Ten Horn, Dutch surgeon)
1. Casas EC: Diccionario Terminologico de Ciencias Medicas. 5th ed. Salvat Editores, SA, 1954

HORNER SIGN, see Spalding sign. (David A. Horner, U.S. obstetrician/gynecologist)

HORNER SYNDROME, HORNER-BERNARD SYNDROME, sympathetic paralysis of the eye with ptosis, miosis, and enophthalmos. Cross-references: Bernard-Horner syndrome; Claude Bernard-Horner syndrome. (Johann F. Horner, 1831-1886, Swiss ophthalmologist; Claude Bernard, 1813-1878, French physiologist)
1. Grinker RR, Sahs AL: Neurology. 6th ed. Springfield: Charles C Thomas, 1966
2. Horner JF: Ueber eine Form von Ptosis. Klin Monatsbl Augenheilkd 7:193-198, 1869

HORNOVÁ SYNDROME, a familial syndrome of swollen eyelids, nodular amyloid deposits in the conjunctiva, congenital cataracts, atrophy of ocular bulb, and amaurosis. (J. Hornová, Czech)
1. Gorlin RJ, Cohen MM Jr: Syndromes of the Head and Neck. 3rd ed. New York: Oxford University Press, 1990
2. Hornová J, Dluhosova O: Primary amyloidosis of gingiva and conjunctiva and mental disorder in a brother and sister. Oral Surg 25:457-464, 1968

HORSLEY OPERATION, a technique for pyloroplasty. (Victor A.H. Horsley (1857-1916, British neurosurgeon) was associated with a group of surgeons working in the area of intracranial neoplasms and their meticulous and careful dissection. He removed the first spinal cord neoplasm more than 90 years ago.)
1. Maffei WE: Os Fundamentos da Medicina. 2nd ed. Livraria Editora Artes Medicas Ltd, 1978
2. Smith RR: Essentials of Neurosurgery. Philadelphia: JB Lippincott

HORSLEY SIGN, the axillary body temperature is higher on the paralyzed side than on the nonparalyzed side in middle meningeal hemorrhage; seen in hemiplegia. (Victor A.H. Horsley)
1. Casas EC: Diccionario Terminologico de Ciencias Medicas. 5th ed. Salvat Editores, SA, 1954

HORTON SYNDROME, migrainous neuralgia and temporal arteritis. Many cases treated with histamine desensitization in the past. Cross-reference: Polymyalgia rheumatica syndrome. (Bayard Horton, 1895-1980, U.S.)
1. Horton BT, Magath TB, Brown GE: Arch Intern Med 53:400-409, 1934

HOSSLIN SIGN, when a paretic muscle is contracted passively, it returns to its usual posture easily; in hysterical paralysis, a paretic muscle remains contracted for a longer time.
1. Casas EC: Diccionario Terminologico de Ciencias Medicas. 5th ed. Salvat Editores, SA, 1954

HOTCHKISS OPERATION, partial resection of the maxilla and mandible, followed by plastic repair; seen in cheek epithelioma.
1. Maffei WE: Os Fundamentos da Medicina. 2nd ed. Livraria Editora Artes Medicas Ltd, 1978

HOUNSFIELD UNIT, an imaging index. (Godfrey Hounsfield, an electronics engineer with the British EMI Research Program, is credited for his work in the development of computed tomography)
1. Smith RR: Essentials of Neurosurgery. Philadelphia: JB Lippincott

HOUSE-BRACKMANN SCALE, a grading system for facial nerve paralysis; Grade VI is complete paralysis.

1. House JW, Brackmann DE: Facial nerve grading system. Otolaryngol Head Neck Surg 93:146-147, 1985

HOUSSAY PHENOMENON, hypoglycemia and a marked increase in sensitivity to insulin, produced by experimental animals that have been hypophysectomized and depancreatized. (Bernardo A. Houssay, 1889-1971, Argentinian physiologist)

1. Dorland's Medical Dictionary. 28th ed. Philadelphia: WB Saunders, 1994

HOWEL-EVANS SYNDROME, diffuse palmoplantar keratoderma occurring between the ages of 5 and 15 years and subsequent development of esophageal cancer later in life. (W. Howel-Evans, British)

1. Howel-Evans W, et al: Q J Med 27:413, 1958

HOWSHIP-ROMBERG SIGN, pressure on the obturator nerve by an obturator hernia produces pain down the inner side of the thigh to the knee. (John Howship, 1781-1841, British surgeon; Moritz Z. Romberg, 1795-1873, German neurologist)

1. Dorland's Medical Dictionary. 28th ed. Philadelphia: WB Saunders, 1994

HOYNE SIGN, the head falls back when the shoulders are elevated; seen in the patient with poliomyelitis. (Archibald Hoyne, 1878-1963, U.S. pediatrician)

1. Dorland's Medical Dictionary. 28th ed. Philadelphia: WB Saunders, 1994

HUCHARD SIGN, paradoxical resonance; seen in pulmonary effusion. (Henri Huchard, 1844-1910, French)

1. Casas EC: Diccionario Terminologico de Ciencias Medicas. 5th ed. Salvat Editores, SA, 1954

HUETER SIGN, lack of bone vibration transmission; seen in the patient with long bone fracture with intervening soft tissue. (Karl Hueter, 1813-1882, German surgeon)

1. Casas EC: Diccionario Terminologico de Ciencias Medicas. 5th ed. Salvat Editores, SA, 1954

HUGH OWEN THOMAS SIGN, see Thomas sign.

HUGHES SYNDROME, progressively coarse acromegaloid facial appearance and thickening of the lips and oral mucosa.

1. Gorlin RJ, Cohen MM Jr: Syndromes of the Head and Neck. 3rd ed. New York: Oxford University Press, 1990
2. Hughes HE, McAlpine PJ, Cox DW, et al: An autosomal dominant syndrome with "acromegaloid" features and thickened oral mucosa. J Med Genet 22:119-125, 1985

HUGHLINGS JACKSON SYNDROME, see Jackson syndrome. (John Hughlings Jackson, 1835-1911, British neurologist)

HUGUIER DISEASE, uterine myeloma. (Pierre C. Huguier, 1804-1873, French surgeon)

1. Casas EC: Diccionario Terminologico de Ciencias Medicas. 5th ed. Salvat Editores, SA, 1954

HUMAN SIGN, the chin and larynx are relaxed during the third stage of anesthesia.

1. Casas EC: Diccionario Terminologico de Ciencias Medicas. 5th ed. Salvat Editores, SA, 1954

HÜNERMANN SYNDROME, see Conradi syndrome. (Carl Hünermann, German)

HUNT NEURAGIA, HUNT SYNDROME, see Ramsay Hunt syndrome. (John Ramsay Hunt, 1874-1937, U.S. neurologist)

HUNT PARADOXICAL PHENOMENON, when an attempt is made at forced plantar flexion of a foot that is in dorsal spasm, the dorsal spasm increases. However, if the patient is asked to extend the foot, plantar flexion occurs; seen in dystonia musculorum deformans. (James Ramsay Hunt)

1. Dorland's Medical Dictionary. 28th ed. Philadelphia: WB Saunders, 1994

HUNTER OPERATION, arterial ligature for treating an aneurysm near the heart. (John Hunter, 1728-1793, Scottish surgeon)

1. Maffei WE: Os Fundamentos da Medicina. 2nd ed. Livraria Editora Artes Medicas Ltd, 1978

HUNTER SYNDROME, mucopolysaccharidosis type II. Severe and mild forms exist. Distinguished from Hurler syndrome by the following: 1) a slower progression with longer survival; 2) a lack of corneal clouding; 3) X-linked rather than autosomal recessive inheritance. (Charles Hunter, 1872-1955, Canadian)

1. Farmer TW: Pediatric Neurology. 2nd ed. Hagerstown: Harper & Row, 1975
2. Hunter C: Proc R Soc Med 10:104-116, 1917

HUNTINGTON CHOREA, HUNTINGON DISEASE, degenerative chorea; a distinctive entity in which dementia associated with chorea appears usually in the 4th or 5th decade of life. The cardinal criteria for diagnosis is hereditary disposition (monohybrid dominant without anticipation or sex-linked inheritance) and choreoathetoid hyperkinesis. In juvenile Huntington disease, two variants are recognized: 1) a hyperkinetic syndrome that culminates in a parkinsonian-like rigidity; 2) progressive rigidity develops in the absence of involuntary movements. Only rarely does torsion dystonia or athetoid hyperkinesis occur. (George S. Huntington, 1850-1916, U.S.)

1. Farmer TW: Pediatric Neurology. 2nd ed. Hagerstown: Harper & Row, 1975
2. Huntington G: On chorea. Med Surg Reporter Phila 26:311-321, 1872

HUNTINGTON COUGHING SIGN, coughing and straining are followed by flexion of the hip and extension of the knee, resulting in elevation of a paretic lower extremity. Cross-reference: Coughing sign. (George S. Huntington)

1. Baker AB, Baker LH: Clinical Neurology. Revised ed. Philadelphia: Harper & Row, 1982

HUPPERT DISEASE, see Kahler disease. (Karl Huppert, 1832-1904, German)

HURLER SYNDROME, mucopolysaccharidosis type I-H; characterized by faulty degradation of dermatan and heparan sulfate with glycosaminoglycan storage in connective tissues due to α-L-iduronidase deficiency. Death is due primarily to congestive heart failure. Transmitted by an X-linked gene. Cross-reference: Pfaundler-Hurler syndrome. (Gertrud Hurler, 1889-1965, German pediatrician)

1. Farmer TW: Pediatric Neurology. 2nd ed. Hagerstown: Harper & Row, 1975
2. Hurler G: Z Kinderheilkd 24:220-234, 1919
3. Rowland LP (ed): Merritt's Textbook of Neurology. 9th ed. Baltimore: Williams & Wilkins, 1995

HURLER-SCHEIE SYNDROME, the patient with a phenotype between the Hurler syndrome and the Scheie syndrome is thought to represent compound heterozygotes, having inherited one Hurler and one Scheie gene from each parent. (Gertrud Hurler; Harold G. Scheie, 1909-1990, U.S. ophthalmologist)

1. McKusick VA: Heritable Disorders of Connective Tissue. 4th ed. St Louis: CV Mosby, 1972
2. Smith DW, Jones KL: Recognizable Patterns of Human Malformations: Genetic, Embryologic, and Clinical Aspects. 3rd ed. Philadelphia: WB Saunders, 1982

HURST ENCEPHALITIS, allergic postviral encephalitis; hyperacute encephalitis with coma lasting for weeks (Edward W. Hurst, Australian)

1. Hurst EW: Med J Australia 2:1-6, 1941

HURST SYNDROME, short stature, delayed bone age, microcephaly, craniosynostosis, small abnormally modeled ears with an atretic external auditory meatus, microstomia, small mandible, slender bones, hooked clavicles, dislocated radial heads, and camptodactyly are features.

1. Gorlin RJ, Cohen MM Jr: Syndromes of the Head and Neck. 3rd ed. New York: Oxford University Press, 1990
2. Hurst JA, Winter RM, Baraitser M: Am J Med Genet 29:107-125, 1988

HÜRTHLE CELL, appears as nests of large pink cells with abundant granular cytoplasm packed with mitochondria; associated with mild thyrotoxicosis. Cross-reference: Askanazy cell. (Karl W. Hürthle, 1860-1945, German histologist)

1. Ballenger JJ: Diseases of the Nose, Throat, Ear, Head and Neck. 12th ed. Philadelphia: Lea & Febiger, 1977
2. Wilson JD, Foster DW, Kronenberg HM, et al (eds): Williams Textbook of Endocrinology. 9th ed. Philadelphia: WB Saunders, 1998

HUTCHINSON FRECKLE, lentigo maligna melanoma; irregularly outlined lesion with scattered melanocytes in the epidermis. Occurs in sun-exposed areas of the skin; often seen in the elderly. Cross-reference: Melanotic freckle.(Sir Jonathan Hutchinson, 1828-1913, British surgeon)

1. Ballenger JJ: Diseases of the Nose, Throat, Ear, Head and Neck. 12th ed. Philadelphia: Lea & Febiger, 1977
2. Hutchinson J: Arch Surg Lond 3:159, 1892

HUTCHINSON PUPIL, dilatation due to compression of the third cranial nerve against the free edge of the tentorium; seen frequently in cases of extradural hematoma, but also occurs in some cases of subdural hematoma. (Sir Jonathan Hutchinson)

1. Lumley JS, Clain A: Hamilton Bailey's Demonstration of Physical Signs in Clinical Surgery. 18th ed. London: Butterworth-Heinemann, 1997

HUTCHINSON SIGN, the presence of interstitial keratitis and a dull-red discoloration of the cornea; seen in the patient with congenital syphilis. (Sir Jonathan Hutchinson)

1. Dorland's Medical Dictionary. 28th ed. Philadelphia: WB Saunders, 1994

HUTCHINSON TEETH, screwdriver teeth; the upper incisors are smaller than normal and broader toward the gum than at their free edge and notches. Only the secondary dentition is affected. Confirmatory evidence of congenital syphilis. (Sir Jonathan Hutchinson)

1. Lumley JS, Clain A: Hamilton Bailey's Demonstration of Physical Signs in Clinical Surgery. 18th ed. London: Butterworth-Heinemann, 1997

HUTCHINSON-GILFORD SYNDROME, progeria; in previously healthy infants who develop premature aging, the cardiovascular complications are primarily those of accelerated atherosclerosis. Hypertension, myocardial infarction, heart failure, cardiovascular accident, and premature death (usually cardiovascular in origin) occur. (Sir Jonathan Hutchinson; Hastings Gilford, 1861-1941, British surgeon)

1. Gilford H: Practitioner 73:188-217, 1904
2. Hutchinson J: Med Chir Trans 69:473-477, 1886

HUTINEL DISEASE, liver cirrhosis caused by tuberculosis. (Victor H. Hutinel, 1849-1933, French pediatrician)

1. Hutinel VH: Rev Mens Mal Enf 11:529-574, 1893

HYALINE MEMBRANE SYNDROME, see Respiratory distress syndrome of newborn.

HYDE DISEASE, urticaria. (James N. Hyde, 1840-1910, U.S. dermatologist)

1. Casas EC: Diccionario Terminologico de Ciencias Medicas. 5th ed. Salvat Editores, SA, 1954

HYDROCEPHALUS-RETINAL DYSPLASIA-ENCEPHALOCELE SYNDROME, see Hare eye syndrome.

HYDROLETHALUS SYNDROME, a lethal syndrome of polyhydramnios, variable degrees of hydrocephalus, crossed polydactyly, talipes, congenital heart anomalies, and severe micrognathia. In nearly all cases, the patient has spontaneously aborted or the fetus is stillborn. Cross-references: Herva syndrome; Salonen-Herva-Norio syndrome.

1. Anyane-Yeboa K, Collins M, Kupsky W, et al: Hydrolethalus (Salonen-Herva-Norio) syndrome: further clinicopathological delineation. Am J Med Genet 26:899-907, 1987
2. Gorlin RJ, Cohen MM Jr: Syndromes of the Head and Neck. 3rd ed. New York: Oxford University Press, 1990
3. Hartikainen-Sorri AL, Kirkinen P, Herva R: Prenatal detection of hydrolethalus syndrome. Prenat Diagn 3:219-224, 1983
4. Salonen R, Herva R, Norio R: Hydrolethalus syndrome. J Med Genet 27:756-759, 1990

HYPERABDUCTION SYNDROME, symptoms similar to thoracic outlet syndrome; caused by compression of the brachial plexus, roots, trunk nerves, and axillary vessels by the pectoralis minor muscle and the coracoid process when the arms are stretched above the head, as during sleep. Cross-reference: Wright syndrome.

1. Wright IS: Am Heart J 29:1-19, 1945

HYPERACTIVE CHILD SYNDROME, attention deficit hyperactivity disorder. Cross-reference: Hyperkinetic syndrome.

1. Dorland's Medical Dictionary. 28th ed. Philadelphia: WB Saunders, 1994

HYPERCALCEMIC SYNDROME, see Milk-alkali syndrome.

HYPEREOSINOPHILIC SYNDROME, a myeloproliferative disorder with persistent, marked eosinophilia (>1500/cu mm) and evidence of organ involvement.

1. Bennett JC, Plum F (eds): Cecil Textbook of Medicine. 20th ed. Philadelphia: WB Saunders, 1996
2. Chusoil MJ, Dale DC, West BC, et al: The hypereosinophilic syndrome: analysis of fourteen cases with review of the literature. Medicine 54:1-27, 1975

HYPERIMMUNOGLOBULINEMIA E SYNDROME, see Job syndrome.

HYPERKINESIS SIGN, see Claude hyperkinesis sign.

HYPERKINETIC HEART SYNDROME, hyperkinemia; commonly observed in the relatively young patient, predominantly a male between 7 and 48 years of age. Characterized by pounding peripheral pulses, systolic ejection clicks, ejection-like systolic murmurs, and possible left ventricular enlargement.

1. Gorlin R: The hyperkinetic heart syndrome. JAMA 182:823-829, 1962

HYPERKINETIC SYNDROME, see Hyperactive child syndrome.

HYPERLUCENT LUNG SYNDROME, see Swyer-James syndrome.

HYPERSOMNIA-BULIMIA SYNDROME, see Kleine-Levin syndrome.

HYPERSOMNIA-SLEEP APNEA SYNDROME, associated with systemic hypertension, cardiac arrhythmia, polycythemia, pulmonary hypertension, cardiac hypertrophy, and occasionally cerebral and myocardial infarcts.

1. Association of Sleep Centers: Diagnostic classification of sleep and arousal disorders. Sleep 2:1-154, 1979
2. Rowland LP (ed): Merritt's Textbook of Neurology. 9th ed. Baltimore: Williams & Wilkins, 1995

HYPERSTIMULATION SYNDROME, marked ovarian enlargement and ascites with possible pleural effusion, hemoconcentration, thromboembolic phenomena, renal failure, and, rarely, death.

1. Engel T, Jewelewicz R, Dyrenforth I, et al: Ovarian hyperstimulation syndrome. Report of a case with notes on pathogenesis and treatment. Am J Obstet Gynecol 112:1052-1060, 1972
2. Gold JJ, Josimovich JB: Gynecologic Endocrinology. 3rd ed. New York: Plenum Medical, 1980

HYPERTELORISM-HYPOSPADIAS SYNDROME, see Opitz syndrome.

HYPERTELORISM-MICROTIA-CLEFTING SYNDROME, hypertelorism, markedly hypoplastic pinnae, short stature, mild psychomotor retardation, and cleft lip/palate are features. Cross-reference: Bixler syndrome.

1. Baraitser M: The hypertelorism microtia clefting syndrome. J Med Genet 19:387-388, 1982
2. Bixler D, Christian JC, Gorlin RJ, et al: Hypertelorism, microtia, and facial clefting. A newly described inherited syndrome. Am J Dis Child 118:495-498, 1969; Birth Defects 5(2):77-81, 1969
3. Gorlin RJ, Cohen MM Jr: Syndromes of the Head and Neck. 3rd ed. New York: Oxford University Press, 1990

HYPERVENTILATION SYNDROME, during an anxiety attack, there is a sensation of tightness in the chest, as though the lungs cannot be adequately filled. The patient responds to this sensation by deep and sighing respirations, sometimes to the point of producing a respiratory alkalosis that adds to the feelings of giddiness, with tingling of the fingertips and even tetany with carpopedal spasm. Cross-reference: Chronic hyperventilation syndrome.

1. Bennett JC, Plum F (eds): Cecil Textbook of Medicine. 20th ed. Philadelphia: WB Saunders, 1996
2. Magarian GJ: Hyperventilation syndromes: infrequently recognized common expression of anxiety and stress. Medicine 61:219-236, 1982

HYPERVISCOSITY SYNDROME, any syndrome associated with increased viscosity of the blood; the myriad of symptoms includes stroke and thrombosis.

HYPNIC HEADACHE SYNDROME, resembles cluster headache as periodicity is strikingly evident. Most commonly occurs in the elderly man who is awakened from sleep, sometimes during a dream, by a diffuse headache and nausea without autonomic symptoms.

HYPOCHONDROPLASIA SYNDROME, short limbs and caudal narrowing of the spine; craniofacial features are nearly normal. An autosomal dominant mutant gene.

1. Smith DW, Jones KL: Recognizable Patterns of Human Malformations: Genetic, Embryologic, and Clinical Aspects. 3rd ed. Philadelphia: WB Saunders, 1982
2. Walker BA, Murdoch JL, McKusick VA, et al: Hypochondroplasia. Am J Dis Child 122:95-104, 1971

HYPOGLOSSIA-HYPODACTYLY SYNDROME, hypoglossia and hypodactyly. The mandible is small and the chin recedes; limb anomalies, normal intelligence, good speech, fused labia majora, unilateral renal agenesis, and congenital occlusion of the superior mesenteric artery may be found. Cross-reference: Hanhart syndrome.

1. Cohen MM Jr, et al: Nosologic and genetic considerations in the aglossyadactyly syndrome. Birth Defects 7(7):237-240, 1971
2. Cosman B, Crikelair GF: Midline branchiogenic syndromes. Plast Reconstr Surg 44:41-48, 1969

HYPOMELANOSIS OF ITO SYNDROME, see Ito disease. (Minor Ito, Japanese dermatologist)

HYPOPHOSPHATASIA SYNDROME, bow legs with irregular metaphyseal rarefaction, early loss of deciduous teeth, and late closure of fontanels with or without craniosynostosis are features. Autosomal recessive inheritance.

1. Macpherson RI, Kroeker M, Houston CS: et al: Hypophosphatasia. J Can Assoc Radiol 23:16-26, 1972
2. Smith DW, Jones KL: Recognizable Patterns of Human Malformations: Genetic, Embryologic, and Clinical Aspects. 3rd ed. Philadelphia: WB Saunders, 1982

HYPOPIGMENTATION-IMMUNODEFICIENCY DISEASE, see Griscelli syndrome.

HYPOPLASTIC LEFT HEART SYNDROME, mitral valve atresia; a constellation of malformations of the heart such as hypoplasia or atresia of the left ventricle and of the aorta or mitral valve or both, and characterized by respiratory distress and extreme cyanosis, with cardiac failure and death in early infancy.

1. Strong WB, et al: Am J Dis Child 120:511-514, 1970

HYPOTHALAMIC HAMARTOBLASTOMA SYNDROME, see Hall syndrome.

HYPOTHALAMIC-PITUITARY-OVARIAN SYNDROME, may present as primary or secondary amenorrhea, oligomenorrhea, polymenorrhea, or menometrorrhagia. Deserves a laboratory validation so that appropriate therapy may be instituted.

1. Buttram VC Jr: Immature HPO axis. J Reprod Med 14:21-25, 1975
2. Gold JJ, Josimovich JB: Gynecologic Endocrinology. 3rd ed. New York: Plenum Medical, 1980

HYPOTONIA SYNDROME, see Floppy mitral valve syndrome.

HYPOTONIC SYNDROME, characterized by a decrease in the ratio of solutes to water in body fluids. Develops when water intake exceeds the sum of renal plus extrarenal water losses.

1. Wilson JD, Foster DW, Kronenberg HM, et al (eds): Williams Textbook of Endocrinology. 9th ed. Philadelphia: WB Saunders, 1998

I-CELL DISEASE, see Leroy syndrome.

ICARD SIGN, when paper soaked in lead acetate is placed inside the nose of a cadaver, the paper becomes black due to products of lung deterioration.

1. Casas EC: Diccionario Terminologico de Ciencias Medicas. 5th ed. Salvat Editores, SA, 1954

ICELAND DISEASE, epidemic neuromyasthenia (benign myalgic encephalomyelitis); has many clinical similarities to early poliomyelitis. Most outbreaks affect hospital staff. Nearly 200 were affected at Los Angeles County Hospital in 1934 and over 300 at the Royal Free Hospital in London in 1955. Cross-references: Akureyri disease; Royal Free disease.

1. Baker AB, Baker LH: Clinical Neurology. Revised ed. Philadelphia: Harper & Row, 1982
2. Bennett JC, Plum F (eds): Cecil Textbook of Medicine. 20th ed. Philadelphia: WB Saunders, 1996

ICHTHYOSIS CONGENITA SYNDROME, an integument that is rough and dry with retained scale but free of erythema suggesting a "fish skin" designation. On close inspection, there may be fine scale with keratin-plugged follicles or large polyhedral scales loosely adherent. The palms and soles may be normal or may be thickened with accentuation of normal creases.

1. Bennett JC, Plum F (eds): Cecil Textbook of Medicine. 20th ed. Philadelphia: WB Saunders, 1996

IDAHO SYNDROME, consists of premature fusion of the sagittal suture, micrognathia, umbilical hernia, anomalous pulmonary venous return, complete anterior dislocation of the tibias, contractures at the proximal interphalangeal joints, and umbilical hernia.

1. Gorlin RJ, Cohen MM Jr: Syndromes of the Head and Neck. 3rd ed. New York: Oxford University Press, 1990

IDIOPATHIC LONG Q-T SYNDROME, characterized by recurrent syncope, a long Q-T interval (usually 0.5-0.7 seconds, sometimes intermittent), ventricular arrhythmias, and sudden and unexpected death. An uncommon condition, first described in deaf siblings, although deafness is not always present.

1. Cheitlin MD, Sokolow M: Clinical Cardiology. 5th ed. Norwalk, Conn: Appleton & Lange, 1993

IDIOPATHIC POSTPRANDIAL SYNDROME, the repeated occurrence of the clinical manifestations of hypoglycemia after meals. No exact etiology found despite investigation.

1. Dorland's Medical Dictionary. 28th ed. Philadelphia: WB Saunders, 1994

IKWA DISEASE, see Trench fever.

ILIESCU SIGN, compression of the phrenic nerve produces pain in the patient with appendicitis.

1. Casas EC: Diccionario Terminologico de Ciencias Medicas. 5th ed. Salvat Editores, SA, 1954

IMERSLÜND SYNDROME, IMERSLÜND-GRÄSBECK SYNDROME, enterocyte cobalamin malabsorption; weakness and anemia beginning in early childhood owing to defective absorption of vitamin B12 in the presence of a normal intrinsic factor. (Olga Imerslünd, Norwegian pediatrician; Ralph Gräsbeck, Finnish pediatrician)

1. Gräsbeck R, Gordin R, Kantero I, et al: Acta Med Scand 167:289-296, 1960
2. Imerslünd O: Idiopathic chronic myeloblastic anemia in children. Acta Paediat 49 (Suppl 119):1-115, 1960
3. McKusick VA: Heritable Disorders of Connective Tissue. 4th ed. St Louis: CV Mosby, 1972

IMMERSION FOOT SYNDROME, effects of prolonged water immersion of the feet; edema, pallor, cyanosis, coldness, and paresthesias are features. Cross-reference: Pernio syndrome.

1. Moschella SL, Hurley HJ: Dermatology. 2nd ed. Philadelphia: WB Saunders, 1985

IMMOBILIZATION SYNDROME, abrupt total immobilization due to casts, traction, or quadriplegia may lead to marked loss of calcium from bone with resultant hypercalciuria. Space travel also causes this syndrome.

1. Campbell MF, Walsh PC: Campbell's Urology. 5th ed. Philadelphia: WB Saunders, 1986

IMMOTILE CILIA SYNDROME, ultrastructurally identifiable abnormalities of the cilia that can be detected in nasal or bronchial mucosal biopsies. In the male with this disorder, motility of sperm is markedly impaired.
1. Bennett JC, Plum F (eds): Cecil Textbook of Medicine. 20th ed. Philadelphia: WB Saunders, 1996
2. Wilson JD, Foster DW, Kronenberg HM, et al (eds): Williams Textbook of Endocrinology. 9th ed. Philadelphia: WB Saunders, 1998

IMPINGEMENT SIGN, demonstrated by the examiner preventing scapular rotation with one hand while the other hand raises the patient's affected arm in forced forward flexion and abduction, thus causing the greater tuberosity to impinge against the acromion.
1. Campbell WC, Crenshaw AH: Campbell's Operative Orthopaedics. 7th ed. St Louis: CV Mosby, 1987
2. Evans RC: Illustrated Essentials in Orthopedic Physical Assessment. St Louis: Mosby Yearbook, 1994

INAPPROPRIATE SECRETION OF ANTIDIURETIC HORMONE, SYNDROME OF, persistent hyponatremia and inappropriately elevated urine osmolality in relation to serum osmolality, with no discernible stimulus for antidiuretic hormone release. Cross-reference: Schwartz-Bartter syndrome.
1. Ballenger JJ: Diseases of the Nose, Throat, Ear, Head and Neck. 12th ed. Philadelphia: Lea & Febiger, 1977
2. Schwartz WB, Bartter F, Curelop S: Am J Med 23:529-542, 1957

INFERIOR NUCLEUS RUBER SYNDROME, INFERIOR RED NUCLEUS SYNDROME, see Claude syndrome.

INFERTILE MALE SYNDROME, the most common disorder of the androgen receptor; in contrast to the other such disorders, not actually a form of male pseudohermaphroditism.
1. Campbell MF, Walsh PC: Campbell's Urology. 5th ed. Philadelphia: WB Saunders, 1986

INSPISSATED BILE SYNDROME, biliary obstruction and jaundice caused by blockage of the bile canaliculi.
1. Dorland's Medical Dictionary. 28th ed. Philadelphia: WB Saunders, 1994

INSULIN RESISTANCE SYNDROME, characterized by obesity, non-insulin dependent diabetes mellitus, hypertension, and dyslipidemia.
1. Haffner SM, Stem MP, et al: Hyperinsulinemia in a population at high risk for non-insulin dependent diabetes mellitus. N Engl J Med 315:220-224, 1986
2. Opara UJ, Levine JH: Southern Med J 90:1162-1167, 1997

INTEROSSEI SIGN, see Finger phenomenon.

INTRAUTERINE PARABIOTIC SYNDROME, see Placental transfusion syndrome.

IRRITABLE BOWEL SYNDROME, IRRITABLE COLON SYNDROME, functional diarrhea; the diagnosis is readily evident from a history of intermittent diarrhea and constipation associated with abdominal pain, and from lack of signs and symptoms of systemic illness.
1. Bennett JC, Plum F (eds): Cecil Textbook of Medicine. 20th ed. Philadelphia: WB Saunders, 1996
2. Snape WJ Jr: Irritable bowel syndrome, in Haubrich WS, Schaffner F, Berk JE (eds): Bockus Gastroenterology. 5th ed. Philadelphia: WB Saunders, 1995, pp 1619-1636

IRUKANDJI SYNDROME, following a mild skin sting by small carybdeid (box) jellyfish, including *Carukia barnesi,* known colloquially as the "Irukandji," a group of delayed (10-40 minutes, mean 30 minutes) severe systemic symptoms occur. Severe toxic heart failure ensues, with admission to intensive care facilities necessary for additional investigation and treatment.
1. Fenner P, Carney I: Aust Fam Phys 28:1131-1137, 1999
2. Martin JC, et al: Med J Aust 153:164-169, 1990

IRVINE-GASS SYNDROME, the most common form of ocular disc swelling, which occurs as part of an ocular inflammatory syndrome following after cataract extraction. Associated with moderately decreased visual acuity and cystoid macular edema. (S.R. Irvine, U.S. ophthalmologist)
1. Irvine SR: Am J Ophthalmol 36:599-619, 1953

ISAACS SYNDROME, ISAACS-MERTENS SYNDROME, continuous muscle fiber activity; a rare syndrome of continuous muscle stiffness, myokymia, and delayed muscle relaxation associated with a polyneuropathy that is usually mild or inapparent and identified only by an electrodiagnostic study. Cross-references: Moersch-Woltmann syndrome; Stiff-man syndrome. (Hyam A. Isaacs, South African neurophysiologist)
1. Isaacs HA: J Neurol Neurosurg Psychiatry 24:319-325, 1961
2. Mertens HB, Zschocke S: Klin Wochenschr 43:917-925, 1965

ISAMBERT DISEASE, acute miliary tuberculosis of the pharynx and larynx. (Emile Isambert, 1827-1876, French)

   1. Casas EC: Diccionario Terminologico de Ciencias Medicas. 5th ed. Salvat Editores, SA, 1954

ISOCHROMOSOME 12P SYNDROME, see Pallister-Killian syndrome.

ISOLATION SYNDROME, the most dramatic variety of aphasia, with normal repetition. Sometimes called "isolation of the speech area."

   1. Baker AB, Baker LH: Clinical Neurology. Revised ed. Philadelphia: Harper & Row, 1982
   2. Geschwind N, et al: Isolation of the speech area. Neuropsychologia 6:327, 1968

ITAI-ITAI SYNDROME, bone pains and signs of chronic nephropathy and gout. (Means "ouch-ouch.")

   1. Thren MJ, et al: Nephropathy in cadmium workers: assessment of risk from airborne occupational exposure to cadmium. Br J Indian Med 46:689-697, 1989

ITARD-CHOLEWA SIGN, anesthesia of the tympanic membrane; seen in the patient with otosclerosis. (Jean Marie G. Itard, 1774-1838, French otologist; Erasmus R. Cholewa, 1845-1931, German)

   1. Casas EC: Diccionario Terminologico de Ciencias Medicas. 5th ed. Salvat Editores, SA, 1954

ITO DISEASE, characteristics include mental deficiencies, seizures, and strabismus, as well as streaked, whorled, or mottled areas of hyperpigmentation on the limbs, usually evident in infancy. Autosomal dominant disorder. Cross-reference: Hypomelanosis of Ito syndrome. (Minor Ito, Japanese dermatologist)

   1. Ito M: Tohoku J Exp Med Suppl 55:51-92, 1952
   2. Schwartz MF Jr, Esterly NB, Fretzin DF, et al: Hypomelanosis of Ito (incontinentia pigmenti achromians): a neurocutaneous syndrome. J Pediatr 90:236-240, 1977

IVEMARK SYNDROME, congenital splenic agenesis; cardiac defects and a partial situs inversus viscerum are features. Cross-references: Asplenia syndrome; Polhemus-Schafer-Ivemark syndrome. (Björn I. Ivemark, Swedish pathologist)

   1. Bhattacharjee M, Friedman AW, Thiagarajan P: Gouty arthritis in a patient with Ivemark syndrome. South Med J 89:834, 1996 (Letter)
   2. Ivemark BI: Acta Paediatar Uppsala 44 (Suppl 104):1-110, 1955
   3. Van Mierop, et al: Asplenia and polysplenia syndromes. Birth Defects 8:74, 1972

IVES-HOUSTON SYNDROME, a lethal syndrome of intrauterine growth retardation, marked microcephaly with craniosynostosis, and severe malformation of the limbs.

   1. Gorlin RJ, Cohen MM Jr: Syndromes of the Head and Neck. 3rd ed. New York: Oxford University Press, 1990
   2. Ives EJ, Houston CS: Am J Med Genet 7:351-360, 1980

IVOR-LEWIS OPERATION, resection and reconstruction of esophageal lesions at all levels.

   1. Schwartz SI: Principles of Surgery. 4th ed. New York: McGraw-Hill, 1983

JACCOUD SYNDROME, chronic arthralgia after recurring bouts of rheumatic fever resulting in fibrous changes in the joint capsules and tendons, leading to deformities that may resemble rheumatoid arthritis; the joints may be painful and rheumatic nodules are often present. (François S. Jaccoud, 1830-1913, French)

   1. Jaccoud S: Leçons de Clinique Médicale Faites a l'Hôpital de la Charité. 2nd ed. Paris: Delahaye, 1869

JACCOUD-OSLER DISEASE, endocarditis.

   1. Casas EC: Diccionario Terminologico de Ciencias Medicas. 5th ed. Salvat Editores, 1954

JACKSON SYNDROME, paralysis of the tongue on one side together with paresis of the contralateral limbs; usually caused by a lesion in the pyramid that interrupts the fibers of the adjacent 12th cranial nerve. (John Hughlings Jackson, 1835-1911, British neurologist)

   1. Baker AB, Baker LH: Clinical Neurology. Revised ed. Philadelphia: Harper & Row, 1982
   2. Grinker RR, Sahs AL: Neurology. 6th ed. Springfield: Charles C Thomas, 1966
   3. Jackson JH: Lancet 1:689-690, 1886

JACKSON-LAWLER SYNDROME, consists of pachyonychia congenita, palmoplantar hyperkeratosis, hyperhidrosis, and follicular keratosis. A variant of the Jadassohn-Lewandowsky syndrome. (A.D.M. Jackson)

   1. Gorlin RJ, Cohen MM Jr, Levin LS: Syndromes of the Head and Neck. 3rd ed. New York: Oxford University Press, 1990
   2. Jackson ADM, Lawler SD: Pachyonychia congenita: a report of six cases in one family. Ann Eugen 16:142-146, 1951

JACKSON-MACKENZIE SYNDROME, see MacKenzie syndrome. (John Hughlings Jackson)

JACKSON-WEISS SYNDROME, craniosynostosis, midfacial hypoplasia, and abnormalities of the feet are characteristics. (C.E. Jackson)

1. Gorlin RJ, Cohen MM Jr, Levin LS: Syndromes of the Head and Neck. 3rd ed. New York: Oxford University Press, 1990
2. Jackson CE, Weiss L, Reynold WA: Craniosynostosis, mid-facial hypoplasia, and foot abnormalities: an autosomal dominant phenotype in a large Amish kindred. J Pediatr 88:963-968, 1976

JACKSONIAN CONVULSIONS, JACKSONIAN SEIZURES, JACKSONIAN EPILEPSY, seizures involving one or more parts of the body on the same side. These differ from ordinary generalized convulsions in many ways. The attacks have a localized origin, often beginning as a twitching in the face or fingers, or less commonly in the foot. (John Hughlings Jackson)

1. Grinker RR, Sahs AL: Neurology. 6th ed. Springfield: Charles C Thomas, 1966
2. Jackson JH: Br Med J 1:773-774, 1875
3. Jackson JH: Med Times Gaz 50:166-167, 1864

JACOBAEUS OPERATION, section of pleural adherent through thoracoscopy. (Hans C. Jacobaeus, 1879-1937, Swedish surgeon)

1. Maffei WE: Os Fundamentos da Medicina. 2nd ed. 1978

JACOBSON PLEXUS, the promontory of the middle ear contains the tympanic plexus, which receives the Jacobson nerve, a branch of the glossopharyngeal nerve arising from the petrosal ganglion below the ear. (Ludwig Jacobson, 1783-1843, Danish anatomist)

1. Ballenger JJ: Diseases of the Nose, Throat, Ear, Head and Neck. 12th ed. Philadelphia: Lea & Febiger, 1977

JACQUET DISEASE, ectodermal dysplasia; features include alopecia and dental anomalies (Leonard M. L. Jacquet, 1860-1914, French)

1. Jacquet L: Presse Med, 1900, pp 8327-8328

JADASSOHN SYNDROME, JADASSOHN SYNDROME OF NEVUS SEBACEOUS, nevus sebaceous with hyperkeratosis. In 1962, Feuerstein and Mims established this neurocutaneous syndrome consisting of the triad of linear sebaceous nevus, seizures, and mental retardation. Cross-reference: CHILD syndrome. (Josef Jadassohn, 1863-1936, German dermatologist in Switzerland)

1. Jadassohn J: Bemerkungen zur Histologie der systematisierten Naevi and über "Talgdrüsen-Naevi." Arch Derm Syph Berl 33:355-394, 1895
2. Monahan RH, et al: Multiple choristomas, convulsions and mental retardation as a new neurocutaneous syndrome. Am J Ophthalmol 64:529-532, 1967

JADASSOHN-LEWANDOWSKY [LEWANDOWSKI] SYNDROME, see Pachyonychia congenita syndrome. (Josef Jadassohn; Felix Lewandowsky [Lewandowski], 1879-1921, German dermatologist)

JADASSOHN-PELLIZARI DISEASE, anetoderma; an eruption consisting of round or oval erythematous macules 5-10 mm in diameter. The most common sites are the trunk and extremities, and to a lesser extent the neck and face. This type of primary macular atrophy occurs mostly in women in the 2nd to 4th decades of life. (Josef Jadassohn; Pietro Pellizari, 1823-1892, Italian dermatologist)

JAESCHE-ARLT OPERATION, see Arlt operation.

JAFFÉ-LICHTENSTEIN SYNDROME, fibrous bone dysplasia characterized by excessive proliferation of fibrous tissues. (Henry L. Jaffé, 1896-1979, U.S. pathologist; Louis Lichtenstein, 1906-1977, U.S.)

1. Jaffé HL, Lichtenstein L: Am J Pathol 18:205-215, 1942

JAHNKE SYNDROME, see Sturge-Weber syndrome.

JAKOB-CREUTZFELDT DISEASE, see Creutzfeldt-Jakob disease.

JAKSCH DISEASE, see Von Jaksch disease.

JANEWAY SPOTS, nontender, macular, hemorrhagic areas usually on the palms or soles; most commonly noted in acute cases of endocarditis. Seen in infective endocarditis.

1. Wyngaarden JB, Smith LH: Cecil's Textbook of Medicine. 17th ed. Philadelphia: WB Saunders, 1985

JANNET DISEASE, neurosis with anxiety.

1. Casas EC: Diccionario Terminologico de Ciencias Medicas. 5th ed. Salvat Editores, 1954

JANSEN OPERATION, resection of the inferior wall of the frontal sinus and curettage of the mucosa. Cross-reference: Kuhnt operation. (Albert Jansen, 1859-1933, German otologist)

1. Maffei WE: Os Fundamentos da Medicina. 2nd ed. 1978

JANSKY-BIELSCHOWSKY DISEASE, see Bielschowsky disease.

JAPANESE B ENCEPHALITIS, caused by a *Flavivirus* first isolated in 1924 and transmitted by the bites of infected mosquitoes. Endemic and epidemic in Asia (Japan, Korea, Taiwan, China, Okinawa, Vietnam, the Philippines, Burma, Malaysia, Bangladesh, east and south India, Thailand, and Indonesia). The morbidity rate is high.

1. Wyngaarden JB, Smith LH: Cecil's Textbook of Medicine. 17th ed. Philadelphia: WB Saunders, 1985

JAPANESE DISEASE, JAPANESE RIVER FEVER, see Tsutsugamushi disease.

JARCHO-LEVIN SYNDROME, spondylothoracic dysplasia; a prominent occiput, a short thorax with diminished ribs and multiple vertebral defects, a short neck, and long digits with camptodactyly and syndactyly. Autosomal recessive inheritance. (Saul W. Jarcho, U.S.; Paul M. Levin, U.S.)

1. Jarcho S, Levin PM: Hereditary malformations of the vertebral bodies. Bull Johns Hopkins Hosp 62:216-226, 1938
2. Hull D, Barnes ND: Children with small chests. Arch Dis Child 47:12-19, 1972

JARVIS OPERATION, extirpation of the hypertrophied concha nasalis with a special device.

1. Maffei WE: Os Fundamentos da Medicina. 2nd ed. 1978

JAW-WINKING PHENOMENON, see Marcus Gunn phenomenon.

JEJUNAL SYNDROME, see Postprandial dumping syndrome.

JELKS OPERATION, surgery for stricture of the rectum by lateral incision of the anus and fibrous perirectal tissue.

1. Maffei WE: Os Fundamentos da Medicina. 2nd ed. 1978

JENDRASSIK SIGN, paralysis of one or many extraocular muscles; seen in Graves disease. (Ernst Jendrassik, 1858-1921, Hungarian)

1. Casas EC: Diccionario Terminologico de Ciencias Medicas. 5th ed. Salvat Editores, SA, 1954

JENSEN DISEASE, retinochoroiditis juxtapapillaris. (Edmund Z. Jensen, 1861-1950, Danish ophthalmologist)

1. Jensen EZ: Graefes Arch Ophthalmol 69:41-48, 1909

JENSEN OPERATION, a compromise of the transposition of the full insertion, similar to the Hummelsheim operation for strengthening of the ocular rectus muscle. (Edmund Z. Jensen)

1. Spaeth GL: Ophthalmic Surgery. Principles and Practice. Philadelphia: WB Saunders, 1982

JERSILD SYNDROME, elephantiasis of the genitals. (Peter Jersild, 1867-1950, Danish)

1. Jersild P: Elephantiasis genito-anorectalis. Derm Wochenschr 96:433-438, 1933

JERVELL AND LANGE-NIELSEN SYNDROME, hereditary prolongation of the QT interval on electrocardiography associated with deaf-mutism, syncope, and sudden death. An autosomal recessive trait. Cross-reference: Lange-Nielsen syndrome. (Anton Jervell, Norwegian; Frederik Lange-Nielsen, Norwegian)

1. Jervell A, Lange-Nielsen F: Am Heart J 54:59-68, 1957

JEUNE SYNDROME, JEUNE THORACIC DYSTROPHY SYNDROME, congenital polychondrodystrophy or asphyxiating thoracic dysplasia; small thorax, short limbs, and hypoplastic iliac wings are characteristics. Autosomal recessive inheritance. (Mathis Jeune, French pediatrician)

1. Campbell MF, Walsh PC: Campbell's Urology. 5th ed. Philadelphia: WB Saunders, 1986
2. Jeune M, Carron R, Beraud C, et al: Polychondrodystrophie avec blocage thoracique d'evolution fatale. Pediatrie 9:380-392, 1954
3. Oberklaid F, Danks DM, Mayne V, et al: Asphyxiating thoracic dystrophy. Clinical radiological, and pathological information on 10 patients. Arch Dis Child 52:758-765, 1977

JIMENEZ-DIAZ SIGN, see Hoffman sign.

JOB SYNDROME, a condition in which reduced neutrophil motility is associated with bacterial respiratory tract infections and cold staphylococcal abscesses, eosinophilia, and greatly increased levels of immunoglobulin E. (Named after Job, from the Book of Job in the Old Testament who suffered from skin disease.) Cross-references: Buckley syndrome; Hyperimmunoglobulinemia E syndrome.

1. Buckley RH, et al: Extreme hyperimmunoglobulinemia E and undue susceptibility to infections. Pediatrics 49:59-70, 1972
2. Wyngaarden JB, Smith LH Jr: Cecil's Textbook of Medicine. 17th ed. Philadelphia: WB Saunders, 1985

JOBERT OPERATION, autoplastic occlusion of a vesicovaginal fistula.
1. Maffei WE: Os Fundamentos da Medicina. 2nd ed. 1978

JOD-BASEDOW SYNDROME, see Graves disease. ("Jod" is German for iodine.) (Karl A. von Basedow, 1799-1854, German)

JOFFROY SIGN, an absence of wrinkling of the forehead when the head is bent down and the patient looks upward; seen in the patient with thyrotoxicosis. (Alexis Joffroy, 1844-1908, French neuropsychiatrist)
1. Bailey H: Physical Signs in Clinical Surgery. 16th ed. Baltimore: Williams & Wilkins, 1983

JOGGER FOOT SYNDROME, see Tarsal tunnel syndrome.

JOHANSON-BLIZZARD SYNDROME, ectodermal dysplasia with endocrine and exocrine insufficiency; hypoplastic alae nasi, hypothyroidism, and deafness are characteristics. Autosomal recessive inheritance.
1. Gorlin RJ, Cohen MM Jr, Levin LS: Syndromes of the Head and Neck. 3rd ed. New York: Oxford University Press, 1990
2. Johanson A, Blizzard RA: J Pediatr 79:982-987, 1971
3. Smith DW, Jones KL: Recognizable Patterns of Human Malformations: Genetic, Embryologic, and Clinical Aspects. 3rd ed. Philadelphia: WB Saunders, 1982

JOHNE DISEASE, pseudotuberculotic enteritis caused by *Mycobacterium paratuberculosi*; seen in cattle and sheep. (H. Albert Johne, 1839-1900, German)
1. Casas EC: Diccionario Terminologico de Ciencias Medicas. 5th ed. Salvat Editores, 1954

JOHNSON SIGN, the inability to contract the frontal muscles when looking upward; seen in a patient with exophthalmic goiter.
1. Casas EC: Diccionario Terminologico de Ciencias Medicas. 5th ed. Salvat Editores, SA, 1954

JOHNSON-STEVENS SYNDROME, see Stevens-Johnson syndrome.

JOLY OPERATION, surgical method for total hysterectomy in cases of prolapse of the uterus.
1. Maffei WE: Os Fundamentos da Medicina. 2nd ed. 1978

JONES CRITERIA, used for guidance in the diagnosis of rheumatic fever.
1. Wyngaarden JB, Smith LH: Cecil's Textbook of Medicine. 17th ed. Philadelphia: WB Saunders, 1985

JONES SYNDROME, cherubism; involves craniosynostosis and the Dandy-Walker malformation. (William A. Jones, U.S. dentist)
1. Gorlin RJ, Cohen MM Jr, Levin LS: Syndromes of the Head and Neck. 3rd ed. New York: Oxford University Press, 1990
2. Jones WA: Am J Cancer 17:946-950, 1933

JONNESCO OPERATION, sympathectomy.
1. Maffei WE: Os Fundamentos da Medicina. 2nd ed. 1978

JORGE LOBO DISEASE, see Lobo disease.

JORISSENNE SIGN, the fetal heart rate in a pregnant woman does not change if the fetal position is changed from horizontal or vertical.
1. Casas EC: Diccionario Terminologico de Ciencias Medicas. 5th ed. Salvat Editores, SA, 1954

JOSEPH DISEASE, striatonigral degeneration; a rare disease of the nervous system inherited as an autosomal dominant disorder in persons of Portuguese or Azorean ancestry. (An Azorean family affected by the disease.) Cross-reference: Machado-Joseph disease.
1. Rosenberg RN, Ivy N, Kirkpatrick J, et al: Joseph disease and Huntington disease: protein patterns in fibroblasts and brain. Neurology 31:1003-1014, 1981
2. Rowland LP: Merritt's Textbook of Neurology. 8th ed. Philadelphia: Lea & Febiger, 1989
3. Wyngaarden JB, Smith LH: Cecil's Textbook of Medicine. 17th ed. Philadelphia: WB Saunders, 1985

JOSSERAND SIGN, a strong metallic sound in the pulmonary area; heard in cases of acute pericarditis.
1. Casas EC: Diccionario Terminologico de Ciencias Medicas. 5th ed. Salvat Editores, SA, 1954

JOSUÉ SYNDROME, myocardial insufficiency causing renal failure.
1. Casas EC: Diccionario Terminologico de Ciencias Medicas. 5th ed. Salvat Editores, 1954

JOUBERT-BOLTSHAUSER SYNDROME, see Váradi syndrome.

JOURDAIN DISEASE, inflammation of the gums and dental alveoli.

1. Casas EC: Diccionario Terminologico de Ciencias Medicas. 5th ed. Salvat Editores, 1954

JOUSSET SIGN, in phrenic neuralgia, pain results if the 5th interspace in the parasternal line is compressed.

1. Casas EC: Diccionario Terminologico de Ciencias Medicas. 5th ed. Salvat Editores, SA, 1954

JUBERG-HAYWARD SYNDROME, see Orocraniodigital syndrome.

JUGULAR FORAMEN SYNDROME, extension of an infection into the jugular bulb or involvement of the bone around it; may result in paralysis of the 9th, 10th, and 11th cranial nerves. Cross-reference: Vernet syndrome.

1. Gorlin RJ, Cohen MM Jr, Levin LS: Syndromes of the Head and Neck. 3rd ed. New York: Oxford University Press, 1990
2. Haymaker W: Bing's Local Diagnosis in Neurological Diseases. 15th ed. St Louis: CV Mosby, 1969

JUGULAR SIGN, see Queckenstedt test.

JÜNGLING DISEASE, multiple cystic tuberculotic osteitis. (Adolph Otto Jüngling, 1884-1944, German surgeon)

1. Jüngling AO: Fortschr Roentgenstr 27:375-383, 1919/1921

JÜRGENSEN SIGN, pulmonary crepitation in acute pneumonia. (Theodor von Jürgensen, 1840-1907, Austrian)

1. Casas EC: Diccionario Terminologico de Ciencias Medicas. 5th ed. Salvat Editores, SA, 1954

JUVENILE PAGET DISEASE, a rare hereditary disorder of bone remodeling. Apparent autosomal recessive inheritance. (James Paget, 1814-1899, British surgeon)

1. Williams' Textbook of Endocrinology. 8th ed. Philadelphia: WB Saunders, 1992

KABUKI MAKE-UP SYNDROME, characterized by mild to moderate mental retardation, postnatal progressive growth retardation, and strikingly unusual facies reminiscent of the make-up used in the Kabuki theater.

1. Braun OH, Schmid E: Kabuki make-up syndrome (Niikawa-Kuroki syndrome) in Europe. J Pediatr 105:849-850, 1984
2. Gorlin RJ, Cohen MM Jr, Levin LS: Syndromes of the Head and Neck. 3rd ed. New York: Oxford University Press, 1990
3. Kaiser-Kupfer MI, Mulvihill JJ, Klein KL, et al: The Niikawa-Kuroki (Kabuki make-up) syndrome in an American black. Am J Ophthalmol 102:667-668, 1986 (Letter)

KADER OPERATION, a method for gastrostomy in which the feeding tube is introduced through a valve-like flap that closes on tube withdrawal. (Bronislaw Kader, 1863-1937, Polish surgeon)

1. Maffei WE: Os Fundamentos da Medicina. 2nd ed. 1978

KAGAMI DISEASE, infectious mononucleosis.

1. Dorland's Pocket Medical Dictionary. 22nd ed. Philadelphia: WB Saunders, 1977

KAHANA DISEASE, see Wolman disease.

KAHLER DISEASE, multiple myeloma. Cross-reference: Huppert disease. (Otto Kahler, 1849-1893, Austrian)

1. Bailey H, Love M: A Short Practice of Surgery. 12th ed. London: HK Lewis & Co, 1962
2. Bodechtel G: Diagnostico Diferencial de las Enfermedades Neurologicas. Madrid, 1967
3. Kahler O: Prag Med Wochenschr 14:33-35, 1889

KALISCHER DISEASE, see Sturge-Kalischer-Weber disease.

KALK SYNDROME, a disorder of bilirubin conjugation in the liver that persists long after clinical remission of hepatitis. This condition may or may not include jaundice.

1. Vannotti A: Clinique et Physiopathologie Médicales. Introduction a la Médecine Clinique. Librairie Maloine, SA, 1973

KALLMANN SYNDROME, the most widely recognized congenital clinical problem involving olfaction, this disorder is usually associated with hypogonadism and may also involve agenesis of the olfactory bulbs and stalks and faulty development of the hypothalamus. Deafness and other symptoms may be present. Cross-reference: Olfactogenital syndrome. (Franz J. Kallmann, 1897-1965, U.S. medical geneticist/psychiatrist)

1. Ballenger JJ: Diseases of the Nose, Throat, Ear, Head and Neck. 12th ed. Philadelphia: Lea & Febiger, 1977 12th ed. Philadelphia, Pa: Lea & Febiger, 1977
2. Campbell MF, Walsh PC: Campbell's Urology. 5th ed. Philadelphia: WB Saunders, 1986

3. Kallmann FJ, Barrera SE: Am J Ment Defic 48:203-236, 1943/44

KANAVEL SIGN, in the patient with infection of the tendon of the palm of the hand, the most painful point is 2 cm distal to the distal crease of the wrist. (Allen B. Kanavel, 1874-1938, U.S. surgeon)
1. Bailey H, Love M: A Short Practice of Surgery. 12th ed. London: HK Lewis, 1962

KANNER SYNDROME, infantile autism; the child appears alert and attractive despite odd behavior. Cross-reference: Asperger syndrome. (Leo Kanner, 1814-1891, Austrian-born U.S. child psychiatrist)
1. Kanner L: Nerve Child 2:217-250, 1943

KANTER SIGN, the absence of movement when the fetal head is palpated; an indication of fetal death.
1. Casas EC: Diccionario Terminologico de Ciencias Medicas. 5th ed. Salvat Editores, SA, 1954

KANTOR SIGN, a thin, string-like shadow in roentgenography of the colon through the filling defect; seen in the patient with colitis and regional ileitis. (John L. Kantor, 1840-1947, U.S. radiologist)
1. Dorland's Medical Dictionary. 28th ed. Philadelphia: WB Saunders, 1994

KAPLAN SIGN, with the arm held straight out, grip strength is checked. The grip strength test is repeated with the examiner encircling the patient's forearm with both hands about an inch below the elbow joint. The sign is positive when initial grip weakness and lateral elbow pain show significant improvement in grip strength and marked lessening of pain upon constriction of the musculature of the upper forearm. Seen in epicondylitis of the elbow.
1. Mazion JM: Illustrated Manual of Orthopedic Signs/Tests/Maneuvers for Office Procedure. 2nd ed. Orlando: Daniels Publishing, 1980

KAPOSI SARCOMA, multiple idiopathic hemorrhagic sarcoma; multiple neoplasms of the skin characterized by dark-colored nodules and plaques with an ulcerative tendency. A nonepithelial cancer which spreads sequentially rather than arising randomly. Disease is still an enigma. (Moritz Kaposi, 1837-1902, Austrian dermatologist)
1. Braunwald E: Heart Disease: A Textbook of Cardiovascular Medicine. 4th ed. Philadelphia: WB Saunders, 1992
2. Howard GM, Jakobioc FA, Devoe AG: Kaposi's sarcoma of the conjunctiva. Am J Ophthalmol 79:420-423, 1975
3. Kaposi M: Arch Derm Syph 4:265-273, 1872

KAPPELER OPERATION, cholecystojejunostomy.
1. Maffei WE: Os Fundamentos da Medicina. 2nd ed. 1978

KARPLUS SIGN, on auscultation over a pleural effusion, the vowel "u" spoken by the patient is heard as "a." (Johann P. Karplus, 1866-1936, Austrian physiologist)
1. Dorland's Medical Dictionary. 28th ed. Philadelphia: WB Saunders, 1994

KARROO SYNDROME, a condition among young Afrikaners in the Karroo region, consisting of high fever, alimentary tract disturbance, and tenderness in the lymph glands of the neck.
1. Dorland's Medical Dictionary. 28th ed. Philadelphia: WB Saunders, 1994

KARTAGENER SYNDROME, .a congenital disorder of the ultrastructure of the tubules of the ciliary axoneme, resulting in impairment of the movement of the mucous blanket of the respiratory mucosa. Characteristics are dextrocardia, situs inversus, sinusitis, and bronchiectasis. An abnormal protein called dynein is present in the cilia microtubules. (Manes Kartagener, 1897-1975, Czech)
1. Campbell MF, Walsh PC: Campbell's Urology. 5th ed. Philadelphia: WB Saunders, 1986
2. Fowler NO: Cardiac Diagnosis and Treatment. 3rd ed. Cambridge: Harper & Row, 1980
3. Kartagener M: Beitr Klin Tuberk 83:489-501, 1933

KASABACH-MERRITT SYNDROME, capillary hemangioma with thrombocytopenia. Approximately 0.3% of infants with hemangiomas, either subcutaneous or visceral, have thrombocytopenia. Cross-reference: Hemangioma-thrombocytopenia syndrome. (Haig H. Kasabach, 1898-1943, U.S. radiologist; Katherine K. Merritt, U.S. pediatrician)
1. Kasabach HH, Merritt KK: Am J Dis Child 59:1063-1070, 1940
2. Moschella SL, Hurley HJ: Dermatology. 2nd ed. Philadelphia: WB Saunders, 1985.
3. Wyngaarden JB, Smith LH Jr: Cecil's Textbook of Medicine. 17th ed. Philadelphia: WB Saunders, 1985

KASHIDA SIGN, the development of hyperesthesia and spasms following the application of either hot or cold packs; an indication of meningeal irritation. Cross-reference: Thermic sign. (K. Kashida, Japanese)
1. Baker AB, Baker LH: Clinical Neurology. Revised ed. Philadelphia: Harper & Row, 1982

KASHIN-BEK DISEASE, see Bek-Kashin disease.

KAST SYNDROME, see Maffucci syndrome.

KATAYAMA DISEASE, schistosomiasis japonica; a parasitic illness appearing mostly in the young Caucasian adult or child and characterized by urticarial swelling, eosinophilia, and a self-limiting course of several weeks. Ova appear in the stool, less often in the urine, and the spleen is palpable. (A town in Japan where the disease is common.) Cross-references: Hankow disease; Kinkiang disease.
  1. Spillane JD: Tropical Neurology. Oxford: Oxford University Press, 1973

KAUFMAN SYNDROME, see Oculocerebrofacial syndrome.

KAULBAUM DISEASE, catatonia.
  1. Casas EC: Diccionario Terminologico de Ciencias Medicas. 5th ed. Salvat Editores, 1954

KAYSER-FLEISCHER RING, a ring caused by copper deposits at the margin of the cornea near the limbus, resulting in golden brown or green discoloration. Occurs in patients with overt neurological symptoms, but not in children with hepatic manifestations alone. (Bernhard Kayser, 1869-1954, German ophthalmologist; Bruno Fleischer, 1874-1965, German ophthalmologist)
  1. Baker AB, Baker LH: Clinical Neurology. Revised ed. Philadelphia: Harper & Row, 1982
  2. Fleischer B: Klin Mbl Augenheilkd 41:489-491, 1903
  3. Kayser B: Klin Mbl Augenheilkd 40:22-25, 1902

KBG SYNDROME, a multiple abnormality syndrome characterized by mild mental retardation, short stature, characteristic facies, macrodontia, and various skeletal anomalies. (K.B.G. are the patient's initials in the first report.)
  1. Gorlin RJ, Cohen MM Jr, Levin LS: Syndromes of the Head and Neck. 3rd ed. New York: Oxford University Press, 1990
  2. Herrmann J, Pallister PD, Tiddy W, et al: The KBG syndrome-a syndrome of short stature, characteristic facies, mental retardation, macrodontia and skeletal anomalies. Birth Defects 11(5):7-18, 1975
  3. Parloir C, Fruns JP, Deroover J, et al: Short stature, craniofacial dysmorphism and dento-skeletal abnormalities in a large kindred. A variant of K.B.G. syndrome or a new mental retardation syndrome. Clin Genet 12:263-266, 1977

KEARNS-SAYRE SYNDROME, myopathy with progressive external ophthalmoplegia and pigmentary degeneration of the retina, with evidence of heart block on the electrocardiogram, and a cerebrospinal fluid protein content of more than 100 mg/dl. More than half of patients also have short stature, hearing loss, and evidence of corticospinal tract or cerebellar disease. Onset before age 15. Cross-references: Barnard-Scholz syndrome; Pearson syndrome. (Thomas P. Kearns, U.S. ophthalmologist; George P. Sayre, U.S. pathologist)
  1. Kearns TP, Sayre GP: Arch Ophthalmol 60:280-289, 1958
  2. Rowland LP (ed): Merritt's Textbook of Neurology. 9th ed. Baltimore: Williams & Wilkins, 1995
  3. Wyngaarden JB, Smith LH Jr: Cecil's Textbook of Medicine. 17th ed. Philadelphia: WB Saunders, 1985

KEDANI DISEASE, see Tsutsugamushi disease.

KEEGAN OPERATION, modification of the Indian method for nasal autoplasty.
  1. Maffei WE: Os Fundamentos da Medicina. 2nd ed. 1978

KEEN OPERATION, omphalotomy. (William W. Keen, 1837-1932, U.S. surgeon)
  1. Maffei WE: Os Fundamentos da Medicina. 2nd ed. 1978

KEEN SIGN, fracture of the distal leg causes increased diameter of the distal tibia. (William W. Keen)
  1. Casas EC: Diccionario Terminologico de Ciencias Medicas. 5th ed. Salvat Editores, SA, 1954

KEETLEY OPERATION, a surgical procedure for radical cure of umbilical hernia.
  1. Maffei WE: Os Fundamentos da Medicina. 2nd ed. 1978

KEHR OPERATION, ablation of the gallbladder and drainage of the hepatic duct.
  1. Maffei WE: Os Fundamentos da Medicina. 2nd ed. 1978

KEHR SIGN, intense pain in the left shoulder; seen in some patients with splenic rupture. (Hans Kehr, 1862-1916; German surgeon)
  1. Casas EC: Diccionario Terminologico de Ciencias Medicas. 5th ed. Salvat Editores, SA, 1954

KEHRER OPERATION, plastic surgery for flat foot.
  1. Maffei WE: Os Fundamentos da Medicina. 2nd ed. 1978

KEHRER SIGN, pain in the cervical spine during coughing and sneezing, due to pressure on the cervical nerves; seen in the patient with increased intracranial pressure.
  1. Bodechtel G: Diagnostico Diferencial De Las Enfermedades Neurologicas. Madrid, 1967

KEIPERT SYNDROME, severe sensorineural hearing loss, unusual facies, and broad terminal phalanges are features. X-linked recessive or autosomal inheritance. (J.A. Keipert, Australian)

  1. Gorlin RJ, Cohen MM Jr, Levin LS: Syndromes of the Head and Neck. 3rd ed. New York: Oxford University Press, 1990

  2. Keipert JA: Austral Pediatr J 9:10-13, 1973

KELLER OPERATION, arthroplasty; most commonly used for bunions. (William L. Keller, 1874-1959, U.S. surgeon)

  1. Schwartz SI: Principles of Surgery. 4th ed. New York: McGraw-Hill, 1983

KELLOCK SIGN, percussion of the ribs while pressing on the chest causes an increase in the vibration of the ribs; an indication of pleural effusion. (T.H. Kellock, U.S.)

  1. Casas EC: Diccionario Terminologico de Ciencias Medicas. 5th ed. Salvat Editores, SA, 1954

KELLY OPERATION, 1) surgical repair of arytenoid cartilage or muscle. Cross-reference: King operation. (Joseph D. Kelly, U.S. otolaryngologist); 2) fixation of the uterus to the anterior abdominal wall in cases of retroversion of the uterus. (Howard A. Kelly, 1858-1943, U.S. surgeon)

  1. Maffei WE: Os Fundamentos da Medicina. 2nd ed. 1978

KELLY SIGN, the ureter contracts like a worm when squeezed with forceps. (Howard A. Kelly)

  1. Casas EC: Diccionario Terminologico de Ciencias Medicas. 5th ed. Salvat Editores, SA, 1954

KENAWY SIGN, upon applying the stethoscope beneath the xiphoid process, auscultation reveals a venous hum that is louder on inspiration. Found frequently with splenomegaly associated with bilharzial fibrosis of the liver (Egyptian splenomegaly) and is probably due to engorgement of the splenic vein. (Mohammed R. Kenawy, Egyptian)

  1. Bailey H: Physical Signs in Clinical Surgery. 16th ed. Baltimore: Williams & Wilkins, 1983

KENNEDY SIGN, bruit heard in the umbilical cord.

  1. Casas EC: Diccionario Terminologico de Ciencias Medicas. 5th ed. Salvat Editores, SA, 1954

KENNEDY SYNDROME, see Foster-Kennedy syndrome.

KENNY SYNDROME, tubular stenosis; proportional growth retardation with macrocephaly, low birth weight, and episodic hypocalcemia with hyperphosphatemia leading to tetany. (Frederic M. Kenny, U.S.)

  1. Caffey J: Congenital stenosis of medullary spaces in tubular bones and calvaria in two proportional dwarfs, mother and son; coupled with transitory hypocalcemic tetany. Am J Roentgenol 100:1-11, 1967

  2. Gorlin RJ, Cohen MM Jr, Levin LS: Syndromes of the Head and Neck. 3rd ed. New York: Oxford University Press, 1990

  3. Kenny FM, Linarelli L: Dwarfism and cortical thickening of the tubular bones: transient hypocalcemia in a mother and son. Am J Dis Child 111:201-207, 1966

KENYA DISEASE, KENYA TICK TYPHUS, see Conor-Bruch disease.

KERANDEL SIGN, pain and hyperesthesia are reduced in the patient with African trypanosomiasis when painful percussion is performed. (Jean F. Kerandel, 1873-1934, French physician in Africa)

  1. Casas EC: Diccionario Terminologico de Ciencias Medicas. 5th ed. Salvat Editores, SA, 1954

KERATODERMA PALMOPLANTAR SYNDROME, see Papillon-Lefèvre syndrome.

KERGARADEC SIGN, uterine bruit seen in pregnancy. (Jean A. le Jameau, Vicomte de Kergaradec, 1788-1877, French gynecologist)

  1. Casas EC: Diccionario Terminologico de Ciencias Medicas. 5th ed. Salvat Editores, SA, 1954

KERNIG SIGN, pains and spasms elicited while lying on the back and flexing the thigh at the hip to a right angle on the abdomen; extending the leg on the thigh is not possible. (Vladimir M. Kernig, 1840-1917, Russian)

  1. Baker AB, Baker LH: Clinical Neurology. Revised ed. Philadelphia: Harper & Row, 1982

  2. Ballenger JJ: Diseases of the Nose, Throat, Ear, Head and Neck. 12th ed. Philadelphia: Lea & Febiger, 1977

KERR SIGN, the texture of the skin is altered distal to the lesion; seen in the patient with spinal cord injury. (Henry H. Kerr, 1881-1963, U.S. surgeon)

  1. Casas EC: Diccionario Terminologico de Ciencias Medicas. 5th ed. Salvat Editores, SA, 1954

KESTENBAUM SIGN, a decrease in the number of arterioles traversing the margin of the optic disc; used as a criterion for diagnosing optic atrophy. (Alfred Kestenbaum, German)

  1. Dorland's Medical Dictionary. 28th ed. Philadelphia: WB Saunders, 1994

KEUTEL SYNDROME, unusual facies, brachytelephalangy, pulmonary stenosis, and diffuse calcification of the cartilages of the pinnae, larynx, trachea, and bronchi, with mixed hearing loss and peripheral pulmonary stenosis are features. (Jürgen Keutel, German)

1. Gorlin RJ, Cohen MM Jr, Levin LS: Syndromes of the Head and Neck. 3rd ed. New York: Oxford University Press, 1990
2. Keutel J, et al: A new autosomal recessive syndrome: peripheral pulmonary stenoses, brachytelephalangism, neural hearing loss and abnormal cartilage calcification/ossification. Birth Defects 8(5):60-68, 1972

KEW GARDENS DISEASE, KEW GARDENS SPOTTED FEVER, rickettsialpox. (Area in New York City where first reported.)

1. Dorland's Pocket Medical Dictionary. 22nd ed. Philadelphia: WB Saunders, 1977

KEY OPERATION, lateral cystotomy using a straight guide.

1. Maffei WE: Os Fundamentos da Medicina. 2nd ed. 1978

KID SYNDROME, *k*eratitis-*i*chthyosis-*d*eafness (KID); see Senter syndrome.

KIENBÖCK DISEASE, a painful disorder of the wrist in which roentgenography shows vascular necrosis of the carpal lunate bone. Most prominent in adult males (ages 15-40) who perform manual labor. (Robert Kienböck, 1871-1953, Austrian radiologist)

1. Kienböck R: Wien Med Wochenschr 51:1346-1348 1901

KIENBÖCK PHENOMENON, the hemidiaphragm falls on expiration and rises on inspiration. (Robert Kienböck)

1. Dorland's Medical Dictionary. 28th ed. Philadelphia: WB Saunders, 1994

KIESEWETTER-REHBEIN OPERATION, utilizes the abdominal approach for correction of a high imperforate anus in infants.

1. Schwartz SI: Principles of Surgery. 4th ed. New York: McGraw-Hill, 1983

KILLIAN OPERATION, 1) resection of the anterior wall of the frontal sinus, curettage of the affected tissue, and formation of a permanent communication with the nose; 2) nasal septal reconstruction. (Gustav Killian, 1860-1921, German laryngologist)

1. Cummings C: Otolaryngology. Head and Neck Surgery. 6th ed. St Louis: CV Mosby, 1986
2. Maffei WE: Os Fundamentos da Medicina. 2nd ed. 1978

KILOH-NEVIN SYNDROME, occurs when the anterior interosseous nerve is compressed or entrapped due to laceration, fracture, hematoma, or repetitive use. Cross-references: Anterior interosseous nerve syndrome; Cubital tunnel syndrome; Parsonage-Turner syndrome. (Leslie G. Kiloh, Australian; Samuel Nevin)

1. Kiloh LG, Nevin S: Br Med J 1:850-851, 1952
2. Spinner M: The anterior interosseous-nerve syndrome. With special attention to its variants. J Bone Joint Surg (Am) 52:84-94, 1970

KIMMELSTIEL-WILSON DISEASE, diabetes mellitus-hypertension-nephrosis; kidney disease often accompanied by severe, refractory hypertension, which undermines renal function and compromises cardiac, cerebral, and peripheral vasculature; seen in the diabetic. (Paul Kimmelstiel, 1900-1970, German pathologist in U.S.; Clifford Wilson, British)

1. Fowler NO: Cardiac Diagnosis and Treatment. 3rd ed. Cambridge: Harper & Row, 1980
2. Kimmelstiel P, Wilson C: Am J Pathol 12:45-81, 1936
3. Ritchie AC: Boyd's Textbook of Pathology. 9th ed. Philadelphia: Lea & Febiger, 1990

KINGSBOURNE SYNDROME, see Dancing eye-dancing foot syndrome.

KINKIANG DISEASE, see Katayama disease.

KINKY-HAIR SYNDROME, see Menkes syndrome.

KIRKLAND DISEASE, acute infection of the face with regional lymphadenitis.

1. Casas EC: Diccionario Terminologico de Ciencias Medicas. 5th ed. Salvat Editores, 1954

KIRMISSON OPERATION, transplantation of the Achilles tendon to the long peroneal muscle in cases of talipes valgus.

1. Maffei WE: Os Fundamentos da Medicina. 2nd ed. 1978

KIRMISSON SIGN, fracture of the distal humerus with dislocation produces an ecchymotic line in the elbow.

1. Casas EC: Diccionario Terminologico de Ciencias Medicas. 5th ed. Salvat Editores, SA, 1954

KIRSCHNER OPERATION, treatment of splenorrhagia by suturing the wound and attaching the epiploon to it.

1. Maffei WE: Os Fundamentos da Medicina. 2nd ed. 1978

KISSING SPINE DISEASE, see Baastrup disease.

KLEBS DISEASE, see Glomerulonephritis syndrome. (Theodor A.E. Klebs, 1834-1913, German bacteriologist)

KLEEBLATTSCHÄDEL SYNDROME, cloverleaf skull; a congenital disorder characterized by synostosis of multiple or all cranial sutures, hydrocephalus, and sometimes associated with facial dysostosis and long bone anomalies.

1. Holtermüller K, Wiedemann HR: Med Monatsschr 14:439-446, 1960

KLEIN-WAARDENBURG SYNDROME, see Waardenburg syndrome. (David Klein, Swiss ophthalmologist; Petras Waardenburg, 1886-1979, Dutch ophthalmologist)

KLEINE-LEVIN SYNDROME, characterized by episodic periods of excessive sleep and overeating, lasting up to several weeks; occurs primarily in adolescent males. There is no specific treatment but the condition remits in adulthood. An extremely rare disorder, now almost never encountered. Cross-reference: Hypersomnia-bulimia syndrome. (William Kleine, German psychiatrist; Max Levin, U.S. neurologist)

1. Kleine W: Monatsschr Psychiatr 57:285-320, 1925
2. Levin M: Brain 59:494-504, 1936
3. Wyngaarden JB, Smith LH Jr: Cecil's Textbook of Medicine. 17th ed. Philadelphia: WB Saunders, 1985

KLEIST SIGN, the fingers of the patient tighten in the examiner's fingers when they are gently elevated; an indication of frontal lobe or thalamic lesions. (Karl Kleist, German neurologist)

KLEMM SIGN, a tympanic sound in the right inferior quadrant, corresponding to gaseous distention of the ascending colon and cecum. (Paul Klemm, 1861-1921, German surgeon)

1. Casas EC: Diccionario Terminologico de Ciencias Medicas. 5th ed. Salvat Editores, SA, 1954

KLEMPERER DISEASE, see Banti syndrome.

KLINEFELTER SYNDROME, a syndrome describing boys with 47,XXY chromosomes who have abnormal physical features such as tall stature, a small penises and testes, and long limbs. Aberrant behavior is frequently noted. Common sex chromosome abnormalities such as this usually are not associated with any congenital malformations. Cross-reference: XXY syndrome. (Harry F. Klinefelter, Jr., U.S.)

1. Caldwell PD, Smith DW: The XXY syndrome in childhood: detection and treatment. J Pediatr 80:250, 1972
2. Klinefelter HR Jr, et al: Syndrome characterized by gynecomastia, aspermatogenesis without A-Leydigism, and increased excretion of follicle stimulating hormone. J Clin Endocrinol 2:615-627, 1942
3. Wilson JD, Foster DW (eds): Williams' Textbook of Endocrinology. 8th ed. Philadelphia: WB Saunders, 1992
4. Wyngaarden JB, Smith LH Jr: Cecil's Textbook of Medicine. 17th ed. Philadelphia: WB Saunders, 1985

KLIPPEL-FEIL SYNDROME, congenital osseous torticollis; usually there is a short webbed neck, limited rotation of the head, and a low hairline. Cross-reference: Cervical-fusion syndrome. (Maurice Klippel, 1858-1942, French neurologist/psychiatrist; André Feil, French neurologist)

1. Campbell MF, Walsh PC: Campbell's Urology. 5th ed. Philadelphia: WB Saunders, 1986
2. Klippel M, Feil A: Nouv Icon Salpetriere 25:223-250, 1912

KLIPPEL-TRÉNAUNAY SYNDROME, KLIPPEL-TRÉNAUNAY-PARKES-WEBER SYNDROME, KLIPPEL-TRÉNAUNAY-WEBER SYNDROME, hemangiectasia hypertrophica; hemangioma of the oral cavity and a port wine stain cutaneous lesion are features. Cross-reference: Sturge-Weber syndrome. (Maurice Klippel; Paul Trénaunay, French neurologist; Frederick Parkes Weber, 1863-1962, British)

1. Klippel M, Trénaunay P: Arch Gen Med 3:641-642, 1900
2. McKusick VA: Heritable Disorders of Connective Tissue. 4th ed. St Louis: CV Mosby, 1972
3. Weber F: Br J Dermatol 19:231-235, 1907
4. Wyngaarden JB, Smith LH Jr: Cecil's Textbook of Medicine. 17th ed. Philadelphia: WB Saunders, 1985

KLIPPEL-WEIL SIGN, consists of involuntary flexion, opposition, and adduction of the thumb on passive extension of the fingers when there is some degree of contracture in flexion. (Maurice Klippel; Adolphe Weil, 1848-1916, German)

1. Baker AB, Baker LH: Clinical Neurology. Revised ed. Philadelphia: Harper & Row, 1982

KLUGE SIGN, blue coloration of the vagina during pregnancy.

1. Casas EC: Diccionario Terminologico de Ciencias Medicas. 5th ed. Salvat Editores, SA, 1954

KLUMPKE SYNDROME, lower brachial plexus palsy. Results from a lesion of the 8th cervical and 1st thoracic nerve roots, and produces paralysis of the muscles supplied by the ulnar nerve and the inner head of the median nerve. Cross-reference: Déjerine-Klumpke syndrome. (Augusta Déjerine-Klumpke, 1859-1927, French neurologist)

1. Déjerine-Klumpke A: Rev Med 5:591-616, 739-790, 1885
2. Grinker RR, Sahs AL: Neurology. 6th ed. Springfield: Charles C Thomas, 1966

KLÜVER-BUCY SYNDROME, behavioral changes following temporal lobectomy, with the patient showing a tendency to touch everything available. Bilateral, large, anterior temporal lobe lesions producing symptoms identical to that seen in animals from which the anterior temporal lobe has been removed. (Heinrich Klüver, 1897-1979, U.S. neurologist; Paul C. Bucy, 1904-1992, U.S. neurosurgeon)

1. Baker AB, Baker LH: Clinical Neurology. Revised ed. Philadelphia: Harper & Row, 1982
2. Bucy PC, Klüver H: Anatomic changes secondary to temporal lobectomy. Arch Neurol Psychiatry 44:1142-1146, 1940
3. Klüver H, Bucy PC: An analysis of certain effects of bilateral temporal lobectomy in rhesus monkeys. J Psychol 5:33-54, 1938

KNAPP OPERATION, 1) peripheral opening of the crystalline lens capsule, without iridectomy, in cataract surgery; 2) evisceration of the globe followed by blepharoplasty. (Herman J. Knapp, 1832-1911, German-born U.S. ophthalmologist)

1. Maffei WE: Os Fundamentos da Medicina. 2nd ed. 1978

KNEE SIGN, unequal dilatation of the pupils in the patient with Graves disease.

1. Dorland's Medical Dictionary. 28th ed. Philadelphia: WB Saunders, 1994

KNIEST SYNDROME, an inherited form of bone dysplasia; flat facies, thick joints, and platyspondylia are features. Cross-reference: Dwarfism Kniest syndrome. (Wilhelm Kniest, German pediatrician)

1. Kniest W: Z Kinderheilkd 70:633-640, 1952
2. McKusick VA: Heritable Disorders of Connective Tissue. 4th ed. St Louis: CV Mosby, 1972
3. Smith DW, Jones KL: Recognizable Patterns of Human Malformations: Genetic, Embryologic, and Clinical Aspects. 3rd ed. Philadelphia: WB Saunders, 1982

KNOBLOCH-LAYER SYNDROME, consists of high myopia, vitreoretinal degeneration, retinal detachment, and occipital encephalocele.

1. Gorlin RJ, Cohen MM Jr, Levin LS: Syndromes of the Head and Neck. 3rd ed. New York: Oxford University Press, 1990
2. Knobloch WA, Layer JM: J Pediatr Ophthalmol 8:181-184, 1971

KNOX OPERATION, ablation of the tongue through a midline incision in the lip and mandibula.

1. Maffei WE: Os Fundamentos da Medicina. 2nd ed. 1978

KÖBNER DISEASE, see Epidermolysis bullosa syndrome. (Heinrich Köbner, 1838-1904, German dermatologist)

KÖBNER PHENOMENON, isomorphic reaction. Among the features of psoriasis is the capacity to reproduce skin lesions at sites of local injury. This reactive phenomenon has intrigued many investigators searching for basic clues to the cause of psoriasis. Described in 1877. (Heinrich Köbner)

1. Greaves MW, Weinstein GD: Treatment of psoriasis. N Engl J Med 332:581-588, 1995
2. Moschella SL, Hurley HJ: Dermatology. 2nd ed. Philadelphia: WB Saunders, 1985

KOCHER OPERATION, 1) resection of the ankle through an incision inferior to the lateral malleolus; 2) excision of the tongue through an incision extending from the mandibular symphysis to the hyoid bone and then to the mastoid process. (Emil Theodore Kocher, 1841-1917, Swiss surgeon)

1. Maffei WE: Os Fundamentos da Medicina. 2nd ed. 1978

KOCHER SIGN, the eyelids raise more quickly than the eyeball when looking upward; seen in the patient with Graves disease. (Emil Theodor Kocher)

KOCHER-DEBRÉ-SÉMÉLAIGNE SYNDROME, see Debré-Sémélaigne syndrome. (Emil Theodore Kocher; Robert Debré, French pediatrician; Georges Sémélaigne, French pediatrician)

KOCK OPERATION, shortening of the broad ligaments through the vagina in cases of retroversion of the uterus.

1. Maffei WE: Os Fundamentos da Medicina. 2nd ed. 1978

KOENIG DISEASE, osteochondritis dissecans. (Franz Kocnig, 1832-1910, German surgeon)
1. Casas EC: Diccionario Terminologico de Ciencias Medicas. 5th ed. Salvat Editores, 1954

KOENIG OPERATION, surgery for congenital luxation of the hip. Cross-reference: Shelving operation.
1. Maffei WE: Os Fundamentos da Medicina. 2nd ed. 1978

KOENIG SYNDROME, local infection of the cecum and terminal ileum; consists of constipation alternating with diarrhea when associated with abdominal pain, meteorism, and gurgling sounds in the right iliac fossa. (Franz Koenig)
1. Dorland's Medical Dictionary. 28th ed. Philadelphia: WB Saunders, 1994

KOERBER-SALUS-ELSCHNIG SYNDROME, see Sylvian syndrome. (Hermann Koerber, German ophthalmologist; Robert Salus, Austrian ophthalmologist; Anton Elschnig, Austrian ophthalmologist)

KOERTE-BALLANCE OPERATION, see Ballance operation.

KÖHLER BONE DISEASE, osteochondrosis of the tarsal navicular bone. (Alban Köhler, 1874-1947, German roentgenologist)
1. Campbell WC, Crenshaw AH: Campbell Operative Orthopaedics. 7th ed. St Louis: CV Mosby, 1987
2. Köhler A: Munch Med Wochenschr 55:1923-1925, 1908

KÖHLER-PELLEGRINI-STIEDA SYNDROME, see Pellegrini disease. (Alban Köhler)

KÖHLMEIER-DEGÓS SYNDROME, vasculitis of the gastrointestinal tract and skin. (W. Köhlmeier, German dermatologist, Robert L. Degós, French dermatologist)
1. Degós R, Delort J, Tricot R: Bull Soc Fr Dermatol Syph 49:148-150, 1942
2. Köhlmeier W: Arch Dermatol Syph 181:783-792, 1941
3. Scully RE, et al: Case records of the Massachusetts General Hospital. N Engl J Med 332:1452-1459, 1995

KOHLSCHÜTTER SYNDROME, amelocerebrohypohidrosis; amelogenesis imperfecta, epilepsy, and mental deterioration are features.
1. Christodolou J, Hall RK, Menahem S, et al: A syndrome of epilepsy, dementia and amelogenesis imperfecta: genetic and clinical features. J Med Genet 25:827-830, 1988
2. Gorlin RJ, Cohen MM Jr, Levin LS: Syndromes of the Head and Neck. 3rd ed. New York: Oxford University Press, 1990
3. Kohlschütter A, Chappuis D, Meier C, et al: Helv Paediatr Acta 29:283-294, 1974

KOJEWNIKOFF EPILEPSY, partial epilepsy; in its typical form includes sudden high fever, loss of consciousness, paralysis, delirium, and generalized convulsions or local spasms. Usually preceded by signs of infection. (Aleksei Y. Kojewnikoff, 1836-1902, Russian neurologist)
1. Grinker RR, Sahs AL: Neurology. 6th ed. Springfield: Charles C Thomas, 1966

KOLOMNIN OPERATION, a method for cauterization of the affected tissue in coxalgia, using incandescent needles.
1. Maffei WE: Os Fundamentos da Medicina. 2nd ed. 1978

KONDOLEON OPERATION, surgical treatment of elephantiasis by extirpation of subcutaneous facial strips. (Emmanuel Kondoleon, 1879-1939, Greek surgeon)
1. Maffei WE: Os Fundamentos da Medicina. 2nd ed. 1978

KONZO DISEASE, an upper motor neuron disease characterized by the abrupt onset of a varying degree of symmetrical, isolated, and permanent but nonprogressive spastic paraparesis. The uniform epidemiological and clinical findings have identified this as a distinct disease entity induced by the combined effects of high cyanide and low sulfur intake from exclusive consumption of insufficiently processed bitter cassava roots. First described in Zaire in 1938 and named after the local designation.
1. Elian M, Dean G: Motor neuron disease and multiple sclerosis among immigrants to England from the Indiana subcontinent, the Caribbean and East and West Africa. J Neurol Neurosurg Psychiatry 56:454-457. 1993
2. Tylleskär T, Howlett WP, Rwiza HT, et al: Konzo: a distinct disease entity with selective upper motor neuron damage. J Neurol Neurosurg Psychiatry 56:638-643, 1993

KOPLIK SIGN, KOPLIK SPOT, small, irregular shaped red spots on the oral mucosa; occurs early in measles. (Henry Koplik, 1858-1927, U.S. pediatrician)
1. Koplik H: Acta Pediatr 13:918-922, 1896

KORÁNYI SIGN, a decrease in sound during percussion of the dorsal spine; seen in the patient with pleural effusion. (Baron Friedrich von Korányi, 1828-1913, Hungarian)

1. Casas EC: Diccionario Terminologico de Ciencias Medicas. 5th ed. Salvat Editores, SA, 1954

KORSAKOFF [KORSAKOV] SYNDROME, amnesia syndrome; a psychiatric condition character-ized by lack of recognition of recently acquired information, retention of material acquired early, and confabulation; encountered in association with transient or permanent lesions (traumatic, toxic, meta-bolic, neoplastic, or infectious) that affect the limbic system mainly from the region of the mammillary bodies rostrally. Cross-reference: Dysmnesic syndrome. (Sergei Korsakoff [Korsakov], 1854-1900, Russian neurologist)
1. Haymaker W: Bing's Local Diagnosis in Neurological Diseases. 15th ed. St Louis: CV Mosby, 1969
2. Korsakoff SS: Vestn Psychiatr (Moska) 4, 1887

KORTZEBORN OPERATION, surgery for median nerve paralysis, consisting of lengthening the extensor muscles of the thumb and their fixation to the ulnar side of the hand.
1. Maffei WE: Os Fundamentos da Medicina. 2nd ed. 1978

KOSHEWNIKOFF EPILEPSY, see Kojewnikoff epilepsy.

KOSTMANN SYNDROME, congenital neutropenia that presents a bone marrow dominated by myeloblasts and promyelocytes that, in isolation, are morphologically indistinguishable from the acute leukemias. (Rolf Kostmann, Swedish)
1. Kostmann R: Acta Paediatr 45 (Suppl 105):1-78, 1956
2. Wyngaarden JB, Smith LH Jr: Cecil's Textbook of Medicine. 17th ed. Philadelphia: WB Saunders, 1985

KOZLOWSKI SPONDYLOMETAPHYSEAL DYSPLASIA SYNDROME, a short spine, irregular metaphyses, and pectus carinatum are features. Autosomal dominant, fresh mutation.
1. Kozlowski K, Maroteaux P, Sprangler G: Presse Med 75:2769-2774, 1967
2. Le Quesne GW, Kozlowski K: Spondylometaphyseal dysplasia. Br J Radiol 46:685-691, 1973
3. Smith DW, Jones KL: Recognizable Patterns of Human Malformations: Genetic, Embryologic, and Clinical Aspects. 3rd ed. Philadelphia: WB Saunders, 1982

KRABBE SYNDROME, globoid cell dystrophy; a rapidly progressive disorder with onset before 6 months of age. Macrocephaly, delay of motor development, pyramidal tract lesions, and opisthotonos are characteristics. Males and females are affected about equally. Autosomal recessive inheritance. (Knud H. Krabbe, 1885-1965, Danish neurologist)
1. Farmer TW: Pediatric Neurology. 2nd ed. Hagerstown: Harper & Row, 1975
2. Krabbe KH: Brain 39:74-114, 1916
3. Wyngaarden JB, Smith LH Jr: Cecil's Textbook of Medicine. 17th ed. Philadelphia, Pa: WB Saunders, 1985

KRAEPELIN-MOREL DISEASE, see Morel-Kraepelin disease.

KRASKE OPERATION, removal of the coccyx and part of the sacrum for gaining access to a rectal carcinoma. (Paul Kraske, 1851-1930, German surgeon)
1. Maffei WE: Os Fundamentos da Medicina. 2nd ed. 1978

KRAUSE OPERATION, see Hartley-Krause operation. (Fedor V. Krause, 1857-1937, German sur-geon)

KRAUSE SYNDROME, encephalo-ophthalmic dysplasia; a constellation of disorders most fre-quently found in premature infants several months after birth. Characterized by malformation of the choroid, retina, and optic nerve, and possible blindness, cataract, coloboma, glaucoma, and microph-thalmos. Cerebral symptoms include aplasia, hyperplasia and hypertrophy of the brain, hydrocephalus, and mental retardation. (Arlington C. Krause, U.S. ophthalmologist)
1. Krause AC: Congenital encephalo-ophthalmic dysplasia. Arch Ophthalmol 36:387-444, 1946

KRAUSS SYNDROME, hyperadrenalism.
1. Casas EC: Diccionario Terminologico de Ciencias Medicas. 5th ed. 1954

KRETSCHMER SYNDROME, see Apallic syndrome. (Ernst Kretschmer, 1888-1964, German psy-chiatrist)

KREYSIG SIGN, see Heim-Kreysig sign. (Friedrich L. Kreysig, 1770-1839, German)

KRIMER OPERATION, uranoplasty.
1. Maffei WE: Os Fundamentos da Medicina. 2nd ed. 1978

KRISHABER DISEASE, a neuropsychiatric disturbance characterized by tachycardia, vertigo, hyper-esthesia, and sensorial hallucinations. (Maurice Krishaber, 1836-1883, Hungarian in France)
1. Casas EC: Diccionario Terminologico de Ciencias Medicas. 5th ed. Salvat Editores, 1954

KRISOVSKI SIGN, scar lines radiating from the mouth in the patient with congenital syphilis. (Max Krisovski, German)
1. Casas EC: Diccionario Terminologico de Ciencias Medicas. 5th ed. Salvat Editores, SA, 1954

KRISTIANSEN SYNDROME, diplopia, seizures, and behavioral alterations and cerebral dysfunction are characteristics.
1. Casas EC: Diccionario Terminologico de Ciencias Medicas. 5th ed. 1954

KRÖNLEIN OPERATION, resection of the lateral wall of the orbit in order to resect a tumor without enucleation of the globe. (Rudolf U. Krönlein, 1847-1910, Swedish surgeon)
1. Maffei WE: Os Fundamentos da Medicina. 2nd ed. 1978

KUFS DISEASE, the adult variety of cerebral sphingolipidosis. Prominent intention myoclonus as well as truncal and facial myoclonus have been described. May be exacerbated by voluntary movement and photic stimulation. (Hugo Kufs, 1871-1955, German psychiatrist)
1. Boehme DH, Cottrell JC, Leonberg SC, et al: A dominant form of neuronal ceroid-lipofuscinosis. Brain 94:745-760, 1971

KUGELBERG-WELANDER SYNDROME, juvenile spinal muscular atrophy. Cross-references: Oppenheimer disease; Werdnig-Hoffmann disease; Wohlfart-Kugelberg-Welander disease. (Eric Kugelberg, 1913-1983, Swedish neurologist; Lisa Welander, Swedish neurologist)

KUGELMASS SIGN, a reddish appearance of the retroauricular region may be an indication of allergy in children.
1. Casas EC: Diccionario Terminologico de Ciencias Medicas. 5th ed. Salvat Editores, SA, 1954

KÜHNE MUSCULAR PHENOMENON, see Porret phenomenon. (Wilhelm F. Kühne, 1837-1900, German physiologist)

KUHNT OPERATION, KUHNT-SZYMANOWSKI PROCEDURE, see Jansen operation.

KÜMMELL DISEASE, spinal compression caused by compression fracture osteoporosis. (Herman Kümmell, 1852-1937, German surgeon)
1. Hamilton & Bailey's Demonstration of Physical Signs Including Surgery. 16th ed. Baltimore: Williams & Wilkins, 1983
2. Kümmell H: Dtsch Med Wochenschr 21:180-181, 1985

KÜNKEL SYNDROME, see Bearn-Künkel syndrome.

KÜNTSCHNER TECHNIQUE, used for open reduction of fracture of the femur. (Gerhard Küntschner, 1902-1972, German surgeon)
1. Schwartz SI: Principles of Surgery. 4th ed. New York: McGraw-Hill, 1983

KÜSSMAUL DISEASE, polyarteritis nodosa; about 0.1% of autopsies show polyarteritis nodosa, and the incidence in the population as a whole is likely considerably lower. May occur at any age, but mostly seen in adults; about 70% of patients are male. Cross-reference: Maier disease. (Adolph Küssmaul, 1822-1902, German)
1. Küssmaul A, Maier R: Dtsch Arch Klin Med 1:484-518, 1866
2. Ritchie AC: Boyd's Textbook of Pathology. 9th ed. Philadelphia: Lea & Febiger, 1990

KÜSSMAUL SIGN, an increase in distention of the jugular veins during inspiration; observed in the patient with pericarditis and mediastinal tumor. (Adolph Küssmaul)
1. Casas EC: Diccionario Terminologico de Ciencias Medicas. 5th ed. Salvat Editores, SA, 1954

KÜSTER OPERATION, opening of the attic, antrum, and tympanum for draining secretions from mastoiditis.
1. Maffei WE: Os Fundamentos da Medicina. 2nd ed. 1978

KÜSTNER SIGN, a cystic tumor located in the midline anterior to the uterus. (Otto E. Küstner, 1849-1931, German gynecologist)
1. Casas EC: Diccionario Terminologico de Ciencias Medicas. 5th ed. Salvat Editores, SA, 1954

KVEIM TEST, consists of an intradermal injection of sarcoid tissue; if positive, a dusky nodule of sarcoid tissue appears within a month. A biopsy of a skin nodule, lymph node, or any accessible tissue is diagnostic. (Morten A. Kveim, Norwegian pathologist)
1. Bailey H, Love M: A Short Practice of Surgery. 12th ed. London: HK Lewis & Co, 1962

LABAND SYNDROME, gingival fibromatosis; abnormalities of the nose and ears as well as hypoplastic changes in the terminal phalanges of the fingers and toes are features. Manifested at birth or within the first few months of life. Autosomal dominant inheritance. Cross-reference: Zimmermann-Laband syndrome. (Peter F. Laband, U.S. dentist)

1. Chodirker BN, Chudley AE, Toffler MA, et al: Zimmerman-Laband syndrome and profound mental retardation. Am J Med Genet 25:543-548, 1986
2. Gorlin RJ, Cohen MM Jr, Levin LS: Syndromes of the Head and Neck. 3rd ed. New York: Oxford University Press, 1990
3. Laband PF, Habib G, Humphreys OS: Oral Surg 17:339-351, 1964
4. Zimmermann KW: Vjschr Zahnheilkd 44:419-434, 1928

LABBÉ OPERATION, gastrotomy through an incision to the level of the left 9th rib. (Léon Labbé, 1832-1916, French surgeon)

1. Maffei WE: Os Fundamentos da Medicina. 2nd ed. Livraria Editora Artes Médicas Ltda, 1978

LABORDE SIGN, see Cloquet sign. (Jean B.V. Laborde, 1830-1903, French)

LACRIMO-AURICULO-DENTO-DIGITAL SYNDROME, lacrimal anomalies consisting of diminished/absent tears, recurrent/chronic tearing, recurrent/chronic conjunctivitis or dacryocystitis, nasolacrimal duct fistulas, and absence/hypoplasia of lacrimal glands or punctata, canaliculi, tear sacs, or nasal ducts. Genitourinary anomalies include congenital obstruction of the duodenum due to peritoneal bands resulting from a malrotated cecum. Digital abnormalities are also found. Cross-reference: Levy-Hollister syndrome.

1. Gorlin RJ, Cohen MM Jr, Levin LS: Syndromes of the Head and Neck. 3rd ed. New York: Oxford University Press, 1990
2. Hollister DW, Klein SH, DeJager HJ, et al: The lacrimo-auriculo-dento-digital syndrome. J Pediatr 83:438-444, 1973
3. Levy WJ: Mesoectodermal dysplasia. A new combination of anomalies. Am J Ophthalmol 63:978-982, 1967

LADIN SIGN, vaginal examination suggests an increase of the elastic zone as pregnancy advances.

1. Casas EC: Diccionario Terminologico de Ciencias Medicas. 5th ed. Salvat Editores, SA, 1954

LAËNNEC SIGN, a round, gelatinous mass observed in the sputum in cases of bronchial asthma. (René T. Laënnec, 1781-1826, French)

1. Casas EC: Diccionario Terminologico de Ciencias Medicas. 5th ed. Salvat Editores, SA, 1954

LAFORA DISEASE, progressive myoclonus epilepsy; diagnosis requires at least three of the following criteria: 1) age of onset between 6 and 15 years; 2) generalized tonic-clonic seizures; 3) electroencephalographic abnormalities; and 4) a progressive clinical course. Often familial, characteristics include seizures and myoclonus; late in the course of the disease, muscular dystrophy, cerebellar ataxia, and mental deterioration are present. Cross-reference: Unverricht disease. (Gonzalo Rodriguez Lafora, 1887-1971, Spanish neurologist)

1. Baker AB, Baker LH: Clinical Neurology. Revised ed. Philadelphia: Harper & Row, 1982
2. Ritchie AC: Boyd's Textbook of Pathology. 9th ed. Philadelphia: Lea & Febiger, 1990

LAFORA SIGN, itching of the nostril; a sign of cerebrospinal meningitis. (Gonzalo Rodriguez Lafora)

1. Casas EC: Diccionario Terminologico de Ciencias Medicas. 5th ed. Salvat Editores, SA, 1954

LAGLEYZE-HIPPLE DISEASE, angioglioma of the retina.

1. Casas EC: Diccionario Terminologico de Ciencias Medicas. 5th ed. Salvat Editores, SA, 1954

LAGRANGE OPERATION, sclerectoiridectomy. (Pierre F. Lagrange, 1857-1928, French ophthalmologist)

1. Maffei WE: Os Fundamentos da Medicina. 2nd ed. Livraria Editora Artes Médicas Ltda, 1978

LAIN DISEASE, erosion and burning sensation of the oral mucosa caused by faradism originating in different metals used for dental prostheses.

1. Casas EC: Diccionario Terminologico de Ciencias Medicas. 5th ed. Salvat Editores, SA, 1954

LAMB SYNDROME, the acronym LAMB (*l*entigines, *a*trial myxoma, *m*ucocutaneous myxomas, and *b*lue nevi) was coined by Rhodes to describe a previously reported cardiocutaneous syndrome (the NAME syndrome). Consists of pigmented macules with lentiginous proliferation of large melanocytes, atrial myomas, cutaneous myxomas, blue nevi, and no neurofibromas. Recognition of this rare syndrome is important so that potentially fatal atrial myxoma can be evaluated and treated surgically. Cross-references: Carney syndrome; NAME syndrome.

1. Atherton DJ, et al: A syndrome of various cutaneous pigmented lesions, myxoid neurofibromata, and atrial myxomas; the NAME syndrome. Br J Dermatol 103:421-429, 1980
2. Gorlin RJ, Cohen MM Jr, Levin LS: Syndromes of the Head and Neck. 3rd ed. New York: Oxford University Press, 1990
3. Rhodes AR: J Am Acad Dermatol 10:72-82, 1984

4. Russell Rees J, Ross FGM, Keen G: Br Heart J 35:874-876, 1973

LAMBERT SYNDROME, LAMBERT-EATON MYASTHENIC SYNDROME, proximal muscle weakness, particularly in the pelvic girdle. The patient initially complains of weakness and fatigability of the legs, with arm weakness being less frequent and milder. Cross-references: Eaton-Lambert syndrome; Myasthenic syndrome. (Edward H. Lambert, U.S. neurophysicist; Lee M. Eaton, 1905-1958, U.S. neurologist)

1. Lambert EH, Eaton LM, Rooke ED: Defect of neuromuscular conduction associated with malignant neoplasm. Am J Physiol 187:612-613, 1956

LAMPERT SYNDROME, craniosynostosis, a long thin face, midface hypoplasia, mild micrognathia, long tapering fingers, postaxial polydactyly, congenital hip dislocation, hallux valgus, and an absent uterus are features.

1. Gorlin RJ, Cohen MM Jr, Levin LS: Syndromes of the Head and Neck. 3rd ed. New York: Oxford University Press, 1990

LAMY-MAROTEAUX SYNDROME, see Diastrophic dysplasia syndrome.

LANCEREAUX-MATHIEU DISEASE, see Weil disease. (Etienne Lancereaux, 1829-1910, French; Albert M. Mathieu, 1855-1917, French)

LANCISI SIGN, heartbeats are muffled; seen in the patient with myocardial myopathy. (Giovanni M. Lancisi, 1654-1720, Italian)

1. Casas EC: Diccionario Terminologico de Ciencias Medicas. 5th ed. Salvat Editores, SA, 1954

LANDOLFI SIGN, pupillary contraction occurs during systole and dilatation occurs during diastole; seen during aortic insufficiency.

1. Casas EC: Diccionario Terminologico de Ciencias Medicas. 5th ed. Salvat Editores, SA, 1954

LANDOLT OPERATION, creation of a lower eyelid using tissue from the upper eyelid. (Edmund Landolt, 1846-1926, ophthalmologist)

1. Maffei WE: Os Fundamentos da Medicina. 2nd ed. Livraria Editora Artes Médicas Ltda, 1978

LANDRY-GUILLAIN-BARRÉ SYNDROME, see Guillain-Barré syndrome. (Jean B.O. Landry de Thézillat, 1826-1865, French; Georges Guillain, 1876-1961, French neurologist; Jean A. Barré, 1880-1967, French neurologist)

LANE DISEASE, chronic intestinal stasis. (Sir William Arbuthnot-Lane, 1856-1943, British surgeon)

1. Lane W: Lancet 1:1193-1194, 1910

LANE OPERATION, ileorectal anastomosis. (Sir William Arbuthnot-Lane)

1. Maffei WE: Os Fundamentos da Medicina. 2nd ed. Livraria Editora Artes Médicas Ltda, 1978

LANGE OPERATION, method for stimulating tissue growth using sterilized silk rings.

1. Maffei WE: Os Fundamentos da Medicina. 2nd ed. Livraria Editora Artes Médicas Ltda, 1978

LANGE-NIELSEN SYNDROME, see Jerville and Lange-Nielsen syndrome. (Frederik Lange-Nielsen, Norwegian)

LANGER MESOMELIC DYSPLASIA SYNDROME, mesomelic dwarfism; rudimentary fibula and micrognathia are features. Autosomal recessive inheritance. (Leonard O. Langer, Jr., U.S.)

1. Langer LO Jr: Mesomelic dwarfism of the hypoplastic ulna, fibula, mandible type. Radiology 89:654, 1967
2. Smith DW, Jones KL: Recognizable Patterns of Human Malformations: Genetic, Embryologic, and Clinical Aspects. 3rd ed. Philadelphia: WB Saunders, 1982

LANGER-GIEDION SYNDROME, multiple exostoses, a bulbous nose with peculiar facies, and loose redundant skin in infancy are features. Etiology unknown. Cross-reference: Trichorhinophalangeal syndrome. (Leonard O. Langer, Jr.)

1. Giedion A: Das tricho-rhino-phalangeal syndrom. Helv Paediatr Acta 21:475-482, 1966
2. Giedion A: Helv Pediatr Acta 28:249-259, 1973
3. Hall BD, Langer LO Jr, Giedion A, et al: Langer-Giedion syndrome. Birth Defects 10(12):147-164, 1974
4. Langer LO Jr: Radiology 91:447-456, 1968

LANGORIA SIGN, relaxation of the extensor muscles of the thigh; an indication of intrascapular fracture of the femoral neck.

1. Casas EC: Diccionario Terminologico de Ciencias Medicas. 5th ed. Salvat Editores, SA, 1954

LANNELONGUE DISEASE, see Osgood-Schlatter disease. (Odilon M. Lannelongue, 1840-1911, French)

LANNELONGUE OPERATION, surgery for microcephaly by removing a strip of parietal bone parallel to the sagittal suture. (Odilon M. Lannelongue)

1. Maffei WE: Os Fundamentos da Medicina. 2nd ed. Livraria Editora Artes Médicas Ltda, 1978

LANNOIS-GRADENIGO SYNDROME, see Gradenigo syndrome.

LANZ OPERATION, insertion of fascia lata patches into an opening on the head of the femur in cases of elephantiasis.

1. Maffei WE: Os Fundamentos da Medicina. 2nd ed. Livraria Editora Artes Médicas Ltda, 1978

LARCHER SIGN, gray spots in the conjunctiva quickly turn blackish; an indication of death.

1. Casas EC: Diccionario Terminologico de Ciencias Medicas. 5th ed. Salvat Editores, SA, 1954

LAROYENNE OPERATION, puncture of the Douglas pouch for drainage of pelvic suppuration. (Lucien Laroyenne, 1831-1902, French surgeon)

1. Maffei WE: Os Fundamentos da Medicina. 2nd ed. Livraria Editora Artes Médicas Ltda, 1978

LARREY SIGN, pain produced in the sacroiliac region of the symphysis when the patient sits abruptly; seen in sacroiliitis. (Dominique J. Larrey, 1766-1842, French surgeon)

1. Casas EC: Diccionario Terminologico de Ciencias Medicas. 5th ed. Salvat Editores, SA, 1954

LARREY-WEIL DISEASE, see Weil disease.

LARSEN SYNDROME, comprised of multiple congenital dislocations with osseous anomalies and unusual facies. The elbows, hips, and knees show dislocation, usually bilaterally. Anterior dislocation of the tibia on the femur is especially characteristic. (Loren Larsen, U.S. orthopedic surgeon)

1. Larsen LJ, Schottstaedt ER, Bost FC: J Pediatr 37:574-581, 1950
2. McKusick VA: Heritable Disorders of Connective Tissue. 4th ed. St Louis: CV Mosby, 1972
3. Smith DW, Jones KL: Recognizable Patterns of Human Malformations: Genetic, Embryologic, and Clinical Aspects. 3rd ed. Philadelphia: WB Saunders, 1982

LARZEL DISEASE, infantile pseudoleukemic anemia.

1. Casas EC: Diccionario Terminologico de Ciencias Medicas. 5th ed. Salvat Editores, SA, 1954

LASÈGUE SIGN, LASÈGUE TEST, while lying supine, the normal patient can raise one leg to almost 90° without pain, but the patient with sciatica experiences pain by elevation of 30° to 40°. Cross-references: Demianoff sign; Straight leg raising test. (Ernest C. Lasègue, 1816-1883, French)

1. Baker AB, Baker LH: Clinical Neurology. Revised ed. Philadelphia: Harper & Row, 1982
2. Campbell WC, Crenshaw AH: Campbell's Operative Orthopaedics. 7th ed. St Louis: CV Mosby, 1987

LATERAL BULBAR SYNDROME, caused by infarction in the retro-olivary area of the medulla oblongata and is present more often in the inferior part of the medulla oblongata than superiorly. Swallowing difficulty and hemianesthesia are features. Cross-reference: Wallenberg syndrome.

1. Alexander L, Suh TH: Arterial supply of the lateral parolivary region. Arch Neurol Psychiatry 38:1243, 1937
2. Baker AB, Baker LH: Clinical Neurology. Revised ed. Philadelphia: Harper & Row, 1982

LATERAL CEREBELLAR SYNDROME, limb ataxia consisting of defective postural fixation of the limbs and errors in rate, range, direction, timing, and force of skilled voluntary movements. Cerebellar astrocytoma and multiple sclerosis are common causes.

1. Baker AB, Baker LH: Clinical Neurology. Revised ed. Philadelphia: Harper & Row, 1982

LATERAL INFERIOR PONTINE SYNDROME, results from occlusion of the anterior inferior cerebellar artery; may cause numbness of the face, hemiparesis, and deafness.

1. Walsh FB, Hoyt EF, Miller NR: Clinical Neuro-Ophthalmology. 4th ed. Baltimore: Williams & Wilkins, 1982

LATERAL MEDULLARY SYNDROME, see Wallenberg syndrome.

LATERAL PONS SYNDROME, in its pure form, this uncommon syndrome is characterized chiefly by ipsilateral cerebellar disturbances owing to involvement of pontocerebellar fibers.

1. Baker AB, Baker LH: Clinical Neurology. Revised ed. Philadelphia: Harper & Row, 1982
2. Haymaker W: Bing's Local Diagnosis in Neurological Diseases. 15th ed. St Louis: CV Mosby, 1969

LATERAL/PERONEAL COMPARTMENT SYNDROME, signs and symptoms are similar to anterior tibial compartment syndrome, but the peroneus longus and peroneus brevis muscles are involved. Pain is usually absent anteriorly, but the muscles of the anterior compartment are paralyzed due to ischemia of the deep peroneal nerve as it passes through the peroneal compartment.

1. Campbell WC, Walsh PC: Campbell's Operative Orthopaedics. 7th ed. St Louis: CV Mosby, 1986
2. Lunceford EM Jr: The peroneal compartment syndrome. South Med J 58:621-623, 1965

LATEROSUPERIOR MIDBRAIN SYNDROME, a syndrome of occlusion consisting chiefly of

contralateral hemihypesthesia and hemihypalgesia; contralateral hypacusis is sometimes present.
1. Haymaker W: Bing's Local Diagnosis in Neurological Diseases. 15th ed. St Louis: CV Mosby, 1969

LATZKO OPERATION, a technique for extraperitoneal cesarean section. (Wilhelm Latzko, 1863-1945, Austrian obstetrician)
1. Maffei WE: Os Fundamentos da Medicina. 2nd ed. Livraria Editora Artes Médicas Ltda, 1978

LAUBRY-SOUCLE SYNDROME, abnormal localized collections of gas in the colon (splenic flexure) and stomach subsequent to occult myocardial infarction; possibly related to pain.
1. Dorland's Medical Dictionary. 28th ed. Philadelphia: WB Saunders, 1994

LAUGIER SIGN, the styloid process of the radius and the ulna are at the same level; seen in the patient with fracture of the distal radius. (Stanislas Laugier, 1799-1872, French surgeon)
1. Casas EC: Diccionario Terminologico de Ciencias Medicas. 5th ed. Salvat Editores, SA, 1954

LAUNOIS SYNDROME, gigantism due to excessive pituitary secretion of growth hormone; headache, perspiration, joint pain, a small penis, and possibly mental retardation are features. (Pierre-Emile Launois, 1856-1914, French)
1. Launois PE, Roy P: Études Biologiques sur les Géants. Paris: Masson, 1904

LAUORY-ROUTIER-VAN BOGAERT SIGN, a third heart sound in diastole; found in the patient with auricular tachycardia.
1. Casas EC: Diccionario Terminologico de Ciencias Medicas. 5th ed. Salvat Editores, SA, 1954

LAURENCE-MOON-BARDET-BIEDL SYNDROME, LAURENCE-MOON-BIEDL SYNDROME, clinically exhibits the pentad of retinal dystrophy, truncal obesity, mild to severe mental retardation, polydactyly, and hypogonadism. An inherited syndrome. Cross-reference: Bardet-Biedl syndrome. (John Z. Laurence; 1830-1874, British ophthalmologist; Robert C. Moon, 1844-1914, British ophthalmologist; Georges Bardet, French; Artur Biedl, 1869-1933, Austrian)
1. Biedl A: Dtsch Med Wochenschr 48:1630, 1922
2. Farmer TW: Pediatric Neurology. 2nd ed. Hagerstown: Harper & Row, 1975
3. Laurence JZ, Moon RC: Ophthalmol Rev 2:32-41, 1866

LAURENS OPERATION, plastic surgery to fill a cavity left by mastectomy.
1. Maffei WE: Os Fundamentos da Medicina. 2nd ed. Livraria Editora Artes Médicas Ltda, 1978

LÄWEN-ROTH SYNDROME, dwarfism with stippled epiphyses and thyroid deficiency; congenital hypothyroidism and cretinism are features.
1. Dorland's Medical Dictionary. 28th ed. Philadelphia: WB Saunders, 1994

LAWFORD SYNDROME, see Sturge-Weber syndrome.

LAWRENCE SYNDROME, see Berardinelli syndrome.

LAWSON-TAIT OPERATION, 1) laparotomy for inflammatory lesions in the uterine area; 2) marsupialization of hydatid cysts of the liver; 3) oophorectomy and salpingectomy. Cross-reference: Tait operation.
1. Maffei WE: Os Fundamentos da Medicina. 2nd ed. Livraria Editora Artes Médicas Ltda, 1978

LAZY LEUKOCYTE SYNDROME, neutropenia with excessive numbers of segmented neutrophils in the marrow, but with a defect in the release of cells. Termed "myelocathexis" when the mature neutrophils in the marrow are morphologically abnormal and "lazy leukocyte syndrome" when they appear normal.
1. Bennett JC, Plum F (eds): Cecil Textbook of Medicine. 20th ed. Philadelphia: WB Saunders, 1996
2. Goldman JM, Foroozanfar N, Gazzard BG, et al: Lazy leukocyte syndrome. J R Soc Med 77:1140-1141, 1984
3. Moschella SL, Hurley HJ: Dermatology. 2nd ed. Philadelphia: WB Saunders, 1985

LE FORT OPERATION, partial colpectomy. (Léon-Clément Le Fort, 1829-1893, French surgeon)
1. Maffei WE: Os Fundamentos da Medicina. 2nd ed. Livraria Editora Artes Médicas Ltda, 1978

LEAK SYNDROME, hemorrhage in a diffuse capillary bed.
1. Baker AB, Baker LH: Clinical Neurology. Revised ed. Philadelphia: Harper & Row, 1982

LEBER DISEASE, hereditary optic atrophy; a rare disorder of visual impairment. A sex-linked recessive trait that usually occurs in males. (Theodor von Leber, 1840-1917, German ophthalmologist)
1. Baker AB, Baker LH: Clinical Neurology. Revised ed. Philadelphia: Harper & Row, 1982
2. Von Leber T: Arch Ophthalmol 17:249-291, 1871

LEBHARDT SIGN, see Jacquemier sign.

LEBRUN OPERATION, a method for cataract extraction.
1. Maffei WE: Os Fundamentos da Medicina. 2nd ed. Livraria Editora Artes Médicas Ltda, 1978

LECENE OPERATION, section of the anterior carpal ligament for treating panaris of the thumb and wrist sheaths.
1. Maffei WE: Os Fundamentos da Medicina. 2nd ed. Livraria Editora Artes Médicas Ltda, 1978

LEDERER DISEASE, acute acquired hemolytic anemia with megaloblastic regeneration and leukocytosis. (Max Lederer, 1885-1952, U.S. pathologist)
1. Lederer M: Am J Med 170:500-501, 1925

LEG SIGN OF RAIMISTE, if the examiner opposes forceful attempts at abduction of the leg on the normal side, the paretic leg carries out a movement identical to that attempted on the normal side. (Johann M. Raimist, German neuropsychiatrist)
1. Baker AB, Baker LH: Clinical Neurology. Revised ed. Philadelphia: Harper & Row, 1982

LEGAL DISEASE, inflammation of the pharyngotympanic region with headache. (Emmo Legal, 1859-1922, German)
1. Legal E: Dtsch Klin Med 40:201-216, 1886

LEGENDRE SIGN, the resistance of the closed eyelid to being raised by the examiner is increased on the contralateral side; seen in the patient with facial hemiplegia. (Gaston J. Legendre, French)
1. Casas EC: Diccionario Terminologico de Ciencias Medicas. 5th ed. Salvat Editores, SA, 1954

LEGG DISEASE, LEGG-CALVÉ-PERTHES DISEASE, LEGG-CALVÉ-WALDENSTRÖM DISEASE, LEGG-PERTHES DISEASE, juvenile osteochondritis deformans; infarction of the head of the femur. Distortion of the femoral head usually becomes evident when the child is between 3 and 10 years old. In 85% of patients, the disease is unilateral. About 80% of patients are boys. Cross-references: Calvé-Perthes disease; Perthes disease; Quilt hip disease. (Arthur Legg, 1874-1939, U.S. surgeon; Jacques Calvé, 1875-1954, French orthopedic surgeon, Georg C. Perthes, 1869-1927, German surgeon)
1. Calvé J: J Radiol Electrol 9:22-27, 1925
2. Campbell WC, Crenshaw AH: Campbell's Operative Orthopaedics. 7th ed. St Louis: CV Mosby, 1987
3. Krugman S, Katz SL: Infectious Diseases of Children. 7th ed. St Louis: CV Mosby, 1981

LEGIONNAIRES DISEASE, appears to occur 2-10 days after inhalation of *Legionella pneumophilia*. The only consistent pathological condition found is in the lung and includes areas of acute fibrinopurulent pneumonia bounded by lobular septa. Cross-reference: Pontiac fever. (First noted at an American Legion convention in 1976.)
1. Bennett JC, Plum F (eds): Cecil Textbook of Medicine. 20th ed. Philadelphia: WB Saunders, 1996
2. Ritchie AC: Boyd's Textbook of Pathology. 9th ed. Philadelphia: Lea & Febiger, 1990

LEGRAND-GEBLEWICS PHENOMENON, a flickering colored light (40-50 pulsations per second) observed indirectly is perceived as a constant white light.
1. Dorland's Medical Dictionary. 28th ed. Philadelphia: WB Saunders, 1994

LEGROUX SIGN, polyadenitis in children due to tuberculosis or other infectious diseases.
1. Casas EC: Diccionario Terminologico de Ciencias Medicas. 5th ed. Salvat Editores, SA, 1954

LEICHTENSTERN SIGN, if a bone is percussed, the patient jumps or grimaces; seen in the patient with encephalitis. (Otto M. Leichtenstern, 1845-1900, German)
1. Casas EC: Diccionario Terminologico de Ciencias Medicas. 5th ed. Salvat Editores, SA, 1954

LEIGH DISEASE, a pyruvate carboxylase deficiency; subacute necrotizing encephalomyelopathy that appears in infancy or early childhood. Characterized by swallowing and feeding difficulty, hypotonia, weakness, ataxia, peripheral neuropathy, external ophthalmoplegia, loss of vision, impaired hearing, and convulsions. An autosomal recessive disorder. (A. Denis Leigh, British neuropathologist)
1. Baker AB, Baker LH: Clinical Neurology. Revised ed. Philadelphia: Harper & Row, 1982
2. Leigh AD: Subacute necrotizing encephalomyelopathy in an infant. J Neurol Neurosurg Psychiatry 14:216-221, 1951
3. Rowland LP (ed): Merritt's Textbook of Neurology. 9th ed. Baltimore: Williams & Wilkins, 1995

LEINER DISEASE, a rare disorder of infants associated with generalized dermatitis and erythroderma, recurrent infections, intractable diarrhea, and failure to thrive. (Karl Leiner, 1871-1930, Austrian pediatrician)
1. Leiner K: Br J Dis Child 5:244-251, 1908

LEISHMANIOSIS SYNDROME, an infection with parasites of the genus *Leishmania*. Usually a zoonosis transmitted by *Phlebotomus* sandflies between wild and peridomestic animals, especially rodents and canines. In humans, the infection is either visceral or cutaneous. Cross-reference: New World syndrome. (Sir William B. Leishman, 1865-1926, Scottish surgeon)

1. Bennett JC, Plum F (eds): Cecil Textbook of Medicine. 20th ed. Philadelphia: WB Saunders, 1996

LELOIR DISEASE, lupus erythematosus. (Henri C. Leloir, 1855-1896, French)

1. Leloir HC: Ann Derm Syph 1:708-709, 1890

LEMIERRE SYNDROME, seen infrequently, it must be considered in the patient with sore throat or dental pain, lateral neck pain, sepsis, and pulmonary symptoms. Diagnosis is based on clinical examination, anaerobic septicemia, radiologic evidence of internal jugular venous thrombosis, and pulmonary septic emboli.

1. Barker J, Winer-Muram HT, Grey SW: Lemierre syndrome. South Med J 89:1021-1023, 1996
2. Lemierre A: On certain septicemias due to anaerobic organisms. Lancet 1:701-703, 1936

LEMPERT OPERATION, fenestration of the lateral semicircular canal for correction of otosclerosis. (Julius Lempert, 1890-1968, U.S. otologist)

1. Maffei WE: Os Fundamentos da Medicina. 2nd ed. Livraria Editora Artes Médicas Ltda, 1978

LENNANDER OPERATION, removal of inguinal and pelvic lymph nodes.

1. Maffei WE: Os Fundamentos da Medicina. 2nd ed. Livraria Editora Artes Médicas Ltda, 1978

LENNERT LYMPHOMA, malignant lymphoma with a high epithelioid histocyte content; resembles the diffuse, mixed cell lymphoma of the Rappaport classification. (Karl Lennert, German histopathologist)

1. Bennett JC, Plum F (eds): Cecil Textbook of Medicine. 20th ed. Philadelphia: WB Saunders, 1996

LENNHOFF SIGN, sulcus felt during inspiration below the last rib in the case of echinococcosis of the liver. (Rudolf Lennhoff, 1866-1933, German)

1. Casas EC: Diccionario Terminologico de Ciencias Medicas. 5th ed. Salvat Editores, SA, 1954

LENNOX SYNDROME, LENNOX-GASTAUT SYNDROME, myoclonic astatic seizures; the essential features are early onset of epilepsy, multiple-seizure types in the same patient including myoclonic jerks, atonic seizures, impaired development and intellect, and generalized slow and spike-and-wave discharge on electroencephalography. (William G. Lennox, 1884-1960, U.S. neurologist; Henri Gastaut, French neurobiologist)

1. Gastaut H, Vigoroux M, Trevisan C, et al: Rev Neurol 97:37-52, 1957
2. Hopkins IJ: Lennox-Gastaut syndrome. Aust Paediatr J 23:269-270, 1986
3. Lennox WG: Clinical correlates of the fast and slow spike wave electroencephalogram. Pediatrics 5:626-627, 1950
4. Rowland LP (ed): Merritt's Textbook of Neurology. 9th ed. Baltimore: Williams & Wilkins, 1995

LENZ MICROPHTHALMIA SYNDROME, consists of microphthalmia, skeletal anomalies of the hands and clavicles, renal anomalies, genital abnormalities, and defects of the dentition. (Widerkind D. Lenz, German)

1. Gorlin RJ, Cohen MM Jr, Levin LS: Syndromes of the Head and Neck. 3rd ed. New York: Oxford University Press, 1990
2. Lenz W: Zschr Kinderheilkd 77:384-390, 1955

LENZ-MAJEWSKI SYNDROME, hyperostotic dwarfism; a large head, characteristic facies, loose skin, mental retardation, and skeletal anomalies are characteristics. (Widerkind D. Lenz)

1. Braham RL: Multiple congenital abnormalities with diaphyseal dysplasia (Camurati-Engelmann's syndrome). Oral Surg 27:20-26, 1969
2. Gorlin RJ, Cohen MM Jr, Levin LS: Syndromes of the Head and Neck. 3rd ed. New York: Oxford University Press, 1990
3. Lenz WD, Majewski FA: A generalized disorder of the connective tissues with progeria, choanal atresia, symphalangism, hypoplasia of dentine and craniodiaphyseal hypostosis. Birth Defects 10(12):133-136, 1974

LEO BUERGER DISEASE, see Buerger disease.

LEOPARD SYNDROME, multiple *l*entigines, *e*lectrocardiographic conduction defects, *o*cular hypertelorism, *p*ulmonary stenosis, *a*bnormalities of the genitalia, *r*etardation of growth, and sensorineural *d*eafness (LEOPARD) are features. Cross-reference: Multiple lentigines syndrome.

1. Gorlin RJ, Anderson RC, Blaw M: Multiple lentigines syndrome. Am J Dis Child 117:652-662, 1969
2. Peter JR, Kemp JS: LEOPARD syndrome: death because of chronic respiratory insufficiency. Am J Med Genet 37:340-341, 1990
3. Smith DW, Jones KL: Recognizable Patterns of Human Malformations: Genetic, Embryologic, and Clinical Aspects.

3rd ed. Philadelphia: WB Saunders, 1982

LEOTTA SIGN, compression of the superior right quadrant if adhesions between the gallbladder and the liver are present.
1. Casas EC: Diccionario Terminologico de Ciencias Medicas. 5th ed. Salvat Editores, SA, 1954

LEPRECHAUNISM SYNDROME, see Donohue syndrome. (A figure in Irish mythology.)

LEREDDE SYNDROME, usually a sequelae of congenital syphilis, with lung dysfunction. Severe dyspnea on exertion dating from early life combined with advanced emphysema and recurrent attacks of acute febrile bronchitis. (Emile Leredde, French dermatologist)
1. Casas EC: Diccionario Terminologico de Ciencias Medicas. 5th ed. 1954

LÉRI DISEASE, pleonosteosis familiaris; the abundance of bone formation characterized by flexion contractures of the fingers, enlarged thumbs and first toes, limited motion, short stature, and mongoloid facies; intelligence is normal. A rare entity of dominant inheritance. (André Léri, 1875-1930, French)
1. Léri A: Presse Med 30:13, 1922
2. McKusick VA: Heritable Disorders of Connective Tissue. 4th ed. St Louis: CV Mosby, 1972

LÉRI SIGN, passive flexion of the hand and wrist results in elbow flexion; seen in the patient with hemiplegia. Cross-reference: Forearm sign. (André Léri)
1. Casas EC: Diccionario Terminologico de Ciencias Medicas. 5th ed. Salvat Editores, SA, 1954

LÉRI-WEILL SYNDROME, dyschondrosteosis; short forearms with the Madelung deformity, with or without a short lower leg, are features. Autosomal dominant inheritance with an excess of affected females. (André Léri; Jean A. Weill, French)
1. Felman AH, Kirkpatrick JA Jr: Dyschondrosteoses. Mesomelic dwarfism of Leri and Weill. Am J Dis Child 120:329, 1970
2. Léri A, Weill J: Bull Soc Med Hop 53:1491-1494, 1929
3. Smith DW, Jones KL: Recognizable Patterns of Human Malformations: Genetic, Embryologic, and Clinical Aspects. 3rd ed. Philadelphia: WB Saunders, 1982

LERICHE OPERATION, periarterial sympathectomy. (René Leriche, 1879-1955, French surgeon)
1. Maffei WE: Os Fundamentos da Medicina. 2nd ed. Livraria Editora Artes Médicas Ltda, 1978

LERICHE SYNDROME, occlusion of the terminal aorta at its bifurcation, which may be produced by traumatic severance, acute aortic dissection, arteriosclerotic thrombosis, or sudden embolism. Cross-reference: Aortic occlusion syndrome. (René Leriche)
1. Leriche R: Presse Med 48, 1940

LERMOYEZ SYNDROME, labyrinthine angiospasm; vertigo, with hearing changes occurring months or years before the first episode. Another form has been described in which vertigo may occur without affecting the cochlear function. Similar to Ménière disease. (Marcel Lermoyez, 1858-1929, French otolaryngologist)
1. Ballenger JJ: Diseases of the Nose, Throat, Ear, Head and Neck. 12th ed. Philadelphia: Lea & Febiger, 1977
2. Lermoyez M: Presse Med 27:1-3, 1919

LEROY SYNDROME, mucolipidosis type II; an inborn metabolic disorder with characteristics of cytoplasmic inclusion in cultured fibroblasts, hypertrophy of the gums, low birth weight, slow psychomotor development, and mental retardation. Progresses to death by age 8 years. Autosomal recessive inheritance. Cross-reference: I-cell disease. (Jules G. Leroy, Belgian geneticist)
1. Kaplan A, Achord DT, Sly WS: Phosphohexosyl components of a lysosomal enzyme are recognized by pinocytosis receptors on human fibroblasts. Proc Natl Acad Sci USA 74:2026, 1977
2. Leroy JG, DeMars RI: Science 157:804-806, 1967

LESCH-NYHAN SYNDROME, a rare disorder characterized by bilateral choreoathetosis, mental retardation, self-mutilation, and hyperuricemia. Features include an abnormality in neurotransmitters, such as dopaminergic function in the basal ganglia, although the abnormality involves all dopaminergic pathways and is not restricted to the basal ganglia. (Michael Lesch, U.S.; William L. Nyhan, U.S. pediatrician)
1. Ernst M, Zametkin AJ, Matochuk JA, et al: Presynaptic dopaminergic deficits in Lesch-Nyhan disease. N Engl J Med 334:1568-1572, 1996
2. Farmer TW: Pediatric Neurology. 2nd ed. Hagerstown: Harper & Row, 1975
3. Lesch M, Nyhan WL: Am J Med 36:561-570, 1964

LESCHKE SYNDROME, LESCHKE-ULLMANN SYNDROME, congenital pigmentary dystrophy; asthenia, hyperglycemia, and pigmentation abnormalities are features. Insulin-resistant diabetes is present in most cases. (Erich F.W. Leschke, 1887-1933, German)

1. Leschke E, Ullmann H: Z Klin Med 102:388-411, 1926

LESER-TRÉLAT SIGN, the sudden appearance of seborrheic keratoses and a rapid increase in the size and number; an indication of an internal malignancy, especially of the gastrointestinal tract. (Edmund Leser, 1853-1916, German surgeon; Ulysses Trélat, Jr., 1828-1890, French surgeon)

1. Casas EC: Diccionario Terminologico de Ciencias Medicas. 5th ed. Salvat Editores, SA, 1954

LESIER SIGN, a decrease in resonance of the right inferior thorax; seen in the patient with typhoid fever.

1. Casas EC: Diccionario Terminologico de Ciencias Medicas. 5th ed. Salvat Editores, SA, 1954

LESIEUR-PRIVEY SIGN, the presence of albumin in the sputum; an indication of lung inflammation.

1. Casas EC: Diccionario Terminologico de Ciencias Medicas. 5th ed. Salvat Editores, SA, 1954

LETIÉVANT OPERATION, resection of ribs in order to create a contact surface between the thoracic wall and the pleura, reducing empyema.

1. Maffei WE: Os Fundamentos da Medicina. 2nd ed. Livraria Editora Artes Médicas Ltda, 1978

LETTERER-SIWE SYNDROME, nonlipid histiocytosis; Letterer described a 6-month-old infant with diffuse purpura, fever, otitis media, lymphadenopathy, and hepatosplenomegaly. Later, Siwe included this case in his series of six similar cases. In all instances, there was diffuse tissue infiltration by histiocytes. Cross-reference: Histiocytosis syndrome. (Erich Letterer, German pathologist; Sturre A. Siwe, 1897-1966, Swedish pediatrician)

1. Bennett JC, Plum F (eds): Cecil Textbook of Medicine. 20th ed. Philadelphia: WB Saunders, 1996
2. Letterer E: Frankf Zschr Pathol 30:377-394, 1924
3. Siwe S: Zschr Kinderheilkd 55:212-247, 1933

LEVASSEUR SIGN, when a suction cup is placed on an open vein and blood is not forthcoming; an indication of death.

1. Casas EC: Diccionario Terminologico de Ciencias Medicas. 5th ed. Salvat Editores, SA, 1954

LEVATOR SIGN, peripheral facial palsy; the patient is asked to look down and then to slowly close the eyes. The sign is present if the upper lid on the paralyzed side moves slightly upward, elevated by the levator palpebrae superioris muscle because its function is no longer counteracted by the orbicularis oculi muscle. Cross-references: Céstan sign; Dutemps-Céstan sign.

1. Baker AB, Baker LH: Clinical Neurology. Revised ed. Philadelphia: Harper & Row, 1982

LEVATOR SYNDROME, coccygodynia; episodic pain and a sensation of fullness and pressure in the perineal area attributed to spasm of the levator ani muscle.

1. Simpson JY: Med Times Gaz 40:1031, 1959

LÉVI-LORAIN DISEASE, pituitary dwarfism. A small, dwarfed body with skin that is thin and wrinkled; the child appears prematurely aged. Occurs when pituitary function is congenitally absent or disabled disease. Cross-reference: Lorain disease. (E. Leopold Lévi, 1868-1933, French endocrinologist, Paul J. Lorain, 1827-1875, French)

1. Grinker RR, Sahs AL: Neurology. 6th ed. Springfield: Charles C Thomas, 1966
2. Lévi EL: Nouv Icon Salpetriere 21:297-324, 1908
3. Lorain PJ: Du Féminisme et de l'Infantilisme chez les Tuberculeux. Paris, 1871 (Thesis)

LEVINE SIGN, the discomfort of angina causes a patient to place a fist over the sternum. (Samuel A. Levine, 1891-1966, U.S. cardiologist)

1. Hurst JW, Schlant RC, Alexander RW, et al: The Heart: Arteries and Veins. 8th ed. New York: McGraw-Hill, 1994

LEVIS OPERATION, injection of 20 drops of phenol into the vaginal sac after drainage of hydrocele fluid.

1. Maffei WE: Os Fundamentos da Medicina. 2nd ed. Livraria Editora Artes Médicas Ltda, 1978

LEVY-HOLLISTER SYNDROME, see Lacrimo-auriculo-dento-digital syndrome. (Walter J. Levy, South African ophthalmologist)

LÉVY-ROUSSY SYNDROME, see Roussy-Lévy syndrome. (Gabrielle Lévy, 1886-1935, French neurologist)

LEWANDOWSKY TUBERCULID, tuberculosis of the skin; characteristics include variable-sized lesions, most frequently on the cheek and forehead. (Felix Lewandowsky, 1879-1921, German dermatologist)

1. Lewandowsky F, Lutz W: Arch Derm Syph 41:193-202, 1922

LEWIS PHENOMENON, hydrophagocytosis.

1. Dorland's Medical Dictionary. 28th ed. Philadelphia: WB Saunders, 1994

LEWIS SYNDROME, asthenia from excessive burning of calories. C.S. Lewis had synostosis involving the first metacarpophalangeal joint and described his own syndrome of manual clumsiness.

1. Lewis CS: Surprised by Joy: The Shape of My Early Life. New York: Harcourt, Brace, and World, 1955

LEXER OPERATION, removal of the gasserian ganglion in trigeminal neuralgia.

1. Maffei WE: Os Fundamentos da Medicina. 2nd ed. Livraria Editora Artes Médicas Ltda, 1978

LEYDEN-MÖBIUS SYNDROME, limb-girdle muscular dystrophy. (Ernst V. von Leyden, 1832-1910, German; Paul J. Möbius, 1853-1907, German neurologist)

1. Von Leyden E: Klinik der Ruckenmarks-Krankheiten. Vol 2. Berlin: Hirschwald, 1876

LHERMITTE SIGN, sudden, transient electric-like shocks that spread down the body into the legs when the patient flexes the head forward; seen in spinal cord compression. (Jean Lhermitte, 1877-1959, French neurologist)

1. Baker AB, Baker LH: Clinical Neurology. Revised ed. Philadelphia: Harper & Row, 1982
2. Grinker RR, Sahs AL: Neurology. 6th ed. Springfield: Charles C Thomas, 1966

LHERMITTE SYNDROME, peduncular hallucinosis; a curious syndrome probably caused by lesions of the posterior diencephalon or midbrain. Consists of nonhorrendous, often pleasurable, colorful visual hallucinations. Cross-reference: McAlpine syndrome. (Jean Lhermitte)

1. Baker AB, Baker LH: Clinical Neurology. Revised ed. Philadelphia: Harper & Row, 1982

LHERMITTE-DUCLOS DISEASE, a peculiar proliferation of abnormal neuronal elements in the cerebellum that has features of hamartoma and neoplasm. (Jean Lhermitte; P. Duclos, French neurologist)

1. Albrecht S, Haber RM, Goodman JC, et al: Cowden syndrome and Lhermitte-Duclos disease. Cancer 70:869-876, 1992
2. Lhermitte J, Duclos P: Bull Assoc Fr Cancer 9:99, 1920
3. Marano SR, Johnson PC, Spetzler RF: Recurrent Lhermitte-Duclos disease in a child. Case report. J Neurosurg 69:599-603, 1988

LIACOPOULOS PHENOMENON, the nonspecific immunosuppression to an antigen that is induced by the administration of large doses of an unrelated antigen.

1. Dorland's Medical Dictionary. 28th ed. Philadelphia: WB Saunders, 1994

LIAN SIGN, percussion of a hydatid cyst producing an echo sound. Cross-reference: Odinet sign.

1. Casas EC: Diccionario Terminologico de Ciencias Medicas. 5th ed. Salvat Editores, SA, 1954

LIBMAN SIGN, hyperesthesia between the angle of the mandible and the styloid process; seen in the patient with angina. (Emanuel Libman, 1872-1946, U.S.)

1. Evans RC: Illustrated Essentials in Orthopedic Physical Assessment. St Louis: Mosby Yearbook, 1994

LIBMAN-SACKS DISEASE, endocarditis associated with systemic lupus erythematosus. (Emmanuel Libman; Benjamin Sacks, 1873-1939, U.S.)

1. Fowler NO: Cardiac Diagnosis and Treatment. 3rd ed. Cambridge: Harper & Row, 1980
2. Libman E, Sacks B: Trans Assoc Am Phys 38:46-61, 1923

LICHTHEIM DISEASE, lesions of the left temporal lobe producing Wernicke-type aphasia. (Ludwig Lichtheim, 1845-1928, German)

1. Lichtheim L: On aphasia. Brain 7:433-484, 1885
2. Pedro-Pons A: Patologia-y-Clinica Medicus. Salvat Editores, SA, 1952

LICHTHEIM SIGN, the patient is unable to talk but can identify the number of syllables in each word he/she is thinking; seen in the patient with subcortical aplasia. Cross-reference: Déjerine-Lichtheim sign. (Ludwig Lichtheim)

1. Casas EC: Diccionario Terminologico de Ciencias Medicas. 5th ed. Salvat Editores, SA, 1954

LICHTHEIM SYNDROME, combined systemic disease and pernicious anemia; onset most frequent in the 4th decade. Common in Nordic blond races. Cross-reference: Dana syndrome. (Ludwig Lichtheim)

1. Dana C: The degenerative diseases of the spinal cord with a description of a new type. J Nerv Ment Dis:205-216, 1891
2. Lichtheim L: Verh Cong Innere Med 6:84-96, 1889

LIDDLE SYNDROME, a rare tubular disorder characterized by hypokalemia, metabolic alkalosis, hypertension, and normal aldosterone secretion rates. (Grant W. Liddle, 1921-1989, U.S. endocrinologist)

1. Bennett JC, Plum F (eds): Cecil Textbook of Medicine. 20th ed. Philadelphia: WB Saunders, 1996
2. Botero-Velez M, Curtis JJ, Warnock DG: Brief report: Liddle's syndrome revisited—a disorder of sodium reabsorption in the distal tubule. N Engl J Med 330:178-181, 1994
3. Liddle GW, Bledsoe T, Coppage WS Jr: Trans Assoc Am Phys 76:199-213, 1963

LIESEGANG PHENOMENON, the unusual formation of a precipitate in the form of concentric banded rings, waves, or spirals, when electrolytes diffuse into and meet in a colloid gel. (Raphael E. Liesegang, 1869-1947, German chemist)

1. Dorland's Medical Dictionary. 28th ed. Philadelphia: WB Saunders, 1994

LIGATURE SIGN, ecchymoses develop in the distal part of a limb to which a ligature has been applied; seen in the patient with hematuria.

1. Dorland's Medical Dictionary. 28th ed. Philadelphia: WB Saunders, 1994

LIGHTWOOD SYNDROME, LIGHTWOOD-ALBRIGHT SYNDROME, renal tubular acidosis. (Reginald Lightwood, British pediatrician; Fuller Albright, 1900-1969, U.S. endocrinologist)

1. Albright F, et al: Metabolic studies and therapy in a case of nephrocalcinosis with rickets and dwarfism. Bull Johns Hopkins Hosp 66:7-33, 1940
2. Lightwood R: Proc Br Paediatr Soc Arch Dis Child 10:205-206, 1935

LIGNAC SYNDROME, LIGNAC-FANCONI DISEASE, see Fanconi anemia. (Georges O.E. Lignac, 1891-1954, Dutch pediatrician; Guido Fanconi, 1882-1979, Swiss pediatrician)

LILLIE-CROWE TEST, retinal vein engorgement results when the contralateral jugular vein is compressed in the presence of lateral sinus thrombosis.

1. Ballenger JJ: Diseases of the Nose, Throat, Ear, Head and Neck. 12th ed. Philadelphia: Lea & Febiger, 1977

LIMB DEFICIENCY-SPLENOGONADAL FUSION SYNDROME, two types are known: 1) a continuous type in which a cord-like structure connects the spleen with the gonadomesonephric structures; 2) a discontinuous type in which the splenogonadal fusion has no structural connection with the spleen itself.

1. Gorlin RJ, Cohen MM Jr, Levin LS: Syndromes of the Head and Neck. 3rd ed. New York: Oxford University Press, 1990

LIN-GETTIG SYNDROME, craniosynostosis, agenesis of the corpus collosum, severe mental deficiency, hypogonadism, and a distinctive facial appearance are features.

1. Gorlin RJ, Cohen MM Jr, Levin LS: Syndromes of the Head and Neck. 3rd ed. New York: Oxford University Press, 1990

LINDAU DISEASE, LINDAU-VON HIPPEL SYNDROME, see Von Hippel-Lindau syndrome.

LINDER SIGN, while lying or sitting with legs outstretched, the patient experiences pain in the leg or the lumbar region caused by flexion of the head; seen in the patient with sciatica.

1. Mazion JM: Illustrated Manual of Orthopedic Signs/Tests/Maneuvers for Office Procedure. 2nd ed. Orlando: Daniels Publishing, 1980

LINEAR NEVUS SEBACEOUS SYNDROME, see Epidermal nevus syndrome.

LIPIDOSES SYNDROME, progressive mental retardation, motor disability, and hypotonia are features.

1. Bennett JC, Plum F (eds): Cecil Textbook of Medicine. 20th ed. Philadelphia: WB Saunders, 1996

LIPSCHÜTZ DISEASE, ulcus vulvae acutum; an acute ulcer of the lower vagina or vulva. (Benjamin Lipschütz, 1878-1931, Austrian)

1. Lipschütz B: Wien Klin Wochenschr 31:461-464, 1918

LISSAUER SYNDROME, dementia paralytica; psychogenic blindness to objects, without agnosia. Symptoms are similar to those caused by lesions in the left occipital lobe and splenium of the corpus callosum. (Heinrich Lissauer, 1861-1891, German psychiatrist)

1. Casas EC: Diccionario Terminologico de Ciencias Medicas. 5th ed. Salvat Editores, SA, 1954

LISSENCEPHALY SYNDROME, a rare congenital malformation with diffuse atrophy of the cerebral cortex associated with dementia paralytica, seizure, hemiplegia, facial paralysis, and hemiplegia.

1. Smith DW, Jones KL: Recognizable Patterns of Human Malformations: Genetic, Embryologic, and Clinical Aspects. 3rd ed. Philadelphia: WB Saunders, 1982
2. Volpe J: Neurology of the Newborn. 3rd ed. Philadelphia: WB Saunders, 1995

LITTEN SIGN, LITTEN PHENOMENON, a horizontal depression of the lateral inferior thorax; seen during respiration. Cross-reference: Diaphragm phenomenon. (Moritz Litten, 1845-1907, German)
1. Casas EC: Diccionario Terminologico de Ciencias Medicas. 5th ed. Salvat Editores, SA, 1954

LITTLE DISEASE, spastic diplegia; various grades of spastic paralysis, mental deficiency, and convulsions have been classified. (William Little, 1810-1894, British surgeon)
1. Grinker RR, Sahs AL: Neurology. 6th ed. Springfield: Charles C Thomas, 1966
2. Little WJ: Trans Obstet Soc Lond 3:293-344, 1862

LITTRÉ OPERATION, inguinal colotomy from the left side through an incision parallel to the Poupart ligament.
1. Maffei WE: Os Fundamentos da Medicina. 2nd ed. Livraria Editora Artes Médicas Ltda, 1978

LIVIERATO SIGN, vasoconstriction due to abdominal sympathetic nerve stimulation by percussion of the xiphoid process in the xiphoumbilical line. (Panagino Livierato, 1860-1936, Italian)
1. Casas EC: Diccionario Terminologico de Ciencias Medicas. 5th ed. Salvat Editores, SA, 1954

LIZARS OPERATION, removal of the maxilla via a curved incision from the angle of the mouth to the malar bone. (John Lizars, 1787-1860, Scottish surgeon)
1. Maffei WE: Os Fundamentos da Medicina. 2nd ed. Livraria Editora Artes Médicas Ltda, 1978

LLOYD SIGN, deep percussion over the kidney produces pain but not a sensation of pressure; a kidney stone is indicated.
1. Casas EC: Diccionario Terminologico de Ciencias Medicas. 5th ed. Salvat Editores, SA, 1954

LOBO DISEASE, keloidal blastomycosis; characterized by polymorphic cutaneous lesions with involvement of the mucosa or internal organs. Caused by *Loboa loboi*, a fungus that has not yet been cultured or classified. In tissues, the fungus grows nodules up to 10 mm in diameter with walls 1 mm thick and often forms branching chains from a single bud. The fungus stains well with silver stains for fungi. A chronic disease with a slow evolution of fresh lesions. Cross-reference: Jorge Lobo disease. (Jorge Lobo, Brazilian)
1. Lobo J: Rev Med 1:763-765, 1931
2. Ritchie AC: Boyd's Textbook of Pathology. 9th ed. Philadelphia: Lea & Febiger, 1990.

LOBSTEIN SYNDROME, see Osteogenesis imperfecta syndrome type I. (Johann F.G. Lobstein, 1777-1835, German)

LOCKED-IN SYNDROME, if occlusion occurs at the midpontine level or below (i.e., the upper brain stem tegmentum being spared), a "locked-in" syndrome may occur. The patient is alert but unable to communicate because of paralysis of all efferent pathways. This must be differentiated from bilateral frontal lobe destruction, which may produce the same clinical picture.
1. Hawkes CH: Locked-in syndrome: report of seven cases. Br Med J 4:379-382, 1976
2. Rowland LP (ed): Merritt's Textbook of Neurology. 9th ed. Baltimore: Williams & Wilkins, 1995

LOCKWOOD SIGN, if the McBurney point is palpated with the left hand, frequent gas is perceived; seen with chronic appendicitis or adhesions.
1. Casas EC: Diccionario Terminologico de Ciencias Medicas. 5th ed. Salvat Editores, SA, 1954

LOEFFLER SYNDROME, endomyocardial disease; thickening of the endocardium with subendocardial, myocardial degeneration, and infiltration by eosinophils leading to heart failure. (Wilhelm Loeffler, 1887-1972, Swiss)
1. Loeffler W: Beitr Klin Tuberculose 79:338-367, 1932
2. Ritchie AC: Boyd's Textbook of Pathology. 9th ed. Philadelphia: Lea & Febiger, 1990

LOMBARDI SIGN, venous varicosities in the area of the cervical and thoracic vertebrae; observed in the beginning stages of pulmonary tuberculosis. (Henri C. Lombardi, 1805-1895, Swiss)
1. Casas EC: Diccionario Terminologico de Ciencias Medicas. 5th ed. Salvat Editores, SA, 1954

LONDON SIGN, the presence of "pattern" bruising of the skin (i.e., an imprint of the clothing is noted on the skin) indicates that a crushing force has been applied sufficient to rupture the bowel against the vertebral column. The presence of this sign is a strong indication that a laparotomy is necessary. (Peter S. London, British surgeon)
1. Lumley JS, Clain A: Hamilton Bailey's Demonstration of Physical Signs in Clinical Surgery. 18th ed. London: Butterworth-Heinemann, 1997

LONGUET OPERATION, transplantation of the testicle in cases of varicocele and hydrocele.

1. Maffei WE: Os Fundamentos da Medicina. 2nd ed. Livraria Editora Artes Médicas Ltda, 1978

LOOP OF HENLE, consists of three anatomically and functionally distinct regions interposed between the proximal and distal tubules: the thick descending limb, the thin ascending limb, and the thick ascending limb. All mammalian nephrons possess this structure.

LOOSER-MILKMAN SYNDROME, see Milkman syndrome. (Emil Looser, 1877-1936, Swiss surgeon; Louisa Milkman, 1895-1951, U.S. radiologist)

LORAIN DISEASE, LORAIN-LÉVI DISEASE, see Lévi-Lorain disease.

LORENZ OPERATION, surgery for congenital dislocation of the hip. Cross-reference: Hoffa-Lorenz operation. (Adolf Lorenz, 1854-1946, Austrian surgeon)

1. Maffei WE: Os Fundamentos da Medicina. 2nd ed. Livraria Editora Artes Médicas Ltda, 1978

LORENZ SIGN, stiffness of the vertebral column, particularly the dorsal and lumbar areas; seen in incipient tuberculosis. (Adolf Lorenz)

1. Pedro-Pons A: Patologia-y-Clinica Medicus. Salvat Editores, SA, 1952

LORETA OPERATION, 1) gastrotomy for pylorus stricture; 2) introduction of a wire into the aneurysmal sac followed by electrolysis.

1. Maffei WE: Os Fundamentos da Medicina. 2nd ed. Livraria Editora Artes Médicas Ltda, 1978

LORIGA DISEASE, circulatory disturbance with paresthesias of the hands in workers who use pneumatic hammers.

1. Casas EC: Diccionario Terminologico de Ciencias Medicas. 5th ed. Salvat Editores, SA, 1954

LOSSEN OPERATION, resection of the maxillary nerve without section of the masseter.

1. Maffei WE: Os Fundamentos da Medicina. 2nd ed. Livraria Editora Artes Médicas Ltda, 1978

LOU GEHRIG DISEASE, amyotrophic lateral sclerosis. Named after Lou Gehrig (1903-1941), a U.S. baseball player with the disease.

LOUIS-BAR SYNDROME, ataxia-telangiectasia; progressive cerebellar ataxia beginning in infancy and progressive telangiectasia of the bulbar conjunctiva and the face are features. Recessive trait inheritance. Cross-references: Boder-Sedgwick syndrome; Paine-Efron syndrome. (Denise Louis-Bar, Belgian neuropathologist)

1. Louis-Barr D: Confin Neurol 4:32-42, 1941
2. Smith DW, Jones KL: Recognizable Patterns of Human Malformations: Genetic, Embryologic, and Clinical Aspects. 3rd ed. Philadelphia: WB Saunders, 1982

LOWE SYNDROME, LOWE-BICKEL SYNDROME, LOWE-TERREY-MACLACHLAN SYNDROME, an X-linked disorder characterized by vitamin D-refractory rickets, hydrophthalmia, congenital glaucoma and cataracts, mental retardation, and tubule reabsorption dysfunction as evidenced by hypophosphatemia, acidosis, and aminoaciduria. Cross-reference: Oculocerebrorenal syndrome. (Charles Lowe, U.S. pediatrician; Mary Terrey, U.S., Elsie MacLachlan)

1. Grinker RR, Sahs AL: Neurology. 6th ed. Springfield, Ill: Charles C Thomas, 1966
2. Lowe C, Terrey M, MacLachlan EA: Am J Dis Child 83:164-184, 1952
3. Scriver CR, Rosenberg LE: Amino Acid Metabolism and Its Disorders. Philadelphia: WB Saunders, 1973

LOWN-GANONG-LEVINE SYNDROME, the patient in whom electrocardiography demonstrates abnormally short PR intervals with normal QRS complexes has been reported to be prone to bouts of supraventricular tachycardia. Cross-reference: Clerc-Levy-Cristeco syndrome. (Bernard Lown, U.S. cardiologist; William F. Ganong, U.S. physiologist; Samuel Levine, 1891-1966, U.S. cardiologist)

1. Clerc A, Levy R, Cristeco C: Arch Mal Coeur 31:569-582, 1938
2. Fowler NO: Cardiac Diagnosis and Treatment. 3rd ed. Cambridge: Harper & Row, 1980
3. Lown B, Ganong W, Levine S: Circulation 8:693-706, 1952

LOWRY SYNDROME, consists of craniosynostosis and bilateral fibular aplasia. (R. Brian Lowry, Irish-Canadian)

1. Gorlin RJ, Cohen MM Jr, Levin LS: Syndromes of the Head and Neck. 3rd ed. New York: Oxford University Press, 1990
2. Lowry RB: J Med Genet 9:227-229, 1972

LOWRY-MACLEAN SYNDROME, mental retardation, ocular proptosis, glaucoma, cleft palate, eventration of the diaphragm, congenital heart defects, growth failure, and craniosynostosis are characteristics. (R. Brian Lowry)

1. Gorlin RJ, Cohen MM Jr, Levin LS: Syndromes of the Head and Neck. 3rd ed. New York: Oxford University Press,

1990
2. Lowry RB, et al: Syndrome of epiphyseal dysplasia, short stature, microcephaly and nystagmus. Clin Genet 8:269-274, 1975

LOWSLEY OPERATION, surgery for correction of hypospadias.
1. Maffei WE: Os Fundamentos da Medicina. 2nd ed. Livraria Editora Artes Médicas Ltda, 1978

LOVE SIGN, placement of two separate spinal needles and injection of procaine; a test of spinal obstruction.
1. Casas EC: Diccionario Terminologico de Ciencias Medicas. 5th ed. Salvat Editores, SA, 1954

LOWY SIGN, administration of adrenaline in the conjunctiva results in notable mydriasis; seen in the patient with pancreatic insufficiency.
1. Casas EC: Diccionario Terminologico de Ciencias Medicas. 5th ed. Salvat Editores, SA, 1954

LSD SYNDROME, symptoms are similar to those experienced on ingestion of D-lysergic acid diethylamide (LSD): light-headedness, giddiness, headache, chilliness, and nausea. Shortly thereafter, visual perception becomes distorted and body image undergoes bizarre changes, while hearing may be keener and visual hallucinations may appear.
1. Baker AB, Baker LH: Clinical Neurology. Revised ed. Philadelphia: Harper & Row, 1982
2. Wikler A: The Relation of Psychiatry to Pharmacology. Baltimore: Williams & Wilkins, 1957

LUBS SYNDROME, see Gilbert-Dreyfus syndrome.

LUC OPERATION, see Caldwell-Luc operation.

LUCAS CHAMPIONNIÈRE DISEASE, chronic pseudomembranous bronchitis. (Justin M.M. Lucas Championnière, 1843-1913, French surgeon)
1. Casas EC: Diccionario Terminologico de Ciencias Medicas. 5th ed. Salvat Editores, SA, 1954

LUCAS SIGN, abdominal distention; seen in the patient with early rickets. (Richard C. Lucas, 1846-1915, British surgeon)
1. Casas EC: Diccionario Terminologico de Ciencias Medicas. 5th ed. Salvat Editores, SA, 1954

LUCATELLO SIGN, the axillary temperature is higher than the oral temperature; seen in the patient with hyperthyroidism.
1. Casas EC: Diccionario Terminologico de Ciencias Medicas. 5th ed. Salvat Editores, SA, 1954

LUCEY-DRISCOL SYNDROME, rapid progressive jaundice occurring after the 7th to 10th day of life, due to defective bilirubin conjugation; apparently the result of an unidentified factor, presumably a steroid in maternal blood transmitted to the infant.
1. Lucey JF, Driscol JJ: Physiological jaundice re-examined, in Saal-Korttsak A (ed): Kernicterus. Toronto: University of Toronto Press, 1961, p 29

LUDER-SHELDON SYNDROME, generalized metabolic disease of amino acids, glucose, and phosphate metabolism. Osteomalacia, polyuria, and fractures are features. Symptoms of Fanconi syndrome have occurred in probands. May result from heavy metal intoxication; rickets is resistant to vitamin D administration. (Joseph Luder, British pediatrician; Wilfred Sheldon, British pediatrician)
1. Luder J, Sheldon W: Familial tubular absorption defect of glucose and amino acids. Arch Dis Child 30:160-164, 1955
2. Scriver CR, Rosenberg LE: Amino Acid Metabolism and Its Disorders. Philadelphia: WB Saunders, 1973

LUDLOFF OPERATION, oblique osteotomy of the first metatarsal bone for correction of the hallux valgus.
1. Maffei WE: Os Fundamentos da Medicina. 2nd ed. Livraria Editora Artes Médicas Ltda, 1978

LUDLOFF SIGN, edema and ecchymosis of the Scarpa triangle; seen in the patient with traumatic separation of the greater trochanter. (Karl Ludloff, 1864-1945, German surgeon)
1. Casas EC: Diccionario Terminologico de Ciencias Medicas. 5th ed. Salvat Editores, SA, 1954

LUDOVICI DISEASE, LUDWIG DISEASE, see Gensoul disease.

LUFT DISEASE, mitochondrial myopathy with euthyroid hypermetabolism; seen in adults. (Rolf Luft, Swedish endocrinologist)
1. Bennett JC, Plum F (eds): Cecil Textbook of Medicine. 20th ed. Philadelphia: WB Saunders, 1996

LUND OPERATION, resection of the astragalus for correction of talipes valgus.
1. Maffei WE: Os Fundamentos da Medicina. 2nd ed. Livraria Editora Artes Médicas Ltda, 1978

LUSCHKA FORAMEN, an area located in the fourth ventricle of the brain. (Hubert von Luschka, 1820-1875, German anatomist)

LUST PHENOMENON, LUST SIGN, if the lateral peroneal nerve is percussed, abduction and flexion of the foot is present; seen in the patient with tetanus. Cross-reference: Peroneal sign. (Franz A. Lust, German pediatrician)

1. Casas EC: Diccionario Terminologico de Ciencias Medicas. 5th ed. Salvat Editores, SA, 1954

LUTEMBACHER SYNDROME, a secundum atrial septal defect with acquired mitral stenosis. Obstruction to the left ventricular inflow aggravates the left-to-right shunt across the atrial sputum. Atrial fibrillation is common. (René Lutembacher, 1884-1936, French cardiologist)

1. Braunwald E: Heart Disease: A Textbook of Cardiovascular Medicine. 4th ed. Philadelphia: WB Saunders, 1992
2. Lutembacher R: Arch Mal Coeur 9:237-253, 1916
3. Ritchie AC: Boyd's Textbook of Pathology. 9th ed. Philadelphia: Lea Febiger, 1990

LUTZ-SPLENDORE-DE ALMEIDA DISEASE, hookworm infection. (Adolfo Lutz, 1855-1940, Brazilian; Alfonso Splendore, 1871-1953, Italian in Brazil; Floriano Paulo de Almeida, Brazilian)

1. Baker AB, Baker LH: Clinical Neurology. Revised ed. Philadelphia: Harper & Row, 1982
2. De Almeida FP: An Fac Med Sci 3:59-64, 1928
3. Lutz A: Impr Med Rio 16:151-163, 1908
4. Splendore A: Bull Soc Pathol Exot Paris 5:313-319, 1912

LYELL DISEASE, see Scalded-skin syndrome. (Alan Lyell, British dermatologist)

LYME DISEASE, a tick-borne bacterial (*Borrelia burgdorferi*, a spirochete) affliction that attacks both sexes and all ages. Skin rash, fatigue, fever, chills, headache, and cervical lymphadenopathy are features; if untreated, results in neurological and arthritic symptoms. Cross-reference: Bannwarth syndrome. (First diagnosed in the town of Lyme, Connecticut.)

1. Ballenger JJ: Diseases of the Nose, Throat, Ear, Head and Neck. 12th ed. Philadelphia: Lea & Febiger, 1977
2. Ritchie AC: Boyd's Textbook of Pathology. 9th ed. Philadelphia: Lea & Febiger, 1990
3. Steere AC, et al: Arthr Rheum 20:7-17, 1977

LYMPHADENOPATHY SYNDROME, a condition occurring in a large number of male homosexuals; characterized by the presence of unexplained lymphadenopathy for 3 or more months involving extrainguinal sites, which on biopsy reveal nonspecific lymphoid hyperplasia. Considered by some authorities to be a prodrome of acquired immunodeficiency syndrome.

1. Dorland's Medical Dictionary. 28th ed. Philadelphia: WB Saunders, 1994

LYON-HORGAN OPERATION, bilateral ligature and section of both superior and inferior thyroid arteries for treating angina pectoris.

1. Maffei WE: Os Fundamentos da Medicina. 2nd ed. Livraria Editora Artes Médicas Ltda, 1978

LYSINE MALABSORPTION SYNDROME, mental and intellectual retardation, excretion of increased amounts of lysine in the urine, convulsions, and hypotonic deep tendon reflexes are characteristics.

1. Omura K, Yamanaka N, Higami S, et al: Lysine malabsorption syndrome: a new type of transport defect. Pediatrics 57:102-105, 1976

MACCLINTOCK SIGN, if the heart rate exceeds 100 beats/minute within 1 hour or more after delivery, hemorrhage is indicated.

1. Casas EC: Diccionario Terminologico de Ciencias Medicas. 5th ed. Salvat Editores, SA, 1954

MACEWEN OPERATION, surgery for cure of a hernia by closing the internal ring with a pad made of a hernial sac. (Sir William Macewen, 1848-1924, Scottish surgeon)

MACEWEN SIGN, a sound similar to that elicited from cracked pottery is obtained upon percussion of the skull; found when there is separation of the cranial sutures. (Sir William Macewen)

1. Grinker RR, Sahs AL: Neurology. 6th ed. Springfield: Charles C Thomas, 1966
2. Pedro-Pons A: Patologia-y-Clinica Medicas. 5th ed. Salvat Editores, SA, 1952

MACHADO-JOSEPH DISEASE, see Joseph disease. (Machado and Joseph are afflicted Azorean families.)

MACKENRODT OPERATION, vaginal fixation of the round ligaments in cases of retroflexion of the uterus. (Alwin K. Mackenrodt, 1859-1925, German gynecologist)

1. Maffei WE: Os Fundamentos da Medicina. 2nd ed. Livraria Editora Artes Médicas Ltda, 1978

MACKENSIE-X DISEASE, hyperkeratosis; aflatoxicosis.

1. Casas EC: Diccionario Terminologico de Ciencias Medicas. 5th ed. Salvat Editores, SA, 1954

MACKENZIE SYNDROME, associated ipsilateral paralysis of the tongue, soft palate, and vocal cord.

Similar to Jackson syndrome with 10th, 11th, and 12th cranial nerve involvement. Cross-reference: Jackson-MacKenzie syndrome. (Sir Stephen MacKenzie, 1844-1909, British)

1. Jackson JH: Lancet 2:770-773, 1872
2. MacKenzie S: Trans Clin Soc Lond 19:317-319, 1886

MACLEAN-MAXWELL DISEASE, chronic inflammation of the calcaneus with edema and pain to pressure. (Charles MacLean, 1788-1824, British in West Africa; James Maxwell, 1836-1921, British in Formosa)

1. Casas EC: Diccionario Terminologico de Ciencias Medicas. 5th ed. Salvat Editores, SA, 1954

MACLEOD SYNDROME, see Swyer-James syndrome. (William M. Macleod, 1911-1977, British)

MACROPHAGE ACTIVATION SYNDROME, peripheral nerve palsy and intrabuccal dysesthesia associated with hypesthesia in the second branch of the trigeminal nerve, hypoacousia, and a tight T8 bank of hypesthesia and optic neuritis. Antibacterial and antiviral serologies, including human immunodeficiency virus, were negative except for Epstein-Barr virus, suggesting a latent infection. Skin rash, weight loss, and fever occur. Bone marrow aspiration establishes the diagnosis. The mortality rate is 50%.

1. J Neurol Neurosurg Psychiatry 62:292, 1997
2. Kaufman DK, Habermann TM, Kurtin PJ, et al: Neurological complications of peripheral and cutaneous T-cell lymphomas. Ann Neurol 36:615-629, 1994

MADELUNG OPERATION, lumbar colotomy. (Otto W. Madelung, 1868-1951, German surgeon)

1. Maffei WE: Os Fundamentos da Medicina. 2nd ed. Livraria Editora Artes Médicas Ltda, 1978

MADELUNG SIGN, the rectal temperature is higher than the axillary temperature; seen in the patient with purulent peritonitis.

1. Casas EC: Diccionario Terminologico de Ciencias Medicas. 5th ed. Salvat Editores, SA, 1954

MADELUNG SYNDROME, benign symmetric lipomatosis; an unusual proliferation of adipose tissue. Characterized by a pronounced deposition of lipomatous masses about the neck and to a lesser extent in the axillae and groin. (Otto W. Madelung)

1. Madelung O: Arch Klin Chir 37:106-130, 1888

MADLENER OPERATION, sterilization by crushing and ligating the middle portion of the fallopian tubes. (Max Madlener, 1868-1951, German surgeon)

1. Maffei WE: Os Fundamentos da Medicina. 2nd ed. Livraria Editora Artes Médicas Ltda, 1978

MADURA FOOT DISEASE, see Ballingall disease.

MAFFUCCI SYNDROME, dyschondroplasia with hemangiomas; characterized by deranged cartilaginous growth in the bones producing multiple cartilaginous enchondrosis within the metaphyses and also by multiple hemangiomas of the skin, mucosa, and internal organs with phlebolith. Patients are normal at birth; hemangiomas and enchondromata develop by adolescence. There is bowing of the long bones, and one limb may be longer than the contralateral one. Cross-reference: Kast syndrome. (Angelo Maffucci, 1847-1903, Italian pathologist)

1. Maffucci A: Di un caso di encondroma ed angioma multiple: contribuzione alla genesi embrionale dei tumori. Movimento Med Chir Nap 13:399-342; 565-575, 1881
2. Smith DW, Jones KL: Recognizable Patterns of Human Malformations: Genetic, Embryologic, and Clinical Aspects. 3rd ed. Philadelphia: WB Saunders, 1982

MAGENDIE SIGN, MAGENDIE-HERTWIG SIGN, ocular deviation; a condition in which one eyeball is deviated upward and outward, the other inward and downward. Cross-reference: Hertwig-Magendie sign. (François Magendie, 1783-1855, French physiologist; Richard C.W.T. von Hertwig, 1850-1937, German zoologist)

1. Grinker RR, Sahs AL: Neurology. 6th ed. Springfield: Charles C Thomas, 1966

MAGITOT DISEASE, osteoperiostitis of the dental alveoli.

1. Casas EC: Diccionario Terminologico de Ciencias Medicas. 5th ed. Salvat Editores, SA, 1954

MAGNAN SIGN, the sensation of foreign bodies under the skin; may be present in cocaine addicts. (Valentin J.J. Magnan, 1835-1916, French psychiatrist)

1. Casas EC: Diccionario Terminologico de Ciencias Medicas. 5th ed. Salvat Editores, SA, 1954

MAGNUS SIGN, if a tourniquet is placed at the base of the finger, no color change is visible. (Rudolph Magnus, 1873-1927, German physiologist)

1. Casas EC: Diccionario Terminologico de Ciencias Medicas. 5th ed. Salvat Editores, SA, 1954

MAGNUSON TEST, a measurement of back pain; the examiner asks the patient to point to the area of back pain and marks the location. The patient is then examined in other parts of the body for a few minutes to divert attention from the area of pain. Examination of the back is resumed. If the patient experiences true local pain, the position of pain remains steadfast. However, if malingering, the patient may not remember the exact location of pain or which areas were identified as tender. (Paul B. Magnuson, 1884-1968, U.S. surgeon)

1. Lumley JS, Clain A: Hamilton Bailey's Demonstration of Physical Signs in Clinical Surgery. 18th ed. London: Butterworth-Heinemann, 1997

MAHLER SIGN, a rapid increase in the heartbeat without a corresponding elevation of temperature; seen in the patient with thrombosis. (Richter A. Mahler, 1863-1941, German obstetrician)

1. Casas EC: Diccionario Terminologico de Ciencias Medicas. 5th ed. Salvat Editores, SA, 1954

MAIER DISEASE, see Kussmaul disease.

MAIGNE SYNDROME, low back pain with radiation to the leg is found in involvement of facet joints and sacroiliac joints. Symptoms can mimic a herniated disc.

1. Maigne: Clin Neurosurg 36:148, 1988

MAISONNEUVE SIGN, hyperextension of the hand; seen in the patient with Colles fracture. (Jules G.F. Maisonneuve, 1809-1897, French surgeon)

1. Casas EC: Diccionario Terminologico de Ciencias Medicas. 5th ed. Salvat Editores, SA, 1954

MAJEWSKI SYNDROME, short rib-polydactyly syndrome type II; the infant is hydropic and there is polyhydramnios, a short and narrow thorax and protuberant abdomen, abbreviated extremities, and pre- and postaxial polysyndactyly with up to nine digits per extremity.

1. Majewski F, Pfeiffer RA, Lenz W, et al: Z Kinderheilkd 11:118-138, 1971

MAJOCCHI-SCHAMBERG DISEASE, a skin disease of uncertain etiology in which there are petechial spots in the skin with surrounding telangiectasia and macules of brownish pigmentation. Occasionally the lesions are itchy, scaly, or thickened. (Domenico Majocchi, 1849-1929, Italian dermatologist; Jay F. Schamberg, 1870-1934, U.S. dermatologist)

1. Kitchens CS: The purpuric disorders. Semin Thromb Hemostat 10:173-189, 1984
2. Majocchi D: Gior Ital Mal Vener 37:242-250, 1896

MAKKA OPERATION, surgery for urinary bladder ectopy, utilizing the cecum as a bladder and the vermiform appendix as a ureter.

1. Maffei WE: Os Fundamentos da Medicina. 2nd ed. Livraria Editora Artes Médicas Ltda, 1978

MALABSORPTION SYNDROME, faulty absorption of proteins, fats, minerals, carbohydrates, and vitamins by the intestine. Weight loss, chronic diarrhea, and abnormal stools that are bulky, light in color, foul smelling, and greasy in appearance and character are symptoms.

1. Bennett JC, Plum F (eds): Cecil Textbook of Medicine. 20th ed. Philadelphia: WB Saunders, 1996
2. Moschella SL, Hurley HJ: Dermatology. 2nd ed. Philadelphia: WB Saunders, 1985

MALASSEZ DISEASE, cyst of the testicles. (Louis Malassez, 1842-1909, French physiologist)

1. Malassez L: Arch Physiol 2:1220-135, 1875

MALE TURNER SYNDROME, seen in phenotypic males in whom the testes are hypoplastic and often undescended; short stature, a webbed neck, and other somatic abnormalities are associated with this syndrome of gonadal dysgenesis. Cross-references: Noonan syndrome; Ullrich syndrome. (Henry H. Turner, 1892-1970, U.S. endocrinologist)

1. Campbell MF, Walsh PC: Campbell's Urology. 5th ed. Philadelphia: WB Saunders, 1986
2. Noonan JA, Ehmke D: J Pediatr 63:468-470, 1963
3. Ranke MB, Heideman P, Knupfer C, et al: Noonan syndrome: growth and clinical manifestations in 144 cases. Eur J Pediatr 148:220-227, 1988

MALGAIGNE SIGN, bulging seen when a patient coughs or blows the nose, usually in thin individuals; seen in the patient with inguinal or femoral hernia. (Joseph F. Malgaigne, 1806-1865, French surgeon)

1. Lumley JS, Clain A: Hamilton Bailey's Demonstration of Physical Signs in Clinical Surgery. 18th ed. London: Butterworth-Heinemann, 1997

MALIGNANT CARCINOID SYNDROME, see Carcinoid syndrome.

MALIN SYNDROME, see Malow syndrome.

MALLET-GUY SIGN, with the patient lying on the right side in the knee-chest position, palpation of the left subcostal region may evoke tenderness not otherwise found. The explanation is that the overlying organs fall to the right in this position, exposing the body and tail of the pancreas to direct palpation. (Pierre Mallet-Guy, French surgeon)

1. Lumley JS, Clain A: Hamilton Bailey's Demonstration of Physical Signs in Clinical Surgery. 18th ed. London: Butterworth-Heinemann, 1997

MALLORY-WEISS SYNDROME, gastroesophageal laceration; massive upper gastrointestinal bleeding caused by a longitudinal tear through or below the esophagogastric junction following alcoholic binges. Retching characteristically precedes the hematemesis. (G. Kenneth Mallory, U.S. pathologist; Soma Weiss, 1898-1942, U.S.)

1. Ballenger JJ: Diseases of the Nose, Throat, Ear, Head and Neck. 12th ed. Philadelphia: Lea & Febiger, 1977
2. Mallory GK, Weiss S: Am J Med Sci 178:506-515, 1929
3. Ritchie AC: Boyd's Textbook of Pathology. 9th ed. Philadelphia: Lea & Febiger, 1990

MALOW SYNDROME, autoerythrophagocytosis and hypersplenism. Cross-reference: Malin syndrome.

1. Casas EC: Diccionario Terminologico de Ciencias Medicas. 5th ed. 1954

MALTA FEVER, brucellosis; an infection with *Brucella* transmissible to man and involving the reticuloendothelial system. (Named after the island of Malta.) Cross-reference: Chipre disease.

1. Casas EC: Diccionario Terminologico de Ciencias Medicas. 5th ed. Salvat Editores, SA, 1954

MANCHESTER-FOTHERGILL OPERATION, a procedure for vaginal hysterectomy/cervicectomy. Cross-reference: Fothergill operation. (William Fothergill, 1865-1926, British gynecologist)

1. Schwartz SI: Principles of Surgery. 4th ed. New York: McGraw-Hill, 1983

MANCHURIA FEVER, hemorrhagic fever with renal syndrome; a type of typhoid fever. (Occurs in South Manchuria.)

1. Casas EC: Diccionario Terminologico de Ciencias Medicas. 5th ed. Salvat Editores, SA, 1954

MANDIBULAR PAIN DYSFUNCTION SYNDROME, see Temporomandibular joint syndrome.

MANGELDORF SIGN, acute dilatation of the stomach; seen in the patient with migraine and seizures.

1. Casas EC: Diccionario Terminologico de Ciencias Medicas. 5th ed. Salvat Editores, SA, 1954

MANN SIGN, 1) a decrease in electrical resistance of the scalp seen in certain traumatic neuroses; 2) the eyes are not on the same horizontal level in exophthalmic goiter. Cross-reference: Dixon Mann sign. (John Dixon Mann, 1840-1912, British)

1. Casas EC: Diccionario Terminologico de Ciencias Medicas. 5th ed. Salvat Editores, SA, 1954

MANN SYNDROME, trauma to the inferior cerebellar peduncle.

1. Casas EC: Diccionario Terminologico de Ciencias Medicas. 5th ed. 1954

MANNABERG SIGN, a decrease in the second heartbeat, such as in appendicitis.

1. Casas EC: Diccionario Terminologico de Ciencias Medicas. 5th ed. Salvat Editores, SA, 1954

MANNKOPF SIGN, an increase in heart rate following pressure on the abdomen; seen in the patient with abdominal pain. (Emil W. Mannkopf, 1836-1918, German)

1. Casas EC: Diccionario Terminologico de Ciencias Medicas. 5th ed. Salvat Editores, SA, 1954

MANSON DISEASE, schistosomiasis mansoni. (Sir Patrick Manson, 1844-1922, British)

1. Casas EC: Diccionario Terminologico de Ciencias Medicas. 5th ed. Salvat Editores, SA, 1954

MANZ DISEASE, retinitis proliferans.

1. Casas EC: Diccionario Terminologico de Ciencias Medicas. 5th ed. Salvat Editores, SA, 1954

MAPLE SYRUP URINE DISEASE, clinical signs usually appearing toward the end of the 1st week of life and consist of lethargy, vomiting, major motor seizures, and increased muscle tone. The urine usually emits a maple syrup odor by the 2nd or 3rd week of life.

1. Baker AB, Baker LH: Clinical Neurology. Revised ed. Philadelphia: Harper & Row, 1982

MARAGLIANO DISEASE, hematic degeneration characterized by formation of vacuoles.

1. Casas EC: Diccionario Terminologico de Ciencias Medicas. 5th ed. Salvat Editores, SA, 1954

MARAÑÓN SIGN, if the skin over the thyroid is scratched, there is a persistent wheal; seen in the patient with hyperthyroidism. (Gregorio Marañón, 1887-1960, Spanish endocrinologist)

1. Casas EC: Diccionario Terminologico de Ciencias Medicas. 5th ed. Salvat Editores, SA, 1954

MARAÑÓN SYNDROME, ovarian insufficiency and osteoporosis. (Gregorio Marañón)

1. Marañón G: Paris Med 1:414-419, 1930

MARBURG VIRUS DISEASE, African hemorrhagic fever. The patient develops congestion of the cerebral and meningeal vessels with some perivascular hemorrhages. Typical glial nodules are present throughout the brain with foci of perivascular cuffing with lymphocytes. Cross-references: Frankfort-Marburg syndrome; Green monkey disease; Vervet monkey disease. (Marburg, Germany where disease first recognized in 1967.)

1. Joynt R, Griggs RC: Clinical Neurology. Revised ed. Philadelphia: Lippincott-Raven, 1997

MARCH DISEASE, exophthalmic goiter.

1. Casas EC: Diccionario Terminologico de Ciencias Medicas. 5th ed. Salvat Editores, SA, 1954

MARCHESANI SYNDROME, see Weill-Marchesani syndrome.

MARCHIAFAVA-BIGNAMI-MICHELI SYNDROME, MARCHIAFAVA-MICHELI SYNDROME, degeneration of the corpus callosum resulting in paroxysmal nocturnal hemoglobinuria. Originally reported in males of Italian descent who consumed excessive amounts of crude red wine, but has since been encountered in patients of varied ancestry and with other alcoholic preferences. (Ettore Marchiafava, 1847-1935, Italian pathologist/neurologist; Amico Bignami, 1862-1929, Italian pathologist; Ferdinando Micheli, 1872-1936, Italian)

1. Heepe P, Nemeth L, Brune F, et al: Marchiafava-Bignami disease. A correlative computed tomography and morphological study. Eur Arch Psychiatr Neurol Sci 237:74-79, 1988
2. Marchiafava E. Bignami A: Sopra un alterazione del corpo calloso osservata in sogeti alcolisti. Riv Patol Nerv Ment 8:544-549, 1903
3. Poser CM: Cental pontine myelinolysis and Marchiafava-Bignami disease. Ann NY Acad Sci 215:373-381, 1973

MARCILLE OPERATION, wrapping the kidney using catgut in cases of rupture not amenable to suturing.

1. Maffei WE: Os Fundamentos da Medicina. 2nd ed. Livraria Editora Artes Médicas Ltda, 1978

MARCKWALD OPERATION, cuneiform excision of two portions of the uterine neck to correct stenosis of the external orifice of the uterus.

1. Maffei WE: Os Fundamentos da Medicina. 2nd ed. Livraria Editora Artes Médicas Ltda, 1978

MARCUS GUNN PHENOMENON, consists of closure of the eye when the mandible is moved. Usually observed in the later stages of peripheral facial palsy. Cross-references: Jaw-winking phenomenon; Marin Amat syndrome; Mueller-Kannberg syndrome. (Robert Marcus Gunn, 1850-1909, British ophthalmologist)

1. Haymaker W: Bing's Local Diagnosis in Neurological Diseases. 15th ed. St Louis: CV Mosby, 1969
2. Marcus Gunn R: Congenital ptosis with peculiar associated movements of the affected lid. Trans Ophthalmol Soc UK 3:283-286, 1883
3. Marin Amat M: Arch Oftalmol Hisp Am 18:70-99, 1918

MARCUS GUNN PUPILLARY SIGN, the pupil reacts paradoxically to light stimulation by dilating slowly, and the consensual reflex may be more active than the direct one. Seen in the patient with optic and retrobulbar neuritis. Cross-references: Gunn sign; Swinging flashlight sign. (Robert Marcus Gunn)

1. Baker AB, Baker LH: Clinical Neurology. Revised ed. Philadelphia: Harper & Row, 1982

MARDEN-WALKER SYNDROME, consists of mental retardation, failure to thrive, characteristic facies, microcephaly, immobility of facial muscles, absent Moro and decreased deep-tendon reflexes, muscle weakness or reduced muscle mass, multiple joint contractures, arachnodactyly, kyphoscoliosis, and transverse palmar creases. (Phillip M. Marden, U.S. pediatrician; William A. Walker, U.S. pediatrician)

1. Gorlin RJ, Cohen MM Jr, Levin LS: Syndromes of the Head and Neck. New York: Oxford University Press, 1990
2. Jaatoul NY, Haddad NE, Khoury LF, et al: The Marden-Walker syndrome. Am J Med Genet 11:259-271, 1982
3. Marden PM, Walker WA: A new generalized connective tissue syndrome. Am J Dis Child 112:225-228, 1966

MAREK DISEASE, a disease of chickens characterized by the infiltration of lymphoid cells into peripheral nerves and other organs, especially the ovary, with resultant enlargement and edema of nerves and paresis, accompanied by lymphoid or other organ tumors. Generally believed to be contagious, but some believe that it is neoplastic. (Josef Marek, 1867-1952, Hungarian veterinarian/pathologist)

1. Hurst JW, Schlant RC, Alexander RW: The Heart: Arteries and Veins. 8th ed. New York: McGraw-Hill, 1994
2. Marek J: Multiple Nervenentzündung (Polyneuritis) bei Hühnern. Duet Tieraztl Wochenschr 15:417-421, 1907

MARFAN SIGN, a purple triangle on the tip of the tongue; an indication of typhoid fever. (Antonin B.J. Marfan, 1858-1942, French pediatrician)

1. Casas EC: Diccionario Terminologico de Ciencias Medicas. 5th ed. Salvat Editores, SA, 1954

MARFAN SYNDROME, congenital mesodermal dystrophy; a connective tissue disease in which hypermobile joints and skeletal deformities, as well as an increased incidence of lens dislocation and disproportionate long bone growth, are features. (Antoine B.J. Marfan)

1. Bennett JC, Plum F (eds): Cecil Textbook of Medicine. 20th ed. Philadelphia: WB Saunders, 1996
2. Marfan AB: Bull Soc Med Hop (Par) 13:220-226, 1896
3. Wilson JD, Foster DW, Kronenberg HM, et al (eds): Williams Textbook of Endocrinology. 9th ed. Philadelphia: WB Saunders, 1998

MARFANOID HYPERMOBILITY SYNDROME, similar to Marfan syndrome but with no involvement of the aorta or displacement of the lenses; believed to be a variant of Marfan syndrome or in some cases of Ehlers-Danlos syndrome. The genetic basis is unclear.

1. Goodman R: Marfan's syndrome and related disorders. N Engl J Med 273:1441, 1965
2. McKusick VA: Heritable Disorders of Connective Tissue. 4th ed. St Louis: CV Mosby, 1972

MARIAN OPERATION, perineal cystostomy.

1. Maffei WE: Os Fundamentos da Medicina. 2nd ed. Livraria Editora Artes Médicas Ltda, 1978

MARIE ATAXIA, MARIE SYNDROME, cerebellar ataxia; the patient presents with combined cerebellar, posterior column, and pyramidal tract features. Lesions of the superior cerebellar peduncle cause ocular paralysis and crossed hemiplegia. Similar to Friedreich ataxia. Cross-reference: Pierre Marie disease. (Pierre Marie, 1853-1940, French neurologist)

1. Baker AB, Baker LH: Clinical Neurology. Revised ed. Philadelphia: Harper & Row, 1982
2. Marie P: Sem Med Paris 13:444-447, 1893

MARIE SIGN, see Charcot-Marie sign.

MARIE-BAMBERGER DISEASE, hypertrophic osteopulmonary arthropathy. Cross-reference: Bamberger-Marie disease. (Pierre Marie; Eugene Bamberger, 1858-1921, Austrian)

1. Marie P, Bamberger E: Rev Med Paris 10:1-36, 1890

MARIE-FOIX SIGN, extreme flexion of the toes or foot which may be the initial response of the flexion spinal defense reflex. Forced flexion of the toes causes the limb to flex in paralysis. Cross-reference: Chiray-Foix-Nicolesco syndrome. (Pierre Marie; Charles Foix, 1882-1927, French neurologist)

1. Baker AB, Baker LH: Clinical Neurology. Revised ed. Philadelphia: Harper & Row, 1982

MARIE-ROBINSON SYNDROME, consists of melancholy, somnolence, and impotence associated with alimentary levulosuria. (Pierre Marie)

1. Casas EC: Diccionario Terminologico de Ciencias Medicas. 5th ed. 1954

MARIE-STRÜMPELL SPONDYLITIS, ankylosing spondylitis with prominent involvement of spinal articulations, sacroiliac joints, and paravertebral soft tissues. Cross-references: Bechterew disease; Strümpell-Marie disease. (Pierre Marie; Ernst A. von Strümpell, 1853-1925, German)

1. Baker AB, Baker LH: Clinical Neurology. Revised ed. Philadelphia: Harper & Row, 1982
2. Marie P, von Strümpell EA: Rev Med Paris 18:285-315, 1898
3. Von Strümpell EA: Arch Psychiatr 10:676-717, 1880

MARIE-TOOTH DISEASE, progressive neuropathic (peroneal) muscular atrophy. (Pierre Marie; Howard Tooth, 1856-1925, British)

1. Marie P, Tooth H: Rev Med Paris 6:97-138, 1886

MARIN AMAT SYNDROME, see Marcus Gunn phenomenon. (Manuel Marin Amat, Spanish)

MARINE-LENHART SYNDROME, hyperthyroidism by multiple toxic adenomas.

1. Gold JJ, Josimovich JB: Gynecologic Endocrinology. 3rd ed. New York: Plenum Medical, 1980

MARINESCO-SJÖGREN SYNDROME, a hereditary disorder consisting of congenital spinocerebellar ataxia accompanied by congenital cataract and oligophrenia. (Georges Marinesco, 1865-1938, Romanian; Karl G.T. Sjögren, Swedish psychiatrist)

1. Marinesco G, Draganesco S, Vasiliu D: Encephale 26:97-109, 1931
2. McKusick VA: Heritable Disorders of Connective Tissue. 4th ed. St Louis: CV Mosby, 1972
3. Sjögren T: Confin Neurol 10:293-308, 1950

MARION DISEASE, an enlarged bladder neck. (Jean Marion, 1869-1960, French neurologist)

1. Bailey H, Love M: A Short Practice of Surgery. 12th ed. London: HK Lewis & Co, 1962
2. Marion J: J Urol Med Chir 23:97-11, 1927

MAROTEAUX-LAMY SYNDROME, mucopolysaccharidosis type VI; pyknodysostosis, osteosclerosis, visual impairment, deafness (recurrent ear infection), short distal phalanges, delayed closure of fontanel, very minimal mental retardation, but scoliosis are features. There is a deficiency of aryl-sulfatase B in all tissues. Increased urinary excretion of mucopolysaccharides consists predominantly of dermatan sulfate. Autosomal recessive (possibly X-linked recessive). (Pierre Maroteaux, French pediatrician; Maurice E.J. Lamy, 1895-1955, French pediatrician)

1. Maroteaux P, Lamy M: Hurler's disease, Morquio's disease and related mucopolysaccharidoses. J Pediatr 67:312-323, 1965
2. Maroteaux P, Lamy M: La pyknodysostosis. Presse Med 70:999-102, 1962
3. Smith DW, Jones KL: Recognizable Patterns of Human Malformations: Genetic, Embryologic, and Clinical Aspects. 3rd ed. Philadelphia: WB Saunders, 1982

MAROTEAUX-MALAMUT SYNDROME, see Acrodysostosis syndrome. (Pierre Maroteaux)

MARSEILLES DISEASE, see Conor-Bruch fever.

MARSHALL SYNDROME, MARSHALL-SMITH SYNDROME, accelerated growth and maturation; shallow orbits, broad middle phalanges, and motor and apparent mental deficiency are characteristics. Etiology unknown. (Richard E. Marshall, U.S.)

1. Marshall RE, Graham CB, Scott CR, et al: Syndrome of accelerated skeletal maturation and relative failure to thrive: a newly recognized clinical growth disorder. J Pediatr 78:95-101, 1971
2. Smith DW, Jones KL: Recognizable Patterns of Human Malformations: Genetic, Embryologic, and Clinical Aspects. 3rd ed. Philadelphia: WB Saunders, 1982

MARSHALL-MARCHETTI-KRANTZ OPERATION, a procedure for vaginal hysterectomy or bladder repair. (Victor F. Marshall-Marchetti, U.S. urologist; Kermit Krantz, obstetrician-gynecologist)

1. Schwartz SI: Principles of Surgery. 4th ed. New York: McGraw-Hill, 1983

MARSHALL-STICKLER SYNDROME, see Stickler syndrome.

MARTIN DISEASE, periosteoarthritis of the feet due to excessive and prolonged walking. (Henry A. Martin, 1824-1884, U.S. surgeon)

1. Casas EC: Diccionario Terminologico de Ciencias Medicas. 5th ed. Salvat Editores, SA, 1954

MARTIN OPERATION, vaginal hysterectomy.

1. Maffei WE: Os Fundamentos da Medicina. 2nd ed. Livraria Editora Artes Médicas Ltda, 1978

MARTIN-BELL SYNDROME, large testes, mental retardation, epilepsy, hyperactivity, and characteristic long facies with big ears are features. Etiology appears to be a fragile X chromosome. Cross-reference: Fragile X syndrome. (J. Purdon Martin, British; J.A. Bell, British)

1. Gorlin RJ, Cohen MM Jr, Levin LS: Syndromes of the Head and Neck. New York: Oxford University Press, 1990
2. Loesch DZ, Hay DA, Sutherland GR, et al: Phenotypic variation in male-transmitted fragile X: genetic inferences. Am J Med Genet 27:401-417, 1987
3. Martin JP, Bell J: J Neurol Neurosurg Psychiatry 6:154-156, 1943

MARTINET DISEASE, pseudoangina caused by nervous dyspepsia.

1. Casas EC: Diccionario Terminologico de Ciencias Medicas. 5th ed. Salvat Editores, SA, 1954

MARTORELL SYNDROME, see Aortic arch syndrome. (Fernando O. Martorell, Spanish cardiologist)

MARTSOLF SYNDROME, unusual facies, severe mental retardation, short stature, cataracts, and hypogonadism are features.

1. Gorlin RJ, Cohen MM Jr, Levin LS: Syndromes of the Head and Neck. New York: Oxford University Press, 1990
2. Harbord MG, Baraitser M, Wilson J: Microcephaly, mental retardation, cataracts, and hypogonadism in sibs: Martsolf's syndrome. Med Genet 26:397-408, 1989
3. Martsolf JT, Hunter AGW, Haworth JC: Am J Med Genet 1:291-299, 1978

MARWEDEL OPERATION, a method of gastrostomy.

1. Maffei WE: Os Fundamentos da Medicina. 2nd ed. Livraria Editora Artes Médicas Ltda, 1978

MASINI SIGN, notable dorsal extension; seen in the child with mental instability. (Giulio Masini, 1874-1937, Italian)

1. Casas EC: Diccionario Terminologico de Ciencias Medicas. 5th ed. Salvat Editores, SA, 1954

MAST SYNDROME, a recessive form of juvenile spastic paraplegia associated with dysarthria and dementia.

1. Farmer TW: Pediatric Neurology. 2nd ed. Hagerstown: Harper & Row, 1975

MASTIN SIGN, pain in the clavicle region; seen in the patient with acute appendicitis.

1. Casas EC: Diccionario Terminologico de Ciencias Medicas. 5th ed. Salvat Editores, SA, 1954

MASTOCYTOSIS SYNDROME, presumably related to histamine release from degranulating mast cells. Usually found in persons with skin lesions, bone lesions, and hepatosplenomegaly; occurs in less than 15% of patients with mastocytosis.

1. Moschella SL, Hurley HJ: Dermatology. 2nd ed. Philadelphia: WB Saunders, 1985

MATERNAL DEPRIVATION SYNDROME, growth failure, autistic behavior, and delayed mental development resulting from loss or absence of the mother or lack of proper mothering are features.

1. Dorland's Medical Dictionary. 28th ed. Philadelphia: WB Saunders, 1994

MATHIEU SIGN, tympanism in the periumbilical region; seen in the patient with bowel obstruction.

1. Casas EC: Diccionario Terminologico de Ciencias Medicas. 5th ed. Salvat Editores, SA, 1954

MATINGNON SIGN, pain in the area of the anus when the patient sits; seen in cases of enterocolitis.

1. Casas EC: Diccionario Terminologico de Ciencias Medicas. 5th ed. Salvat Editores, SA, 1954

MAURIAC SYNDROME, a disturbance of glycogen metabolism in infants with diabetes in association with dwarfism, hepatomegaly, obesity, liver with content glycopenia, hypopituitarism, hypersecretion of corticosteroid, and low insulin tolerance. Cross-reference: Wolcott-Rallison syndrome. (Pierre Mauriac, 1832-1905, French)

1. Guest GM: The Mauriac syndrome. Diabetes 2:415-417, 1953
2. Mauriac P: Gaz Hedb Sci Med Bordeaux 51:402-404, 1930

MAXCY DISEASE, an endemic form of typhus in the southwestern U.S. (Kenneth F. Maxcy, U.S. bacteriologist)

1. Maxcy KF: US Publ Health Rep 41:1213-1220, 1926

MAY SIGN, the administration of an adrenaline solution produces mydriasis; seen in the patient with glaucoma.

1. Casas EC: Diccionario Terminologico de Ciencias Medicas. 5th ed. Salvat Editores, SA, 1954

MAYER-ROKITANSKY-KÜSTER-HAUSER SYNDROME, congenital absence of a vagina and a rudimentary uterus, with normal uterine tubes, ovaries, and secondary female sex characteristics and normal growth. Cross-reference: Rokitansky syndrome. (August Mayer, 1787-1865, German; Karl von Rokitansky, 1804-1878, Austrian pathologist; Hermann Küster, German gynecologist; G.A. Hauser, Swiss)

1. Campbell MF, Walsh PC: Campbell's Urology. 5th ed. Philadelphia: WB Saunders, 1986
2. Hauser GA, Keller M, Koller T, et al: Gynaecologia 151:111-112, 1961
3. Küster H: Z Geburtshife Gynaekol 67:692-718, 1910
4. Mayer CAJ: J Chir Augenheilkd 13:525-564, 1829
5. Von Rokitansky KF: Med Jahrb Obstet Staat 26:39-77, 1838

MAYNIHAN METHOD, see Murphy "kidney punch" sign.

MAYO SIGN, the inferior mandibular muscle relaxes, signifying that the patient is in a state of deep anesthesia.

1. Casas EC: Diccionario Terminologico de Ciencias Medicas. 5th ed. Salvat Editores, SA, 1954

MAYOR SIGN, the presence of a fetal heart murmur during pregnancy.

1. Casas EC: Diccionario Terminologico de Ciencias Medicas. 5th ed. Salvat Editores, SA, 1954

McALPINE SYNDROME, see Lhermitte syndrome.

McARDLE DISEASE, McARDLE-SCHMID-PEARSON DISEASE, glycogen storage disease type V; due to a deficiency of muscle phosphorylase and characterized by pain, weakness, and stiffness of muscles after exercise. The rarest of the glycogen storage diseases, this disorder is probably underrecognized because the patient is functional and usually asymptomatic until adolescence or early adulthood. (Brian McArdle, British neurologist)

1. Grinker RR, Sahs AL: Neurology. 6th ed. Springfield: Charles C Thomas, 1966
2. McArdle B: Clin Soc Lond 10:13-35, 1951
3. Pearson CM: Am J Med 30:502-517, 1961
4. Schmid R, Hammaker L: N Engl J Med 264:223-225, 1961

McARTHUR OPERATION, catheterization of the bile duct for injection of contrast media into the duodenum.

1. Maffei WE: Os Fundamentos da Medicina. 2nd ed. Livraria Editora Artes Médicas Ltda, 1978

McBRIDE OPERATION, procedure for repair of hallux valgus or bunions. (Earl D. McBride, U.S. orthopedic surgeon)

1. Schwartz SI: Principles of Surgery. 4th ed. New York: McGraw-Hill, 1983

McBURNEY OPERATION, incision for appendectomy or Meckel diverticulitis. (Charles McBurney, 1845-1913, U.S. surgeon)
1. Schwartz SI: Principles of Surgery. 4th ed. New York: McGraw-Hill, 1983

McBURNEY POINT, a point of tenderness between the umbilicus and the anterosuperior iliac spine; seen in the patient with acute appendicitis. (Charles McBurney)
1. Dorland's Medical Dictionary. 28th ed. Philadelphia: WB Saunders, 1994

McBURNEY SIGN, pain on palpation of the right lower quadrant; an indication of appendicitis. (Charles McBurney)
1. Lumley JS, Clain A: Hamilton Bailey's Demonstration of Physical Signs in Clinical Surgery. 18th ed. London: Butterworth-Heinemann, 1997

McCUNE-ALBRIGHT SYNDROME, see Albright syndrome. (Donovan J. McCune, U.S.)

McDOWELL OPERATION, oophorectomy through an abdominal incision.
1. Maffei WE: Os Fundamentos da Medicina. 2nd ed. Livraria Editora Artes Médicas Ltda, 1978

McKISSOCK OPERATION, a technique used for reduction mammaplasty.
1. Schwartz SI: Principles of Surgery. 4th ed. New York: McGraw-Hill, 1983

McKUSICK METAPHYSEAL CHONDRODYSPLASIA SYNDROME, mild bowing of the legs, wide irregular metaphyses, fine sparse hair, small stature, incomplete extension of the elbow, and loose-jointed "limp" hands and feet are features. Autosomal recessive inheritance.
1. Smith DW, Jones KL: Recognizable Patterns of Human Malformations: Genetic, Embryologic, and Clinical Aspects. 3rd ed. Philadelphia: WB Saunders, 1982

McLEOD SYNDROME, limb weakness, acanthocytes, and very elevated creatine kinase level in the blood are features. First discovered in blood banks because the donors lacked Kell antigen. The condition is related to Xp21.
1. Rowland LP (ed): Merritt's Textbook of Neurology. 9th ed. Baltimore: Williams & Wilkins, 1995

McMURRAY SIGN, a cartilage click during manipulation of the knee; meniscal injury is indicated. (Thomas P. McMurray, 1887-1949, British orthopedic surgeon)
1. Mazion JM: Illustrated Manual of Orthopedic Signs/Tests/Maneuvers for Office Procedure. 2nd ed. Orlando: Daniels Publishing, 1980

McQUARRIE SYNDROME, see Harris syndrome.

McVAY OPERATION, operation for abdominal wall hernias. (Chester B. McVay, U.S. surgeon)
1. Schwartz SI: Principles of Surgery. 4th ed. New York: McGraw-Hill, 1983

MEAN SIGN, lag of the eyeball on upward gaze; seen in the patient with Graves disease. (James H. Mean, 1885-1967, U.S. endocrinologist)
1. Dorland's Medical Dictionary. 28th ed. Philadelphia: WB Saunders, 1994

MECKEL CAVE, a hiatus present at the petrous apex between the tentorium and the petrosa, which forms a canal for the passage of the 5th cranial nerve. (Johann F. Meckel, 1724-1774, German anatomist)
1. Ballenger JJ: Diseases of the Nose, Throat, Ear, Head and Neck. 12th ed. Philadelphia: Lea & Febiger, 1977

MECKEL SYNDROME, MECKEL-GRUBER SYNDROME, dysencephalia splanchnocystica; multiple cyst formation of the kidneys with functional and clinical sequelae that are encountered in several malformation syndromes. Encephalocele, polydactyly, and polycystic kidneys are characteristics. Autosomal recessive inheritance; prenatal diagnosis may be possible. Cross-reference: Gruber syndrome. (Johann F. Meckel; Georg B. Gruber, 1884-1977, German pathologist)
1. Gruber GB: Beitr Pathol Anat 93:459-476, 1934
2. Meckel JF: Beschreibung zweier durch sehr ähnliche Bildungsabweichung entsteller Geschwister. Dtsch Arch Physiol 7:99-172, 1822
3. Smith DW, Jones KL: Recognizable Patterns of Human Malformations: Genetic, Embryologic, and Clinical Aspects. 3rd ed. Philadelphia: WB Saunders, 1982

MECONIUM BLOCKAGE SYNDROME, MECONIUM PLUG SYNDROME, a plug of neonatal meconium obstruction of the rectum or colon; removal of the plug results in cure. Does not usually accompany fibrocystic disease of the pancreas.
1. Ritchie AC: Boyd's Textbook of Pathology. 9th ed. Philadelphia: Lea & Febiger, 1990
2. Van Leeuwen G, Riley WC, Glenn L, et al: Meconium plug syndrome with aganglionosis. Pediatrics 40:665-666, 1967

MEDIAL INFERIOR PONTINE SYNDROME, results from occlusion of a paramedian branch of the basilar artery.
1. Walsh FB, Hoyt EF, Miller NR: Clinical Neuro-Ophthalmology. 4th ed. Baltimore: Williams & Wilkins, 1982

MEDIAL MIDPONTINE SYNDROME, occlusion of a paramedian branch of the midbasilar artery. Results in ataxia of the ipsilateral limbs and contralateral paresis of the face, arm, and leg with variable contralateral sensory loss.
1. Baker AB, Baker LH: Clinical Neurology. Revised ed. Philadelphia: Harper & Row, 1982

MEDIAL PONTINE (PARAMEDIAN) SYNDROME, may result from small vessel occlusion or from occlusion of the entire basilar artery. Unilateral or bilateral signs are possible.
1. Walsh FB, Hoyt EF, Miller NR: Clinical Neuro-Ophthalmology. 4th ed. Baltimore: Williams & Wilkins, 1982

MEDIAL SUPERIOR PONTINE SYNDROME, results from occlusion of the paramedian branches of the upper basilar artery.
1. Walsh FB, Hoyt EF, Miller NR: Clinical Neuro-Ophthalmology. 4th ed. Baltimore: Williams & Wilkins, 1982

MEDIAN CLEFT FACIAL SYNDROME, a primary defect in midfacial development with features of incomplete anterior appositional alignment of the eyes, medial cleft palate, and double frenulum. Etiology unknown.
1. DeMyer W: The median cleft face syndrome. Differential diagnosis of cranium bifidum occultum, hypertelorism, and median cleft nose, lip, and palate. Neurology 17:961-971, 1967
2. Smith DW, Jones KL: Recognizable Patterns of Human Malformations: Genetic, Embryologic, and Clinical Aspects. 3rd ed. Philadelphia: WB Saunders, 1982

MEDIOPLANTAR REFLEX, see Guillain-Barré sign.

MEDITERRANEAN DISEASE, see Cooley anemia.

MEESMANN SYNDROME, see Meretoja syndrome.

MEGACYSTITIS-MEGAURETER SYNDROME, chronic ureteral dilatation (megaureter) associated with hypotonia and dilatation of the bladder (megacystiti) and gaping of ureteral orifices, permitting vesicoureteral reflux of urine and resulting in chronic pyelonephritis.
1. Dorland's Medical Dictionary. 28th ed. Philadelphia: WB Saunders, 1994

MEGAW DISEASE, see Tsutsugamushi disease.

MEIBOMIAN CYST, chalazion cyst of the meibomian gland of the eye. (Heinrich Meibomian, 1638-1700, German anatomist)
1. Lumley JS, Clain A: Hamilton Bailey's Demonstration of Physical Signs in Clinical Surgery. 18th ed. London: Butterworth-Heinemann, 1997

MEIGE SYNDROME, a focal form of facial and mandibular dystonia. Causes long-lasting facial movements (sustained dystonic movements) compared to the rapid, brief and repetitive movements of tardive dyskinesia. Cross-reference: Brueghel syndrome. (Henri Meige, 1866-1940, French)
1. Meige H: Rev Neurol 20:437-443, 1910
2. Rowland LP (ed): Merritt's Textbook of Neurology. 9th ed. Baltimore: Williams & Wilkins, 1995

MEIGS SYNDROME, MEIGS-CASS SYNDROME, transudative ascites associated with ovarian fibroma or cystadenoma, struma ovarii, and "ovarian overstimulation" syndrome. Removal of the tumor usually cures the ascites. Cross-reference: Demons-Meigs syndrome. (Joseph V. Meigs, 1892-1963, U.S. obstetrician/gynecologist)
1. Meigs JV, Cass JW: Am J Obstet Gynecol 33:249-267, 1937
2. O'Flanagan SJ, Tighe BF, Egans TJ, et al: Meigs' syndrome and pseudo-Meigs syndrome. J R Soc Med 80:252-253, 1987
3. Sleisenger MH, Fordtran JS: Gastrointestinal Disease: Pathophysiology, Diagnosis, Management. 2nd ed. Philadelphia: WB Saunders, 1978

MELANOTIC FRECKLE, see Hutchinson freckle.

MELEDA DISEASE, endemic familial keratoderma on the Meleda island in the Adriatic Sea.
1. Casas EC: Diccionario Terminologico de Ciencias Medicas. 5th ed. Salvat Editores, SA, 1954

MELKERSSON SYNDROME, MELKERSSON-ROSENTHAL SYNDROME, a rare form of recurrent facial paralysis. Signs and symptoms include facial edema, facial paralysis, and furrowed tongue. Associated ophthalmic symptoms may include lagophthalmos, burning sensation of the eyes, blepharochalasis, swelling of the eyelids, corneal opacities, retrobulbar neuritis, and bilateral recurrent exophthalmos. (Ernst Melkersson, 1898-1932, Swedish; Curt Rosenthal, German neurologist/psychiatrist)

1. Farmer TW: Pediatric Neurology. 2nd ed. Hagerstown: Harper & Row, 1975
2. Melkersson E: Ett fall av recidiverande facialspares I samband med angioneurotisk ödem. Hygeia 90:737-741, 1928
3. Rosenthal C: Z Ges Neurol Psychol 131:475-501, 1931

MELNICK-FRASER SYNDROME, see Branchio-oto-renal syndrome.

MELNICK-NEEDLES SYNDROME, osteodysplasty; prominent eyes, bowing of the long bones, ribbon-like ribs, osteodysplasia, and a small thoracic cape, short clavicle, and short upper arms are features. Autosomal dominant inheritance. (John Charles Melnick, U.S. radiologist)

1. Melnick JC, Needles CF: An undiagnosed bone dysplasia. A two family study of four generations and three generations. Am J Roentgenol 97:39-48, 1966
2. Smith DW, Jones KL: Recognizable Patterns of Human Malformations: Genetic, Embryologic, and Clinical Aspects. 3rd ed. Philadelphia: WB Saunders, 1982

MELTZER SIGN, pain at the McBurney point on pressure and on elevation of the leg with the knee in extension; seen in the patient with chronic appendicitis. (Samuel J. Meltzer, 1851-1920, U.S. physiologist)

1. Casas EC: Diccionario Terminologico de Ciencias Medicas. 5th ed. Salvat Editores, SA, 1954

MENDEL REFLEX, MENDEL-BECHTEREW SIGN, to elicit the toe flexor reflex (latent deep plantar muscle reflex), the examiner taps the lateral aspect of the dorsum of the patient's foot. Cross-references: Bechterew-Mendel reflex; Dorsocuboidal sign. (Kurt Mendel, 1874-1946, German neurologist; Vladimir M. von Bechterew, 1857-1927, Russian neurologist)

1. Haymaker W: Bing's Local Diagnosis in Neurological Diseases. 15th ed. St Louis: CV Mosby, 1969

MENDEL SIGN, pain on percussion of the epigastric region; seen in the patient with gastric or duodenal ulcer.

1. Pedro-Pons A: Patologia-y-Clinica Medicas. 5th ed. Salvat Editores, SA, 1952

MENDELSOHN SIGN, the heart rate does not change with exertion; an indication of cardiac asthenia.

1. Casas EC: Diccionario Terminologico de Ciencias Medicas. 5th ed. Salvat Editores, SA, 1954

MENDELSON SYNDROME, see Pulmonary acid aspiration syndrome. (Curtis L. Mendelson, U.S. obstetrician/gynecologist)

MENDENHALL DISEASE, characterized by a mutation in the insulin receptor gene with consequent life-long uncontrolled hyperglycemia. A sural nerve biopsy from a patient with this disease showed a gross loss of myelinated fibers that was comparable with the degree of fiber loss in a case-matched diabetic patient with established neuropathy. (E.N. Mendenhall, U.S.)

1. Malik RA, Kumer S, Boulton AJM: Mendenhall's syndrome: clues to the aetiology of human diabetic neuropathy. J Neurol Neurosurg Psychiatry 58:493-495, 1995
2. Mendenhall EN: J Indiana Med 43:32-36, 1950

MENDES DA COSTA SYNDROME, macular epidermolysis bullosa dystrophica. The infant appears normal at birth; after several months, tense bullae appear on the trunk and extremities, hair loss occurs, and coarse-meshed reticulated hyperpigmentation along with macular atrophy develops on the face and extremities. Inherited in a sex-linked recessive manner. (Samuel Mendes da Costa, Dutch)

1. Mendes da Costa S: Acta Dermatol Vener 6:255-261, 1925
2. Moschella SL, Hurley HJ: Dermatology. 2nd ed. Philadelphia: WB Saunders, 1985

MÉNÉTRIER DISEASE, giant hypertrophic gastritis characterized by gastric mucosal hypertrophy, hyposecretion of gastric acid, increased loss of protein from the stomach, edema, weight loss, and, occasionally pain, nausea, and vomiting. (Pierre E. Ménétrier, 1859-1935, French)

1. Bennett JC, Plum F (eds): Cecil Textbook of Medicine. 20th ed. Philadelphia: WB Saunders, 1996
2. Ménétrier PE: Arch Physiol Norm Pathol 1:32-55, 1888

MENGERT SHOCK SYNDROME, a condition resembling shock that sometimes occurs when a pregnant woman in the late antepartum period lies in the supine position; caused by pressure of the uterus on the vena cava.

MÉNIÈRE DISEASE, MÉNIÈRE SYNDROME, labyrinthine vertigo; sudden attacks of vertigo, tinnitus, vomiting, prostration, and progressive deafness, in addition to distention of the endolymphatic system. In 1848, Ménière described this symptom complex, citing the case of a young girl who died from labyrinthine hemorrhage to illustrate the anatomic origin of the symptoms. He likened the disease to glaucoma. (Prosper Ménière, 1799-1862, French ear, nose, throat specialist)

1. Ballenger JJ: Diseases of the Nose, Throat, Ear, Head and Neck. 12th ed. Philadelphia: Lea & Febiger, 1977
2. Farmer TW: Pediatric Neurology. 2nd ed. Hagerstown: Harper & Row, 1975
3. Ménière P: Gaz Med Paris (3rd Ser) 16:29, 1861

MENISCUS SIGN, see Crescent sign.

MENKES SYNDROME, an X-linked recessive inherited disorder of connective tissue characterized by intestinal malabsorption of copper, low serum copper ceruloplasmin concentration, severe copper deficiency growth retardation, and kinky or "steely" hair. Cross-references: Kinky-hair syndrome; Steely-hair syndrome. (John H. Menkes, U.S. pediatrician/neurologist)

1. Gupta A, Arora NK, Desai N, et al: Menkes disease. Indian J Pediatr 55:445-447, 1988
2. McKusick VA: Heritable Disorders of Connective Tissue. 4th ed. St Louis: CV Mosby, 1972
3. Menkes JH, Alter M, Steigeeder GK, et al: Pediatrics 29:764-769, 1962

MENNELL SIGN, the examiner places a thumb over the posterosuperior iliac spine, exerts pressure, and then slides the thumb outward and upward. The sign is positive if tenderness is increased, which helps to determine that the tenderness is due to strained superior sacroiliac ligaments. (James B. Mennell, 1880-1957, British)

1. Evans RC: Illustrated Essentials in Orthopedic Physical Assessment. St Louis: Mosby Yearbook, 1994

MENOPAUSAL SYNDROME, a term used to describe a group of symptoms experienced by some women during the climacteric period; the most frequent characteristics are vasomotor disturbances consisting of hot flashes which are often accompanied by sweats and chills. Other less specific nervous system symptoms include irritability, depression, headaches, and insomnia. Cross-reference: Climacteric syndrome.

1. Campbell MF, Walsh PC: Campbell's Urology. 5th ed. Philadelphia: WB Saunders, 1986
2. Gold JJ, Josimovich JB: Gynecologic Endocrinology. 3rd ed. New York: Plenum Medical, 1980

MENTAL RETARDATION-OVERGROWTH SYNDROME, see Simpson-Golabi-Behmel syndrome.

MERCIER OPERATION, transurethral prostatectomy. (Louis Mercier, 1811-1882, French urologist)

1. Maffei WE: Os Fundamentos da Medicina. 2nd ed. Livraria Editora Artes Médicas Ltda, 1978

MEREDITH OPERATION, cholecystectomy.

1. Maffei WE: Os Fundamentos da Medicina. 2nd ed. Livraria Editora Artes Médicas Ltda, 1978

MERETOJA SYNDROME, systemic amyloidosis with corneal lattice dystrophy, cranial nerve palsy, and cutis laxa of the facial skin. Cross-references: Biber-Haab-Dimmer syndrome; Meesmann syndrome. (J. Meretoja, Finnish)

1. Gorlin RJ, Cohen MM Jr, Levin LS: Syndromes of the Head and Neck. New York: Oxford University Press, 1990
2. Meretoja J: Ann Clin Rep 1:314-324, 1969
3. Meretoja J: Clin Genet 4:173-185, 1973

MERRF SYNDROME, *m*yoclonus with *e*pilepsy with *r*agged *r*ed *f*ibers (MERRF), an example of a maternally inherited disorder. An encephalomyopathy first described by Fukuhara et al. Cross-references: Fukuhara syndrome; Ophthalmoplegia syndrome.

1. Rosing HS, et al: maternally inherited mitochondrial myopathy and myoclonic epilepsy. Ann Neurol 17:228-237, 1985

METACARPAL SIGN, normally a line drawn tangentially to the distal ends of the heads of the fourth and fifth metacarpal bones extends distal to the third metacarpal bone. A positive metacarpal sign is present when the line passes through the head of the third metacarpal. When the line is tangential to the head of the third metacarpal, the sign is considered to be borderline. A positive sign is most often bilateral.

1. Gold JJ, Josimovich JB: Gynecologic Endocrinology. 3rd ed. New York: Plenum Medical, 1980

METAMERIC SYNDROME, see Segmentary syndrome.

METASTATIC CARCINOID SYNDROME, see Carcinoid syndrome.

METATROPIC DWARFISM SYNDROME, a small thorax, thoracic kyphoscoliosis, and metaphyseal flaring are features. Both autosomal dominant and autosomal recessive inheritance.

1. Maroteaux P, Spranger J, Wiedemann H: Der metatropische Zwergwuchs. Arch Kinderheilkd 173:211-226, 1966

METHIONINE MALABSORPTION SYNDROME, a disorder of methionine absorption in which the urine has a characteristic odor resembling that of the interior of an oasthouse (a building for drying hops) due to á-hydroxybutyric acid formed by bacterial action on the unabsorbed methionine; charac-

terized by white hair, mental retardation, convulsions, and attacks of hyperpnea. Autosomal recessive inheritance. Cross-reference: Oasthouse disease.
1. Smith AJ, Strang LB: An inborn error of metabolism with the urinary excretion of a a-hydroxy-butyric acid and phenylpyruvic acid. Arch Dis Child 33:109-113, 1958

MEUNIER SIGN, in measles, daily weight loss after the incubation period but before the appearance of a rash.
1. Casas EC: Diccionario Terminologico de Ciencias Medicas. 5th ed. Salvat Editores, SA, 1954

MEYER SIGN, paresthesias of the hands and feet; occurs during the time of rash in the patient with scarlet fever.
1. Casas EC: Diccionario Terminologico de Ciencias Medicas. 5th ed. Salvat Editores, SA, 1954

MEYNERT SYNDROME, see Wernicke syndrome.

MIBELLI DISEASE, porokeratosis. (Vittorio Mibelli, 1860-1910, Italian dermatologist)
1. Mibelli V: Gior Ital Mal Vener 28:313-355, 1893

MICHAELIS SIGN, a low fever postpartum or postoperatively with no apparent cause; can indicate thrombotic disease.
1. Casas EC: Diccionario Terminologico de Ciencias Medicas. 5th ed. Salvat Editores, SA, 1954

MICHEL DEFORMITY, a congenital hereditary hearing loss with a complete lack of development of the inner ear. (E.M. Michel, French)
1. Ballenger JJ: Diseases of the Nose, Throat, Ear, Head and Neck. 12th ed. Philadelphia: Lea & Febiger, 1977
2. Gorlin RJ, Cohen MM Jr, Levin LS: Syndromes of the Head and Neck. 3rd ed. New York: Oxford University Press, 1990

MICHELON-WEISS SIGN, otitis in the middle ear in the patient with tuberculosis; the patient hears his/her own respiration.
1. Casas EC: Diccionario Terminologico de Ciencias Medicas. 5th ed. Salvat Editores, SA, 1954

MICHELS SYNDROME, consists of craniofacial anomalies including anterior chamber eye abnormalities and skeletal defects.
1. Gorlin RJ, Cohen MM Jr, Levin LS: Syndromes of the Head and Neck. New York: Oxford University Press, 1990
2. Michels VV, Hittner HM, Beaudet AL: J Pediatr 93:444-446, 1978

MICROCELLULAR STRIATAL SYNDROME, profound pathological alterations in the caudate and lenticular nuclei, which are severely shrunken in the later stages. The small cells of the caudate nucleus and the putamen are more affected.
1. Grinker RR, Sahs AL: Neurology. 6th ed. Springfield: Charles C Thomas, 1966

MIDBRAIN TEGMENTUM SYNDROME, a syndrome that results from occlusion of branches penetrating the lateral part of the tegmentum at caudal midbrain levels.
1. Haymaker W: Bing's Local Diagnosis in Neurological Diseases. 15th ed. St Louis: CV Mosby, 1969

MIDDLE LOBE SYNDROME, chronic pneumonitis associated with atelectasis of the right middle lobe. Cross-references: Brock syndrome; Right middle lobe syndrome.
1. Brock RC: Guys Hosp Rep 87:295-317, 1937

MIDDLE RADICULAR SYNDROME, injury to the 7th cervical nerve root or the middle primary nerve trunk that causes paralysis of the muscles enervated by the radial nerve, with the exception of the brachioradialis muscle.
1. Rowland LP (ed): Merritt's Textbook of Neurology. 9th ed. Baltimore: Williams & Wilkins, 1995

MIETENS SYNDROME, MIETENS-WEBER SYNDROME, marked growth retardation and mild mental retardation; corneal opacity, narrow nose, and flexion contracture at elbow are features. Etiology undetermined. Questionable autosomal recessive inheritance. (Carl Mietens, German)
1. Gorlin RJ, Cohen MM Jr, Levin LS: Syndromes of the Head and Neck. New York: Oxford University Press, 1990
2. Mietens C, Weber H: A syndrome characterized by corneal opacity, nystagmus, flexion contracture of the elbows, growth failure, and mental retardation. J Pediatr 69:624-629, 1966

MIKULICZ DISEASE, chronic bilateral parotid and lacrimal gland enlargement, usually associated with dryness of the mouth and absence of tears. (Johannes von Mikulicz-Radecki, 1850-1905, Polish surgeon)
1. Lumley JS, Clain A: Hamilton Bailey's Demonstration of Physical Signs in Clinical Surgery. 18th ed. London: Butterworth-Heinemann, 1997
2. Ritchie AC: Boyd's Textbook of Pathology. 9th ed. Philadelphia: Lea & Febiger, 1990

MIKULICZ OPERATION, 1) ablation of the sternocleidomastoid muscle in cases of torticollis; 2) tarsectomy with resection of the calcaneum, astragalus, and cuboid, scaphoid, and articular surfaces of the tibia and fibula. Cross-reference: Vladimiroff-Mikulicz operation. (Johannes von Mikulicz-Radecki)
1. Maffei WE: Os Fundamentos da Medicina. 2nd ed. Livraria Editora Artes Médicas Ltda, 1978

MILIAN SIGN, see Saint Anthony's fire. (Gaston Milian, 1871-1945, French dermatologist)

MILK-ALKALI SYNDROME, prolonged metabolic alkalosis due to alkali loading; occurs because of the prolonged ingestion of calcium and absorbable alkali in the patient with peptic ulcer. In patients with impaired renal function, hypercalcemic nephropathy may progress to renal failure. Cross-references: Burnett syndrome; Hypercalcemic syndrome.
1. Bennett JC, Plum F (eds): Cecil Textbook of Medicine. 20th ed. Philadelphia: WB Saunders, 1996
2. Burnett C, Commons RR, Albright F, et al: N Engl J Med 240:787-794, 1949

MILKMAN SYNDROME, persistent fractures due to osteomalacia; a generalized bone disease marked by multiple transparent stripes of absorption in the long and flat bones. Cross-reference: Looser-Milkman syndrome. (Louis A. Milkman, 1895-1951, U.S. radiologist)
1. Looser E: Zentralbl Chir 47:1470-1474, 1920
2. Milkman LA: Am J Roentgenol 24:29-37, 1930

MILL DISEASE, progressive ascendent hemiplegia.
1. Casas EC: Diccionario Terminologico de Ciencias Medicas. 5th ed. Salvat Editores, SA, 1954

MILLAR DISEASE, laryngeal stridor. (John Millar, 1733-1805, Scottish)
1. Casas EC: Diccionario Terminologico de Ciencias Medicas. 5th ed. Salvat Editores, SA, 1954

MILLARD-GUBLER SYNDROME, crossed paralysis affecting the limbs on one side of the body and the face on the opposite side, together with paralysis of outward movement of the eye; due to infarction of the pons, involving the 6th and 7th cranial nerves and the fibers of the corticospinal tract. Cross-references: Foville syndrome; Gubler syndrome. (Auguste L.J. Millard, 1830-1915, French; Adolphe M. Gubler, 1821-1879, French)
1. Foville ALF: Note sur une paralysie peu connue des certains muscles de l'oeil, et la liasion avec quelques pints de l'anatomie et la physiologie de la protubérance annulaire. Bull Soc Anat (2nd ser) 33:393-414, 1858
2. Grinker RR, Sahs AL: Neurology. 6th ed. Springfield: Charles C Thomas, 1966
3. Gubler AM: De l'hémiplégie alterne envisagée comme sign de lésion de la protubérance annulaire et comme preuve de al décussation des nerfs faciaux. Gaz Hebd Med (Par) 3:749-788, 811, 1856

MILLER FISHER SYNDROME, see One-and-a-half syndrome. (Miller Fisher, U.S. neurologist)

MILLER SYNDROME, malar hypoplasia, micrognathia, cleft lip and/or cleft palate, cup-shaped ears, and limb deficiencies are features. Autosomal recessive inheritance. Cross-references: Genée-Wiedmann syndrome; Wildervanck-Smith syndrome. (Marvin Miller, U.S. pediatrician)
1. Miller M, Fineman R, Smith DW: Postaxial acrofacial dysostosis syndrome. J Pediatr 95:970-975, 1979
2. Smith DW, Jones KL: Recognizable Patterns of Human Malformations: Genetic, Embryologic, and Clinical Aspects. 3rd ed. Philadelphia: WB Saunders, 1982

MILLER-DIEKER SYNDROME, a specific "lissencephaly syndrome" in siblings. Craniofacial anomaly, bitemporal hollowing, a small jaw, and a short nose with upturned nares are due to a deletion in the region of chromosome 17. (James Q. Miller, U.S.)
1. Dieker H, Edwards RH, Zurhein GM, et al: The lissencephaly syndrome. N. F. March of Dimes. New York, 1969, pp 53-64
2. Grinker RR, Sahs AL: Neurology. 6th ed. Springfield: Charles C Thomas, 1966
3. Miller JQ: Lissencephaly in two siblings. Neurology 13:841-850, 1963
4. Volpe J: Neurology of the Newborn. 3rd ed. Philadelphia: WB Saunders, 1995

MILLINGEN OPERATION, surgery for trichiasis using the mucosa of the lip to cover the wound.
1. Maffei WE: Os Fundamentos da Medicina. 2nd ed. Livraria Editora Artes Médicas Ltda, 1978

MILLS MANEUVER, pain is elicited by pronation of the forearm with the elbow straight and the wrist flexed; seen in cases of tennis elbow.
1. Lumley JS, Clain A: Hamilton Bailey's Demonstration of Physical Signs in Clinical Surgery. 18th ed. London: Butterworth-Heinemann, 1997

MILLS-REINCKE PHENOMENON, due to water purification, a corresponding decrease in mortality rate is seen in all diseases. (Hiram F. Mills, 1836-1921, U.S. engineer; John J. Reincke, German)
1. Dorland's Medical Dictionary. 28th ed. Philadelphia: WB Saunders, 1994

MILROY SYNDROME, familial congenital lymphedema; a hereditary defect in the lymphatic vessels that causes severe lymphedema of one or both legs. The age at onset and the severity tend to be similar in a family. Cross-reference: Nonne-Milroy syndrome. (William F. Milroy, 1855-1942, U.S.)

1. Mason PB, Allen EV: Congenital lymphangiectasis (lymphedema). Am J Dis Child 50:945-953, 1935
2. Meige H: Dystrophic oedematose hereditaire. Presse Med 6:341-343, 1898
3. Milroy WF: Undescribed variety of hereditary oedema. NY Med J 56:505-508. 1892

MINAMATA DISEASE, a toxic neurological syndrome caused by the consumption of fish and shell-fish containing methylmercury. Between 1952 and 1958, an epidemic disease affecting all ages, but predominantly children under the age of 10 years, appeared in Minamata City in southern Japan. The disease also affected infants born to apparently healthy mothers. Its chief manifestations were numbness of the limbs and lips, concentric constriction of visual fields, dysarthria, hearing defects, truncal and limb ataxia, intention and resting tremor, and slight mental retardation. The cause was traced to factory effluent discharged into Minamata Bay.

1. Farmer TW: Pediatric Neurology. 2nd ed. Hagerstown: Harper & Row, 1975
2. Kurland LH, et al: World Neurol 1:370-395, 1961
3. Ritchie AC: Boyd's Textbook of Pathology. 9th ed. Philadelphia: Lea & Febiger, 1990

MINGAZZINI-FOERSTER OPERATION, see Foerster operation.

MINKOWSKI-CHAUFFARD SYNDROME, hereditary spherocytosis. (Oskar Minkowski, 1858-1931, Lithuanian; Anatole M.E. Chauffard, 1855-1932, French)

1. Chauffard AM: Sem Med 27:25-29, 1907
2. Minkowski O: Verh Dtsch Kongr Inn Med 18:316-319, 1900

MINOR SIGN, the patient stands from a seated position with one hand supporting the lumbar region and weightbearing on the contralateral leg; seen in the patient with sciatica. (Lazar S. Minor, 1855-1942, Russian neurologist)

1. Casas EC: Diccionario Terminologico de Ciencias Medicas. 5th ed. Salvat Editores, SA, 1954

MINOT DISEASE, a hemorrhagic disease of the newborn with spontaneous healing. (George Minot, 1885-1950, U.S. pathologist)

1. Casas EC: Diccionario Terminologico de Ciencias Medicas. 5th ed. Salvat Editores, SA, 1954

MINOT-VON WILLEBRAND DISEASE, see Von Willebrand disease. (Francis Minot, 1821-1899, U.S.; Erik A. von Willebrand, 1870-1949, Finnish)

MIRANDA SYNDROME, cerebral dysgenesis with renal malformations.

1. Campbell MF, Walsh PC: Campbell's Urology. 5th ed. Philadelphia: WB Saunders, 1986

MIRCHAMP SIGN, a sour substance applied to the mucous membrane of the tongue causes painful secretion; seen in cases of parotiditis.

1. Casas EC: Diccionario Terminologico de Ciencias Medicas. 5th ed. Salvat Editores, SA, 1954

MIRIZZI SYNDROME, results from extrinsic compression of the common hepatic or common bile duct by a large stone passing through the cystic duct. Obstructive jaundice may develop. Calcification of the gallbladder ("porcelain gallbladder") is uncommon but of special significance because of its frequent association with carcinoma of the gallbladder.

1. Bennett JC, Plum F (eds): Cecil Textbook of Medicine. 20th ed. Philadelphia: WB Saunders, 1996
2. Mirizzi PL: G Intern Chir 8:731-777, 1948

MITCHELL DISEASE, erythromelalgia; a vasomotor disorder marked by the sudden onset of irritative lesions and red, glossy, perspiring skin. (Silas Weir Mitchell, 1829-1914, U.S. neurologist)

1. Mitchell SW: Am J Med Sci 76:17-36, 1878

MITRAL CLICK SYNDROME, see Floppy mitral valve syndrome.

MITRAL VALVE PROLAPSE SYNDROME, exists when one or both leaflets of the valve abnormally protrude into the left atrium during systole. Mitral regurgitation, nonspecific abnormality of S-T and T waves on the electrocardiogram, noninjection systolic click, a systolic murmur chest pain, and cardiac arrhythmia may be present. Cross-references: Barlow syndrome; Blue valve syndrome; Click syndrome.

1. Barlow JB: Am Heart J 66:442-452, 1963

MIXTER-BARR OPERATION, prolapse of the intervertebral disc as a source of back pain; first delineated in 1934. Cross-reference: Barr operation. (William J. Mixter, U.S.; Jason S. Barr, U.S.)

MÖBIUS SIGN, the inability to keep the eyeballs converged due to insufficiency of the internus rectus muscles; seen in the patient with Graves disease. (Paul J. Möbius, 1853-1907, German neurologist)

1. Bodechtel G: Diagnostico Diferential de las Enfermedades Neurologicas. Madrid: Pas Montalvo Editorial, 1967

MÖBIUS SYNDROME, an infantile nuclear syndrome. In this condition, a peripheral type of bilateral facial paralysis is usually associated with abduction weakness of the eyes and congenital abnormalities. (Paul J. Möbius)

1. Grinker RR, Sahs AL: Neurology. 6th ed. Springfield: Charles C Thomas, 1966
2. Kumar D: Moebius syndrome. J Med Genet 27:122-126, 1990
3. Möbius PJ: Ueber angeborene doppelseitige Abducens-Facialis-Laehmung. Munch Med Wochenschr 35:91-94, 108-111, 1888

MODELUNG DISEASE, massive diffuse lipoma of the neck with symmetrical lipomas of the shoulders and proximal limbs; often associated with peripheral neuropathy.

1. Chalk CH, Mills KR, Jacobs JM, Familial multiple symmetric lipomatosis with peripheral neuropathy. Neurology 40:1246-1250,1990

MOERSCH-WOLTMANN SYNDROME, see Isaacs syndrome. (Frederick Moersch, U.S.; Henry W. Woltmann, 1889-1964, U.S.)

MOHS OPERATION, chemosurgery for carcinomas of the facial-orbital area. (Frederick Mohs, U.S. surgeon)

1. Spaeth GL: Ophthalmic Surgery. Principles and Practice. Philadelphia: WB Saunders, 1982

MOLLARET SYNDROME, a rare, recurrent viral meningitis characterized by repeated attacks of headache, fever, and nuchal rigidity. Each attack is abrupt in onset and lasts for 2-3 days. (Pierre Mollaret, French neurologist)

1. Bennett JC, Plum F (eds): Cecil Textbook of Medicine. 20th ed. Philadelphia: WB Saunders, 1996
2. Mollaret P: Rev Neurol 76:57-76, 1944

MÖLLER-BARLOW DISEASE, subperiosteal hematoma in rickets caused by vitamin C deficiency in newborns. Cross-reference: Cheadle disease. (Julius O.L. Möller, 1819-1887, German surgeon; Thomas Barlow, 1845-1945, British)

1. Barlow T: Med Chir Trans Lond 66:159-219, 1883
2. Bodechtel G: Diagnostico Diferencial de las Enfermedades Neurologicas. Madrid: Pas Montalvo Editorial, 1967
3. Möller JOL: Konigsberg Med Jb 1:377, 1859

MONAKOW SYNDROME, contralateral hemiplegia, hemianesthesia, and hemianopsia due to occlusion of the anterior choroidal artery. (Constantin von Monakow, 1853-1930, Russian-born neurologist in Switzerland)

1. Casas EC: Diccionario Terminologico de Ciencias Medicas. 5th ed. 1954

MÖNCKEBERG ARTERIOSCLEROSIS, senile aortic stenosis and sclerosis. (Johann Mönckeberg, 1877-1925, German pathologist)

1. Hurst JW, Schlant RC, Alexander RW: The Heart: Arteries and Veins. 8th ed. New York: McGraw-Hill, 1994
2. Mönckeberg J: Virchows Arch Pathol 171:141-167, 1903

MONDAY MORNING DISEASE, byssinosis (from the Greek for flax) or cotton-mill fever. Occurs in cotton workers; a shortness of breath and tightness in the chest appears on Monday mornings, when the workers return to the mill after a weekend free of exposure.

1. Popendorf W, Donham KJ, Easton DN, et al: A synopsis of agricultural respiratory hazards. Am Ind Hyg Assoc J 46:154-161, 1985
2. Ritchie AC: Boyd's Textbook of Pathology. 9th ed. Philadelphia: Lea & Febiger, 1990

MONDINI DISEASE, congenital hereditary hearing loss, due to only a primitive single curved tube representing the cochlea with similar maldevelopment of the vestibular system. (C. Mondini, 1729-1803, Italian)

1. Mondini C: Banoniae 7:419-431, 1791

MONDOR DISEASE, superficial thrombophlebitis of the thoracoepigastric veins; a rare, benign type of thrombophlebitis (the so-called string phlebitis), which may be related to direct mechanical or surgical trauma or to physical muscle strain from work or sports. (Henri Mondor, 1885-1962, French surgeon)

1. Hurst JW, Schlant RC, Alexander RW: The Heart: Arteries and Veins. 8th ed. New York: McGraw-Hill, 1994
2. Mondor H, Bertrand I: Presse Med 59:1533-1535, 1951

MONGE DISEASE, pulmonary hypertension of chronic mountain sickness; reversible with a descent to lower altitudes. (Carlos Monge, 1884-1970, Peruvian pathologist)

1. Braunwald E: Heart Disease: A Textbook of Cardiovascular Medicine. 4th ed. Philadelphia: WB Saunders, 1992

2. Fowler No: Cardiac Diagnosis and Treatment. 3rd ed. Cambridge: Harper & Row, 1980
3. Monge C: Arch Intern Med 59:32-40, 1937

MONIZ OPERATION, see Egas Moniz operation.

MONKEY DISEASE, in some cases the entire body is covered with hair that in conjunction with blackening of the skin and atrophic hands produces a monkey-like appearance.
1. Farmer TW: Pediatric Neurology. 2nd ed. Hagerstown: Harper & Row, 1975

MONOSOMY 21 SYNDROME, characteristics of the infant usually are hypertonicity, a small size and failure to thrive (death is usually within the first year of life), head circumference is markedly reduced (between the 3rd and 10th percentiles), the occiput is prominent.
1. Carpenter NJ, et al: Partial deletion 21: case report with biochemical studies and review. J Med Genet 24:706-708, 1987
2. Gorlin RJ, Cohen MM Jr, Levin LS: Syndromes of the Head and Neck. New York: Oxford University Press, 1990

MONTEVERDE SIGN, subcutaneous injection of an ammonia solution fails to produce a response; an indication of death.
1. Casas EC: Diccionario Terminologico de Ciencias Medicas. 5th ed. Salvat Editores, SA, 1954

MOON TURRETED MOLARS, dome-shaped first molars seen in congenital syphilis. (Henry Moon, 1845-1892, British dental surgeon)
1. Lumley JS, Clain A: Hamilton Bailey's Demonstration of Physical Signs in Clinical Surgery. 18th ed. London: Butterworth-Heinemann, 1997

MOORE OPERATION, introduction of a coil into an aneurysmal sac in order to coagulate the aneurysm.
1. Maffei WE: Os Fundamentos da Medicina. 2nd ed. Livraria Editora Artes Médicas Ltda, 1978

MOORE SYNDROME, paroxysmal abdominal pain epilepsy. There may be cardiorespiratory genito-urinary involvement. (Matthew T. Moore, U.S. neurologist)
1. Moore MT: Paroxysmal abdominal pain: a form of focal symptomatic epilepsy. JAMA 124:561-563, 1944

MOORE-CORRADI OPERATION, treatment of aneurysms using galvanic current. Cross-reference: Corradi operation.
1. Maffei WE: Os Fundamentos da Medicina. 2nd ed. Livraria Editora Artes Médicas Ltda, 1978

MOORE-FEDERMAN SYNDROME, a dominantly inherited form of dwarfism with ocular and perhaps cardiac abnormalities. The proband has retinal detachment, glaucoma, and hyperopia; the skin of the forearms is taut and "bound down." Asthmatic bronchitis is frequent in affected persons. (W.T. Moore, U.S.)
1. McKusick VA: Heritable Disorders of Connective Tissue. 4th ed. St Louis: CV Mosby, 1972
2. Moore WT, Federman DD: Familial dwarfism and "stiff joints." Report of a kindred. Arch Intern Med 115:398-404, 1965

MOOSA FEVER, see Trench fever.

MORAN OPERATION, an otologist in 1768 reported an infection of the mastoid process that had spread to the dura. He entered the cranial cavity and drained the abscess. Antibiotics were not available yet and he used water and turpentine to rinse the abscess cavity.

MORAND DISEASE, paresis of the distal part of a limb.
1. Casas EC: Diccionario Terminologico de Ciencias Medicas. 5th ed. Salvat Editores, SA, 1954

MORDEN SYNDROME, scleroderma.
1. Casas EC: Diccionario Terminologico de Ciencias Medicas. 5th ed. 1954

MOREAU OPERATION, 1) resection of the elbow using a posterior H-shaped incision; 2) resection of the patella using an anterior H-shaped incision.
1. Maffei WE: Os Fundamentos da Medicina. 2nd ed. Livraria Editora Artes Médicas Ltda, 1978

MOREL SYNDROME, a combination of internal frontal hyperostosis, obesity, and virilism. Glucos-uria and polyuria may also occur. Cross-references: Morgagni syndrome; Stewart-Morel syndrome. (Bénédikt A. Morel, 1809-1873, French psychiatrist)
1. Bodechtel G: Diagnostico Diferential de las Enfermedades Neurologicas. Madrid: Pas Montalvo Editorial, 1967
2. Morgagni GB: De Sedibus et Causis Morborum. Venezia: Typographia Romondiniani, 1761

MOREL-KRAEPELIN DISEASE, dementia praecox or schizophrenia. Cross-reference: Kraepelin-Morel disease. (Bénédikt A. Morel; Emil Kraepelin, 1856-1926, German psychiatrist)
1. Casas EC: Diccionario Terminologico de Ciencias Medicas. 5th ed. Salvat Editores, SA, 1954

MOREL-LAVALLÉE DISEASE, see Perrin-Ferraton disease.

MORESTIN OPERATION, disarticulation of the patella through a condylotomy of the femur.
1. Maffei WE: Os Fundamentos da Medicina. 2nd ed. Livraria Editora Artes Médicas Ltda, 1978

MORGAGNI DISEASE, MORGAGNI-ADAMS-STOKES SYNDROME, see Adams-Stokes syndrome. (Giovanni B. Morgagni, 1682-1771, Italian anatomist and pathologist)

MORGAGNI SYNDROME, MORGAGNI-MOREL SYNDROME, MORGAGNI-STEWART SYNDROME, see Morel syndrome. (Giovanni B. Morgagni)

MORGAGNI-TURNER-ALBRIGHT SYNDROME, see Turner syndrome. (Giovanni B. Morgagni)

MORGAN LINE, a crease in the lower eyelids; seen in atropic dermatitis. Cross-reference: Dennie sign.
1. Dorland's Medical Dictionary. 28th ed. Philadelphia: WB Saunders, 1994

MORISCHI OPERATION, circumcision of the leg for the treatment of varices.
1. Maffei WE: Os Fundamentos da Medicina. 2nd ed. Livraria Editora Artes Médicas Ltda, 1978

MORLAN REFLEX, very similar to the Babinski reflex but is elicited by scratching the triangular area at the base of the big toe near the ball of the foot. Described by Edgar Morales at the June 1994 International Pediatric Surgery Meeting in Lima, Peru.
1. Casas EC: Diccionario Terminologico de Ciencias Medicas. 5th ed. Salvat Editores, SA, 1954

MORNING GLORY SYNDROME, a type of optic disc dysplasia consisting of a unilaterally enlarged, funnel-shaped, excavated, and distorted optic disc surrounded by an elevated annulus of chorioretinal pigment.
1. Itakura T, Miyamoto K, Uematsu Y, et al: Bilateral morning glory syndrome associated with sphenoid encephalocele. Case report. J Neurosurg 77:949-951, 1992
2. Kindlier P: Morning glory syndrome: unusual congenital optic disk anomaly. Am J Ophthalmol 69:376-384, 1970
3. Manshot WA: Morning glory syndrome: a histopathologic study. Br J Ophthalmol 74:560-580, 1990

MORQUIO SIGN, when lying flat, the patient cannot rise to a sitting position unless the knees are bent; seen in cases of epidemic poliomyelitis. (Luis Morquio, 1867-1935, Uruguayan pediatrician)
1. Casas EC: Diccionario Terminologico de Ciencias Medicas. 5th ed. Salvat Editores, SA, 1954

MORQUIO SYNDROME, MORQUIO-BRAILSFORD SYNDROME, mucopolysaccharidosis type IVA; the predominant clinical features relate to skeletal abnormalities and to symptoms of spinal cord compression resulting from instability of the neck. Intelligence capability is normal. Dwarfism, knock-knees, coarse broad mouth, spaced teeth, and very loose unstable joints are features. Cross-references: Brailsford-Morquio syndrome; Morquio-Ullrich syndrome. (Luis Morquio; James F. Brailsford, 1888-1961, British radiologist)
1. Brailsford JF: Am J Surg 7:404-410, 1929
2. Farmer TW: Pediatric Neurology. 2nd ed. Hagerstown: Harper & Row, 1975
3. Morquio L: Sur une forme de dystrophie osseuse familiale. Bull Soc Pediatr (Par) 27:145-152, 1929
4. Vannotti A: Clinique et Physiopathologie Médicales. Introduction a la Médecine Clinique. Libraire Maloine, SA, 1973

MORQUIO-BARRAQUER-SIMONS DISEASE, see Barraquer disease. (Luis Morquio)

MORQUIO-LIKE SYNDROME, mucopolysaccharidosis type IVB; a form of mucopolysaccharidosis with ß-galactosidase deficiency. Short stature, mild pectus carinatum, corneal clouding, odontoid hypoplasia with cervical instability, mild dysostosis multiplex, moderate lumbar kyphosis, and mild genu valgum have been found. (Luis Morquio)
1. Bennett JC, Plum F (eds): Cecil Textbook of Medicine. 20th ed. Philadelphia: WB Saunders, 1996

MORQUIO-ULLRICH SYNDROME, see Morquio syndrome. (Luis Morquio; Otto Ullrich, 1894-1959, German)

MORRIS SIGN, pressure on the Morris point in the abdomen is painful; seen in the patient with appendicitis.
1. Casas EC: Diccionario Terminologico de Ciencias Medicas. 5th ed. Salvat Editores, SA, 1954

MORT D'AMOUR SYNDROME, sudden death during sexual intercourse ("death by love").
1. Heggveit HA: La mort d'amour. Am Heart J 69:287-294, 1965

MORTIMER DISEASE, lupus vulgaris without ulceration. (Named for Hutchinson's patient, Mrs. Mortimer.)
1. Hutchinson J: Arch Surg Lond 9:307-314, 1898

MORTOLA SIGN, the intensity of pain provoked by pinching a relaxed abdominal wall indicates the degree of intra-abdominal inflammation.

1. Casas EC: Diccionario Terminologico de Ciencias Medicas. 5th ed. Salvat Editores, SA, 1954

MORTON SYNDROME, a malformation of the first metatarsal segment of the foot; characterized by metatarsalgia due to shortening or relaxation of the segment. Cross-reference: Short first metatarsal syndrome. (Dudley J. Morton, 1884-1960, U.S. orthopedic surgeon)

1. Morton DJ: J Bone Joint Surg 9:531-544, 1927

MORTON TOE, a disease of the foot most often found in overweight women; the tibial nerve is relatively secure from trauma, but when injured, a causalgia may develop. Pain is sometimes bilateral and occurs beneath the heads of the third and fourth metatarsals, extending to the third and fourth toes and at times up the posterior aspect of the leg, thigh, and hip, associated with cramping of the muscles and paresthesias of the affected toes. (Thomas G. Morton, 1835-1903, U.S. surgeon)

1. Baker AB, Baker LH: Clinical Neurology. Revised ed. Philadelphia: Harper & Row, 1982
2. Morton TG: Am J Med Sci 71:37-45, 1876

MORVAN CHOREA, myoclonus involving muscles of the calves, posterior parts of the thighs, and sometimes the trunk. Cross-reference: Fibrillaris syndrome. (Augustin M. Morvan, 1819-1897, French)

1. Morvan AM: Gaz Hebd Med 27:173-176, 1890

MORVAN DISEASE, analgesic paralysis; manifestation of syringomyelia marked by thickening of the subcutaneous tissues of the hands, which become edematous, soft, swollen, cyanotic, and cold (main succulent or Marinesco succulent hand); associated with analgesic ulceration of the tips of the fingers and paresthesias and atrophy of the hands and forearms. (Augustin M. Morvan)

1. Baker AB, Baker LH: Clinical Neurology. Revised ed. Philadelphia: Harper & Row, 1982
2. Morvan AM: De la paresie analgesique a panaris des extremities superieures ou pareso-analgesie des extremities superieures. Gaz Hebd Med 20:580-583, 590-594, 624-626, 1883

MOSCHCOWITZ [MOSKOWICZ] SIGN, the restoration of color compared to the other side after short compression of a limb; a sign of vascular gangrene. (Eli Moschcowitz [Moskowicz], 1879-1964, U.S.)

1. Casas EC: Diccionario Terminologico de Ciencias Medicas. 5th ed. Salvat Editores, SA, 1954

MOSCHCOWITZ [MOSKOWICZ] SYNDROME, thrombotic thrombocytopenic purpura; an acute, diffuse disorder of the microcirculation characterized by thrombocytopenic purpura, microangiopathic hemolytic anemia, transient and fluctuating neurological signs, renal dysfunction, and a febrile course. Cross-reference: Baehr-Schiffrin syndrome. (Eli Moschcowitz [Moskowicz])

1. Bennett JC, Plum F (eds): Cecil Textbook of Medicine. 20th ed. Philadelphia: WB Saunders, 1996
2. Moschcowitz E: Arch Intern Med 36:89-93, 1925

MOSLER SIGN, sternal tenderness in acute myeloblastic leukemia. (Karl F. Mosler, 1831-1911, German)

1. Dorland's Medical Dictionary. 28th ed. Philadelphia: WB Saunders, 1994

MOSSE SYNDROME, cirrhosis of the liver accompanied by polycythemia vera. (Max Mosse, German)

1. Mosse M: Dtsch Med Wochenschr 33:2175-2176, 1907

MOSSMAN DISEASE, endemic disease among sugar cane plantation workers in Mossman (Queensland, Australia); characterized by edema of the axillary and inguinal lymph nodes.

1. Casas EC: Diccionario Terminologico de Ciencias Medicas. 5th ed. Salvat Editores, SA, 1954

MOULAGE SIGN, a waxy-cast appearance of the bowel segments; seen in the patient with celiac disease. ("Moulage" is French for molding.)

1. Dorland's Medical Dictionary. 28th ed. Philadelphia: WB Saunders, 1994

MOUNIER-KUHN SYNDROME, tracheobronchomegaly; emphysema and spontaneous pneumothorax are features. In rare instances, hemoptysis is a complication. (Pierre Mounier-Kuhn, French)

1. McKusick VA: Heritable Disorders of Connective Tissue. 4th ed. St Louis: CV Mosby, 1972
2. Mounier-Kuhn P: Ann Otolaryngol 12:387-404, 1945
3. Mounier-Kuhn P: Lyon Med 150:106-109, 1932

MOUNT FUJI SIGN, is seen in subdural tension pneumocephalus. On CT scan the subdural air separates and compresses the frontal lobes, creating a widened interhemispheric space between the

tips of the frontal lobes that mimics the silhouette of Mt. Fuji.
1. Ishiwata Y, Fujitsu K, Sekino T, et al: J Neurosurg 68:58-61, 1988
2. Pop M, Thompson JR, Zinke DR, et al: Tension pneumocephalus. J Comput Assist Tomogr 6:894-901, 1982

MOUTARD-MARTIN SIGN, pain of the affected limb when the opposite limb is flexed firmly in sciatica.
1. Casas EC: Diccionario Terminologico de Ciencias Medicas. 5th ed. Salvat Editores, SA, 1954

MOVIE SIGN, a dull aching discomfort, well localized to the anterior part of the knee, and most prominent after sitting in one position for a long time; seen in cases of chondromalacia.
1. Campbell WC, Crenshaw AH: Campbell's Operative Orthopaedics. 7th ed. St Louis: CV Mosby, 1987

MOYAMOYA DISEASE, a cerebrovascular disorder of basal occlusion with telangiectasia. The occlusive lesion involves the arteries at the base of the brain, but there is also marked telangiectasia in the region of the basal ganglia. More common in girls and usually progressive and bilateral. (First reported in Japanese children; the radiographic presentation was described by the Japanese expression "moyamoya" or something hazy.")
1. Farmer TW: Pediatric Neurology. 2nd ed. Hagerstown: Harper & Row, 1975

MOYNAHAN SYNDROME, consists of multiple symmetrical lentigines, congenital mitral stenosis, dwarfism, genital hypoplasia, and mental deficiency. (E.J. Moynahan, British)
1. Moschella SL, Hurley HJ: Dermatology. 2nd ed. Philadelphia: WB Saunders, 1985
2. Moynahan EJ: Proc R Soc Med 55:959-960, 1962

MOZER DISEASE, myosclerosis in adults.
1. Casas EC: Diccionario Terminologico de Ciencias Medicas. 5th ed. Salvat Editores, SA, 1954

MU (m) CHAIN DISEASE, secretion of free m heavy chains into the plasma; a rare occurrence in chronic lymphocytic leukemia.
1. Bennett JC, Plum F (eds): Cecil Textbook of Medicine. 20th ed. Philadelphia: WB Saunders, 1996

MUCHA-HABERMANN DISEASE, an acute polymorphous eruption of the skin that heals with superficial scarring and pigmentation. The cause is unknown and there is no associated underlying disease. (Viktor Mucha, 1887-1919, Austrian dermatologist; Rudolf H. Habermann, 1884-1941, German dermatologist)
1. Habermann R: Derm Zschr 45:2-8, 1925
2. Moschella SL, Hurley HJ: Dermatology. 2nd ed. Philadelphia: WB Saunders, 1985
3. Mucha V: Arch Derm Syph 123:586-592, 1916

MUCKLE-WELLS SYNDROME, characterized by amyloidosis involving the kidneys and causing nephritis, recurrent urticaria, deafness, and pain in the extremities. Premature loss of libido with relative infertility. Autosomal dominant inheritance. (Thomas J. Muckle, Canadian pediatrician; Michael V. Wells, British)
1. Muckle TJ, Wells M: Urticaria, deafness and amyloidosis: a new heterofamilial syndrome. Q J Med 31:235-248, 1962

MUCOCUTANEOUS LYMPH NODE SYNDROME, see Kawasaki disease.

MUCOEPITHELIAL DYSPLASIA SYNDROME, multiple abnormalities involving the skin and various mucous membranes, eyes, and lungs. Cross-reference: Witkop syndrome.
1. Gorlin RJ, Cohen MM Jr, Levin LS: Syndromes of the Head and Neck. New York: Oxford University Press, 1990
2. Witkop CJ Jr: Am J Genet 31:414-427, 1979

MUCOSAL NEUROMAS SYNDROME, multiple endocrine neoplasia (MEN) type III; differs from MEN type II in four respects: 1) the medullary carcinoma of the thyroid and the pheochromocytomas may be accompanied by striking and disfiguring neuromas of the lips, buccal mucosa, and tongue as well as by ganglioneuroma of the gastrointestinal tract, thickened corneal nerves visible upon slit-lamp examination, and café-au-lait spots, neuromas, or neurofibromas of the skin; 2) the body habitus may resemble that seen in the patient with Marfan syndrome; 3) parathyroid hyperplasia is rare, if it occurs at all; 4) mean survival time is considerably shorter than that in MEN type II (30 vs. 60 years).
1. Bennett JC, Plum F (eds): Cecil Textbook of Medicine. 20th ed. Philadelphia: WB Saunders, 1996

MUELLER-KANNBERG SYNDROME, see Marcus Gunn phenomenon.

MUIR-TORRE SYNDROME, a rare disorder resulting in multiple adenocarcinomas and epidermoid carcinomas in multiple organs, in association with a large number of sebaceous cysts. Cross-reference: Torre syndrome. (E.G. Muir, British; Douglas P. Torre, U.S. dermatologist)

1. Gorlin RJ, Cohen MM Jr, Levin LS: Syndromes of the Head and Neck. 3rd ed. New York: Oxford University Press, 1990
2. Householder MS, Zeligman I: Sebaceous neoplasms associated with visceral carcinomas. Arch Dermatol 116:61-64, 1980
3. Muir EG, Bell AY, Barlow KA: Br J Surg 54:191-195, 1967
4. Torre D: Arch Dermatol 98:549-551, 1968

MULIBREY-NANISM SYNDROME, *mu*scle-*li*ver-*br*ain-*ey*e (MULIBREY)-nanism; small stature, pericardial constriction, and yellow dots in the fundus are features. Autosomal recessive inheritance. Cross-reference: Perheentupa syndrome.

1. Perheentupa J, Antio S, Leisti S, et al: Mulibrey-Nanism dwarfism with muscles, liver, brain and eye involvement. Acta Paediatr Scand 59 (Suppl 206):74, 1970
2. Smith DW, Jones KL: Recognizable Patterns of Human Malformations: Genetic, Embryologic, and Clinical Aspects. 3rd ed. Philadelphia: WB Saunders, 1982

MÜLLER OPERATION, 1) method of hysterectomy by division of the uterus into two lateral halves; 2) method of cesarean section in which the uterus is opened only after being extracted from the abdomen. Cross-reference: Sanger operation.

1. Maffei WE: Os Fundamentos da Medicina. 2nd ed. Livraria Editora Artes Médicas Ltda, 1978

MÜLLER SIGN, aortic insufficiency that consists of pulsation of the uvula and redness of the tonsils and velum palati; occurs synchronously with action of the heart. (Friedrich von Müller, 1858-1941, German)

1. Hurst JW, Schlant RC, Alexander RW: The Heart: Arteries and Veins. 8th ed. New York: McGraw-Hill, 1994

MÜLLERIAN DISEASE, the müllerian ducts normally give rise to the fallopian tubes, the uterus, the cervix, and the upper vagina in genetic females. For unknown reasons, one or more of the derivatives may not develop and this failure may go unrecognized until puberty. The anomalies vary in severity, from an imperforate hymen to complete aplasia of all müllerian duct derivatives with vaginal atresia. (Johannes P. Müller, 1801-1858, German physiologist)

1. Bennett JC, Plum F (eds): Cecil Textbook of Medicine. 20th ed. Philadelphia: WB Saunders, 1996

MÜLLERIAN DUCT SYNDROME, defects in synthesis, secretion, or response to müllerian-inhibiting substances. More than 80 men and boys have been described with relatively normal testicular morphology and male external genitalia who possess well-developed müllerian structures in addition to male ducts. (Johannes P. Müller)

1. Bennett JC, Plum F (eds): Cecil Textbook of Medicine. 20th ed. Philadelphia: WB Saunders, 1996
2. Wilson JD, Foster DW, Kronenberg HM, et al (eds): Williams Textbook of Endocrinology. 9th ed. Philadelphia: WB Saunders, 1998

MULTIPLE EPIPHYSEAL DYSPLASIA SYNDROME, hereditary epiphyseal dysplasia; small, irregular epiphyses, pain and stiffness in the hips, and short stature are features. Autosomal dominant inheritance.

1. Hoefnagel D, Sycamore LK, Russell SW, et al: Hereditary multiple epiphyseal dysplasia. Ann Hum Genet 30:201, 1967

MULTIPLE EXOSTOSES SYNDROME, multiple cartilaginous exostoses; diaphyseal outgrowths lead to limb deformity, with or without short metacarpal bones. Autosomal dominant inheritance, with a 60% chance of being familial.

1. Smith DW, Jones KL: Recognizable Patterns of Human Malformations: Genetic, Embryologic, and Clinical Aspects. 3rd ed. Philadelphia: WB Saunders, 1982
2. Solomon L: Hereditary multiple exostosis. Am J Hum Genet 16:351-363, 1964

MULTIPLE GLANDULAR DEFICIENCY SYNDROME, multiple endocrine deficiency; primary failure of any combination of the endocrine glands, including the adrenal, thyroid, and parathyroid glands and the endocrine pancreas, as well as the gonads. Often accompanied by nonendocrine autoimmune abnormalities.

1. Dorland's Medical Dictionary. 28th ed. Philadelphia: WB Saunders, 1994

MULTIPLE HAMARTOMA SYNDROME, see Cowden disease.

MULTIPLE LENTIGINES SYNDROME, see LEOPARD syndrome.

MULTIPLE NEUROMA SYNDROME, multiple neuromas of the tongue and lips, medullary thyroid carcinoma, and pheochromocytoma. Autosomal dominant inheritance.

1. Smith DW, Jones KL: Recognizable Patterns of Human Malformations: Genetic, Embryologic, and Clinical Aspects.

3rd ed. Philadelphia: WB Saunders, 1982

MULTIPLE ODONTOMA-ESOPHAGEAL STENOSIS SYNDROME, huge tumors of the maxilla and mandible.
1. Gorlin RJ, Cohen MM Jr, Levin LS: Syndromes of the Head and Neck. New York: Oxford University Press, 1990
2. Herrmann M: Über von Zahnsystem ausgehende Tumoren bei Kindem. Fortschr Kiefer Gesichtschir 4:226-229, 1958

MULTIPLE SYNOSTOSES SYNDROME, see Acrocephalo-synankie syndrome.

MUNCHAUSEN SYNDROME, seen in malingerers, some of whom are self-mutilating patients or remarkably pathological liars, who travel from hospital to hospital gaining admission by means of dramatic pretensions of illness. (Baron Karl F.H. von Munchausen, 1720-1797, German)
1. Asher R: Munchausen syndrome. Lancet 1:339-341, 1951
2. Bennett JC, Plum F (eds): Cecil Textbook of Medicine. 20th ed. Philadelphia: WB Saunders, 1996

MÜNCHMEYER DISEASE, myositis ossificans progressiva; a connective tissue disorder in which there is progressive ossification adjacent to striated muscle. (Ernst Münchmeyer, 1846-1880, German)
1. McKusick VA: Heritable Disorders of Connective Tissue. 4th ed. St Louis: CV Mosby, 1972
2. Münchmeyer E: Zschr Ration Med 34:1, 1869

MUNK DISEASE, lipoid nephrosis. (Fritz Munk, German)
1. Munk F: Zschr Klin Med 78:1-52, 1913

MUNSON SIGN, unusual bulging of the lower eyelid when the eye is rolled downward; due to abnormal curvature of the cornea. (Edward S. Munson, U.S. ophthalmologist)
1. Dorland's Medical Dictionary. 28th ed. Philadelphia: WB Saunders, 1994

MURAT SIGN, if the patient speaks loudly, a vibration is felt on the affected side of the chest; seen in the patient with tuberculosis. (Louis Murat, French)
1. Casas EC: Diccionario Terminologico de Ciencias Medicas. 5th ed. Salvat Editores, SA, 1954

MURCHISON-PEL-EBSTEIN DISEASE, see Pel-Ebstein disease. (Charles M. Murchison, 1830-1879, British; Pieter Pel, 1852-1919, Dutch; Wilhelm Ebstein, 1836-1912, German)

MURPHY "KIDNEY PUNCH" SIGN, MURPHY SIGN, the patient sits up with folded arms. The examiner's thumb is then placed under the 12th rib, and short, jabbing movements are made. At first the movements are very gentle, but their force is increased if pain is not experienced. This sign is of great value in determining deep-seated tenderness; an indication of gallbladder disease. Cross-reference: Maynihan method. (John B. Murphy, 1857-1916, U.S. surgeon)
1. Lumley JS, Clain A: Hamilton Bailey's Demonstration of Physical Signs in Clinical Surgery. 18th ed. London: Butterworth-Heinemann, 1997

MURRAY VALLEY ENCEPHALITIS, similar to Japanese B encephalitis in pathogenesis and clinical features; caused by closely related flaviviruses. (Occurred in small epidemics in the Murray and Darling River Valleys of Victoria and New South Wales, Australia.) Cross-reference: Rocio encephalitis.
1. Bennett JC, Plum F (eds): Cecil Textbook of Medicine. 20th ed. Philadelphia: WB Saunders, 1996

MURRAY-PURETIC-DRESCHER SYNDROME, gingival fibromatosis with juvenile hyaline fibromatosis. (John Murray, British)
1. Drescher E, et al: J Pediatr Surg 2:427-436, 1967
2. Murray J: On three peculiar cases of molluscum fibrosum in children. Med Chir Trans Lond 56:235-238, 1873
3. Puretic S, et al: Br J Dermatol 74:8-19, 1962

MUSCLE PHENOMENON, the tendency of striated muscle to contract in hard lumps upon percussion.
1. Dorland's Medical Dictionary. 28th ed. Philadelphia: WB Saunders, 1994

MUSSET SIGN, rhythmic head motion synchronized with the heartbeat; seen in aortic insufficiency or aneurysm. Cross-reference: De Musset sign. (Alfred De Musset, 1810-1857, French poet)
1. Casas EC: Diccionario Terminologico de Ciencias Medicas. 5th ed. Salvat Editores, SA, 1954

MUSTARDÉ OPERATION, an effective method of eradicating epicanthic folds by breaking up the tight vertical line in the fold.
1. Spaeth GL: Ophthalmic Surgery. Principles and Practice. Philadelphia: WB Saunders 1982

MYASTHENIA GRAVIS SYNDROME, a defect in acetylcholine resynthesis and packaging due to the presence of antibodies to acetylcholine receptors at the neuromuscular junction. Occurs at all ages but affects females twice as often as males. The peak incidence for females is in the third decade. The onset is usually subacute or insidious; 90% of patients develop weakness of the ocular muscles. Cross-reference: Erb disease.

1. Greer M, Schotland M: Myasthenia gravis in the newborn. Pediatrics 26:101-108, 1960
2. Kase NG, Weingold AB: Principles and Practice of Clinical Gynecology. New York: John Wiley & Sons, 1983

MYASTHENIC SYNDROME, see Lambert syndrome.

MYELODYSPLASTIC SYNDROME, a preneoplastic disorder in which an abnormal clone of hematopoietic cells causes changes in the bone marrow and the blood that progress to leukemia. Most patients are over 50 years old and have refractory anemia. Cross-reference: Preleukemic syndrome.

1. Antin JH, Rosenthal DS: Acute leukemias, myelodysplasia and lymphomas. Clin Geriatr Med 1:795-826, 1985
2. Ritchie AC: Boyd's Textbook of Pathology. 9th ed. Philadelphia: Lea & Febiger, 1990

MYELOFIBROSIS-OSTEOSCLEROSIS SYNDROME, MYELOPROLIFERATIVE SYNDROME, a variation of myeloproliferative disease characterized by fibrosis of the bone marrow, splenomegaly, extramedullary hematopoiesis, and leukoerythroblastosis.

1. Dorland's Medical Dictionary. 28th ed. Philadelphia: WB Saunders, 1994

MYER SIGN, paresthesias and numbness of the hand in a patient with scarlet fever.

1. Casas EC: Diccionario Terminologico de Ciencias Medicas. 5th ed. Salvat Editores, SA, 1954

MYERSON SIGN, a persistent response in the patient with extrapyramidal disease. Best tested by using the thumb and index finger to pull back a fold of skin on the temple lateral to the external canthus and then applying a brisk tap to the thumb. (Abraham Myerson, 1881-1948, U.S. neurologist)

1. Baker AB, Baker LH: Clinical Neurology. Revised ed. Philadelphia: Harper & Row, 1982

MYOFASCIAL PAIN SYNDROME, fibrositis-fibromyalgia; prolonged tonic contraction of skeletal muscles which has an underlying pathogenesis of psychological tension, resentment, and anxiety, and may produce pain in which the cause is not immediately apparent to the patient.

1. Bennett JC, Plum F (eds): Cecil Textbook of Medicine. 20th ed. Philadelphia: WB Saunders, 1996

NAEGELE DISEASE, fever associated with urticaria; found in South Africa.

1. Casas EC: Diccionario Terminologico de Ciencias Medicas. 5th ed. Salvat Editores, SA, 1954

NAEGELI SYNDROME, see Franceschetti-Jadassohn syndrome. (Oskar Naegeli, 1885-1959, Swiss dermatologist)

NAFFZIGER AND VIETS TEST, a measurement of increased intracranial or intraspinal pressure by digital compression of the jugular veins. Pressure should be maintained until the patient complains of a feeling of fullness in the head and the test should not be considered negative until venous return has been impeded for at least 2 minutes. Jugular compression is carried out with a sphygmomanometer cuff, maintaining a pressure of 40 mm mercury for 10 minutes. (Howard C. Naffziger, 1884-1961, U.S. neurosurgeon)

1. Baker AB, Baker LH: Clinical Neurology. Revised ed. Philadelphia: Harper & Row, 1982
2. Pedro-Pons A: Patologia-y-Clinica Medicas. 5th ed. Salvat Editores, SA, 1952

NAFFZIGER SYNDROME, see Scalenus anticus syndrome. (Howard C. Naffziger)

NAGER SYNDROME, NAGER-de REYNIER SYNDROME, radial limb hypoplasia, malar hypoplasia, and ear defects are features. Etiology unknown. (Félix R. Nager, 1877-1959, Swiss otorhinolaryngologist)

1. Nager FR, de Reynier JP: Das Gehörorgan bei den angeborenen Kopfmissbildung. Pract Otorhinolaryngol 10 (Suppl 2):1-128, 1948
2. Smith DW, Jones KL: Recognizable Patterns of Human Malformations: Genetic, Embryologic, and Clinical Aspects. 3rd ed. Philadelphia: WB Saunders, 1982

NAIL-PATELLA SYNDROME, onycho-osteodysplasia; a disorder of mesenchymal tissue characterized by atrophic or absent fingernails, hypoplasia or aplasia of the patella, accessory conical iliac horns, thickening of the scapula, and subluxation of the radial heads at the elbow. In 40% of patients, the kidneys may be involved. Autosomal dominant trait.

1. McKusick VA: Heritable Disorders of Connective Tissue. 4th ed. St Louis: CV Mosby, 1972
2. Trauner R, Rieger H: Arch Klin Chir 137:659-666, 1925

NAME SYNDROME, *n*evi, *a*trial myxoma, *m*yxoid neurofibromatosis, and *e*phelides (NAME); see LAMB syndrome.

NANCE-HORAN SYNDROME, a congenital syndrome characterized by cataracts and dental abnormalities. (Walter E. Nance, U.S.; M.B. Horan, Australian)
1. Gorlin RJ, Cohen MM Jr, Levin LS: Syndromes of the Head and Neck. New York: Oxford University Press, 1990
2. Horan MB, Billson FH: Austral Paediatr J 10:98-102, 1974
3. Nance WE, Warburg M, Bixler D: Birth Defects 10:285-291, 1974

NARATH OPERATION, fixation of the epiploon to the subcutaneous tissue of the abdominal wall to provide collateral circulation in cases of portal vein obstruction.
1. Maffei WE: Os Fundamentos da Medicina. 2nd ed. Livraria Editora Artes Médicas Ltda, 1978

NARCOLEPSY-CATALEPSY SYNDROME, a distinct clinical syndrome of unknown cause that has well-defined symptoms, age of onset, and natural history. The two major symptoms are recurrent episodes of excessive and uncontrollable daytime somnolence and sleep during the normal waking part of the day, and cataplexy, which is characterized by brief, sudden episodes of muscle weakness without loss of consciousness.
1. Rowland LP (ed): Merritt's Textbook of Neurology. 9th ed. Baltimore: Williams & Wilkins, 1995

NARSAROFF PHENOMENON, the difference in rectal temperature before and after a cold bath gradually decreases as cold baths are repeated.
1. Dorland's Medical Dictionary. 28th ed. Philadelphia: WB Saunders, 1994

NASOPALPEBRAL LIPOMA-COLOBOMA SYNDROME, see Penchaszadeh syndrome.

NASSILOV OPERATION, provides access to the thoracic portion of the esophagus through the mediastinum via resection of several ribs.
1. Maffei WE: Os Fundamentos da Medicina. 2nd ed. Livraria Editora Artes Médicas Ltda, 1978

NAUMOFF SYNDROME, short rib-polydactyly syndrome type III; a syndrome of short rib-poly-dactylous dwarfism with less severe changes in the ilia and long bones. (Peter Naumoff, U.S.)
1. Naumoff P: Radiology 122:443-447, 1977

NAUNYN SIGN, pressure under the ribs producing pain; seen in cholecystitis.
1. Dorland's Medical Dictionary. 28th ed. Philadelphia: WB Saunders, 1994

NAVICULOCAPITATE FRACTURE SYNDROME, fracture of the scaphoid bone, with axial compression of the dorsiflexed wrist forcing further dorsiflexion; after the scaphoid fracture, the dorsal lip of the radius forcefully impacts the head of the capitate, causing it to fracture.
1. Campbell WC, Crenshaw AH: Campbell's Operative Orthopedics. 7th ed. St Louis: CV Mosby, 1987
2. Rowland LP (ed): Merritt's Textbook of Neurology. 9th ed. Baltimore: Williams & Wilkins, 1995

NEAPOLITAN FEVER, see Bang disease.

NECK-TONGUE SYNDROME, consists of pain in the neck and altered sensation in the ipsilateral half of the tongue, aggravated by neck movement. Has been attributed to damage to lingual afferent fibers traveling from the hypoglossal nerve to the C2 spinal roots.
1. Lance JW, Anthony M: J Neurol Neurosurg Psychiatry 43:97-101, 1980

NEFTEL DISEASE, the patient is unable to move, including sitting or walking, without pain in the shoulders and head, but pain is relieved when the patient lies down.
1. Casas EC: Diccionario Terminologico de Ciencias Medicas. 5th ed. Salvat Editores, SA, 1954

NEGRO PHENOMENON, the patient is asked to look up. The eyeball on the paralyzed side deviates outward and goes higher owing to overreaction of the superior rectus and inferior oblique muscles; a sign of cogwheel rigidity. Cross-reference: Cogwheel phenomenon. (Camillo Negro, 1861-1927, Italian neurologist)
1. Baker AB, Baker LH: Clinical Neurology. Revised ed. Philadelphia: Harper & Row, 1982
2. Pedro-Pons A: Patologia-y-Clinica Medicas. 5th ed. Salvat Editores, SA, 1952

NÉLATON OPERATION, 1) disarticulation of the shoulder through a transverse incision; 2) rhino-plasty utilizing lateral grafts from the cheeks; 3) prerectal lithotomy; 4) amputation of the foot via a subastragalar disarticulation; 5) ablation of nasopharyngeal polyps via the mouth.
1. Maffei WE: Os Fundamentos da Medicina. 2nd ed. Livraria Editora Artes Médicas Ltda, 1978

NELSON SYNDROME, increased pigmentation of the skin and mucosa after bilateral adrenalectomy for adrenocorticotrophic hormone-producing pituitary tumors for Cushing syndrome. Cross-reference: Addisonian syndrome. (D.H. Nelson, U.S.)
1. Addison T: Anaemia-disease of the supra-renal capsules. Lond Hosp Gaz 43:517-518, 1849
2. Kasperlik-Zaluska AA, Nielubowicz J, Wislawski J, et al: Nelson's syndrome: incidence and prognosis. Clin Endo-

crinol 19:693-698, 1983
3. Moschella SL, Hurley HJ: Dermatology. 2nd ed. Philadelphia: WB Saunders, 1985
4. Nelson DH, Meakin JW, Thorn GW: Ann Intern Med 52:560-569, 1960

NÉRI SIGN, combined flexion of the thigh and leg. While in a standing position, the patient is asked to flex the hips and lean forward as far as possible. Normally the knees remain in extension, but in a patient with pyramidal paresis, there is flexion of the knees. (Vincenzo Néri, Italian neurologist)
1. Baker AB, Baker LH: Clinical Neurology. Revised ed. Philadelphia: Harper & Row, 1982
2. Pedro-Pons A: Patologia-y-Clinica Medicas. 5th ed. Salvat Editores, SA, 1952

NERVE PRESSURE SIGN, tension on the sciatic nerve is increased when the tibial nerve is compressed in the popliteal space.
1. Baker AB, Baker LH: Clinical Neurology. Revised ed. Philadelphia: Harper & Row, 1982

NETHERTON SYNDROME, ichthyosiform lesions of the trunk and limbs with flexural disposition and sparse brittle hair. Cross-reference: Comél syndrome. (Earl W. Netherton, U.S. dermatologist)
1. Comél M: Dermatologica 98:122-136, 1949
2. Netherton EW: A unique case of trichorrhexis nodosa: bamboo hairs. Arch Dermatol 78:483-487, 1958
3. Ritchie AC: Boyd's Textbook of Pathology. 9th ed. Philadelphia: Lea & Febiger, 1990

NETTLESHIP DISEASE, urticaria pigmentosa; a chronic skin disease characterized by pigmented macules or nodules. (Edward Nettleship, 1845-1913, British ophthalmologist and dermatologist)
1. Nettleship E: Br Med J 2:435, 1869

NEU-LAXOVÁ SYNDROME, a lethal syndrome of marked intrauterine growth retardation, marked microcephaly, characteristic facies, and flexion deformities. (Richard L. Neu, U.S.)
1. Gorlin RJ, Cohen MM Jr, Levin LS: Syndromes of the Head and Neck. New York: Oxford University Press, 1990
2. Laxová R, Ohara PT, Timothy JAD: A further example of a lethal autosomal recessive condition in sibs. J Ment Defic Res 16:139-143, 1972
3. Meguid NA, Temtamy SA: Neu-Laxova syndrome in two Egyptian families. Am J Med Genet 41:30-31, 1991
4. Neu RL, Kajii T, Gardener LI, et al: Pediatrics 47:611-612, 1971

NEUBER OPERATION, filling of an osseous cavity using cutaneous grafts from the edges of the wound.
1. Maffei WE: Os Fundamentos da Medicina. 2nd ed. Livraria Editora Artes Médicas Ltda, 1978

NEUMANN DISEASE, pemphigus vegetans. (Isidor Neumann, 1837-1906, Austrian)
1. Casas EC: Diccionario Terminologico de Ciencias Medicas. 5th ed. Salvat Editores, SA, 1954

NEURAL CREST SYNDROME, a familial dysautonomia consisting of loss of deep or superficial pain sensibility, with autonomic dysfunction manifested by the following: pupillary abnormalities ranging from partial to complete bilateral Horner syndrome, neurogenic anhidrosis with otherwise normal sweat glands, and vasomotor instability with abnormal vanillylmandelic and homovanillic acid urine assays. Other signs include aplasia of dental enamel and meningeal thickening and cystic changes. Patients tend to have blond hair, blue-green eyes, and a fair complexion.
1. Brown WJ, Podosin R: Arch Neurol 15:294-301, 1966

NEUROCUTANEOUS SYNDROME, see Sturge-Weber syndrome.

NEUROFIBROMATOSIS SYNDROME, see Von Recklinghausen disease.

NEUROLEPTIC MALIGNANT SYNDROME, a complication of antipsychotic drug therapy; seen in a patient in whom a therapeutic dose of haloperidol or another neuroleptic drug causes muscular contraction, pyrexia, and often coma. Autonomic dysfunction causes sweating, tachycardia, dyspnea, and incontinence.
1. Caroff SN, Mann SC: Neuroleptic malignant syndrome. Med Clin North Am 77:185-201, 1993
2. Ritchie AC: Boyd's Textbook of Pathology. 9th ed. Philadelphia: Lea & Febiger, 1990

NEVIN-JONES DISEASE, see Creutzfeldt-Jakob disease.

NEVO SYNDROME, see Sotos syndrome.

NEVOCUTANEOUS MELANOSIS SYNDROME, melanosis of the skin and pia arachnoid. Central nervous system function may be initially normal but progressive seizures and mental deficiency develop.
1. Ritchie AC: Boyd's Textbook of Pathology. 9th ed. Philadelphia: Lea & Febiger, 1990

NEVOID BASAL CELL EPITHELIOMA SYNDROME, see Basal cell nevus syndrome.

NEW WORLD SYNDROME, see Leishmaniosis syndrome.

NEWCASTLE DISEASE, an acute systemic disease of chickens, intransmissible to humans, caused by a paramyxovirus. (First reported in Newcastle-Upon Tyne, England.) Cross-reference: Ranikhet disease.
1. Baker AB, Baker LH: Clinical Neurology. Revised ed. Philadelphia: Harper & Row, 1982
2. Kroneveld FC: Over een in nod-India hurschende ziekte ondes het plumes. Ned Indisch Bl Diergeneesk, 1926

NEZELOF SYNDROME, cellular immunodeficiency with abnormal immunoglobulin synthesis; characterized by lymphopenia, diminished lymphoid tissue, abnormal thymus architecture, and normal or increased levels of most of the five immunoglobulin classes. Unlike the patient with DiGeorge syndrome, the child with this disease has no endocrine or cardiovascular anomalies. (Christian Nezelof, French pediatrician)
1. Bennett JC, Plum F (eds): Cecil Textbook of Medicine. 20th ed. Philadelphia: WB Saunders, 1996
2. Moschella SL, Hurley HJ: Dermatology. 2nd ed. Philadelphia: WB Saunders, 1985

NICHE SIGN, see Haudek sign.

NICOLADONI SIGN, see Branham sign.

NICOLAS-FAVRE DISEASE, see Durand-Nicolas-Favre disease.

NIEMANN-PICK TYPE A DISEASE, transient neonatal jaundice is followed by progressive hepatosplenomegaly, developmental regression, and weight loss leading to death by age 2 years. The most common and most severe form occurs more frequently in individuals of Ashkenazi background. (Albert Niemann, 1880-1921, German pediatrician; Ludwig Pick, 1868-1944, German)
1. Gal AE, Brady RO, Barranger JA, et al: The diagnosis of type A and type B Niemann-Pick disease and detection of carriers using leukocytes and a chromogenic analogue of sphingomyelin. Clin Chim Acta 104:129-132, 1980
2. Rowland LP (ed): Merritt's Textbook of Neurology. 9th ed. Baltimore: Williams & Wilkins, 1995

NIEMANN-PICK TYPE B DISEASE, a familial disorder occurring in infants. More common in the Jewish race and in females. The disease is characterized by the accumulation of lipids, mainly sphingomyelin, in the reticuloendothelial cells of the liver and spleen. (Albert Niemann; Ludwig Pick)
1. Farmer TW: Pediatric Neurology. 2nd ed. Hagerstown: Harper & Row, 1975

NIEMANN-PICK TYPE C DISEASE, patients are normal in infancy but after 1-2 years develop progressive dementia, seizures, spasticity, vertical gaze paresis, and ataxia. Hepatosplenomegaly is less prominent than in other types. (Albert Niemann; Ludwig Pick)
1. Pentchev PG, Comly ME, Kruth HS, et al: A defect in cholesterol esterification in Niemann-Pick disease (Type C) patients. Proc Natl Acad Sci USA 82:8247-8251, 1985
2. Pentchev PG, et al: Group C Niemann-Pick disease: faulty regulation of low-density lipoprotein uptake and cholesterol storage in cultured fibroblast. FASEB J 1:40-45, 1987
3. Rowland LP (ed): Merritt's Textbook of Neurology. 9th ed. Baltimore: Williams & Wilkins, 1995

NIEVERGELT SYNDROME, a bone disease characterized by hearing loss, deformed great toes, subluxation of radial or ulnar heads, and clubfeet. Onset from birth. (Kurt Nievergelt, Swiss orthopedic surgeon)
1. Nievergelt K: Arch Julius Klaus Stift 19:157-160, 1944

NIKOLSKY SIGN, normal epidermis rubs off easily from the surrounding skin; produced by minor trauma including pemphigus and other hereditary blistering skin diseases. (Pyotr V. Nikolsky [Nokolsky], 1858-1940, Russian dermatologist)
1. Casas EC: Diccionario Terminologico de Ciencias Medicas. 5th ed. Salvat Editores, SA, 1954

NISSEN OPERATION, fundoplication for repair of hiatal hernia; can be done either transabdominally or transthoracically. (Rudolf Nissen, German surgeon)
1. Schwartz SI: Principles of Surgery. 4th ed. New York: McGraw-Hill, 1983

NISSL-ALZHEIMER ENTERITIS, characterized by internal proliferation in the absence of inflammatory reaction. (Franz Nissl, 1860-1919, German neuropathologist; Alois Alzheimer, 1864-1915, German neurologist)
1. Baker AB, Baker LH: Clinical Neurology. Revised ed. Philadelphia: Harper & Row, 1982
2. Nissl F, Alzheimer A: Histol Histopathol Arb 1:315-494, 1904

NOACK SYNDROME, acrocephalopolysyndactyly type I; see Pfeiffer-type syndrome. (Margot Noack, German)

NOGUES-SIRAL DISEASE, see Steinert disease.

NOKOLSKY SIGN, see Nikolsky sign. (Pyotr V. Nikolsky [Nokolsky])

NONNE SYNDROME, hereditary cerebellar ataxia. (Max Nonne, 1861-1959, German neurologist)
1. Nonne M: Dtsch Z Nervenheilkd 27:169-216, 1904

NONNE-MILROY SYNDROME, see Milroy syndrome. (Max Nonne; William F. Milroy, 1855-1942, U.S.)

NOONAN SYNDROME, see Male Turner syndrome.

NORDAU DISEASE, degeneration of the powers of the body and mind (sense latum). (Max S. Nordau, 1849-1923, German)
1. Nordau MS: Dégénérescence. Paris: Alcan, 1894

NORRIE DISEASE, hereditary disorder consisting of bilateral blindness due to retinal malformation, mental retardation, and deafness. (Gordon Norrie, 1855-1941, Danish ophthalmologist)
1. Norrie G: Acta Ophthalmol 5:363-364, 1927

NORTHCOTT OPERATION, stimulation of vascular endothelium through an electrolytic current to promote increased production of sex hormones.
1. Maffei WE: Os Fundamentos da Medicina. 2nd ed. Livraria Editora Artes Médicas Ltda, 1978

NOTHNAGEL SIGN, poor emotional response of the facies; seen in the patient with hypothalamic tumor.
1. Casas EC: Diccionario Terminologico de Ciencias Medicas. 5th ed. Salvat Editores, SA, 1954

NOTHNAGEL SYNDROME, contralateral ataxia with or without signs of ipsilateral cerebellar deficiency, paralysis of gaze (either upward or contralateral), and variable ipsilateral internal and external ophthalmoplegia (due to involvement of the third nucleus). Cross-references: Brun syndrome; Claude-Nothnagel syndrome; Pretectal syndrome. (Carl W.H. Nothnagel, 1841-1905, Austrian)
1. Baker AB, Baker LH: Clinical Neurology. Revised ed. Philadelphia: Harper & Row, 1982
2. Nothnagel H: Topische Diagnostik der Gehirnkrankheiten: Eine Klinische Studie. Berlin: Hirschwald, 1879, p 220

NUFTAL-SANTANA DISEASE, see South African tick-bite fever.

NUMB CHIN SYNDROME, typical mentalis neuropathy seen in women with a lytic jaw mass, lymphadenopathy, splenomegaly, and a multifocal neurological disorder. Suggests local involvement of the inferior alveolar nerve or the mental nerve.
1. Calverley JR, Mohnac AM: Syndrome of the numb chin. Arch Intern Med 112:819-821, 1963
2. Lossos A, Siegal T: Correspondence: Case 27-1994: the numb chin syndrome. N Engl J Med 331:1460, 1994
3. Rowland LP (ed): Merritt's Textbook of Neurology. 9th ed. Baltimore: Williams & Wilkins, 1995

NYSTAGMUS BLOCKAGE SYNDROME, NYSTAGMUS COMPENSATION SYNDROME, infantile esotropia; abnormal head posture toward the adducted fixing eye. The patient is often blind.
1. Von Noorden GK: The nystagmus compensation (blockage) syndrome. Am J Ophthalmol 82:287-289, 1976

OASTHOUSE SYNDROME, OASTHOUSE URINE DISEASE, see Methionine malabsorption syndrome.

OAT CELL CARCINOMA, a small cell undifferentiated carcinoma that is rare in the larynx, even though it comprises approximately 10%-15% of lung tumors. The male-to-female ratio is 3:1 and the tumor is found more commonly in smokers. The most common location is the subglottis.
1. Ballenger JJ: Diseases of the Nose, Throat, Ear, Head and Neck. 12th ed. Philadelphia: Lea & Febiger, 1977

OAV SYNDROME, oculoauriculovertebral (OAV) dysplasia; see Goldenhar syndrome.

OBER TEST, while positioned in the left lateral decubitus position, the patient's right leg is abducted and flexed and dropped, causing contraction of the fascia lata. (Frank R. Ober, 1881-1960, U.S. orthopedic surgeon)
1. Casas EC: Diccionario Terminologico de Ciencias Medicas. 5th ed. Salvat Editores, SA, 1954

OBERST OPERATION, insertion of a cutaneous graft into the abdomen for draining ascites.
1. Maffei WE: Os Fundamentos da Medicina. 2nd ed. Livraria Editora Artes Médicas Ltda, 1978

O'BRIEN OPERATION, facial nerve block over the mandibular condyle, inferior to the posterior zygomatic process, to achieve akinesia.
1. Spaeth GL: Ophthalmic Surgery. Principles and Practice. Philadelphia: WB Saunders, 1982

OBTURATUR SIGN, see Hefke-Turner sign.

OCCIPITAL HORN SYNDROME, occipital exostoses, soft easily bruisable skin, hyperextensible joints, and widening and bowing of multiple long bones are features. Cross-reference: Ehlers-Danlos syndrome type IX.

1. Blackston RD, et al: Ehlers-Danlos syndrome (EDS), type IX: biochemical evidence for X-linkage. Am J Hum Genet 41(3):A49, 1987 (Abstract)
2. Gorlin RJ, Cohen MM Jr, Levin LS: Syndromes of the Head and Neck. New York: Oxford University Press, 1990

OCHOA SYNDROME, see Urofacial syndrome.

OCHSNER CLASPING TEST, a measurement for medial nerve injury; the patient is asked to clasp the hands together firmly. If the medial nerve has been interrupted above the level at which the flexor digitorum sublimis muscle is innervated (the crease of the elbow joint), the index finger fails to flex. (Albert J. Ochsner, 1858-1925, U.S. surgeon)

1. Lumley JS, Clain A: Hamilton Bailey's Demonstration of Physical Signs in Clinical Surgery. 18th ed. London: Butterworth-Heinemann, 1997

O'CONNELL TEST, a measurement of low back pain following lumbosacral radiation. The is first carried out on the sound limb, and the angle of flexion and site of pain are recorded. Pain may be on the opposite side (Fajersztajn crossed sciatic sign); the test is then carried out on the affected limb, and the flexion angle and site of pain are again noted. Both thighs are then flexed simultaneously while extension is maintained at the knee.

1. Baker AB, Baker LH: Clinical Neurology. Revised ed. Philadelphia: Harper & Row, 1982

OCULAR HISTOPLASMOSIS SYNDROME, a focal chorioretinitis in the macular area believed to be related to a hypersensitivity response to products of *Histoplasma capsulatum*. No direct relationship to fungal infection has been proved.

1. Bennett JC, Plum F (eds): Cecil Textbook of Medicine. 20th ed. Philadelphia: WB Saunders, 1996

OCULAR ISCHEMIC SYNDROME, a progressive disorder resulting from hypoperfusion of the eye.

1. Walsh FB, Hoyt EF, Miller NR: Clinical Neuro-Ophthalmology. 4th ed. Baltimore: Williams & Wilkins, 1982

OCULAR-MUCOUS MEMBRANE SYNDROME, see Stevens-Johnson syndrome.

OCULOCEREBRAL-HYPOPIGMENTATION SYNDROME, see Cross syndrome.

OCULOCEREBROCUTANEOUS SYNDROME, orbital cysts, cerebral malformations, accessory skin tags, and focal cutaneous hypoplasia are features. Cross-reference: Delleman syndrome.

1. Delleman JW, Oorthuys JWE: Clin Genet 19:191-198, 1981

OCULOCEREBROFACIAL SYNDROME, mental retardation, microbrachycephaly, a long narrow face, sparse eyebrows, preauricular tags, upward-slanting palpebral fissures, microcornea, strabismus, pale optic discs, myopia, and micrognathia are features. Cross-reference: Kaufman syndrome.

1. Kaufman RL, et al: Birth Defects 7:135-138, 1971

OCULOCEREBRORENAL SYNDROME, see Lowe disease.

OCULODENTODIGITAL SYNDROME, OCULODENTO-OSSEOUS SYNDROME, microphthalmos, microcornea, short palpebral fissures, enamel hypoplasia, syndactyly of the 4th and 5th fingers and 3rd and 4th toes, camptodactyly of the 5th fingers, broad tubular bones, and a mandible with wide alveolar ridge are features. Autosomal dominant inheritance. Cross-references: Dysplasia oculodentodigitalis syndrome; Peter syndrome.

1. Gorlin RJ, Chaudhry KP, Moss ML: J Pediatr 56:778-785, 1960
2. Judisch GF, Martin-Casals A, Hanson J, et al: Oculodentodigital dysplasia. Arch Ophthalmol 97:878, 1979
3. Smith DW, Jones KL: Recognizable Patterns of Human Malformations: Genetic, Embryologic, and Clinical Aspects. 3rd ed. Philadelphia: WB Saunders, 1982

OCULODENTO-OSSEOUS SYNDROME, see Oculodentodigital syndrome.

OCULOMANDIBULOFACIAL SYNDROME, see Hallermann-Streiff syndrome.

ODIENET SIGN, see Lian sign.

ODONTOTRICHOMELIC SYNDROME, a form of ectodermal dysplasia with tetramelic deficiency.

1. Freire-Maia N, Pinheiro M: Ectodermal Dysplasias: A Clinical and Genetic Study. New York: Alan R Liss, 1984, pp 106-108
2. Gorlin RJ, Cohen MM Jr, Levin LS: Syndromes of the Head and Neck. New York: Oxford University Press, 1990

OEFELEIN SIGN, with the patient in the prone position, percussion of the muscles from the 7th to the 12th thoracic vertebrae produces a unilateral reflex of these muscles; seen in the case of peptic ulcer.

1. Casas EC: Diccionario Terminologico de Ciencias Medicas. 5th ed. Salvat Editores, SA, 1954

OGILVIE SYNDROME, false colonic obstruction; abdominal distention simulating colonic obstruction, with persistent contraction of intestinal musculature but without evidence of organic disease of the colon. Occurs as a result of a defect in the sympathetic nerve supply. Has been reported to occur following lumbar laminectomy. (Sir William H. Ogilvie, 1887-1971, British surgeon)

1. Nanni G, Garbini A, Luchetti P, et al: Ogilvie's syndrome (acute colonic pseudo-obstruction): review of literature and report of 4 additional cases. Dis Colon Rectum 55:157-177, 1982
2. Ogilvie H: Large-intestine colic due to sympathetic deprivation: a new clinical syndrome. Br Med J 2:671-673, 1948

OGSTON OPERATION, 1) resection of the lateral condyles of the femur in cases of genu valgum; 2) resection of a cuneiform portion of the tarsus in cases of flat foot to correct the plantar arch.

1. Maffei WE: Os Fundamentos da Medicina. 2nd ed. Livraria Editora Artes Médicas Ltda, 1978

OGUCHI DISEASE, a form of hereditary night blindness occurring in Japan. (Chuta Oguchi, 1875-1945, Japanese ophthalmologist)

1. Oguchi C: Graefes Arch Ophthalmol 81:109-117, 1912

OGURA AND BILLER OPERATION, supraglottic laryngectomy and hemilaryngectomy.

1. Schwartz SI: Principles of Surgery. 4th ed. New York: McGraw-Hill, 1983

OHARA DISEASE, tularemia. (Shoichiro Ohara, Japanese)

1. Casas EC: Diccionario Terminologico de Ciencias Medicas. 5th ed. Salvat Editores, SA, 1954

OLDFIELD SYNDROME, familial polyposis of the colon associated with extensive sebaceous cysts. A possible variant of Gardner syndrome. (Michael C. Oldfield, British)

1. Ingram JT, Oldfield MC: Hereditary sebaceous cysts. Br Med J 1:960-963, 1937
2. Oldfield MC: The association of familial polyposis of the colon with multiple sebaceous cyst. Br J Surg 41:534-541, 1954

OLFACTOGENITAL SYNDROME, see Kallmann syndrome.

OLIVER-CARDARELLI-OLSHAUSEN SIGN, a tumor (usually dermoid) on a portion of the uterus; seen in young, single women. Cross-reference: Porter sign. (William S. Oliver, 1836-1906, British; Antonio Cardarelli, 1831-1927, Italian)

1. Casas EC: Diccionario Terminologico de Ciencias Medicas. 5th ed. Salvat Editores, SA, 1954

OLIVOPONTOCEREBELLAR ATROPHY SYNDROME, chronic progressive ataxia; a disorder characterized by impaired cerebellar functions and impairment of or reduction in neurons in the inferior olivary nuclei of the medulla, in the basis pontes, in the cerebellar cortex, and in the deep cerebellar nuclei.

1. Konigsmark BW, Weiner LP: The olivopontocerebellar atrophy: a review. Medicine 49:227-241, 1970

OLLIER SYNDROME, see Osteochondromatosis syndrome. (Louis Ollier, 1830-1900, French surgeon)

OLMER DISEASE, Mediterranean exanthematous fever.

1. Casas EC: Diccionario Terminologico de Ciencias Medicas. 5th ed. Salvat Editores, SA, 1954

OMBRÉDANNE SYNDROME, a hypermetabolic syndrome characterized by pale skin, hyperthermia, and seizures in infants. (Louis Ombrédanne, 1871-1956, French)

1. Ombrédanne L: Rev Neurol, 1929, p 617

OMM SYNDROME, *o*phthalmo-*m*andibulo-*m*elic (OMM) dysplasia; see Pillay syndrome.

OMSK HEMORRHAGIC FEVER, see Kyasanur Forest disease. (Found in central Russia.)

ONDINE CURSE, see Central alveolar hypoventilation syndrome.

ONE-AND-A-HALF SYNDROME, a varying degree of paralysis of the ipsilateral gaze and failure of adduction on gaze to the opposite side, with nystagmus in the abducting eye. Cross-references: Fisher syndrome; Miller Fisher syndrome.

1. Fisher M: N Engl J Med 255:57-65, 1956
2. Fross RD, Daube JR: Neuropathy in the Miller-Fisher syndrome: clinical and electrophysiologic findings. Neurology 37:1493-1498, 1987
3. Rowland LP (ed): Merritt's Textbook of Neurology. 9th ed. Baltimore: Williams & Wilkins, 1995

O'NYONG-NYONG DISEASE, this disease was first recognized in 1959 when a major epidemic affecting almost 2 million people broke out in East Africa. Resembles Chikungunya disease, with lymphadenitis as a differentiating feature. (O'nyong-nyong means severe joint pain in the language of the Acholi people in East Africa.)

1. Baker AB, Baker LH: Clinical Neurology. Revised ed. Philadelphia: Harper & Row, 1982
2. Davies, CW, et at: O'Nyong-Nyong fever: an epidemic virus disease in East Africa: introduction. Trans R Soc Rop Med Hyg 54:517, 1960

O'ORMOND SYNDROME, retroperitoneal liposclerosis; impairment of renal venous return, partial ureteric obstruction, and proteinuria are present.

1. Vannotti A: Clinique et Physiopathologie Médicales. Introduction a la Médecine Clinique. Librairie Maloine SA, 1973

OPERCULUM SYNDROME, see Foix-Chavany-Marie syndrome.

OPHTHALMOMANDIBULOMELIC DYSPLASIA SYNDROME, see Pillay syndrome.

OPHTHALMOPLEGIA SYNDROME, see MERRF syndrome.

OPHTHALMOSCOPIC SIGN, blood in the retinal vessels gradually ceases to move and the column of blood splits into fragments; seen as death approaches.

1. Dorland's Medical Dictionary. 28th ed. Philadelphia: WB Saunders, 1994

OPITZ SYNDROME, OPITZ BBB/G COMPOUND SYNDROME, OPITZ-FRIAS (G) SYNDROME, OPITZ-OCULO-GENITO-LARYNGEAL SYNDROME, hypertelorism and hypospadias. Swallowing problem with recurrent aspiration. Autosomal dominant inheritance. Cross-references: G syndrome; Hypertelorism-hypospadias syndrome. (John M. Opitz; German-born U.S. pediatrician)

1. Opitz JM: "G" syndrome (hypertelorism with esophageal abnormalities and hypospadia, or hypospadias-dysphagia, or Opitz-Frias or the "Opitz G" syndrome). Perspective in 1987 and bibliography. Am J Med Genet 28:275-285, 1987 (Editorial)
2. Opitz JM, Frias JL, Gutenberger JE, et al: Birth Defects 5:95-103, 1969
3. Opitz JM, Summit RL, Smith DW: Birth Defects 2:86-94, 1969
4. Smith DW, Jones KL: Recognizable Patterns of Human Malformations: Genetic, Embryologic, and Clinical Aspects. 3rd ed. Philadelphia: WB Saunders, 1982

OPITZ TRIGONOCEPHALY SYNDROME, see C syndrome.

OPPEL OPERATION, adrenalectomy.

1. Maffei WE: Os Fundamentos da Medicina. 2nd ed. Livraria Editora Artes Médicas Ltda, 1978

OPPENHEIM DISEASE, congenital flaccid weakness, a nonfamilial history, and a nonprogressive course are the usual features. Undoubtedly some cases can be placed in the group of congenital myopathies. In infants, there is weakness and hypotonia. Originally described as a syndrome in which there was a marked degree of muscular flaccidity. Cross-reference: Schwalbe-Ziehen-Oppenheim disease. (Hermann Oppenheim, 1858-1919, German neurologist)

1. Campbell WC, Crenshaw AH: Campbell's Operative Orthopaedics. 7th ed. St Louis: CV Mosby, 1987
2. Grinker RR, Sahs AL: Neurology. 6th ed. Springfield: Charles C Thomas, 1966
3. Oppenheim H: Monatsschr Psych 8:232-233, 1900

OPPENHEIM REFLEX, dorsiflexion of the great toe is elicited by applying heavy pressure with the thumb and index finger to the anterior surface of the tibia, mainly on its medial aspect, and stroking down the infrapatellar region to the ankle; seen in the patient with pyramidal tract disease. (Hermann Oppenheim)

1. Baker AB, Baker LH: Clinical Neurology. Revised ed. Philadelphia: Harper & Row, 1982

OPPOIZER SIGN, the beat at the cardiac apex changes according to the patient's position; seen in serofibrinous pericarditis.

1. Casas EC: Diccionario Terminologico de Ciencias Medicas. 5th ed. Salvat Editores, SA, 1954

OPTIC-CEREBRAL SYNDROME, OPTICO-PYRAMIDAL SYNDROME, the patient with carotid artery disease may experience the simultaneous occurrence of cerebral infarction and ipsilateral ischemic optic neuropathy.

1. Walsh FB, Hoyt EF, Miller NR: Clinical Neuro-Ophthalmology. 4th ed. Baltimore: Williams & Wilkins, 1982

ORAL-FACIAL-DIGITAL SYNDROME, characterized by a short upper lip, hypertrophied frenula of the lips and tongue, a multilobed tongue, clefts of the hard and soft palate, sparse hair, numerous milia, polycystic kidneys and liver, dental caries, and brachydactyly and syndactyly. A 50% incidence of mental retardation.

1. Bennett JC, Plum F (eds): Cecil Textbook of Medicine. 20th ed. Philadelphia: WB Saunders, 1996

ORBELI PHENOMENON, when the response of a cultured nerve-muscle preparation is diminishing because of fatigue, stimulation of the sympathetic nerve increases the height of the contractions. (Leon A. Orbeli, 1882-1958, Russian physiologist)

1. Dorland's Medical Dictionary. 28th ed. Philadelphia: WB Saunders, 1994

ORBICULARIS SIGN, the inability to close the eye on the paralyzed side without closing the other eye; seen in hemiplegia. Cross-reference: Revilliod sign.
1. Dorland's Medical Dictionary. 28th ed. Philadelphia: WB Saunders, 1994

ORD OPERATION, rupture of recent articular adherents.
1. Maffei WE: Os Fundamentos da Medicina. 2nd ed. Livraria Editora Artes Médicas Ltda, 1978

ORGANIC ANXIETY SYNDROME, an organic mental syndrome characterized by prominent, recurrent panic attacks or generalized anxiety caused by a specific organic factor and not associated with delirium. Causes may include hyperthyroidism, hypothyroidism, pheochromocytoma, fasting hypoglycemia, hypercortisolism, or the use of psychoactive substances.
1. Dorland's Medical Dictionary. 28th ed. Philadelphia: WB Saunders, 1994

ORGANIC BRAIN SYNDROME, see Organic mental syndrome.

ORGANIC DELUSIONAL SYNDROME, an organic mental syndrome characterized by the presence of delusions caused by a specific organic factor and not associated with delirium. Causes include ingestion of substances such as amphetamines, cannabis, and hallucinogens, and diseases such as temporal lobe epilepsy, head trauma or cerebral lesions, and Huntington chorea. The substance-induced syndromes are named as "disorder" (e.g., cannabis delusional disorder).
1. Dorland's Medical Dictionary. 28th ed. Philadelphia: WB Saunders, 1994

ORGANIC MENTAL SYNDROME, a group of psychological or behavioral signs and symptoms associated with one or more specific organic etiological factors. The *Diagnostic and Statistical Manual, 3rd Ed., Revised,* includes six specific organic brain syndromes: delirium and dementia; amnestic syndrome or organic hallucinosis; organic delusional syndrome, organic mood syndrome, and organic anxiety syndrome; organic personality syndrome; intoxication and withdrawal; and a residual category, organic mental syndrome not otherwise specified. Cross-references: Acute brain-acute organic syndrome; Chronic brain syndrome; Organic brain syndrome.
1. Dorland's Medical Dictionary. 28th ed. Philadelphia: WB Saunders, 1994

ORGANIC MOOD SYNDROME, an organic mental syndrome characterized by the presence of manic or depressive mood disturbance caused by a specific organic factor and not associated with delirium. Common causes are ingestion of psychoactive substances (notably reserpine, methyldopa, and certain hallucinogens), endocrine disorders (notably Cushing syndrome, Addison disease, hypothyroidism, and hyperparathyroidism), and viral infections. The substance-induced syndromes are named as "disorders" (e.g., hallucinogen mood disorder).
1. Dorland's Medical Dictionary. 28th ed. Philadelphia: WB Saunders, 1994

ORGANIC PERSONALITY SYNDROME, an organic mental syndrome characterized by lability, marked apathy, impaired impulse control, and paranoid ideation, caused by a specific organic factor and not associated with delirium or dementia. The most common causes are space-occupying lesions of the brain, head trauma, and cerebrovascular disease.
1. Dorland's Medical Dictionary. 28th ed. Philadelphia: WB Saunders, 1994

O'RIAIN TEST, the patient's fingers are placed in warm water for approximately 30 minutes and then removed. In normal fingers, the skin is wrinkled; in denervated fingers, it is not. Valid only in the first few months after an injury.
1. Evans RC: Illustrated Essentials in Orthopedic Physical Assessment. St Louis: Mosby Yearbook, 1994

ORMOND DISEASE, retroperitoneal fibrosis. (John K. Ormond, U.S. urologist)
1. Dorland's Pocket Medical Dictionary. 22nd ed. Philadelphia: WB Saunders, 1977

OROCRANIODIGITAL SYNDROME, cleft lip/palate, mild microcephaly, hypoplastic and distally positioned thumbs, limited extension of the elbows due to anterior displacement of the radial head, and short stature are features. Cross-reference: Juberg-Hayward syndrome.
1. Juberg RC, Hayward JR: J Pediatr 74:755-762, 1969

OROMANDIBULAR SYNDROME, see Hanhart syndrome.

OROYA FEVER, an acute, febrile, hemolytic anemia with appreciable mortality; the second stage, verruga peruana, is a benign cutaneous eruption of hemangiomatous papules and nodules, caused by *Bartonella bacilliformis* and transmitted by the bite of sandflies. Cross-reference: Carrión disease. (Named for Oroya, Peru, where the first cases were reported in 1885.)

1. Bennett JC, Plum F (eds): Cecil Textbook of Medicine. 20th ed. Philadelphia: WB Saunders, 1996

ORTNER SYNDROME, hoarseness with cardiovascular lesions. A heart disease associated with a left laryngeal nerve palsy from compression between aorta pulmonary artery. Cross-reference: Cardiovocal syndrome. (Norbert Ortner, 1867-1935, German)

1. Braunwald E: Heart Disease: A Textbook of Cardiovascular Medicine. 4th ed. Philadelphia: WB Saunders, 1992
2. Ortner N: Wien Klin Wochenschr 10:753-755, 1897

ORTOLANI CLICK, ORTOLANI SIGN, the presence of a click on movement of the hip; seen in congenital dislocation of the hip. (Marius Ortolani, Italian orthopedic surgeon)

1. Mazion JM: Illustrated Manual of Orthopedic Signs/Tests/Maneuvers for Office Procedure. 2nd ed. Orlando: Daniels Publishing, 1980

OSGOOD-SCHLATTER DISEASE, osteochondrosis of the tibial tuberosity; apophyseal osteitis of the tibia. Occurs in children 8-15 years old and mainly in athletes. Named after American and Swiss surgeons who described it independently in 1903. Cross-references: Lannelongue disease; Schlatter-Osgood disease. (Robert Osgood, 1873-1956, U.S. orthopedic surgeon; Carl Schlatter, 1864-1934, Swiss surgeon)

1. Campbell WC, Crenshaw AH: Campbell's Operative Orthopaedics. 7th ed. St Louis: WB Saunders, 1987
2. Green NE, Edwards K: Bone and joint infections in children. Orthop Clin North Am 18:555-576, 1987

OSIANDER SIGN, vaginal pulsation; an indication of pregnancy.

1. Casas EC: Diccionario Terminologico de Ciencias Medicas. 5th ed. Salvat Editores, SA, 1954

OSLER DISEASE, OSLER-VAQUEZ DISEASE, characterized by an overabundance of circulating red cells, granulocytes, and often platelets. Cross-reference: Vaquez disease. (Sir William Osler, 1849-1919, Canadian-U.S.; Louis Vaquez, 1860-1936, French)

1. Baker AB, Baker LH: Clinical Neurology. Revised ed. Philadelphia: Harper & Row, 1982
2. Grinker RR, Sahs AL: Neurology. 6th ed. Springfield: Charles C Thomas, 1966

OSLER NODES, small, tender nodules associated with infective endocarditis. Most frequently found on the finger or toe pads, and persist for hours to days. (Sir William Osler)

1. Bennett JC, Plum F (eds): Cecil Textbook of Medicine. 20th ed. Philadelphia: WB Saunders, 1996

OSLER-WEBER-RENDU SYNDROME, hereditary hemorrhagic telangiectasia; a disorder resulting from a widespread developmental abnormality of the vasculature. Dilatation and convolution of venules and capillaries give rise to telangiectatic lesions in the skin and mucous membranes. (Sir William Osler; Frederick Parkes Weber, 1863-1962, British; Henri J.L. Rendu, 1844-1902, French)

1. Moschella SL, Hurley HJ: Dermatology. 2nd ed. Philadelphia: WB Saunders, 1985
2. Osler W: Q J Med (Oxf) 1:53-8, 1907
3. Rendu HJL: Bull Soc Med Hop 13:731-733, 1896
4. Weber FP: Edinburgh Med J, 1904, pp 346-349

OSTEOCHONDROMATOSIS SYNDROME, a disorder of the growing ends of long bones, characterized by asymmetric enchondromas with local growth deficiency. Etiology unknown. Cross-reference: Ollier syndrome.

1. Ollier L: De la dyschondroplasia. Bull Soc Chir 3:22-27, 1899
2. Smith DW, Jones KL: Recognizable Patterns of Human Malformations: Genetic, Embryologic, and Clinical Aspects. 3rd ed. Philadelphia: WB Saunders, 1982

OSTEOGENESIS IMPERFECTA SYNDROME, an inherited disorder characterized by a variety of phenotypic abnormalities, the most significant being osseous fragility and fractures. Type I (dominant form) is characterized by fragile bones, blue sclera, hyperextensibility and hypoplasia of dentin. Cross references: Adair-Dighton syndrome; Eddowes syndrome; Lobstein syndrome; Spurway-Eddowes syndrome; van der Hoeve syndrome. Type II (recessive form) patients usually die in infancy; survivors have hydrocephalus. Cross-reference: Vrolik disease.

1. Eddowes A: Br Med J 2:222, 1900
2. Freda VJ, Vosburgh GJ, Di Liberti C: Osteogenesis imperfecta congenita. A presentation of 16 cases and review of the literature. Obstet Gynecol 18:535, 1961
3. Spurway J: Br Med J:844, 1896
4. Wyngaarden JB, Smith LH Jr: Cecil's Textbook of Medicine. 17th ed. Philadelphia: WB Saunders, 1985

OSTRUM-FURST SYNDROME, congenital fusion of the vertebrae of the neck, platybasia, and Sprengel deformity. (Herman Ostrum, U.S.; William Furst, U.S.)

1. Furst W, Ostrum HW: Am J Roentgenol 47:588-590, 1942

OTODENTAL SYNDROME, disease characterized by dental anomalies and sensorineural hearing loss.
1. Chen RJ, et al: "Otodental" dysplasia. Oral Surg Oral Med Oral Pathol 66:353-358, 1988
2. Gorlin RJ, Cohen MM Jr, Levin LS: Syndromes of the Head and Neck. 3rd ed. New York: Oxford University Press, 1990

OTO-ONYCHO-PERONEAL SYNDROME, minor craniofacial malformations, multiple contractures, dysplastic pinnae, hypoplasia of the nails, and fibular hypoplasia are features.
1. Gorlin RJ, Cohen MM Jr, Levin LS: Syndromes of the Head and Neck. New York: Oxford University Press, 1990
2. Leiba S, et al: Oculo-otonasal malformations associated with osteo-onychodysplasia. Birth Defects 11(2):67-73, 1975

OTOPALATODIGITAL SYNDROME, deafness, cleft palate, and broad distal digits with short nails are features X-linked semidominant inheritance. Cross-reference: Taybi syndrome.
1. Gorlin RJ, Poznanski AK, Hendon I: The oto-palato-digital (OPD) syndrome in females. Oral Surg 35:218, 1973
2. Smith DW, Jones KL: Recognizable Patterns of Human Malformations: Genetic, Embryologic, and Clinical Aspects. 3rd ed. Philadelphia: WB Saunders, 1982
3. Taybi H: Am J Roentgenol 88:450-457, 1962

OTT SIGN, while lying in the left lateral decubitus position, there is a sensation of painful stretching inside the abdomen; an indication of appendicitis.
1. Casas EC: Diccionario Terminologico de Ciencias Medicas. 5th ed. Salvat Editores, SA, 1954

OTTO DISEASE, osteoarthritis of the acetabulum. (Adolph Otto, 1785-1845, German surgeon)
1. Casas EC: Diccionario Terminologico de Ciencias Medicas. 5th ed. Salvat Editores, SA, 1954

OUTLET SYNDROME, see Thoracic outlet syndrome.

OVARIAN VEIN SYNDROME, on the right side, the relationship of the gonadal vessels to the ureter accounts for those rare circumstances in which ovarian vein dilatation results in interference with ureteral drainage.
1. Campbell MF, Walsh PC: Campbell's Urology. 5th ed. Philadelphia: WB Saunders, 1986
2. Dure-Smith P: Ovarian vein syndrome: is it a myth? Urology 13:355, 1979
3. Dykhuizen RF, Roberts JA: The ovarian vein syndrome. Surg Gynecol Obstet 130:443-452, 1970

OVARIAN-REMNANT SYNDROME, cyclical pelvic pain, typically occurring several weeks or months after oophorectomy and usually associated with a pelvic mass, most frequently a corpus luteum cyst, which sometimes leads to unilateral ureteral obstruction. Due to the survival of an ovarian fragment after the operation.
1. Dorland's Medical Dictionary. 28th ed. Philadelphia: WB Saunders, 1994

OVERLAY SYNDROME, characterized by the appearance of some or many of the classic features of periarteritis nodosa and allergic granulomatosis in the same patient.
1. Moschella SL, Hurley HJ: Dermatology. 2nd ed. Philadelphia: WB Saunders, 1985

PAAS DISEASE, familial osseous dystrophy characterized by skeletal deformities, scoliosis, spondylitis, and coxa valga. (H.R. Paas, German)
1. Casas EC: Diccionario Terminologico de Ciencias Medicas. 5th ed. Salvat Editores, SA, 1954

PACHYDERMOPERIOSTOSIS SYNDROME, see Touraine-Solente-Golé syndrome.

PACHYONYCHIA CONGENITA SYNDROME, thick nails, hyperkeratosis, foot blisters, epidermal cysts filled with loose keratin on the face, neck, and upper chest and leukokeratosis of the mouth and tongue are features. Autosomal dominant inheritance. Cross-reference: Jadassohn-Lewandowsky syndrome.
1. Gorlin RJ, Cohen MM Jr, Levin LS: Syndromes of the Head and Neck. 3rd ed. New York: Oxford University Press, 1990
2. Jadassohn J, Lewandowsky F, Neisser A, et al: Pachyonychia congenita, in Neisser A, Jacobi E (eds): Ikonographia Dermatologica. Berlin: Urbach and Schwarzenberg, 1906
3. Young lL, Lenox JA: Pachyonychia congenita. A long-term evaluation. Oral Surg 36:663, 1973

PACI OPERATION, a modification of the Lorenz operation.
1. Maffei WE: Os Fundamentos da Medicina. 2nd ed. Livraria Editora Artes Médicas Ltda, 1978

PADGETT OPERATION, reconstruction of the lips using transplantation of tubular grafts from the neck and scalp. (Earl C. Padgett, 1893-1946, U.S. surgeon)
1. Maffei WE: Os Fundamentos da Medicina. 2nd ed. Livraria Editora Artes Médicas Ltda, 1978

PAGE DISEASE, traumatic neurosis.
1. Casas EC: Diccionario Terminologico de Ciencias Medicas. 5th ed. Salvat Editores, SA, 1954

PAGENSTECHER OPERATION, surgery for correction of upper eyelid ptosis using the occipitofrontalis muscle. (Alexander Pagenstecher, 1828-1879, German ophthalmologist)

1. Maffei WE: Os Fundamentos da Medicina. 2nd ed. Livraria Editora Artes Médicas Ltda, 1978

PAGET DISEASE, 1) disordered bone remodeling, often familial and seen in older patients; 2) in older women, Paget disease of the breast is almost invariably associated with underlying intraductal adenocarcinoma. Dusky papules arising on a persistently edematous upper extremity following radical mastectomy are assumed to be lymphangiosarcoma until proved otherwise. The lesions may occur singly or at multiple sites. Cross-reference: Stewart-Treves syndrome. (James Paget, 1814-1899, British surgeon)

1. Hurst JW, Schlant RC, Alexander RW: The Heart: Arteries and Veins. 8th ed. New York: McGraw-Hill, 1994
2. McKusick VA: Heritable Disorders of Connective Tissue. 4th ed. St Louis: CV Mosby, 1972
3. Stewart FW, Treves N: Lymphangiosarcoma in postmastectomy lymphedema. Report of six cases of elephantiasis chirurgica. Cancer 1:64-81, 1948

PAGET-SCHRÖTTER SYNDROME, PAGET-VON SCHRÖTTER SYNDROME, thrombosis and thrombophlebitis of the supraclavicular fossa. Cross-reference: Schrötter syndrome. (James Paget; K.L. von Schrötter, 1837-1908, Austrian)

1. Paget J: Clinical Lectures and Essays. London, 1875
2. Von Schrötter L: Erkrankungen der Gefasse, in Nothnagel's Handbuch der Pathologie und Therapie. Wien, 1884

PAGNIELLO SIGN, intense pain on compression of the left 9th intercostal space in the mid-axillary line; seen in malaria.

1. Casas EC: Diccionario Terminologico de Ciencias Medicas. 5th ed. Salvat Editores, SA, 1954

PAHVANT VALLEY DISEASE, tularemia. (Named for Pahvant Valley, Utah, where some of the first cases were reported.)

1. Casas EC: Diccionario Terminologico de Ciencias Medicas. 5th ed. Salvat Editores, SA, 1954

PAINE-EFRON SYNDROME, see Louis-Bar syndrome.

PAINFUL ARC SYNDROME, shoulder pain occurring at a particular portion of the arc of motion during abduction as a result of inflammation or tear of the tendons of the supraspinatus muscle.

1. Dorland's Medical Dictionary. 28th ed. Philadelphia: WB Saunders, 1994

PAINFUL BRUISING SYNDROME, see Gardner-Diamond syndrome.

PAINFUL FAT SYNDROME, lipedema; atypical chronic symmetric swelling and aching of the legs are features. Cross-reference: Dercum disease.

1. Moschella SL, Hurley HJ: Dermatology. 2nd ed. Philadelphia: WB Saunders, 1985

PALATODIGITAL SYNDROME, see Catel-Manzke syndrome.

PALEOSTRIATAL SYNDROME, juvenile paralysis agitans; one of the disorders known as the Ramsay Hunt syndrome.

1. Dorland's Medical Dictionary. 28th ed. Philadelphia: WB Saunders, 1994

PALLIDAL SYNDROME, PALLIDOMESENCEPHALIC SYNDROME, a syndrome consisting of rigidity, poverty of movement, and bradykinesia, amounting to a parkinsonian state.

1. Dorland's Medical Dictionary. 28th ed. Philadelphia: WB Saunders, 1994

PALLISTER-HALL SYNDROME, see Hall syndrome. (Philip D. Pallister, U.S.)

PALLISTER-KILLIAN SYNDROME, mosaic tetrasomy 12p; mental retardation, postnatal growth deficiency, slow-growing hair, and a distinctive facies are features. Cross-reference: Isochromosome 12p syndrome. (Philip D. Pallister; Wolfgang Killian, Austrian)

1. Gorlin RJ, Cohen MM Jr, Levin LS: Syndromes of the Head and Neck. 3rd ed. New York: Oxford University Press, 1990
2. Pallister PD, et al: The Pallister mosaic syndrome. Birth Defects 13(3B):103-110, 1977

PALM-CHIN REFLEX, see Radovici sign.

PALMOPLANTAR SIGN, see Filipovitch sign.

PALTAULF-STERNBERG DISEASE, see Hodgkin disease. (Richard Paltauf, 1858-1924, Austrian pathologist; Carl von Sternberg, 1872-1935, German)

PANAMA DISEASE, see Chagres disease.

PANAS OPERATION, insertion of the upper eyelid into the frontalis muscle in cases of blepharoptosis.

1. Maffei WE: Os Fundamentos da Medicina. 2nd ed. Livraria Editora Artes Médicas Ltda, 1978

PANCOAST OPERATION, section of the second division of the trigeminal nerve when it is outside of the cranial cavity.

1. Maffei WE: Os Fundamentos da Medicina. 2nd ed. Livraria Editora Artes Médicas Ltda, 1978

PANCOAST SYNDROME, neoplasms at the extreme apex of the lung may invade contiguous structures. Pain is the most common initial complaint, usually in the shoulder, scapular, or interscapular area, upper anterior chest, arm and neck, or axilla. Cross-references: Hare syndrome; Superior sulcus tumor syndrome. (Henry K. Pancoast, 1875-1939, U.S. radiologist)

1. Bennett JC, Plum F (eds): Cecil Textbook of Medicine. 20th ed. Philadelphia: WB Saunders, 1996
2. Pancoast HK: Superior pulmonary sulcus tumor. JAMA 99:1391-1396, 1932

PANCREATIC CHOLERA SYNDROME, see Verner-Morrison syndrome.

PANCREATICOHEPATIC SYNDROME, see Zieve syndrome.

PANCYTOPENIA-DYSMELIA SYNDROME, see Fanconi anemia.

PANDY TEST, PANDY REACTION, a measurement to determine the presence of proteins in the spinal fluid. (Kalman Pandy, Hungarian neurologist)

1. Stedman's Medical Dictionary. 26th ed. Baltimore: Williams & Wilkins, 1995

PANNER DISEASE, juvenile metatarsophalangeal deformans osteochondritis. (Hans Panner, 1871-1930, Danish radiologist)

1. Köhler A: Munch Med Wochenschr 87:1289-1290, 1920

PAPATASI FEVER, phlebotomus fever; an acute, self limiting, flu-like illness of 2-4 days' duration which is transmitted by the bite of infected *Phlebotomus* sandflies. Cross-reference: Sandfly fever.

1. Bennett JC, Plum F (eds): Cecil Textbook of Medicine. 20th ed. Philadelphia: WB Saunders, 1996

PAPILLON-LEFÈVRE SYNDROME, congenital palmoplantar keratosis; a rare autosomal recessive trait manifested by psoriasiform hyperkeratosis of the palms and soles, gingival inflammation that destroys the periodontal ligaments to produce almost complete absence of teeth, and ectopic calcification in the skull. Cross-references: Haim-Munk syndrome; Keratoderma palmoplantar syndrome. (M.M. Papillon, French dermatologist; Paul Lefèvre, French dermatologist)

1. Gorlin RJ, Cohen MM Jr, Levin LS: Syndromes of the Head and Neck. 3rd ed. New York: Oxford University Press, 1990
2. Haim S, Munk J: Br J Dermatol 77:42-54, 1965
3. Papillon MM; Lefèvre P: Deux cas de kératodermie palmaire et plantaire symétrique familiale. Bull Soc Fr Dermatol Syph 31:82-87, 1924

PARACENTRAL LOBULE SYNDROME, includes a spastic paresis or paralysis of both lower extremities and urinary incontinence. May be mistaken for a spinal cord injury and is generally due to a meningioma arising from the falx and extending laterally into the right and left paracentral lobes.

1. Baker AB, Baker LH: Clinical Neurology. Revised ed. Philadelphia: Harper & Row, 1982

PARADOXICAL ANKLE REFLEX, tapping the anterior aspect of the ankle joint produces plantar flexion of the foot.

1. Baker AB, Baker LH: Clinical Neurology. Revised ed. Philadelphia: Harper & Row, 1982

PARADOXICAL BABINSKI SIGN, plantar flexion of the great toes in response to stimulation of the soles of the feet. (Joseph F.F. Babinski, 1857-1932, French neurologist)

1. Grinker RR, Sahs AL: Neurology. 6th ed. Springfield: Charles C Thomas, 1966

PARADOXICAL DIAPHRAGM PHENOMENON, the diaphragm on the affected side rises during inspiration and falls during expiration; seen in the patient with phrenic nerve paralysis and eventration.

1. Dorland's Medical Dictionary. 28th ed. Philadelphia: WB Saunders, 1994

PARAMEDIAN BULBAR SYNDROME, occlusion of the paramedian branches of the vertebral artery or of the anterior spinal artery or its branches; results in paralysis of the ipsilateral side of the tongue and hemiplegia involving the contralateral side of the body, with predominant involvement of the upper limb.

1. Baker AB, Baker LH: Clinical Neurology. Revised ed. Philadelphia: Harper & Row, 1982
2. Division C: Syndrome of the anterior spinal artery of the medulla oblongata. Arch Neurol Psychiatry 37:91, 1937

PARAMEDIAN MIDBRAIN SYNDROME, the vessels of concern here are predominantly the proximal branches of the posterior cerebral artery that reach the paramedian midbrain by penetrating the posterior perforated substance.

1. Baker AB, Baker LH: Clinical Neurology. Revised ed. Philadelphia: Harper & Row, 1982
2. Haymaker W: Bing's Local Diagnosis in Neurological Diseases. 15th ed. St Louis: CV Mosby, 1969

PARAMEDIAN PONS SYNDROME, in the field supplied by the paramedian arteries, focal lesions due to vascular disease are common and are often limited to the more dorsal part of the pars basilaris pontes. Rarely, a lesion thus induced is more or less limited to pyramidal bundles (in the form of a large lacuna), giving rise contralaterally to paresis, then spasticity, of the limbs and paresis of the tongue.

1. Haymaker W: Bing's Local Diagnosis in Neurological Diseases. 15th ed. St Louis: CV Mosby, 1969

PARAMETHADIONE SYNDROME, see Fetal trimethadione syndrome.

PARANEOPLASTIC SYNDROME, the systemic effects of cancer, including cachexia, cutaneous manifestations, neuromyopathies, ectopic hormone production, hypertrophic osteoarthropathy, hematologic-hemostatic abnormalities, renal manifestations, and fever. Some tumor markers have been identified.

1. Bennett JC, Plum F (eds): Cecil Textbook of Medicine. 20th ed. Philadelphia: WB Saunders, 1996
2. Campbell MF, Walsh PC: Campbell's Urology. 5th ed. Philadelphia: WB Saunders, 1986

PARAPHILIAC SYNDROME, men with severe sexual deviance who experience recurrent fantasies about deviant sex, intense sexual cravings, and stereotyped behavioral responses who act out their fantasies. These individuals most often engage in homosexual or heterosexual pedophilia or exhibitionism.

1. Wilson JD, Foster DW, Kronenberg HM, et al (eds): Williams Textbook of Endocrinology. 9th ed. Philadelphia: WB Saunders, 1998

PARASELLAR SYNDROME, lesions causing this can stem from a neoplasm (primary intracranial tumor or metastatic tumor), arterial aneurysm, or inflammation (herpes zoster, Tolosa-Hunt syndrome, temporal arteritis, Wegener granulomatosis, or syphilis).

1. Rowland LP (ed): Merritt's Textbook of Neurology. 9th ed. Baltimore: Williams & Wilkins, 1995

PARATRIGEMINAL SYNDROME, see Raeder syndrome.

PARDEE SIGN, changes in ST and RT waves or downward deflection of the T wave; seen in recovery from myocardial infarction.

1. Casas EC: Diccionario Terminologico de Ciencias Medicas. 5th ed. Salvat Editores, SA, 1954

PARÉ OPERATION, for cleft lip, using sutures in the form of a figure eight. (Ambroise Paré, 1510-1590, French surgeon)

1. Maffei WE: Os Fundamentos da Medicina. 2nd ed. Livraria Editora Artes Médicas Ltda, 1978

PARIETAL LOBE SYNDROME, lesions of the left parietal operculum lead to conduction aphasia, often associated with facial apraxia and bilateral limb apraxia. This term is applied in the literature to an astonishing array of remarkable clinical pictures.

1. Bennett JC, Plum F (eds): Cecil Textbook of Medicine. 20th ed. Philadelphia: WB Saunders, 1996

PARINAUD OCULOGLANDULAR SYNDROME, a general term applied to conjunctivitis, most often unilateral and of the follicular type, and followed by tenderness and enlargement of the preauricular lymph nodes; often caused by infection with a lepothrix, or may be associated with other infections, such as cat-scratch fever, lymphogranuloma venereum, or tularemia. (Henri Parinaud, 1844-1905, French)

1. Parinaud H, Galezowski X: Ann Ocul 101:252-253, 1889

PARINAUD SYNDROME, when afferent pathways from the light reflex and the cerebral eye fields are blocked by lesions impinging on the pretectal area and the midbrain tegmentum, wide light-fixed pupils and loss of upward gaze are noted. Nystagmus and hydrocephalus is common. (Henri Parinaud)

1. Baker AB, Baker LH: Clinical Neurology. Revised ed. Philadelphia: Harper & Row, 1982
2. Grinker RR, Sahs AL: Neurology. 6th ed. Springfield: Charles C Thomas, 1966
3. Parinaud H: Paralisie des mouvements associes des yeux. Arch Neurol 5:145-172, 1883

PARIS DISEASE, acrodynia.

1. Casas EC: Diccionario Terminologico de Ciencias Medicas. 5th ed. Salvat Editores, SA, 1954

PARKE SYNDROME, hyperammonemia acidosis, causing vomiting, in children.

1. Casas EC: Diccionario Terminologico de Ciencias Medicas. 5th ed. Salvat Editores, SA, 1954

PARKINSON DISEASE, a major manifestation characterized by tremor, muscular rigidity, and loss of postural reflexes. One of the most frequently encountered of all the basal ganglia disorders and a

193

leading cause of neurological disability in individuals older than 60 years. No definable cause has been uncovered. (James Parkinson, 1755-1824, British)

1. Grinker RR, Sahs AL: Neurology. 6th ed. Springfield: Charles C Thomas, 1966
2. Parkinson J: An Essay on the Shaking Palsy. London: Sherwood, Neeley-Jones, 1817
3. Ritchie AC: Boyd's Textbook of Pathology. 9th ed. Philadelphia: Lea & Febiger, 1990

PARKINSON SIGN, masked facies; seen in the patient with Parkinson disease. (James Parkinson)

1. Casas EC: Diccionario Terminologico de Ciencias Medicas. 5th ed. Salvat Editores, SA, 1954

PARROT FEVER, psittacosis; an infection of birds produced by the obligate intracellular bacterium *Chlamydia psittaci.* When transmitted to humans, it can produce asymptomatic infection, a transient influenza-like illness, or a serious pneumonia-like disease characterized by high fever, headache, cough, myalgia, pulmonary infiltrates, and significant mortality.

1. Bennett JC, Plum F (eds): Cecil Textbook of Medicine. 20th ed. Philadelphia: WB Saunders, 1996

PARROT SIGN, dilatation of the pupils when the neck skin is pinched; seen in the patient with meningitis. (Joseph M.J. Parrot, 1829-1883, French)

1. Casas EC: Diccionario Terminologico de Ciencias Medicas. 5th ed. Salvat Editores, SA, 1954

PARRY DISEASE, see Graves disease. (Caleb Parry, 1755-1822, British)

PARRY-ROMBERG SYNDROME, see Romberg syndrome. (Caleb Parry; Moritz H. Romberg, 1795-1873, German)

PARSONAGE-TURNER SYNDROME, slow, painless weakness and wasting of the muscles of the shoulder girdle, due to denervation of the affected muscles. An unusual chronic and painless variant of idiopathic brachial plexus neuropathy.

1. J Neurol Neurosurg Psychiatr 46, 1983
2. Parsonage MJ, Turner JWA: Neuralgic amyotrophy, the shoulder-girdle syndrome. Lancet 1:973-978, 1948

PARTIAL TRISOMY 10Q SYNDROME, trisomy 10q24-qter; affects the distal segment of the long arm of chromosome 10. Ptosis, short palpebral fissures, and camptodactyly are features.

1. Smith DW, Jones KL: Recognizable Patterns of Human Malformations: Genetic, Embryologic, and Clinical Aspects. 3rd ed. Philadelphia: WB Saunders, 1982
2. Yunis JJ, et al: A new syndrome resulting from partial trisomy for the distal third of the long arm of chromosome 10. J Pediatr 84:567-570, 1974

PARTINGTON SYNDROME, see Russell-Silver syndrome.

PASCHUTIN DISEASE, neural degeneration in diabetics.

1. Casas EC: Diccionario Terminologico de Ciencias Medicas. 5th ed. Salvat Editores, SA, 1954

PASQUALINI SYNDROME, see Female eunich syndrome.

PASSAVANT OPERATION, staphylopharyngorrhaphy.

1. Maffei WE: Os Fundamentos da Medicina. 2nd ed. Livraria Editora Artes Médicas Ltda, 1978

PASTIA SIGN, areas of hyperpigmentation occur, occasionally with tiny petechiae, in the creases or folds of the joints, particularly in the antecubital fossae; seen in the patient with scarlet fever rash. Cross-reference: Thomson sign. (Chessec Pastia, Romanian)

1. Krugman S, Katz SL: Infectious Disease of Children. 7th ed. St Louis: CV Mosby, 1981

PATAU SYNDROME, see Trisomy 13 syndrome. (Klaus Patau, U.S. geneticist)

PATELLA DISEASE, pyloric stenosis in a patient with tuberculosis. (Vincenzo Patella, 1856-1928, Italian)

1. Casas EC: Diccionario Terminologico de Ciencias Medicas. 5th ed. Salvat Editores, SA, 1954

PATELLAR TAP, a pathognomonic sign; while in the horizontal position, a considerable amount of excessive synovial fluid gravitates into the suprapatellar pouch. With one hand placed above the patella, downward and backward pressure is exerted on the suprapatellar pouch, and the fluid is driven into the knee joint proper. With the index finger of the other hand, the patella with a sharp, jerky movement is depressed. Should the characteristic tap be felt, it is proof of the existence of excessive fluid in the joint.

1. Lumley JS, Clain A: Hamilton Bailey's Demonstration of Physical Signs in Clinical Surgery. 18th ed. London: Butterworth-Heinemann, 1997

PATERSON-BROWN-KELLY SYNDROME, see Plummer-Vinson syndrome. (Donald Paterson, 1863-1939, British ear, nose, throat surgeon; Adam Brown-Kelly, 1865-1941, British ear, nose, throat surgeon)

PATINO-MAYER SIGN, when more than 30% lymphocytes are found in the blood without fever, syphilis may be suspected.

    1. Casas EC: Diccionario Terminologico de Ciencias Medicas. 5th ed. Salvat Editores, SA, 1954

PATON SYNDROME, see Foster-Kennedy syndrome.

PATRICK SIGN, consists of pain in the hip when the heel or the external malleolus of the painful extremity is placed upon the opposite knee and the thigh is pressed downward. (Hugh T. Patrick, 1860-1938, U.S. neurologist)

    1. Baker AB, Baker LH: Clinical Neurology. Revised ed. Philadelphia: Harper & Row, 1982

PAUL SIGN, pain following pressure on the inside of the foot; occurs if postoperative thrombosis is imminent. (Constantin C.T. Paul, 1833-1896)

    1. Casas EC: Diccionario Terminologico de Ciencias Medicas. 5th ed. Salvat Editores, SA, 1954

PAUZAT DISEASE, periostitis of the bones of the feet. (Jean Pauzat, French)

    1. Pauzat JE: Arch Med Pharm Milit 10:337-353, 1887

PAVY DISEASE, cyclic albuminuria. (Frederick Pavy, 1829-1911, British)

    1. Pavy F: Lancet 2:706-708, 1885

PAXTON DISEASE, tinea caused by *Trichorrhexis nodosa*. (Francis V. Paxton, 1840-1924, British)

    1. Paxton F: J Cutan Med 3:133-136, 1869

PAYR SIGN, 1) with the patient in the Turkish seated position, the examiner applies downward pressure on the knee joint. If pain is on the medial side of the joint, the sign is positive, indicating a lesion of the posterior horn of the medial meniscus; 2) a pilomotor reflex caused by irritation of the skin in adrenal failure. (Erwin Payr, 1871-1946, German surgeon)

    1. Evans RC: Illustrated Essentials in Orthopedic Physical Assessment. St Louis: Mosby Yearbook, 1994

PEARSON SYNDROME, see Kearns-Sayre syndrome.

PEDUNCULAR SYNDROME, results from occlusion of a branch artery to the basis pedunculi that passes through the decussation of the brachium conjunctivum to reach the tegmentum, the oculomotor nucleus, and the medial longitudinal fasciculus. Hemiataxia and hemiasynergia ipsilaterally, coarse tremor contralaterally, and conjugate ocular palsies of variable degree are features.

    1. Baker AB, Baker LH: Clinical Neurology. Revised ed. Philadelphia: Harper & Row, 1982

PEELING SKIN SYNDROME, the disease has been associated marked erythema with scaling, serpiginous borders, and hairs that are easily removed from the scalp. Autosomal recessive inheritance.

    1. Moschella SL, Hurley HJ: Dermatology. 2nd ed. Philadelphia: WB Saunders, 1985

PEET OPERATION, for arterial hypertension; subdiaphragmatic ablation of the splanchnic nerves and 9th, 10th, 11th, and 12th thoracic ganglia.

    1. Maffei WE: Os Fundamentos da Medicina. 2nd ed. Livraria Editora Artes Médicas Ltda, 1978

PEL-EBSTEIN DISEASE, irregular episodes of pyrexia of several days' duration, with intervening periods in which the temperature is normal; often seen in Hodgkin disease. Cross-references: Ebstein-Pel disease; Murchison-Pel-Ebstein disease. (Pieter Pel, 1852-1919, Dutch; Wilhelm Ebstein, 1836-1912, German)

    1. Ebstein W: Berl Klin Wochenschr 22:31-37, 1885; 24:565-568, 1887

PELGER-HUËT NUCEAR ANOMALY, neutrophils showing abnormalities in nuclear segmentation, most frequently in the bilobed nucleus. (Karel Pelger, 1885-1931, Dutch; G.J. Huët, 1879-1970, Dutch)

    1. Pelger K: Ned Tschr Geneeskd 72:1179, 1928

PELIZAEUS-MERZBACHER DISEASE, a rare variety of leukodystrophy, distinguished by its onset early in infancy with prominent nystagmus and cerebellar signs, its exceedingly slow rate of progression, and a characteristic pattern of inheritance. X-linked recessive trait. (Friedrich Pelizaeus, 1850-1917, German neurologist; Ludwig Merzbacher, 1875-1942, German physician in Argentina)

    1. Garg BP, Markand ON, DeMyer WE: Usefulness of BAER studies in early diagnosis of Pelizaeus-Merzbacher disease. Neurology 33:955-956, 1983

    2. Merzbacher L: Med Klin Berl 4:1952-1955, 1908

    3. Pelizaeus F: Arch Psychiatr Berl 16:698-710, 1885

PELLEGRINI DISEASE, PELLEGRINI-STIEDA SYNDROME, calcification of the medial collateral ligament of the knee. Cross-references: Köhler-Pellegrini-Stieda syndrome; Stieda syndrome.

(Augusto Pellegrini, Italian surgeon; Alfred Stieda, 1869-1945, German surgeon)

1. Brantigan OC, Voshell AF: The tibial collateral ligament: its function, its bursae, and its relation to the medial meniscus. J Bone Joint Surg 25:121-131, 1943
2. Pellegrini A: Ossificazione traumatica del legamento collaterale tibiale dell'articulazione del ginocchio sinistro. Clin Mod Firenze 11:433-439, 1905

PELLETIER-LEISTI SYNDROME, a congenital condition characterized by unusual facies, short stature, and a hypoplastic penis. Cross-reference: Floating-harbor syndrome.

1. Gorlin RJ, Cohen MM Jr, Levin LS: Syndromes of the Head and Neck. 3rd ed. New York: Oxford University Press, 1990
2. Leisti J, et al: Case report 12. Syndrome Ident 2(1):3-5, 1974

PELLIZZI SYNDROME, see Epiphyseal syndrome. (G.B. Pellizzi, Italian)

PELVIC CONGESTION SYNDROME, an ill-defined syndrome marked by the presence of consistent lower abdominal pain accentuated at the time of the menses and associated with low back pain, dyspareunia, and discomfort on prolonged sitting or standing. Also often associated with varying degrees of premenstrual tension and systemic signs and symptoms.

1. Kase NG, Weingold AB: Principles and Practice of Clinical Gynecology. New York: John Wiley & Sons, 1983

PEMBERTON SIGN, if the size of the thoracic inlet is already reduced by a retrosternal goiter, raising both arms until they touch the sides of the head further narrows the thoracic inlet and causes venous congestion in the face; seen in mediastinal obstruction lymphoma secondary to lymphoma or tumor. (John J. de Pemberton, 1887-1967, U.S. surgeon)

1. Wilson JD, Foster DW, Kronenberg HM, et al (eds): Williams Textbook of Endocrinology. 9th ed. Philadelphia: WB Saunders, 1998

PEMPHIGUS, a disease of the skin and mucosa. The vulgaris and vegetans forms affect the oral mucosa. The former occurs primarily in middle age and is said to be more frequent in those of Jewish, Italian, Greek, and Arab heritage, possibly being related to an immunological mechanism.

1. Ballenger JJ: Diseases of the Nose, Throat, Ear, Head and Neck. 12th ed. Philadelphia: Lea & Febiger, 1977

PEN-TOUCHING TEST, a measurement of the abductor pollicis brevis muscle. The patient places the affected hand flat upon a table, palm uppermost with the thumb straight and resting on the table or as near to the table as possible. While holding a pen or pencil, the examiner rests a hand upon the patient's outstretched fingers (to keep them flat). Patient is told to touch the pen with the edge of his thumb.

1. Lumley JS, Clain A: Hamilton Bailey's Demonstration of Physical Signs in Clinical Surgery. 18th ed. London: Butterworth-Heinemann, 1997

PENA-SHOKEIR SYNDROME, Type I: neurogenic arthrogryposis, pulmonary hypoplasia, and hypertelorism are features. Type II: neurogenic arthrogryposis, microcephaly, microphthalmia, and/or cataract are features. Autosomal recessive inheritance. Cross-reference: Cerebro-oculo-facial-skeletal syndrome. (Sergio D.J. Pena, Canadian; M.H.K. Shokeir, Canadian)

1. Pena SDJ, Shokeir MKH: Autosomal recessive cerebro-oculo-facio-skeletal (COFS) syndrome. Clin Genet 5:285-293, 1974
2. Pena SDJ, Shokeir MKH: Syndrome of camptodactyly, multiple ankyloses, facial anomalies, and pulmonary hypoplasia: a lethal condition. J Pediatr 85:373-375, 1974
3. Smith DW, Jones KL: Recognizable Patterns of Human Malformations: Genetic, Embryologic, and Clinical Aspects. 3rd ed. Philadelphia: WB Saunders, 1982

PENCHASZADEH SYNDROME, consists of striking facies characterized by congenital symmetrical, round to ovoid lipomas of the upper eyelids, lipomas of the nasopalpebral region, and bilateral symmetrical coloboma of both upper and lower eyelids at the junction of the inner and middle third of the lids. In addition, the upper and, less often, the lower lacrimal puncta are malpositioned or occasionally absent, with resultant epiphora. Autosomal dominant inheritance. Cross-reference: Nasopalpebral lipoma-coloboma syndrome.

1. Gorlin RJ, Cohen MM Jr, Levin LS: Syndromes of the Head and Neck. 3rd ed. New York: Oxford University Press, 1990
2. Penchaszadeh VB, et al: The nasopalpebral lipoma-coloboma syndrome: a new autosomal dominant dysplasia-malformation syndrome with congenital nasopalpebral lipomas, eyelids coloboma, telecanthus and maxillary hypoplasia. Am J Med Genet 11:397-410, 1982

PENDE OPERATION, resection of the left splanchnic nerves for treatment of hypertension in cases of suprarenalism.

1. Maffei WE: Os Fundamentos da Medicina. 2nd ed. Livraria Editora Artes Médicas Ltda, 1978

PENDE SIGN, see André Thomas sign.

PENDRED SYNDROME, a familial disorder in which there is congenital hearing loss and goiter. A pool of intrathyroid iodine may be discharged by thiocyanate or perchlorate. Physical and mental development is normal. (Vaughan Pendred, 1869-1946, British)

1. Farmer TW: Pediatric Neurology. 2nd ed. Hagerstown: Harper & Row, 1975
2. Pendred V: Deaf-mutism and goiter. Lancet 2:532, 1896
3. Wilson JD, Foster DW, Kronenberg HM, et al (eds): Williams Textbook of Endocrinology. 9th ed. Philadelphia: WB Saunders, 1998

PENTA-X SYNDROME, a hereditary syndrome characterized by the presence of 49,XXXXX chromosones; severe prenatal and postnatal growth retardation and mental retardation are invariable findings. Cross-reference: XXXXX syndrome.

1. Smith DW, Jones KL: Recognizable Patterns of Human Malformations: Genetic, Embryologic, and Clinical Aspects. 3rd ed. Philadelphia: WB Saunders, 1982
2. Wilson JD, Foster DW, Kronenberg HM, et al (eds): Williams Textbook of Endocrinology. 9th ed. Philadelphia: WB Saunders, 1998

PERCUSSION (TAP) SIGN, with the patient erect, the fingers of the examiner's left hand are placed just below the saphenous vein opening. The main bundle of varicosities is percussed once with the right middle finger. When valves within the segment under review are incompetent, there is no barrier to the upward wave of blood and an impulse is felt by the fingers overlying the long saphenous vein above.

1. Lumley JS, Clain A: Hamilton Bailey's Demonstration of Physical Signs in Clinical Surgery. 18th ed. London: Butterworth-Heinemann, 1997

PÉREZ SIGN, a friction-like sound in the sternum when the patient gets up and puts one arm by the side; seen in the patient with mediastinal tumor or aortic arch aneurysm. (Jorjen V. Pérez, 1851-1920, Spanish)

1. Casas EC: Diccionario Terminologico de Ciencias Medicas. 5th ed. Salvat Editores, SA, 1954

PERHEENTUPA SYNDROME, see MULIBREY-nanism syndrome. (Jaakko Perheentupa, Finnish)

PERICOLIC MEMBRANE SYNDROME, symptoms resemble those of chronic appendicitis such as symptoms due to the pressure of pericolic membranes.

1. Dorland's Medical Dictionary. 28th ed. Philadelphia: WB Saunders, 1994

PERIER OPERATION, eversion and resection of the uterus using an elastic ligature.

1. Maffei WE: Os Fundamentos da Medicina. 2nd ed. Livraria Editora Artes Médicas Ltda, 1978

PERNIO SYNDOME, see Immersion foot syndrome.

PERONEAL SIGN, see Lust sign.

PERREACTIVE SPLEEN SYNDROME, see Tropical splenomegaly syndrome.

PERRET SIGN, see Parrot sign.

PERRIN-FERRATON DISEASE, coxarthropathy or snapping hip. Cross-reference: Morel-Lavallée disease. (Maurice Perrin, 1826-1889, French surgeon; Louis Ferraton, French surgeon)

1. Casas EC: Diccionario Terminologico de Ciencias Medicas. 5th ed. Salvat Editores, SA, 1954

PERRONCITO SIGN, tympanism and pain upon palpation of the duodenal region; seen in the patient with hookworm. (Aldo Perroncito, 1882-1929, Italian histologist)

1. Casas EC: Diccionario Terminologico de Ciencias Medicas. 5th ed. Salvat Editores, SA, 1954

PERSISTENT MÜLLERIAN DUCT SYNDROME, the patient has bilateral fallopian tubes, a uterus, and an upper vagina, with variable development of the vas deferens; penile development is normal and cryptorchidism common. The patient commonly presents with inguinal hernia that contains the uterus.

1. Campbell MF, Walsh PC: Campbell's Urology. 5th ed. Philadelphia: WB Saunders, 1986
2. Nilson O: Hernia uteri inguinalis. Acta Chir Scand 83:231-249, 1939

PERTHES DISEASE, see Legg disease. (Georg Perthes, 1869-1927, German surgeon)

PERTUSSIS SYNDROME, PERTUSSIS-LIKE SYNDROME, a syndrome indistinguishable from pertussis, but in which there is no infection with *Bordetella pertussis* or *B. parapertussis*; evidence of other infectious agents, such as adenoviruses types 1, 2, 3, 5, and 6, can be demonstrated.

1. Dorland's Medical Dictionary. 28th ed. Philadelphia: WB Saunders, 1994

PETER SYNDROME, see Oculodentodigital syndrome.

PETERSEN OPERATION, a method for suprapubic lithotomy.
1. Maffei WE: Os Fundamentos da Medicina. 2nd ed. Livraria Editora Artes Médicas Ltda, 1978

PETIT DISEASE, diaphragmatic eventration.
1. Casas EC: Diccionario Terminologico de Ciencias Medicas. 5th ed. Salvat Editores, SA, 1954

PETRUSCHKI [PETRUSCHKY] SIGN, pain on percussion of the 1st thoracic vertebra; seen in the patient with tracheobronchial adenopathy. (Johannes Petruschki [Petruschky], German bacteriologist)
1. Casas EC: Diccionario Terminologico de Ciencias Medicas. 5th ed. Salvat Editores, SA, 1954

PEUTZ-JEGHERS SYNDROME, PEUTZ-JEGHERS-TOURAINE SYNDROME, a rare familial disorder associated with recurrent abdominal pain and characterized by intestinal polyposis and mucocutaneous pigmentation. Autosomal dominant transmission. (John L.A. Peutz, 1866-1957, Dutch; Harold J. Jeghers, U.S.)
1. Bennett JC, Plum F (eds): Cecil Textbook of Medicine. 20th ed. Philadelphia: WB Saunders, 1996
2. Jeghers H, McKusick VA, Katz KH: Generalized intestinal polyposis and melanin spots of the oral mucosa lips and digits: syndrome of clinical significance. N Engl J Med 241:993-1005, 1031-1036, 1949
3. Peutz JLA: Ned Monatsschr Genesk 10:134-136, 1921

PEYRONIE DISEASE, penile fibromatosis; affects middle-aged men and consists of a fibrous mass localized on the dorsum of the penis but may also involve the ventral or lateral surfaces. Painful erections, with deformities, result from the abnormal curvature caused by the mass. (François de la Peyronie, 1678-1747, French surgeon)
1. Campbell MF, Walsh PC: Campbell's Urology. 5th ed. Philadelphia: WB Saunders, 1986
2. De la Peyronie F: Mem Acad Chir 1:42, 1743

PFANNENSTIEL DISEASE, familial jaundice in the newborn. (Hermann J. Pfannenstiel, 1862-1909, German gynecologist)
1. Casas EC: Diccionario Terminologico de Ciencias Medicas. 5th ed. Salvat Editores, SA, 1954

PFANNENSTIEL INCISION, an incision used in gynecological operations, mostly on young patients, for better cosmetic results. (Hermann J. Pfannenstiel)
1. Schwartz SI: Principles of Surgery. 4th ed. New York: McGraw-Hill, 1983

PFAUNDLER-HURLER SYDNROME, see Hurler syndrome. (Meinhard von Pfaundler, 1872-1947, German pediatrician; Gertrud Hurler, 1889-1965, German)

PFEIFFER-TYPE CARDIOCRANIAL SYNDROME, sagittal synostosis, facial dysmorphism, and complex cardiovascular malformations are features.
1. Gorlin RJ, Cohen MM Jr, Levin LS: Syndromes of the Head and Neck. 3rd ed. New York: Oxford University Press, 1990

PFEIFFER-TYPE DOLICHOCEPHALOSYNDACTYLY SYNDROME, sagittal synostosis, facial dysmorphism, genitourinary anomalies, and limb defects are features.
1. Gorlin RJ, Cohen MM Jr, Levin LS: Syndromes of the Head and Neck. 3rd ed. New York: Oxford University Press, 1990

PFEIFFER-TYPE SYNDROME, acrocephalosyndactyly type V or acrocephalopolysyndactyly type I; brachycephaly, mild syndactyly, broad short thumbs, and big toes are features. Autosomal recessive inheritance. Cross-reference: Noack syndrome. (Rudolf A. Pfeiffer, German)
1. Noack M: Arch Kinderheilkd 160:168-171, 1959
2. Pfeiffer RA: Z Kinderheilkd 90:301-320, 1964

PFUHL SIGN, PFUHL-JAFFÉ SIGN, in the patient with a subphrenic abscess, liquid is expelled under pressure during inspiration, but not in the case of pyopneumothorax. Only valid in the nonparalyzed diaphragm. Cross-reference: Jaffé sign. (Eduard Pfuhl, 1852-1905, German; Max Jaffé, 1841-1911, German physiological chemist)
1. Casas EC: Diccionario Terminologico de Ciencias Medicas. 5th ed. Salvat Editores, SA, 1954

PHALEN SIGN, the patient is instructed to flex both wrists to an extreme degree and maintain this position for 1 minute. In instances of compression neuropathy, there is usually prompt exacerbation of the numbness and paresthesias in the median distribution of the hand. Cross-reference: Prayer sign.
1. Evans RC: Illustrated Essentials in Orthopedic Physical Assessment. St Louis: Mosby-Yearbook, 1994
2. Grinker RR, Sahs AL: Neurology. 6th ed. Springfield: Charles C Thomas, 1966

PHARYNGEAL POUCH SYNDROME, see DiGeorge syndrome.

PHC SYNDROME, *p*remature *h*ereditary *c*anities (PHC); see Böök syndrome.

PHENOMENON OF GRASSET AND GAUSSEL, a patient with pyramidal lesions may be able to raise either leg separately but cannot raise both simultaneously. If the paretic leg is raised first, it falls back heavily as soon as the patient attempts to raise the normal one or if the normal is passively raised; this is the result of an inability to steady the pelvic muscles on the paretic side. If the patient first raises the normal leg and then the paretic leg is raised passively, the sound leg remains elevated and is held in place by the fixed pelvic muscles on that side. (Joseph Grasset, 1849-1918, French; Amans Gaussel, 1871-1937, French)
    1. Baker AB, Baker LH: Clinical Neurology. Revised ed. Philadelphia: Harper & Row, 1982

PHI PHENOMENON, the sequential flashing of a stationary row of light is perceived as moving.
    1. Dorland's Medical Dictionary. 28th ed. Philadelphia: WB Saunders, 1994

PHILAGRIUS OPERATION, ligation and extirpation of aneurysms. Cross-reference: Purmann method.
    1. Maffei WE: Os Fundamentos da Medicina. 2nd ed. Livraria Editora Artes Médicas Ltda, 1978

PHILLIPS-GRIFFITHS SYNDROME, cleft palate, macular coloboma, short stature, and skeletal abnormalities are features. (C.I. Phillips, British ophthalmologist)
    1. Phillips CI, Griffiths DL: Macular coloboma and skeletal abnormalities. Br J Ophthalmol 53:346-349, 1969

PHILLIPSON REFLEX, stimulation of the foot or leg on one side causes flexion of that extremity with an extension response on the contralateral side; an indication of a partial or incomplete spinal lesion. Cross-reference: Crossed extensor reflex.
    1. Baker AB, Baker LH: Clinical Neurology. Revised ed. Philadelphia: Harper & Row, 1982

PHOCAS DISEASE, see Tillaux disease. (B. Gerasime Phocas, 1861-1937, French surgeon)

PHRENIC PHENOMENON, see Litten sign.

PHYSICK OPERATION, extirpation of a circular portion of the iris using special sharpened instruments.
    1. Maffei WE: Os Fundamentos da Medicina. 2nd ed. Livraria Editora Artes Médicas Ltda, 1978

PICCHINI SYNDROME, polyserositis caused by trypanosomiasis.
    1. Casas EC: Diccionario Terminologico de Ciencias Medicas. 5th ed. Salvat Editores, SA, 1954

PICK DISEASE, a degenerative disorder of the cerebral cortex that produces dementia in middle and late life. Distinguishable from Alzheimer disease by its morbid anatomy. (Arnold Pick, 1851-1924, Czech psychiatrist)
    1. Grinker RR, Sahs AL: Neurology. 6th ed. Springfield: Charles C Thomas, 1966
    2. Pick A: Prag Med Wochenschr 17:165-167, 1892
    3. Rowland LP (ed): Merritt's Textbook of Neurology. 9th ed. Baltimore: Williams & Wilkins, 1995

PICK-HERXHEIMER DISEASE, chronic atrophic dermatitis. Cross-reference: Taylor disease. (Phillipp J. Pick, 1834-1910, Czech; Karl Herxheimer, 1861-1944, German)
    1. Herxheimer K, Hartmann K: Arch Derm Syph 61:57-76, 1902

PICKWICKIAN SYNDROME, in some individuals, chronic cardiopulmonary insufficiency is related to obesity and shares many essential features with hypersomnia-sleep apnea syndrome. (Named after Mr. Pickwick from Charles Dickens' "Pickwick Papers." First applied by William Osler.)
    1. Baker AB, Baker LH: Clinical Neurology. Revised ed. Philadelphia: Harper & Row, 1982
    2. Ritchie AC: Boyd's Textbook of Pathology. 9th ed. Philadelphia: Lea & Febiger, 1990

PIEDALLU SIGN, indicates an abnormality in the torsion movement of the sacroiliac joint.
    1. Evans RC: Illustrated Essentials in Orthopedic Physical Assessment. St Louis: Mosby Yearbook, 1994

PIERE OPERATION, vagotomy.
    1. Maffei WE: Os Fundamentos da Medicina. 2nd ed. Livraria Editora Artes Médicas Ltda, 1978

PIERRE MARIE DISEASE, see Marie's ataxia.

PIERRE ROBIN SYNDROME, micrognathia-glossoptosis; the single initiating defect of this disorder may be hypoplasia of the mandibular area prior to 9 weeks in utero, allowing the tongue to be posteriorly located and thereby impairing the closure of the posterior palatal shelves that must "grow over" the tongue to meet in the midline. Cross-reference: Robin syndrome. (Pierre Robin, 1867-1950, French dental surgeon)
    1. Moschella SL, Hurley HJ: Dermatology. 2nd ed. Philadelphia: WB Saunders, 1985

2. Robin P: La glossoptose; son diagnostic, ses consequences, son traitement. J Med (Par) 43:235-237, 1923
3. Smith DW, Jones KL: Recognizable Patterns of Human Malformations: Genetic, Embryologic, and Clinical Aspects. 3rd ed. Philadelphia: WB Saunders, 1982

PIERRET-ROUGIER SYNDROME, psychoses in conjunction with tabes; hallucinations and paranoia are common.

1. Rimbaud L: Compendo de Neurologia. Livraria Editora Freitas Bastos, 1940

PIGMENT DISPERSION SYNDROME, see Alezzandrini syndrome.

PILLAY SYNDROME, consists of corneal opacities, short forearms due to radiohumeral and proximal radioulnar dislocations, and aplasia of the lateral humeral condyle, the head of the radius, and the lower third of the ulna. Cross-reference: Ophthalmomandibulomelic dysplasia syndrome. (V.K. Pillay, orthopedic surgeon in Singapore)

1. Gorlin RJ, Cohen MM Jr, Levin LS: Syndromes of the Head and Neck. 3rd ed. New York: Oxford University Press, 1990
2. Pillay VK, Orth MC: Ophthalmo-mandibulomelic dysplasia. An hereditary syndrome. J Bone Joint Surg (Am) 46:858-862, 1964

PILLORE OPERATION, surgery for reconstruction of an artificial anus, suturing the cecum to the abdominal wall.

1. Maffei WE: Os Fundamentos da Medicina. 2nd ed. Livraria Editora Artes Médicas Ltda, 1978

PILTZ SIGN, PILTZ-WESTPHAL PHENOMENON, contraction of the pupils followed by dilatation after vigorous closure of the eyes. Cross-reference: Westphal-Piltz phenomenon. (Jan Piltz, 1870-1931, Polish neurologist; Alexander K.O. Westphal, 1863-1941, German neurologist)

1. Casas EC: Diccionario Terminologico de Ciencias Medicas. 5th ed. Salvat Editores, SA, 1954

PINARD SIGN, if pain at the fundus of the uterus is present after the 6th month of pregnancy, a buttock presentation is indicated. (Adolphe Pinard, 1844-1934, French obstetrician)

1. Casas EC: Diccionario Terminologico de Ciencias Medicas. 5th ed. Salvat Editores, SA, 1954

PINEAL SYNDROME, see Epiphyseal syndrome.

PINK DISEASE, caused by poisoning with inorganic salts of mercury in infancy. Common when mercurous chloride, calomel, and other inorganic mercurial compounds were administered to infants, but now is rare.

1. Mahaffey KR: Toxicity of lead, cadmium and mercury: consideration for total parenteral nutritional support. Bull NY Acad Med 60:196-209, 1984
2. Ritchie AC: Boyd's Textbook of Pathology. 9th ed. Philadelphia: Lea & Febiger, 1990

PINKUS SIGN, lymphocytosis.

1. Casas EC: Diccionario Terminologico de Ciencias Medicas. 5th ed. Salvat Editores, SA, 1954

PINS SIGN, see Ewart sign.

PIORGOFF OPERATION, disarticulation and amputation of the foot, leaving a portion of the calcaneus.

1. Maffei WE: Os Fundamentos da Medicina. 2nd ed. Livraria Editora Artes Médicas Ltda, 1978

PIOTROWSKI SIGN, if percussion of the anterior tibial muscle produces exaggerated flexion and inversion of the foot, a lesion of the central nervous system is indicated. (Alexander Piotrowski, German neurologist)

1. Casas EC: Diccionario Terminologico de Ciencias Medicas. 5th ed. Salvat Editores, SA, 1954

PIRIFORMIS MUSCLE SYNDROME, the maneuver is reproduced by having the patient lie with the painful side up, the painful leg flexed, and the knee resting on the table. Buttock pain is produced when the patient lifts and holds the knee several inches off the table. Can be diagnosed in the examining room.

1. Beatty RA: The piriformis muscle syndrome: a simple diagnostic maneuver. Neurosurgery 34:512-514, 1994
2. Papadopoulos SM, et al: Unusual cause of "piriformis muscle syndrome." Arch Neurol 47:1144:1990

PISKACEK SIGN, an asymmetric increase in size of the uterus; an indication of pregnancy. (Ludwig Piskacek, 1854-1933, Austrian obstetrician)

1. Casas EC: Diccionario Terminologico de Ciencias Medicas. 5th ed. Salvat Editores, SA, 1954

PITFIELD SIGN, a vibration is perceived by the opposite hand when the abdomen is flicked on one side; an indication of ascites.

1. Casas EC: Diccionario Terminologico de Ciencias Medicas. 5th ed. Salvat Editores, SA, 1954

PITRES SIGN, the absence of a deep pain sensation on squeezing the scrotum and testes; may indicate neurosyphilis. (Jean A. Pitres, 1848-1927, French)

1. Baker AB, Baker LH: Clinical Neurology. Revised ed. Philadelphia: Harper & Row, 1982

PITT-ROGERS-DANKS SYNDROME, features include intrauterine growth retardation, unusual facies, microcephaly, epilepsy, hyperactive behavior, and moderate to severe mental retardation (IQ 35-49). (D.B. Pitt, Australian)

1. Gorlin RJ, Cohen MM Jr, Levin LS: Syndromes of the Head and Neck. 3rd ed. New York: Oxford University Press, 1990
2. Pitt DB, Rogers JG, Danks DM: Mental retardation, unusual facies and intrauterine growth retardation—a new recessive syndrome? Am J Med Genet 19:307-313, 1984

PITTS OPERATION, stretching of the inferior dental nerve through an intraoral incision parallel to the anterior edge of the ascending branch of the mandible.

1. Maffei WE: Os Fundamentos da Medicina. 2nd ed. Livraria Editora Artes Médicas Ltda, 1978

PIZA-MEYER-GOMES DISEASE, exanthematous typhus.

1. Casas EC: Diccionario Terminologico de Ciencias Medicas. 5th ed. Salvat Editores, SA, 1954

PLACENTAL DYSFUNCTION SYNDROME, malnutrition and hypoxia of the fetus due to degenerative changes in the placenta. In the full-blown condition, the nails, skin, and vernix are bright yellow and the umbilical cord is yellow-green.

1. Dorland's Medical Dictionary. 28th ed. Philadelphia: WB Saunders, 1994

PLACENTAL SIGN, endometrial bleeding.

1. Dorland's Medical Dictionary. 28th ed. Philadelphia: WB Saunders, 1994

PLACENTAL TRANSFUSION SYNDROME, the birth of one anemic and one plethoric twin due to forcing of the blood of one fetal twin into the circulation of the other via interconnections between their blood vessels. Cross-references: Intrauterine parabiotic syndrome; Transfusion syndrome.

1. Dorland's Medical Dictionary. 28th ed. Philadelphia: WB Saunders, 1994

PLASTER CAST SYNDROME, see Cast syndrome.

PLATYSMA SIGN, a failure of the platysma muscle to contract on the involved side when the mouth is opened.

1. Mazion JM: llustrated Manual of Neurological Reflexes/Signs/Tests of Office Procedure. 2nd ed. Orlando: Daniels Publishing, 1980

PLAUT DISEASE, PLAUT-VINCENT DISEASE, necrotizing ulcerative gingivostomatitis. Cross-reference: Vincent disease. (Hugo Plaut, 1858-1928, German)

1. Bennett JC, Plum F (eds): Cecil Textbook of Medicine. 20th ed. Philadelphia: WB Saunders, 1996
2. Lumley JS, Clain A: Hamilton Bailey's Demonstration of Physical Signs in Clinical Surgery. 18th ed. London: Butterworth-Heinemann, 1997

PLUMB-LINE SIGN, displacement of the sternum determined using a plumb-line; seen in the diagnosis of pleuritic effusion.

1. Dorland's Medical Dictionary. 28th ed. Philadelphia: WB Saunders, 1994

PLUMMER DISEASE, toxic multinodular goiter, a disease of aging that arises in a simple goiter of long standing. (Henry S. Plummer, 1874-1937, U.S.)

1. Ballenger JJ: Diseases of the Nose, Throat, Ear, Head and Neck. 12th ed. Philadelphia: Lea & Febiger, 1977
2. Plummer HS: Am J Med Sci 146:790-795, 1913

PLUMMER NAILS, a term applied to separation of the distal margin of the nail from the nail bed with irregular recession of the junction (onycholysis).

1. Wilson JD, Foster DW, Kronenberg HM, et al (eds): Williams Textbook of Endocrinology. 9th ed. Philadelphia: WB Saunders, 1998

PLUMMER SIGN, the inability to step up (as in walking up stairs or stepping onto a chair) due to myopathy; seen in the patient with Graves disease. (Henry S. Plummer)

1. Dorland's Medical Dictionary. 28th ed. Philadelphia: WB Saunders, 1994

PLUMMER-VINSON SYNDROME, a syndrome usually occurring in middle-aged women with hypochromic anemia, chiefly characterized by cracks or fissures at the corners of the mouth, painful tongue with atrophy of the filiform and later the fungiform papillae, and dysphagia due to esophageal stenosis or webs. Cross-references: Paterson-Brown-Kelly syndrome; Vinson syndrome. (Henry S. Plummer; Porter P. Vinson, 1890-1959, U.S.)

1. Paterson DR: J Laryngol Otol 34:285-291, 1919
2. Plummer HS: Diffuse dilatation of the esophagus without anatomic stenosis (cardiospasm). A report of ninety-one cases. JAMA 58:2013-2015, 1912
3. Vinson PP: Med Clin North Am 3:623-627, 1919

POEMS SYNDROME, *p*olyneuropathy, *o*rganomegaly, endocrinopathy, *m*onoclonal gammopathy, and *s*kin changes (POEMS). A multisystem syndrome that may include diabetes mellitus, primary gonadal failure, plasma cell dyscrasia, and sclerotic bone lesions. Cross-reference: Crow-Fukase syndrome.

1. Kase NG, Weingold AB: Principles and Practice of Clinical Gynecology. New York: John Wiley & Sons, 1983
2. Wilson JD, Foster DW, Kronenberg HM, et al (eds): Williams Textbook of Endocrinology. 9th ed. Philadelphia: WB Saunders, 1998

POFAIN SYNDROME, dyspepsia with dilatation of the right ventricle and an increase in pulmonary sounds.

1. Casas EC: Diccionario Terminologico de Ciencias Medicas. 5th ed. Salvat Editores, SA, 1954

POINTING TEST, a sign of great value in diagnosing a ruptured intestine. The examiner asks the patient to point with one finger to where the pain is most acute or where it started. The patient may locate accurately the site of the perforation.

1. Lumley JS, Clain A: Hamilton Bailey's Demonstration of Physical Signs in Clinical Surgery. 18th ed. London: Butterworth-Heinemann, 1997

POLAND ANOMALY, POLAND SYNDROME, unilateral absence of the sternocostal head of the pectoralis major muscle and ipsilateral syndactyly. (Alfred Poland, 1820-1872, British surgeon)

1. Poland A: Deficiency of the pectoral muscles. Guys Hosp Rep 6:191-193, 1841

POLHEMUS-SCHAFER-IVEMARK SYNDROME, see Ivemark syndrome.

POLITZER OPERATION, 1) formation of a permanent opening in the tympanic membrane by incision and electrocautery; 2) division of the anterior ligament of the hamate bone.

1. Maffei WE: Os Fundamentos da Medicina. 2nd ed. Livraria Editora Artes Médicas Ltda, 1978

POLLITZER DISEASE, suppurative adenitis.

1. Casas EC: Diccionario Terminologico de Ciencias Medicas. 5th ed. Salvat Editores, SA, 1954

POLLOCK OPERATION, disarticulation of the knee using a posterior short graft and anterior long graft, leaving the patella intact.

1. Maffei WE: Os Fundamentos da Medicina. 2nd ed. Livraria Editora Artes Médicas Ltda, 1978

POLYCYSTIC OVARY SYNDROME, grossly, the ovaries are sometimes enlarged, with a glistening surface and a cortex thickened by excessive collagen deposition. This is the most frequent cause of secondary amenorrhea; it is associated with increased steroid hormone production and comprises a number of different entities. Cross-reference: Stein-Leventhal syndrome.

1. Gold JJ, Josimovich JB: Gynecologic Endocrinology. 3rd ed. New York: Plenum Medical, 1980
2. Leventhal ML: Amenorrhea associated with bilateral polycystic ovaries. Am J Obstet Gynecol 29:181-191, 1935
3. Stein IF: N Engl J Med 259:420-423, 1958

POLYMICROGYRIA SYNDROME, see Zellweger syndrome.

POLYMYALGIA RHEUMATICA SYNDROME, see Horton syndrome.

POLYSPLENIA SYNDROME, multiple splenic masses (two or more), ambiguous abdominal situs, and bilateral left-sidedness are features; while cardiovascular abnormalities are frequent, they are not as severe as seen in Ivemark syndrome.

1. Bennett JC, Plum F (eds): Cecil Textbook of Medicine. 20th ed. Philadelphia: WB Saunders, 1996
2. Moller JH, Nekib A, Anderson RC, et al: Circulation 36:789-799, 1967
3. Smith DW, Jones KL: Recognizable Patterns of Human Malformations: Genetic, Embryologic, and Clinical Aspects. 3rd ed. Philadelphia: WB Saunders, 1982

POLYSYNDACTYLY SYNDROME, consists of preaxial polydactyly and syndactyly. Autosomal dominant inheritance.

1. Anderson CE, Fernhoff PM, Quan L: Dominant polysyndactyly: a report of two families. J Pediatr 90:961, 1977
2. Smith DW, Jones KL: Recognizable Patterns of Human Malformations: Genetic, Embryologic, and Clinical Aspects. 3rd ed. Philadelphia: WB Saunders, 1982

POMPE DISEASE, glycogen storage disease type II; a severe form of glycogen storage disease characterized by the generalized deposition of normal glycogen in the tissues and severe cardiomegaly.

(Johann C. Pompe, Dutch)
1. Bennett JC, Plum F (eds): Cecil Textbook of Medicine. 20th ed. Philadelphia: WB Saunders, 1996
2. Farmer TW: Pediatric Neurology. 2nd ed. Hagerstown: Harper & Row, 1975
3. Pompe JC: Ned Tijdschr Geneeskd 76:304-305, 1932

PONCET OPERATION, 1) stretching of the Achilles tendon to treat foot deformities; 2) perineal urethrostomy.
1. Maffei WE: Os Fundamentos da Medicina. 2nd ed. Livraria Editora Artes Médicas Ltda, 1978

PONCET SIGN, if the patient's saliva is rubbed on a silver coin and smells like garlic, the patient has iodoform poisoning.
1. Casas EC: Diccionario Terminologico de Ciencias Medicas. 5th ed. Salvat Editores, SA, 1954

PONTIAC FEVER, see Legionnaires disease. (Named for Pontiac, Michigan, where an outbreak occurred among occupants of a single building in 1968.)

PONTILE TEGMENTUM SYNDROME, occlusion of the branches of the superior cerebellar artery that penetrate the lateral surface of the midbrain and extend into the rostral pontile tegmentum. Ipsilateral conjugate ocular palsies and cerebellar disturbance are characteristics.
1. Baker AB, Baker LH: Clinical Neurology. Revised ed. Philadelphia: Harper & Row, 1982
2. Haymaker W: Bing's Local Diagnosis in Neurological Diseases. 15th ed. St Louis: CV Mosby, 1969

PONTINE SYNDROME, see Raymond-Céstan syndrome.

POOL PHENOMENON, POOL-SCHLESINGER SIGN, tension on the brachial plexus by forceful elevation and abduction of the arm while the forearm is extended; followed by tetanic spasm of the muscles of the forearm, hand, and fingers (arm phenomenon). Tension on the sciatic nerve by forceful flexion of the thigh on the trunk with the leg in extension is followed by spasm of the muscles of the foot and leg (leg phenomenon). Cross-reference: Schlesinger sign. (Eugene H. Pool, 1874-1949, U.S. surgeon; Hermann Schlesinger, 1868-1934, Austrian)
1. Baker AB, Baker LH: Clinical Neurology. Revised ed. Philadelphia: Harper & Row, 1982

POPLITEAL PTERYGIUM SYNDROME, POPLITEAL WEB SYNDROME, compression of the popliteal artery; symptoms include low birth weight, mental retardation, mild growth retardation, microcephaly, filiform adhesions of the eyelids, corneal ulceration, a hypoplastic nasal tip, microstomia, cleft lip/palate, soft tissue syngnathia, micrognathia, supernumerary nipples, aplastic labia majora, bicornuate uterus, and lanugo hair. Autosomal recessive inheritance. Cross-references: Facio-genito-popliteal syndrome; Fèvre-Languepin syndrome.
1. Fèvre M, Languepin A: Presse Med 70:615-618, 1962
2. Gorlin RJ, et al: Popliteal pterygium syndrome. Pediatrics 41:503-509, 1968

PORRET PHENOMENON, the passage of a continuous current through a living muscle fiber causes undulation proceeding from the positive toward the negative pole. Cross-reference: Kühne muscular phenomenon.
1. Dorland's Medical Dictionary. 28th ed. Philadelphia: WB Saunders, 1994

PORRO-VEIT OPERATION, technique in which the stump is ligated and put back in place.
1. Maffei WE: Os Fundamentos da Medicina. 2nd ed. Livraria Editora Artes Médicas Ltda, 1978

PORTER SIGN, see Oliver-Cardarelli-Olshausen sign. (William H. Porter, 1853-1933, U.S.)

POSADAS DISEASE, POSADAS-WERNICKE DISEASE, coccidioidomycosis. (Alejandro Posadas, 1870-1920, Argentine pathologist; Robert Wernicke, 1854-1922, Argentine pathologist)
1. Casas EC: Diccionario Terminologico de Ciencias Medicas. 5th ed. Salvat Editores, SA, 1954

POSNER-SCHLOSSMAN SYNDROME, characterized by a mild recurrent anterior uveitis associated with an out-of-proportion intraocular pressure spike in the same eye. The cause is unclear. This syndrome affects persons aged between 20-50 years. Some have tried to connect it with primary open-angled glaucoma.
1. Harrington Jr JA: Optom Assoc 70:715-723, 1999
2. Narang SK, et al: Indian J Ophthalmol 70:25-27, 1972

POSTAXIAL POLYDACTYLY-DENTAL-VERTEBRAL SYNDROME, bilateral broad halluces, postaxial polydactyly of the hands and feet, short middle phalanges of the hands, short pointed distal phalanges, and abnormal vertebral bodies are characteristics.
1. Gorlin RJ, Cohen MM Jr, Levin LS: Syndromes of the Head and Neck. 3rd ed. New York: Oxford University Press, 1990

2. Rogers JG, et al: A postaxial polydactyly-dental-vertebral syndrome. J Pediatr 90:230-235, 1977
3. Temtamy S, McKusick V: The genetics of hand malformations. Birth Defects 14(3):411-413, 1978

POSTCARDIOTOMY SYNDROME, a group of symptoms consisting of anxiety, confusion, and perceptual disturbances occurring 2 to 5 days after an operation using cardiopulmonary bypass. Cross-references: Postcommissurotomy syndrome; Postpericardiotomy syndrome.

1. Khan AM: The postcardiac injury surgery. Clin Cardiol 15:67-72, 1992
2. Ritchie AC: Boyd's Textbook of Pathology. 9th ed. Philadelphia: Lea & Febiger, 1990
3. Soloff LA, Zatuchni J, Janton OH, et al: Circulation 8:481-493, 1953

POSTCHOLECYSTECTOMY SYNDROME, the presence of significant abdominal symptoms after cholecystectomy. In the majority of patients, this probably means that the sole gallstone disease was not the cause of their preoperative complaints.

1. Bennett JC, Plum F (eds): Cecil Textbook of Medicine. 20th ed. Philadelphia: WB Saunders, 1996

POSTCOMMISSUROTOMY SYNDROME, see Postcardiotomy syndrome.

POSTCONCUSSION SYNDROME, a constellation of symptoms following head injury, usually including headache, irritability, and a feeling of lightheadedness or dizziness but not true vertigo. Other complaints include difficulty with concentration, worry and apprehension, a preoccupation with self, a lack of interest in others' affairs, mild difficulty with memory, intolerance to loud noises and alcohol, insomnia, and loss of sexual interest. Cross-references: Concussion syndrome; Posttraumatic syndrome.

1. Baker AB, Baker LH: Clinical Neurology. Revised ed. Philadelphia: Harper & Row, 1982
2. Bennett JC, Plum F (eds): Cecil Textbook of Medicine. 20th ed. Philadelphia: WB Saunders, 1996

POSTERIOR CORD SYNDROME, sensory and ataxic phenomena deriving from a lesion of the posterior column of the spinal cord, as in locomotor ataxia.

1. Bennett JC, Plum F (eds): Cecil Textbook of Medicine. 20th ed. Philadelphia: WB Saunders, 1996

POSTERIOR INFERIOR CEREBELLAR ARTERY SYNDROME, see Wallenberg syndrome.

POSTERIOR SPINAL ARTERY SYNDROME, because of damage to the posterior column, vibratory and position sense is likely to be affected, out of proportion to other sensory alterations, and paralysis may be transient and less profound. Clinically, infarctions are much less common but do occur.

1. Baker AB, Baker LH: Clinical Neurology. Revised ed. Philadelphia: Harper & Row, 1982
2. Perier O, Demanet J, Henneaux J, et al: Existe-t-il un syndrome des artères spinales postérieures? A propos de deux observations anatomo-cliniques. Rev Neurol 103:396, 1960

POSTERIOR-THALAMIC SYNDROME, see Déjerine-Roussy syndrome.

POSTEROLATERAL SYNDROME, an ataxic and spasmodic condition due to lesions of the posterolateral elements of the spinal cord.

1. Dorland's Medical Dictionary. 28th ed. Philadelphia: WB Saunders, 1994

POSTGASTRECTOMY SYNDROME, see Afferent loop syndrome.

POSTIRRADIATION SYNDROME, a symptom complex caused by massive radiation exposure, with hemorrhage, anemia, and malnutrition.

1. Dorland's Medical Dictionary. 28th ed. Philadelphia: WB Saunders, 1994

POSTLUMBAR PUNCTURE SYNDROME, several hours after lumbar puncture, headache occurs while the patient is in the erect posture; nuchal pain, nausea, vomiting, diaphoresis, and malaise may also occur and are relieved by recumbency and lasting a few days. Symptoms are similar to those seen in low-pressure headache caused by leakage of cerebrospinal fluid through the needle tract.

1. Dorland's Medical Dictionary. 28th ed. Philadelphia: WB Saunders, 1994

POSTMATURITY SYNDROME, placental dysfunction syndrome occurring in postmature fetuses.

1. Dorland's Medical Dictionary. 28th ed. Philadelphia: WB Saunders, 1994

POSTMYOCARDIAL INFARCTION SYNDROME, see Dressler syndrome.

POSTPARTUM PITUITARY NECROSIS SYNDROME, see Sheehan syndrome.

POSTPERFUSION SYNDROME, a complication occurring about 3 to 6 weeks after extracorporeal circulation or multiple blood transfusions during open heart or other surgical procedures; characteristics include fever, lymphenopathy, and a macular papular rash. Cross-reference: Posttransfusion syndrome.

1. Reyman TA: Postperfusion syndrome. Am Heart J 72:116-123, 1966

POSTPERICARDIOTOMY SYNDROME, see Postcardiotomy syndrome.

POSTPHLEBITIC SYNDROME, about 5% of patients with thrombophlebitis develop venous insufficiency with stasis dermatitis. Cross-reference: Postthrombotic syndrome.
1. Bennett JC, Plum F (eds): Cecil Textbook of Medicine. 20th ed. Philadelphia: WB Saunders, 1996
2. Moschella SL, Hurley HJ: Dermatology. 2nd ed. Philadelphia: WB Saunders, 1985

POSTPOLIO SYNDROME, a patient who had paralytic poliomyelitis early in life and whose neurological deficit had been stable notes increasing weakness years or decades after the initial attack. Often must be differentiated from amyotrophic lateral sclerosis. Over the long term, a patient seem to slowly lose strength, most likely from the additional loss of motor units that had become enlarged and functionally more important with reinnervation.
1. Dalakas MC, Bartfeld H, Kurland G: The post-polio syndrome: advances in the pathogenesis and treatment. Ann NY Acad Sci 753:1-320, 1995
2. Rowland LP (ed): Merritt's Textbook of Neurology. 9th ed. Baltimore: Williams & Wilkins, 1995

POSTPRANDIAL DUMPING SYNDROME, can occur whenever the pyloric mechanism is disrupted either by pyloroplasty, gastroduodenostomy (Billroth I), or gastrojejunostomy (Billroth II). Occurs most often after truncal vagotomy and antrectomy; rarely develops after proximal gastric vagotomy. Cross-reference: Dumping syndrome.
1. Bennett JC, Plum F (eds): Cecil Textbook of Medicine. 20th ed. Philadelphia: WB Saunders, 1996
2. Ritchie AC: Boyd's Textbook of Pathology. 9th ed. Philadelphia: Lea & Febiger, 1990

POSTTACHYCARDIA T-WAVE SYNDROME, the characteristic T wave in versions seen sometimes after tachycardia.
1. Katz AM: N Engl J Med 332:161, 1995

POSTTHROMBOTIC SYNDROME, see Postphlebitic syndrome.

POSTTRANSFUSION SYNDROME, see Postperfusion syndrome.

POSTTRAUMATIC PERICARDITIS, pericarditis that develops after either penetrating or nonpenetrating injury to the chest.
1. Bennett JC, Plum F (eds): Cecil Textbook of Medicine. 20th ed. Philadelphia: WB Saunders, 1996
2. Rowland LP (ed): Merritt's Textbook of Neurology. 9th ed. Baltimore: Williams & Wilkins, 1995

POSTTRAUMATIC SYNDROME, POSTTRAUMATIC BRAIN SYNDROME, see Postconcussion syndrome.

POTAIN SIGN, a dull sound heard from the aortic region to the third intercostal space on the right; seen in the patient with aortitis. (Pierre C. Potain, 1825-1901, French)
1. Casas EC: Diccionario Terminologico de Ciencias Medicas. 5th ed. Salvat Editores, SA, 1954

POTT DISEASE, tuberculous spondylitis. Cross-reference: David disease. (Sir Percivall Pott, 1713-1788, British surgeon)
1. Haymaker W: Bing's Local Diagnosis in Neurological Diseases. 15th ed. St Louis: CV Mosby, 1969
2. Pott P: Remarks on that kind of palsy of the lower limbs which is frequently found to accompany a curvature of the spine and is supposed to be caused by it, together with its methods of cure. London: Johnson, 1779

POTTENGER SIGN, intercostal muscle rigidity in pleural and pulmonary inflammation. (Francis M. Pottenger, 1869-1961, U.S.)
1. Casas EC: Diccionario Terminologico de Ciencias Medicas. 5th ed. Salvat Editores, SA, 1954

POTTER SYNDROME, renofacial dysplasia; renal agenesis occurs in the first 31 days of fetal development, limiting the amount of amniotic fluid and thus resulting in additional anomalies. The primary defect is oligohydramnios. Infants die shortly after birth. (Edith L. Potter, U.S.)
1. Potter EL: Ipsilateral renal agenesis. J Pediatr 29:68-76, 1946
2. Smith DW, Jones KL: Recognizable Patterns of Human Malformations: Genetic, Embryologic, and Clinical Aspects. 3rd ed. Philadelphia: WB Saunders, 1982

POTTS OPERATION, 1) side-to-side anastomosis used in infants and small children; 2) an aortopulmonary shunt. (Willis Potts, 1895-1968, U.S. surgeon)
1. Schwartz SI: Principles of Surgery. 4th ed. New York: McGraw-Hill, 1983

PÖTZL SYNDROME, difficulty in naming colors, in association with homonymous hemianopsia and agnosia.
1. Bordas LB (ed): Neurologia Fundamental. 2nd ed. Toray, 1968

POULET DISEASE, rheumatic osteoperiostitis.
1. Casas EC: Diccionario Terminologico de Ciencias Medicas. 5th ed. Salvat Editores, SA, 1954

POURFOUR DU PETIT SYNDROME, a hyperactive cervical sympathetic state following damage to the cervical sympathetic nerves, causing ipsilateral Horner syndrome. (Francois Pourfour du Petit, 1664-1741, French)
1. Teeple E, et al: Pourfour du Petit syndrome-hypersympathetic dysfunctional state following a direct nonpenetrating injury to the cervical sympathetic chain and brachial plexus. Anesthesiology 55:591-592, 1981

POWER OPERATION, extirpation of a leukoma followed by transplantation of a rabbit cornea.
1. Maffei WE: Os Fundamentos da Medicina. 2nd ed. Livraria Editora Artes Médicas Ltda, 1978

POZZI OPERATION, bilateral artificial laceration of the uterine neck followed by suturing in order to correct anteflexion of the uterus. (Samuel J. de Pozzi, 1846-1918, French gynecologist)
1. Maffei WE: Os Fundamentos da Medicina. 2nd ed. Livraria Editora Artes Médicas Ltda, 1978

POZZI SYNDROME, leukorrhea, anal pain, and endometriosis are features. (Samuel J. de Pozzi)
1. Casas EC: Diccionario Terminologico de Ciencias Medicas. 5th ed. Salvat Editores, SA, 1954

PRADER-WILLI SYNDROME, in this not uncommon condition, infants are born with severe hypotonia and feeding difficulties. Boys exhibit a small penis and cryptorchidism, and hypoplastic labia are seen in girls. Small hands and feet, almond-shaped eyes, and fish mouth are seen in both sexes. (Andrea Prader, Swiss pediatrician; Heinrich Willi, 1900-1971, Swiss pediatrician)
1. Farmer TW: Pediatric Neurology. 2nd ed. Hagerstown: Harper & Row, 1975
2. Prader A, Labhart A, Willi H: Schweiz Med Wochenschr 86:1260-1261, 1956

PRAT SIGN, muscle rigidity with gangrene or wound necrosis, an indication of the need for surgery.
1. Casas EC: Diccionario Terminologico de Ciencias Medicas. 5th ed. Salvat Editores, SA, 1954

PRAYER SIGN, see Phalen sign.

PRECHTL SYNDROME, chorea associated with dyslexia.
1. Baker AB, Baker LH: Clinical Neurology. Revised ed. Philadelphia: Harper & Row, 1982
2. Money: Reading Disability, Progress and Research Needs in Dyslexia. Baltimore: Johns Hopkins Press, 1962
3. Prechtl HFR: The choreatifom syndrome in children. Dev Med Child Neurol 4:119-127, 1962

PRE-ECLAMPSIA SYNDROME, proteinuria, edema, overactive tendon reflexes, and headache are features; more common in poorly nourished young primiparous women with advanced extrauterine pregnancy.
1. Rowland LP (ed): Merritt's Textbook of Neurology. 9th ed. Baltimore: Williams & Wilkins, 1995

PRE-EXCITATION SYNDROME, refers to a variety of cardiac situations whereby an accessory pathway "bypasses" some portion of the normal conduction system, with two important consequences: 1) the presence of such an accessory pathway may allow the normal physiological delaying mechanism of the arteriovenous node to be bypassed; 2) the presence of a parallel conduction system at some level of the heart provides a route for re-entry. The most common of these is Wolff-Parkinson-White syndrome.
1. Bennett JC, Plum F (eds): Cecil Textbook of Medicine. 20th ed. Philadelphia: WB Saunders, 1996
2. Cheitlin MD, Sokolow M: Clinical Cardiology. 5th ed. Norwalk, Conn: Appleton & Lange, 1993

PREHN SIGN, painful elevation of the scrotum except in cases of torsion of the testicle; seen in epididymitis. (D.T. Prehn, U.S.)
1. Casas EC: Diccionario Terminologico de Ciencias Medicas. 5th ed. Salvat Editores, SA, 1954

PREISSER DISEASE, posttraumatic osteoporosis. (George Preisser, 1879-1913, German orthopedic surgeon)
1. Casas EC: Diccionario Terminologico de Ciencias Medicas. 5th ed. Salvat Editores, SA, 1954

PRELEUKEMIC SYNDROME, see Myelodysplastic syndrome.

PREMENSTRUAL SYNDROME, PREMENSTRUAL TENSION SYNDROME, includes depression or anxiety, fatigue, irritability, swelling of the legs and abdomen, breast tenderness, weight gain, and acneiform eruptions; occurs 1 week before and 1 day after menstruation.
1. Wilson JD, Foster DW, Kronenberg HM, et al (eds): Williams Textbook of Endocrinology. 9th ed. Philadelphia: WB Saunders, 1998

PREMOLAR APLASIA-HYPERHIDROSIS-PREMATURE CANITIES SYNDROME, premolar aplasia, hyperhidrosis, and premature canities are features. Autosomal dominant inheritance with complete penetrance. Cross-reference: Böök syndrome.
1. Böök JA: Am J Hum Genet 2:240-263, 1950
2. Gorlin RJ, Cohen MM Jr, Levin LS: Syndromes of the Head and Neck. 3rd ed. New York: Oxford University Press, 1990

PREMOTOR SYNDROME, the presence of spastic hemiplegia with increased reflexes, disturbances of skilled movements, forced grasping, and transient vasomotor disturbances; occurs in lesions of the premotor cortex.

1. Dorland's Medical Dictionary. 28th ed. Philadelphia: WB Saunders, 1994

PRERENAL SYNDROME, the major classes of prerenal disorders are: 1) renal hypoperfusion secondary to a reduction in effective circulating volume; 2) renal ischemia because of occlusive disease in one or both renal arteries. Both sets of disorders are associated with hyperreninemia.

1. Bennett JC, Plum F (eds): Cecil Textbook of Medicine. 20th ed. Philadelphia: WB Saunders, 1996

PRETECTAL SYNDROME, see Nothnagel syndrome.

PREVEL SIGN, acceleration of the cardiac rate when one's position is changed from sitting to standing.

1. Casas EC: Diccionario Terminologico de Ciencias Medicas. 5th ed. Salvat Editores, SA, 1954

PRÉVOST SIGN, conjugate deviation of the head and eyes toward the hemiplegic side. (Jean L. Prévost, 1838-1927, Swiss)

1. Casas EC: Diccionario Terminologico de Ciencias Medicas. 5th ed. Salvat Editores, SA, 1954

PRÉVOT OPERATION, ablation of a ruptured uterus through laparotomy.

1. Maffei WE: Os Fundamentos da Medicina. 2nd ed. Livraria Editora Artes Médicas Ltda, 1978

PRIBRAM OPERATION, thermoelectrocauterization of the gallbladder.

1. Maffei WE: Os Fundamentos da Medicina. 2nd ed. Livraria Editora Artes Médicas Ltda, 1978

PRIEWALSKY SIGN, difficulty in maintaining hip extension; seen in the patient with appendicitis or swelling of the groin caused by lymphadenitis.

1. Casas EC: Diccionario Terminologico de Ciencias Medicas. 5th ed. Salvat Editores, SA, 1954

PRINGLE DISEASE, see Bourneville disease. (John J. Pringle, 1855-1922, British dermatologist)

PRINZMETAL ANGINA, an angina pectoris variant; defined as chest pain at rest in association with S-T segment deviation without affecting heart rate or blood pressure. Related to coronary artery spasm. Cross-reference: Anterior chest wall syndrome. (Myron Prinzmetal, U.S. cardiologist)

1. Prinzmetal M, Ekme K, Keimamer R, et al: JAMA 174:1794-1800, 1960
2. Prinzmetal M, Massumi R: The anterior chest wall syndrome. JAMA 159:177-184, 1955
3. Zipes DP, Jalife J: Cardiac Electrophysiology: From Cell to Bedside. 2nd ed. Philadelphia: WB Saunders, 1995

PRION SYNDROME, see Gerstmann-Sträussler syndrome.

PROFICHET SYNDROME, the appearance of calcium nodules near big joints, with irritability and trophic alteration. (Georges C. Profichet, French)

1. Profichet GC: Sur une Variété de Concrétion Phosphatiques Subcutanée. Paris, 1890

PROGRESSIVE HEMIFACIAL ATROPHY SYNDROME, see Romberg syndrome.

PRONATION SIGN, see Strümpell sign, def. 2.

PROTEUS SYNDROME, proteiform syndrome; includes partial gigantism of the hands and/or feet, asymmetry of the limbs, plantar hyperplasia, hemangiomas, lipomas, lymphangiomas, varicosities, verrucous epidermal nevi, macrocephaly, cranial hyperostoses, and long bone overgrowth. It is now known that Joseph Merrick, the famous "elephant man," had Proteus syndrome and not neurofibromatosis. (Named after the Greek god Proteus, who was polymorphous and could change his shape at will to avoid capture.) Cross-reference: Thanos syndrome.

1. Cohen MM Jr: Craniosynostosis update 1987. Am J Med Genet Suppl 4:99-148, 1988
2. Gorlin RJ, Cohen MM Jr, Levin LS: Syndromes of the Head and Neck. 3rd ed. New York: Oxford University Press, 1990
3. Thanos C: Syndrome Indent 5:19-21, 1977

PROTRACTED ABSTINENCE SYNDROME, characterized by tremulousness, agitation, and insomnia, the low-grade withdrawal symptoms of acute alcoholism. Can last up to 6 months.

1. Bennett JC, Plum F (eds): Cecil Textbook of Medicine. 20th ed. Philadelphia: WB Saunders, 1996

PRUNE BELLY SYNDROME, the most common term for the congenital absence, deficiency, or hypoplasia of the abdominal musculature accompanied by a large hypotonic bladder, dilated and tortuous ureters, and bilateral cryptorchidism. Cross-reference: Eagle-Barrett syndrome.

1. Eagle JF Jr: Pediatrics 6:721, 1950
2. Greskovich FJ, Myberg LM Jr: The prune belly syndrome: a review of its etiology, defects, treatment and prognosis. J Urol 140:707-713, 1988

PSEUDO-ACHONDROPLASIA SYNDROME, spondyloepiphyseal dysplasia; small, irregular, mushroom-shaped metaphyses, with flattening and/or anterior breaking of vertebrae and normal craniofacial appearance. Autosomal dominant inheritance.
1. Rubin P: Achondroplasia versus pseudoachondroplasia. Radiol Clin North Am 1:621, 1963
2. Smith DW, Jones KL: Recognizable Patterns of Human Malformations: Genetic, Embryologic, and Clinical Aspects. 3rd ed. Philadelphia: WB Saunders, 1982

PSEUDO-BABINSKI SIGN, the Babinski reflex is modified so that only the big toe is extended; all the foot muscles except the dorsiflexors of the big toe are paralyzed. Seen in the patient with poliomyelitis. (Joseph F.F. Babinski, 1857-1932, French neurologist)
1. Dorland's Medical Dictionary. 28th ed. Philadelphia: WB Saunders, 1994

PSEUDO-BARTTER SYNDROME, a metabolic disorder with symptomatology mimicking the Bartter syndrome. Difficult to treat because of the patient's psychological dependence on vomiting, diuretics, or cathartics. (Frederick C. Bartter, 1919-1983, U.S.)
1. Bennett JC, Plum F (eds): Cecil Textbook of Medicine. 20th ed. Philadelphia: WB Saunders, 1996

PSEUDOCLAUDICATION SYNDROME, a condition in which symptoms similar to those of intermittent claudication result from compression of the cauda equina owing to hypertrophic ridging or a herniated lumbar disc or spinal stenosis. Sitting down in the flexed position relieves the symptoms, whereas in true vascular claudication, symptoms improve by just resting.
1. Dorland's Medical Dictionary. 28th ed. Philadelphia: WB Saunders, 1994

PSEUDO-DOUBLE ELEVATOR PALSY SYNDROME, may occur due to a tight inferior rectus muscle in thyroid-related eye diseases. Mimics chronic 6th nerve paresis.
1. Smith JL: Neuro-Ophthalmology, Volume 6. St Louis: CV Mosby, 1972

PSEUDO-GRAEFE PHENOMENON, eyelid retraction similar to the von Graefe sign, but a slow descent of upper eyelid on looking downward and quick ascent on looking up. (Albrecht von Graefe, 1828-1870, German ophthalmologist)
1. Dorland's Medical Dictionary. 28th ed. Philadelphia: WB Saunders, 1994

PSEUDO-HURLER POLYDYSTROPHY SYNDROME, mucolipidosis type III or pseudopolydystrophy; an inborn metabolic disorder with mild Hurler-like symptoms and the characteristics of coarse facies, stiff joints by 2-4 years of age, no mucopolysacchariduria, aortic valve disease, mild corneal opacities, mild mental deficiency, and mild platyspondylia are features. Similar to I-cell disease but with neither hepatosplenomegaly nor mucopolysacchariduria. Stiffness of the joints may develop early. Autosomal recessive inheritance. (Gertrud Hurler, 1889-1965, Austrian pediatrician)
1. McKusick VA: Heritable Disorders of Connective Tissue. 4th ed. St Louis: CV Mosby, 1972
2. Smith DW, Jones KL: Recognizable Patterns of Human Malformations: Genetic, Embryologic, and Clinical Aspects. 3rd ed. Philadelphia: WB Saunders, 1982

PSEUDO-TURNER SYNDROME, characteristic facies includes a narrow maxilla, small mandible, triangular mouth, epicanthic eye folds with downward slant of the eyes, prominent low-set ears, and webbing of the neck. Patients with normal chromosomes probably fall within the poorly delimited spectrum of Noonan syndrome. Mental retardation is occasionally severe. Pulmonic stenosis and other forms of congenital heart disease may be present. Cross-reference: Male Turner syndrome. (Henry H. Turner, 1892-1970, U.S. endocrinologist)
1. Bennett JC, Plum F (eds): Cecil Textbook of Medicine. 20th ed. Philadelphia: WB Saunders, 1996
2. Wilson JD, Foster DW, Kronenberg HM, et al (eds): Williams Textbook of Endocrinology. 9th ed. Philadelphia: WB Saunders, 1998

PSOAS SIGN, see Cope sign.

PTERYGOPALATINE SYNDROME, sphenomaxillary fossa; usually a metastatic growth, involving either neoplastic growth to this space or invasion directly from a palatal or maxillary sinus tract. Presenting signs may include blindness (which clearly differentiates this syndrome from Trotter syndrome) and pterygoid muscle paralysis with trismus. Cross-reference: Behr syndrome.
1. Ballenger JJ: Diseases of the Nose, Throat, Ear, Head and Neck. 12th ed. Philadelphia: Lea & Febiger, 1977
2. Gorlin RJ, Cohen MM Jr, Levin LS: Syndromes of the Head and Neck. 3rd ed. New York: Oxford University Press, 1990

PTOSIS-AORTIC COARCTATION SYNDROME, characterized by congenital bilateral ptosis, sensorineural hearing deficit, coarctation of the aorta, and asthma. Autosomal dominant inheritance.
1. Cornel G, et al: Familial coarctation of the aortic arch with bilateral ptosis. A new syndrome? J Pediatr Surg 22:724-

726, 1987

2. Gorlin RJ, Cohen MM Jr, Levin LS: Syndromes of the Head and Neck. 3rd ed. New York: Oxford University Press, 1990

PUDDLE SIGN, a method for detecting the presence of free liquid in the abdominal cavity; used during the examination for ascites.

1. Dorland's Medical Dictionary. 28th ed. Philadelphia: WB Saunders, 1994

PUENTE DISEASE, cheilitis.

1. Casas EC: Diccionario Terminologico de Ciencias Medicas. 5th ed. Salvat Editores, SA, 1954

PULMONARY ACID ASPIRATION SYNDROME, a disorder produced as a complication of anesthesia administration by inhalation of gastric contents with a pH of less than 2.5, which causes bronchoconstriction and destruction of tracheal mucosa progressing to a syndrome resembling the acute form of respiratory distress syndrome. Cross-reference: Mendelson syndrome.

1. Mendelson CL: Aspiration of stomach contents into the lungs during obstetric anesthesia. Am J Obstet Gynecol 52:191-205, 1946

PULMONARY DYSMATURITY SYNDROME, see Wilson-Mikity syndrome.

PULSELESS DISEASE, see Aortic arch syndrome.

PUNCH DRUNK SYNDROME, repeated mild traumas with short periods of unconsciousness; known to produce definite permanent mental and neurological changes.

1. Baker AB, Baker LH: Clinical Neurology. Revised ed. Philadelphia: Harper & Row, 1982

PUPILLOTONIC PSEUDOTABES SYNDROME, complete bilateral oculomotor nuclear palsy, with bilateral ptosis and paralysis of eye movement in the vertical plane. Divergence of the globes with inability to adduct or converge the eyes and pupillary mydriasis with lack of response to light. Cross-reference: Holmes-Adie syndrome.

1. Baker AB, Baker LH: Clinical Neurology. Revised ed. Philadelphia: Harper & Row, 1982

PURKINJE PHENOMENON, as the eye adapts to light and the region of brightness shifts from red-yellow to blue-green, the reds become less luminous and the blues become more luminous. (Johannes E. Purkinje, 1787-1869, Czech physiologist)

1. Casas EC: Diccionario Terminologico de Ciencias Medicas. 5th ed. Salvat Editores, SA, 1954

PURMANN METHOD, see Philagrius operation. (Matthias Purmann, 1648-1721, German surgeon)

PURTSCHER DISEASE, traumatic angiopathy of the retina with lymphorrhagia. (Otmar Purtscher, 1852-1927, German ophthalmologist)

1. Purtscher O: Graefes Arch Ophthalmol 82:347-371, 1912

PUTNAM SIGN, widening of gait in hysterical thigh pain.

1. Casas EC: Diccionario Terminologico de Ciencias Medicas. 5th ed. Salvat Editores, SA, 1954

PUTNAM SYNDROME, paresthesias and pain in arm occurring in middle-aged women exclusively while patient lies down. Stiffness in the nondominant hand but improves with massage. (James J. Putnam, 1846-1918, U.S. neurologist)

1. Putnam J: A series of cases of paresthesia, mainly of the hand, of periodical recurrence, and possibly, of vasomotor origin. Arch Med NY 4:147-162, 1880

PUTRAM SYNDROME, sclerosis of the posterior column combined with systemic disease.

1. Casas EC: Diccionario Terminologico deCiencias Medicas. 5th ed. 1954

PUUSEPP OPERATION, incision of the posterior median sulcus of the spinal cord for treating syringomyelia. (Lyudvig Puusepp, 1875-1942, Estonian neurosurgeon)

1. Maffei WE: Os Fundamentos da Medicina. 2nd ed. Livraria Editora Artes Médicas Ltda, 1978

PYLE DISEASE, metaphyseal dysplasia; despite bizarre roentgenographic changes, this disorder has few clinical findings other than genu valgum. The craniofacial bones are at the most only mildly affected, thus distinguishing this disease from the craniometaphyseal dysplasias. (Edwin Pyle, 1891-1961, U.S.)

1. Pyle E: J Bone Joint Surg 13:874-876, 1931

QT PROLONGATION SYNDROME, on electrocardiography, a combination of a prolonged QT interval and torsade de pointes; may be congenital or acquired. The acquired form is usually the result of drug administration.

1. Dorland's Medical Dictionary. 28th ed. Philadelphia: WB Saunders, 1994

QUAGLINO OPERATION, sclerotomy.
1. Maffei WE: Os Fundamentos da Medicina. 2nd ed. Livraria Editora Artes Médicas Ltda, 1978

QUAIN DISEASE, fibrotic degeneration of the myocardium. (Richard Quain, 1816-1898, British)
1. Casas EC: Diccionario Terminologico de Ciencias Medicas. 5th ed. Salvat Editores, SA, 1954

QUANT SIGN, a T-shaped depression in the occipital bone; seen at times in the patient with rickets. (C.A.J. Quant, Dutch)
1. Casas EC: Diccionario Terminologico de Ciencias Medicas. 5th ed. Salvat Editores, SA, 1954

QUECKENSTEDT TEST, a measurement of bilateral simultaneous compression of the jugular veins causes increased intracranial pressure; helpful in determining the presence of lateral sinus thrombosis. Cross-reference: Jugular sign. (Hans H.G. Queckenstedt, 1876-1918, German neurologist)
1. Ballenger JJ: Diseases of the Nose, Throat, Ear, Head and Neck. 12th ed. Philadelphia: Lea & Febiger, 1977

QUEEN SQUARE DISEASE, described as a unique familial case characterized by a variable combination of developmental delay, retinitis pigmentosa, dementia, seizures, ataxia, proximal weakness, and sensory neuropathy. (Queen Square, London, England)

QUEENSLAND TICK TYPHUS, tick-borne rickettsiae of the eastern hemisphere (also African and North Asian tick). Each is a zoonosis, with humans an accidental dead-end host, and is transmitted by the bite of one or more species of ixodid ticks. Cross-reference: Australian tick typhus.
1. Bennett JC, Plum F (eds): Cecil Textbook of Medicine. 20th ed. Philadelphia: WB Saunders, 1996

QUÉNU-MAYO OPERATION, extirpation of the rectum and adjacent lymph nodes in cases of rectal carcinoma. (Eduard A. Quénu, 1852-1933, French surgeon)
1. Maffei WE: Os Fundamentos da Medicina. 2nd ed. Livraria Editora Artes Médicas Ltda, 1978

QUÉNU-MURET SIGN, when an aneurysm on the main artery of a limb is compressed, good collateralization may be indicated if there is blood distally. (Eduard A. Quénu; Paul L. Muret, French surgeon)
1. Casas EC: Diccionario Terminologico de Ciencias Medicas. 5th ed. Salvat Editores, SA, 1954

QUERVAIN DISEASE, see De Quervain disease.

QUICKERT-DRYDEN OPERATION, indwelling silicone intubation for dilating a stenotic canaliculus.
1. Spaeth GL: Ophthalmic Surgery. Principles and Practice. Philadelphia: WB Saunders, 1982

QUILT HIP DISEASE, see Legg disease.

QUINCKE SIGN, QUINCKE PULSE, capillary pulsation; a sign of arteriolar dilatation especially seen in the patient with severe aortic insufficiency. (Heinrich I. Quincke, 1842-1922, German)

QUINQUAUD SIGN, trembling of the fingers with the hands in semipronation; seen in tremors and a sign of alcoholism. (Charles E. Quinquaud, 1842-1894, French)
1. Casas EC: Diccionario Terminologico de Ciencias Medicas. 5th ed. Salvat Editores, SA, 1954

QUINTAN FEVER, see Trench fever. (Recurring every fifth day.)

RABBIT SYNDROME, is a movement disorder associated with neuroleptic drugs which causes a movement that resembles those of a rabbit's mouth and nose. It has been treated in the past with Botulin injections.
1. Jus A, Jus K, Fontaine P: Long term treatment of tardive dyskinesia. J Clin Psychiatry 40:72-77, 1979
2. Southern Med J 83:854, 1990

RADIAL APLASIA-THROMBOCYTOPENIA SYNDROME, thrombocytopenia with absence or hypoplasia of the radius, often with associated hypoplasia of the ulna, hands, legs, and/or feet, as well as leukemoid granulocytosis or anemia. Autosomal recessive inheritance. Cross-reference: Thrombocytopenia-absent radius syndrome.
1. Hall JG, et al: Thrombocytopenia with absent radius (TAR). Medicine 48:441, 1969
2. Smith DW, Jones KL: Recognizable Patterns of Human Malformations: Genetic, Embryologic, and Clinical Aspects. 3rd ed. Philadelphia: WB Saunders, 1982

RADIALIS SIGN, see Strümpell sign, def. 1.

RADIATION SYNDROME, typically seen after exposure of most or all of the body to external sources of penetrating ionizing radiation; high doses of phosphorus-32, iodine-131, and gold-198 have also evoked it.
1. Bennett JC, Plum F (eds): Cecil Textbook of Medicine. 20th ed. Philadelphia: WB Saunders, 1996

RADICULAR SYNDROME, a group of syndromes resulting from lesions of the spinal nerve roots, consisting of restricted mobility of the spine and nerve root pain and paresthesia.

1. Dorland's Medical Dictionary. 28th ed. Philadelphia: WB Saunders, 1994

RADOVICI SIGN, no response following stimulation of the chin with a pin; seen in peripheral paralysis. Cross-reference: Palm-chin reflex. (André Radovici, French physiologist)

1. Casas EC: Diccionario Terminologico de Ciencias Medicas. 5th ed. Salvat Editores, SA, 1954

RAEDER SIGN, see Reder sign.

RAEDER SYNDROME, paratrigeminal neuralgia; the paratrigeminal space is a small area containing components of the 5th cranial nerve, including the gasserian ganglion, and the third is characterized by retro-orbital pain although sensation is intact. Dilated pupils, ptosis, enophthalmos, and sometimes exophthalmos are features. Cross-reference: Paratrigeminal syndrome. (Johann G. Raeder, 1889-1956, Norwegian neuro-ophthalmologist)

1. Baker AB, Baker LH: Clinical Neurology. Revised ed. Philadelphia: Harper & Row, 1982
2. Ballenger JJ: Diseases of the Nose, Throat, Ear, Head and Neck. 12th ed. Philadelphia: Lea & Febiger, 1977
3. Raeder JG: Brain 47:149-158, 1924

RAMDOHR OPERATION, enterorrhaphy.

1. Maffei WE: Os Fundamentos da Medicina. 2nd ed. Livraria Editora Artes Médicas Ltda, 1978

RAMON SYNDROME, gingival fibromatosis, hypertrichosis, cherubism, mental and somatic retardation, and epilepsy are features. (Yochanon Ramon, Israeli dentist)

1. Gorlin RJ, Cohen MM Jr, Levin LS: Syndromes of the Head and Neck. 3rd ed. New York: Oxford University Press, 1990
2. Ramon Y, Berman W, Bubis JJ, et al: Gingival fibromatosis combined with cherubism. Oral Surg 24:436-448, 1967

RAMOND SIGN, rigidity of the erector spinae muscle; disappears when pus is present. Seen in the patient with pleural effusion. (Louis Ramond, 1879-1952, French internist)

1. Casas EC: Diccionario Terminologico de Ciencias Medicas. 5th ed. Salvat Editores, SA, 1954

RAMSAY HUNT SYNDROME, geniculate ganglion neuralgia and herpes zoster oticus. In this rarely encountered syndrome the infecting herpes zoster virus invades, variously, the geniculate ganglion or the 7th and 8th cranial nerves (or both). The most obvious symptom is intense, deep, boring ear pain. Cross-references: Cephalic zoster syndrome; Geniculate ganglion syndrome; Hunt neuralgia. (John Ramsay Hunt, 1874-1937, U.S. neurologist)

1. Ballenger JJ: Diseases of the Nose, Throat, Ear, Head and Neck. 12th ed. Philadelphia: Lea & Febiger, 1977
2. Hunt JR: J Nerv Ment Dis 34:73-96, 1907

RAMSDEN OPERATION, ligation of the subclavian artery through a transverse incision in the posterior triangle of the neck, 2 cm above the clavicle.

1. Maffei WE: Os Fundamentos da Medicina. 2nd ed. Livraria Editora Artes Médicas Ltda, 1978

RANDALL SIGN, an exaggerated response to dipping the arms in cold water; in a pregnant woman, indicates the possibility of toxemia.

1. Casas EC: Diccionario Terminologico de Ciencias Medicas. 5th ed. Salvat Editores, SA, 1954

RANGPUR DISEASE, see Forrest disease.

RANIKHET DISEASE, see Newcastle disease.

RANKIM OPERATION, two-stage abdominal-peritoneal resection of rectal carcinoma.

1. Maffei WE: Os Fundamentos da Medicina. 2nd ed. Livraria Editora Artes Médicas Ltda, 1978

RANSOHOFF OPERATION, multiple cross incisions in the pleura in cases of empyema.

1. Maffei WE: Os Fundamentos da Medicina. 2nd ed. Livraria Editora Artes Médicas Ltda, 1978

RANZIER DISEASE, bluish edema of a limb in an hysterical person.

1. Casas EC: Diccionario Terminologico de Ciencias Medicas. 5th ed. Salvat Editores, SA, 1954

RAPP-HODGKIN SYNDROME, ectodermal dysplasia; variable growth deficiency and thin skin with hypohidrosis, hypodontia, a small mouth with variable cleft lip/palate, a bifid uvula, and hypospadias genitalia are features. Autosomal dominant inheritance.

1. Rapp RS, Hodgkin WE: Anhidrotic ectodermal dysplasia. Autosomal dominant inheritance with palate and lip anomalies. J Med Genet 5:269-272, 1968
2. Smith DW, Jones KL: Recognizable Patterns of Human Malformations: Genetic, Embryologic, and Clinical Aspects. 3rd ed. Philadelphia: WB Saunders, 1982

RASCH SIGN, a measurement of amniotic fluid in early pregnancy. (Herman Rasch, German obstetrician)

1. Casas EC: Diccionario Terminologico de Ciencias Medicas. 5th ed. Salvat Editores, SA, 1954

RASIN SIGN, see Jellinek sign.

RASMUSSEN ENCEPHALITIS, usually has onset in childhood; cytomegalovirus has been found in seven of 10 biopsies. Focal encephalitis with progressive hemiparesis and intractable epilepsy are commonly seen.

1. Adams RD, Victor M: Principles of Neurosurgery. 2nd ed. New York: McGraw-Hill, 1981

RAT-BITE FEVER, a single designation for two clinically somewhat similar but etiologically distinct diseases that usually follow the bite of a rat or other rodent. One form is bacillary caused by *Streptobacillus moniliformis* and the other form is spirillary caused by *Spirrilum* minus.

1. Bennett JC, Plum F (eds): Cecil Textbook of Medicine. 20th ed. Philadelphia: WB Saunders, 1996

RAVITCH OPERATION, corrective surgery for pectus excavatum.

1. Schwartz SI: Principles of Surgery. 4th ed. New York: McGraw-Hill, 1983

RAYER DISEASE, xanthomatosis, vitiligoideas of the skin, chronic jaundice, splenomegaly, and hepatomegaly are features. (Pierre F. Rayer, 1793-1867, French)

1. Rayer PF: Traité des Maladies de la Peau. 1835

RAYMOND-CÉSTAN SYNDROME, lesions of the pontine region caused by obstruction of twigs of the basilar artery. Contralateral anesthesia or hypesthesia with symmetrical or dissociated conjugate ocular paralysis on attempted ipsilateral gaze occurs. Ocular nystagmus can sometimes be elicited. May also be sensory deficit in the ipsilateral side of the face. Cross-references: Céstan-Raymond syndrome; Pontine syndrome. (Fulgence Raymond, 1844-1910, French neurologist; Raymond Céstan, 1872-1934, French neurologist)

1. Grinker RR, Sahs AL: Neurology. 6th ed. Springfield: Charles C Thomas, 1966
2. Raymond F, Céstan R: Rev Neurol 9:70-77, 1901

RAYNAUD DISEASE, the skin of the digits becomes thickened or atrophic and the tips of the fingers or toes eventually become gangrenous. A severe and long-standing disorder. If the syndrome is secondary to some other condition, it is called Raynaud phenomenon. Cause unknown. (A.G. Maurice Raynaud, 1834-1881, French)

1. Haymaker W: Bing's Local Diagnosis in Neurological Diseases. 15th ed. St Louis: CV Mosby, 1969
2. Raynaud A: De L'Asphyxie Locale et de la Gangrèna Symetrique des Extrémités. Paris: Rignoux, 1862
3. Ritchie AC: Boyd's Textbook of Pathology. 9th ed. Philadelphia: Lea & Febiger, 1990

RAYNAUD SIGN, acrocyanosis. (A.G. Maurice Raynaud)

1. Casas EC: Diccionario Terminologico de Ciencias Medicas. 5th ed. Salvat Editores, SA, 1954

REBOUND PHENOMENON, loss of coordination between groups of antagonistic muscles of the extremities in cerebellar dysfunction.

1. Dorland's Medical Dictionary. 28th ed. Philadelphia: WB Saunders, 1994

RECKLINGHAUSEN DISEASE, RECKLINGHAUSEN NEUROFIBROMATOSIS, see Von Recklinghausen disease.

RECKLINGHAUSEN-APPLEBAUM DISEASE, hemochromatosis. (Friedrich D. von Recklinghausen; L. Applebaum, German)

1. Casas EC: Diccionario Terminologico de Ciencias Medicas. 5th ed. Salvat Editores, SA, 1954

RECLOTTING PHENOMENON, thixotropy.

1. Dorland's Medical Dictionary. 28th ed. Philadelphia: WB Saunders, 1994

RECLUS DISEASE, see Schimmelbusch disease. (Paul Reclus, 1847-1914, French surgeon)

RECLUS OPERATION, surgical creation of an iliac artificial anus in cases of rectal carcinoma.

1. Maffei WE: Os Fundamentos da Medicina. 2nd ed. Livraria Editora Artes Médicas Ltda, 1978

REDER SIGN, a painful point above and to the right of the O'Beirne sphincter (a band of fibers at the rectosigmoid junction); seen in the patient with appendectomy. Cross-reference: Raeder sign.

1. Casas EC: Diccionario Terminologico de Ciencias Medicas. 5th ed. Salvat Editores, SA, 1954

REDLICH-FLATAU DISEASE, acute disseminated encephalomyelopathy usually with a benign, although protracted, course. (Emil Redlich, 1866-1930, Austrian neurologist; Edward Flatau, 1869-1932, Polish neurologist)

1. Redlich E: Dtsch Med Wochenschr 55:562-563, 1929

REED CELLS, REED-STERNBERG CELLS, abundant cytoplasm virtually pathognomonic of

Hodgkin disease. Cross-reference: Sternberg cells. (Dorothy Reed, 1874-1964, U.S. pathologist; Karl von Sternberg, 1872-1935, Austrian pathologist)
1. Ballenger JJ: Diseases of the Nose, Throat, Ear, Head and Neck. 12th ed. Philadelphia: Lea & Febiger, 1977

REED OPERATION, ligation of veins in cases of tubo-ovarian varicocele.
1. Maffei WE: Os Fundamentos da Medicina. 2nd ed. Livraria Editora Artes Médicas Ltda, 1978

REED-HODGKIN DISEASE, see Hodgkin disease. (Dorothy Reed; Thomas Hodgkin, 1798-1866, British)

REES SIGN, contraction of the pectoralis major muscle fixates a tumor attached to the pectoralis fascia.
1. Casas EC: Diccionario Terminologico de Ciencias Medicas. 5th ed. Salvat Editores, SA, 1954

REFLEX OF PROTROWSKI, antagonistic anterior tibial reflex; characterized by plantar flexion of the ankle and sometimes of the toes when the belly of the anterior tibial muscle is tapped.
1. Baker AB, Baker LH: Clinical Neurology. Revised ed. Philadelphia: Harper & Row, 1982

REFLEX SYMPATHETIC DYSTROPHY, classic features are pain and tenderness of the distal extremities with signs and symptoms of vasomotor instability, trophic skin changes, and swelling. A form of sympathetically mediated pain; allodynia is an important feature.
1. Bennett JC, Plum F (eds): Cecil Textbook of Medicine. 20th ed. Philadelphia: WB Saunders, 1996
2. Moschella SL, Hurley HJ: Dermatology. 2nd ed. Philadelphia: WB Saunders, 1985

REFSUM DISEASE, heredopathia atactica polyneuritiformis; an extremely rare condition in which features of a chronic polyneuropathy are combined with ataxia, retinitis pigmentosa, ichthyosis, and other defects. All cases to date are in Caucasians, many of Scandinavian origin. (Sigvald Refsum, Norwegian neurologist)
1. Rowland LP (ed): Merritt's Textbook of Neurology. 9th ed. Baltimore: Williams & Wilkins, 1995

REHN OPERATION, resection of prolapsed rectal mucosa followed by suturing.
1. Maffei WE: Os Fundamentos da Medicina. 2nd ed. Livraria Editora Artes Médicas Ltda, 1978

REICHMANN SYNDROME, an excessive increase in gastric juice production. (Mikolaj Reichmann, 1851-1918, Polish)
1. Casas EC: Diccionario Terminologico de Ciencias Medicas. 5th ed. Salvat Editores, SA, 1954

REIFENSTEIN SYNDROME, familial incomplete pseudohermaphroditism; seen in a heterogeneous group of 46XY individuals with partial androgen resistance. The external genitalia are predominantly male or ambiguous. Cross-reference: Rosewater syndrome. (Edward C. Reifenstein, Jr., 1908-1975, U.S.)
1. Campbell MF, Walsh PC: Campbell's Urology. 5th ed. Philadelphia: WB Saunders, 1986
2. Reifenstein EC Jr: Recent Prog Horm Res 3:224, 1948
3. Rosewater S, Gwinup G, Hamwi G: Familial gynecomastia. Ann Intern Med 63:377-385, 1965

REIMAN SYNDROME, periodic fever associated with abdominal symptoms.
1. Maffei WE: OS Fundamentos da Medicina. 2nd ed. Livraria Editora Artes Médicas Ltda, 1978

REINKE DISEASE, diffuse vocal polyposis, caused by persistent vocal cord overuse along with smoking. Untreated hypothyroidism can also be associated with vocal fold edema and diffuse laryngeal polyposis. (Friedrich Reinke, German)
1. Reinke F: Fortschr Med 13:469-478, 1895

REISS SIGN, a cardiac murmur audible in the stomach; seen in the patient with pericardial effusion.
1. Casas EC: Diccionario Terminologico de Ciencias Medicas. 5th ed. Salvat Editores, SA, 1954

REITER SYNDROME, although the association of arthritis, urethritis, and conjunctivitis was recorded early in the 19th century, this triad of clinical manifestations bears the name of the physician who described a patient with nongonococcal urethritis, conjunctivitis, and arthritis after an episode of diarrhea. Other manifestations include fever, oral and genital mucous membrane lesions, cutaneous keratosis, and iritis. The majority of patients are young males; rarely seen in women regardless of age. Cross-reference: Fiessinger-Leroy-Reiter syndrome. (Hans C. Reiter, 1881-1969, German bacteriologist)
1. Bennett JC, Plum F (eds): Cecil Textbook of Medicine. 20th ed. Philadelphia: WB Saunders, 1996
2. Campbell MF, Walsh PC: Campbell's Urology. 5th ed. Philadelphia: WB Saunders, 1986
3. Reiter H: Dtsch Med Wochenschr 42:1535-1536, 1916

RELEASE SIGN, see Blumberg sign.

REMAK SIGN, the double sensation of pain produced by a needle in the patient with tabes dorsalis. (Robert Remak, 1815-1865, German physiologist)

1. Bodechtel G: Diagnostico Diferential de las Enfermedades Neurologicas. Madrid: Pas Montalvo Editorial, 1967

REMLINGER SIGN, trembling and difficulty stretching the tongue; seen in the patient with typhoid fever.

1. Casas EC: Diccionario Terminologico de Ciencias Medicas. 5th ed. Salvat Editores, SA, 1954

RENAL PARENCHYMAL SYNDROME, see Glomerulonephritis syndrome.

RENDU-OSLER-WEBER DISEASE, a hereditary hemorrhagic telangiectasia that occurs in all parts of the body but particularly the oral and nasal mucosa. Characterized by dilatation of the arterioles, capillaries, and venules, which form into small angiomas, particularly on the oral and nasal mucosa and where slight trauma leads to multiple sites of bleeding that is difficult to control. (Henri J.L.M. Rendu, 1844-1902, French; William Osler, 1849-1919, Canadian; Frederick Parkes Weber, 1863-1962, British)

1. Osler W: Q J Med 1:53-58, 1907
2. Rendu H: Bull Soc Med Hop 13:731-733, 1896
3. Weber PF: Edinburgh Med J, 1904, pp 346-349

RESISTANT OVARY SYNDROME, see Savage syndrome.

RESPIRATORY DISTRESS SYNDROME OF NEWBORN, a severe complication in a newborn of generalized sepsis due to enteric bacteria. Frequently associated with severe hypoxia and thrombocytopenia. Cross-reference: Hyaline membrane syndrome.

1. Bennett JC, Plum F (eds): Cecil Textbook of Medicine. 20th ed. Philadelphia: WB Saunders, 1996

RESTLESS LEGS SYNDROME, burning feet or an intolerable discomfort or feeling of weariness in the legs which obliges the patient to move or walk about to obtain relief. Cross-reference: Ekbom syndrome.

1. Bennett JC, Plum F (eds): Cecil Textbook of Medicine. 20th ed. Philadelphia: WB Saunders, 1996
2. Ekbom KA: Akroparestesier och restless legs under graviditet. Lakartidningen 57:2597-2603, 1960
3. Moschella SL, Hurley HJ: Dermatology. 2nd ed. Philadelphia: WB Saunders, 1985

RETINAL CONE DYSTROPHY SYNDROME, see Cone syndrome.

RETINO-OTODIABETIC SYNDROME, see Alström syndrome.

RETRACTION SYNDROME, see Duane syndrome.

RETROPAROTID SPACE SYNDROME, see Villaret syndrome.

RETT SYNDROME, after normal initial infant development of up to 7-18 months, there is a progressive disorder of the brain; occurs principally in females. Characterized by autistic behavior, ataxia, dementia, seizures, and loss of purposeful use of the hands, with cerebral atrophy, mild hyperammonemia, and decreased levels of biogenic amines. (Andreas Rett, Austrian)

1. Moeschler JB, et al: Rett syndrome: natural history and management. Pediatrics 82:1-10, 1988
2. Rett A: Monatsschr Kinderheilkd 116:310-311, 1968

REUSNER SIGN, strong pulsation of the uterine arteries heard at the fundus after the 4th month of pregnancy.

1. Casas EC: Diccionario Terminologico de Ciencias Medicas. 5th ed. Salvat Editores, SA, 1954

REVILLIOD SIGN, see Orbicularis sign. (Jean L.A. Revilliod, 1835-1919, Swiss)

REWARD DEFICIENCY SYNDROME, addictive, impulsive, and compulsive behavior are characteristics.

1. Blum K, et al: Reward deficiency syndrome. Am Scientist 84:132-145, 1996

REYE SYNDROME, an acute disease affecting infants and young children and characterized by fatty degeneration of the encephalopathy. Salicylate use during a viral illness has been ascribed to be an important factor in precipitating this condition. The pathological features consist of fatty changes in the liver, kidneys, myocardium, and other viscera in association with acute cerebral edema. Progressive increase in intracranial pressure leads to coma. Most occurrences are sporadic and it is particularly common in Thailand. (Ralph Douglas K. Reye, 1912-1977, Australian)

1. Farmer TW: Pediatric Neurology. 2nd ed. Hagerstown: Harper & Row, 1975
2. Krugman S, Katz SI: Infectious Diseases of Children. 7th ed. St Louis: CV Mosby, 1981
3. Reye RDK, Morgan G, Baral J: Encephalopathy and fatty degeneration of the viscera: a disease entity in childhood. Lancet 2:749-752, 1963

REYE-SHEEHAN SYDNROME, see Sheehan syndrome.

REYNOLDS SYNDROME, acrofacial dysostosis. The craniofacial manifestations are those of mild mandibulofacial dysostosis and include an unusual facies that resembles that of maxillofacial dysostosis. Mild congenital mixed-type of hearing loss and variable acral abnormalities are present.

1. Bodechtel G: Diagnostico Diferential de las Enfermedades Neurologicas. Madrid: Pas Montalvo Editorial, 1967
2. Gorlin RJ, Cohen MM Jr, Levin LS: Syndromes of the Head and Neck. 3rd ed. New York: Oxford University Press, 1990
3. Reynolds JF, et al: A new autosomal dominant acrofacial dysostosis syndrome. Am J Med Genet Suppl 2:143-150, 1986

RH$_{NULL}$ SYNDROME, chronic hemolytic anemia affecting individuals who lack all Rh factors (Rh$_{null}$); marked by spherocytosis, stomatocytosis, and increased osmotic fragility.

1. Dorland's Medical Dictionary. 28th ed. Philadelphia: WB Saunders, 1994

RHEA BARTON OPERATION, cunciform osteotomy of the inferior portion of the diaphysis of the femur in cases of ankylosis of the knee. Cross-reference: Barton operation. (John Rhea Barton, 1794-1871, U.S. surgeon)

1. Maffei WE: Os Fundamentos da Medicina. 2nd ed. Livraria Editora Artes Médicas Ltda, 1978

RHIZOMELIC CHONDRODYSPLASIA PUNCTATA SYNDROME, see Conradi syndrome.

RHODESIAN SLEEPING SICKNESS, trypanosomiasis; a disease of eastern Africa spread by tsetse flies (*Glossina morsitans*), which live in open savanna with enough vegetation to provide shade and resting places. Primarily an occupational illness, occurring mainly in those whose work takes them into areas where wild game, especially bushbuck, survives. Hunters, fishermen, honey-gatherers, and tourists are all at risk.

1. Bennett JC, Plum F (eds): Cecil Textbook of Medicine. 20th ed. Philadelphia: WB Saunders, 1996

RIB-GAP SYNDROME, see Cerebrocostomandibular syndrome.

RIBAS-TORRES DISEASE, variola minor; a mild form of smallpox.

1. Casas EC: Diccionario Terminologico de Ciencias Medicas. 5th ed. Salvat Editores, SA, 1954

RICHARDS-RUNDLE SYNDROME, a condition characterized by ketoaciduria, mental retardation, underdevelopment of secondary sex characteristics, deafness, ataxia, and peripheral muscular wasting which progresses but eventually becomes static. (B.W. Richards, British; A.T. Rundle, British)

1. Richards BW, Rundle AT: J Ment Def 3:33-55, 1959

RICHARDSON SIGN, when a tourniquet is placed on the arm and there is no filling of the peripheral veins, the patient is considered dead.

1. Casas EC: Diccionario Terminologico de Ciencias Medicas. 5th ed. Salvat Editores, SA, 1954

RICHET-NETTE SIGN, contraction of the adductor muscle of the thigh; seen in the patient with appendicitis.

1. Casas EC: Diccionario Terminologico de Ciencias Medicas. 5th ed. Salvat Editores, SA, 1954

RICHNER-HANHART SYNDROME, oculocutaneous tyrosinemia; a rare autosomal recessive disease with painful punctate erosive and hyperkeratotic changes on the palms and soles. Eye involvement and mental retardation may be present. (Herman R. Richner, Swiss; Ernst Hanhart, 1891-1973, Swiss)

1. Hanhart E: Dermatologica 94:286-308, 1990
2. Moschella SL, Hurley HJ: Dermatology. 2nd ed. Philadelphia: WB Saunders, 1985
3. Richner H: Klin Monatsbl Augenheilkd 100:580-588, 1938

RICHTER HERNIA, parietal hernia; strangulation of a portion of the circumference of the intestine. (August G. Richter, 1742-1812, German surgeon)

1. Lumley JS, Clain A: Hamilton Bailey's Demonstration of Physical Signs in Clinical Surgery. 18th ed. London: Butterworth-Heinemann, 1997

RICHTER SYNDROME, chronic lymphocytic leukemia with diffuse histiocytic lymphoma. (Maurice Richter, U.S. pathologist)

1. Richter MN: Am J Pathol 4:285-292, 1928

RIDDOCH SYNDROME, see Verger-Déjerine syndrome.

RIDLEY SYNDROME, tachycardia with asthma.

1. Casas EC: Diccionario Terminologico deCiencias Medicas. 5th ed. 1954

RIEDEL OPERATION, choledochoduodenostomy.

1. Maffei WE: Os Fundamentos da Medicina. 2nd ed. Livraria Editora Artes Médicas Ltda, 1978

RIEDEL STRUMA, invasive fibrous thyroiditis; a rare presentation of thyroiditis in which there is irreversible, profound hypothyroidism and a stony, hard, irregular, fibrous gland. Symptoms can include cough, dyspnea, and difficulty swallowing. (Bernhard Riedel, 1846-1916, German surgeon)
1. Ballenger JJ: Diseases of the Nose, Throat, Ear, Head and Neck. 12th ed. Philadelphia: Lea & Febiger, 1977
2. Riedel B: Verh Dtsch Ges Chir 25:101-105, 1896

RIEGER PHENOMENON, see Brake phenomenon.

RIEGER SYNDROME, a structural defect of the anterior ocular chamber, consisting of dysplasia of the iris, hypodontia, and hypospadias. Autosomal dominant inheritance. Cross-reference: Anterior chamber cleavage syndrome. (Herwigh Rieger, 1898-1986, German ophthalmologist)
1. Jorgenson RJ, et al: The Rieger syndrome. Am J Med Genet 2:307, 1978
2. Rieger H: Graefes Arch Ophthalmol 133:602-635, 1935
3. Smith DW, Jones KL: Recognizable Patterns of Human Malformations: Genetic, Embryologic, and Clinical Aspects. 3rd ed. Philadelphia: WB Saunders, 1982

RIEHL MELANOSIS, patchy facial melanodermas associated with inflammatory, probably photosensitivity related, reactions. Cosmetic ingredients have been commonly suspected as being causative agents. Some scaling and follicular plugs tend to accompany the facial pigmentation. (Gustav Riehl, 1855-1943, Austrian dermatologist)
1. Riehl G: Wien Klin Wochenschr 30:780-781, 1917

RIESMAN SIGN, a bruit in the globe is audible; seen in the patient with exophthalmic goiter. Cross-reference: Snellen sign. (David Riesman, 1867-1940, U.S.)
1. Casas EC: Diccionario Terminologico de Ciencias Medicas. 5th ed. Salvat Editores, SA, 1954

RINMAN SIGN, cutaneous striae in the beginning of pregnancy.
1. Casas EC: Diccionario Terminologico de Ciencias Medicas. 5th ed. Salvat Editores, SA, 1954

RIFT VALLEY FEVER, an acute viral illness, usually of short duration; characterized by high fever, headache, retro-orbital pain, myalgia, prostration, photophobia, and conjunctival injection. Humans generally acquire the disease by contact with infected domestic animals, although the virus may also be mosquito-borne. (Named for a valley in Kenya where the first case was described in 1931.)
1. Bennett JC, Plum F (eds): Cecil Textbook of Medicine. 20th ed. Philadelphia: WB Saunders, 1996

RIGA DISEASE, aphthosis in cachexia. (Antonio Riga, 1832-1919, Italian)
1. Casas EC: Diccionario Terminologico de Ciencias Medicas. 5th ed. Salvat Editores, SA, 1954

RIGAUD OPERATION, autoplasty for urethral fistula.
1. Maffei WE: Os Fundamentos da Medicina. 2nd ed. Livraria Editora Artes Médicas Ltda, 1978

RIGGS DISEASE, see Fauchard disease. (John M. Riggs, 1810-1885, U.S. dentist)

RIGHT MIDDLE LOBE SYNDROME, see Middle lobe syndrome.

RILEY-DAY SYNDROME, congenital autonomic dysfunction commencing in infancy. Usually affects Ashkenazi Jewish children; in rare instances, a similar disorder is seen in adulthood. Autonomic disturbances prevail in this kalcidoscopic disorder. (Conrad M. Riley, U.S. pediatrician; Richard L. Day, U.S. pediatrician)
1. Farmer TW: Pediatric Neurology. 2nd ed. Hagerstown: Harper & Row, 1975
2. Riley CM, Day RL, Greeley DM, et al: Pediatrics 3:468-478, 1949

RILEY-SMITH SYNDROME, see Bannayan-Zonana syndrome. (Harris D. Riley, Jr., U.S. pediatrician; William R. Smith, U.S.)

RINNE TEST, a measurement of hearing. The examiner places a vibrating tuning fork on the mastoid process, with the limbs of the fork sloping backward. The patient is instructed to signal when no sound is heard. The still-vibrating fork is then held close to the external auditory meatus. If vibrations are still audible, air conduction is better than bone conduction. This is the finding when hearing is normal or in perceptive deafness, and in these circumstances the Rinne test is said to be positive. (Heinrich A. Rinne, 1819-1868, German otologist)
1. Lumley JS, Clain A: Hamilton Bailey's Demonstration of Physical Signs in Clinical Surgery. 18th ed. London: Butterworth-Heinemann, 1997

RIO GRANDE DISEASE, brucellosis.
1. Casas EC: Diccionario Terminologico de Ciencias Medicas. 5th ed. Salvat Editores, SA, 1954

RIPAULT SIGN, pressure on the eye causes no alteration of the pupil; an indication of death. (Louis H.A. Ripault, 1807-1856, French)

1. Casas EC: Diccionario Terminologico de Ciencias Medicas. 5th ed. Salvat Editores, SA, 1954

RIPPLE SIGN, a cortical "ripple" or pattern due to alterations in normal sulci and gyri, described by Heinz and Cooper. Seen in the intermediate phase in good-quality films of arteriograms.
1. Baker AB, Baker LH: Clinical Neurology. Revised ed. Philadelphia: Harper & Row, 1982

RISQUES SIGN, blood pigments seen in the peripheral smear in cases of malaria.
1. Casas EC: Diccionario Terminologico de Ciencias Medicas. 5th ed. Salvat Editores, SA, 1954

RITTER DISEASE, generalized exfoliative dermatitis in newborn infants with staphylococcal scalded-skin syndrome. (Gottfried Ritter von Rittershain, 1820-1883, German)
1. Ritter von Rittershain G: Osterr Jb Pediatr 1:23-24, 1870

RITTER-ROLLET PHENOMENON, flexion of the foot upon gentle electric stimulation and its extension upon energetic stimulation. (Johann W. Ritter, 1776-1810, German physicist; Alexander Rollet, 1834-1903, Austrian physiologist)
1. Dorland's Medical Dictionary. 28th ed. Philadelphia: WB Saunders, 1994

RIVALTA DISEASE, actinomycosis.
1. Casas EC: Diccionario Terminologico de Ciencias Medicas. 5th ed. Salvat Editores, SA, 1954

RIVIERE SIGN, a dull sound heard at the level of T5-7; an indication of tuberculosis. (Clive Riviere, 1873-1929, British)
1. Casas EC: Diccionario Terminologico de Ciencias Medicas. 5th ed. Salvat Editores, SA, 1954

ROBERTS OPERATION, surgical method for correcting deviation of the nasal septum.
1. Maffei WE: Os Fundamentos da Medicina. 2nd ed. Livraria Editora Artes Médicas Ltda, 1978

ROBERTS SYNDROME, an inherited syndrome of imperfect development of the long bones of the limbs associated with the left palate and lip. Hypomelia, midfacial defects, severe growth deficiency, severe mental defects, cleft lip, and cryptorchidism are features. Autosomal recessive inheritance. (John B. Roberts, 1852-1924, U.S. surgeon)
1. Roberts JB: Ann Surg 70:252-254, 1919
2. Smith DW, Jones KL: Recognizable Patterns of Human Malformations: Genetic, Embryologic, and Clinical Aspects. 3rd ed. Philadelphia: WB Saunders, 1982
3. Waldenmaier C, Aldenhoff P, Klemm T: The Roberts syndrome. Hum Genet 40:345, 1978

ROBERTSON SIGN, 1) fibrillary contraction of the pectoralis muscle over the cardiac area, due to heart disease; seen in approaching death; 2) the absence of pupillary dilatation upon pressure over allegedly painful areas in malingering; 3) fullness and tension of the patient's flanks, felt by the examiner with the patient supine; seen in ascites. (William E. Robertson, 1869-1956, U.S.)
1. Casas EC: Diccionario Terminologico de Ciencias Medicas. 5th ed. Salvat Editores, SA, 1954

ROBIN SYNDROME, see Pierre Robin syndrome.

ROBINOW SYNDROME, dwarfism associated with a flat facial profile, short forearms, and hypoplastic genitalia. Autosomal dominant inheritance. Cross-reference: Fetal face syndrome. (Meinhard Robinow, U.S.)
1. Robinow M, Silverman FN, Smith HD: A newly recognized dwarfing syndrome. Am J Dis Child 17:645-651, 1969
2. Smith DW, Jones KL: Recognizable Patterns of Human Malformations: Genetic, Embryologic, and Clinical Aspects. 3rd ed. Philadelphia: WB Saunders, 1982

ROBINSON DISEASE, hidrocystoma. (Andrew R. Robinson, 1845-1924, U.S.)
1. Robinson AR: J Cutan Dis 11:293-303, 1893

ROBINSON OPERATION, surgery for varices.
1. Maffei WE: Os Fundamentos da Medicina. 2nd ed. Livraria Editora Artes Médicas Ltda, 1978

ROBLES DISEASE, onchocerciasis; infection by nematodes of the genus *Onchocerca*. Marked by fever with moderate symptoms of 2 to 3 weeks' duration; found mainly in Africa and the Western Hemisphere. (Rudolfo Robles, 1879-1939, Guatemalan dermatologist)
1. Casas EC: Diccionario Terminologico de Ciencias Medicas. 5th ed. Salvat Editores, SA, 1954

ROCHE SIGN, the inability to distinguish the epididymis from the body of the testis; seen in the patient with torsion of the testicle. (Henri G.L. Roche, French surgeon)
1. Casas EC: Diccionario Terminologico de Ciencias Medicas. 5th ed. Salvat Editores, SA, 1954

ROCHON-DUVIGNEAUD SYNDROME, see Tolosa-Hunt syndrome.

ROCIO ENCEPHALITIS, see Murray Valley encephalitis.

ROCKLEY TEST, a measurement for malar fracture.
1. Casas EC: Diccionario Terminologico de Ciencias Medicas. 5th ed. Salvat Editores, SA, 1954

ROCKY MOUNTAIN DISEASE, ROCKY MOUNTAIN SPOTTED FEVER, infection with *Rickettsia*, transmitted by ticks in dogs, rodents, and foxes and marked by fever with muscle pain and weakness followed by a macular petechial eruption that begins on the hands and feet and spreads to the trunk and face. There is involvement of the central nervous system. Occurs in North and South America.
1. Bennett JC, Plum F (eds): Cecil Textbook of Medicine. 20th ed. Philadelphia: WB Saunders, 1996

ROD SYNDROME, characterized by the complaint of night blindness (i.e., prolonged adjustment to conditions of dim illumination). May be documented by abnormality of the rod branch of the dark adaptation curve.
1. Smith JL: Neuro-Ophthalmology, Volume 6. St Louis: CV Mosby, 1972

RODMAN OPERATION, ablation of the breast and lymph nodes in cases of carcinoma of the breast.
1. Maffei WE: Os Fundamentos da Medicina. 2nd ed. Livraria Editora Artes Médicas Ltda, 1978

ROEMHELD SYNDROME, see Gastrocardiac syndrome. (Ludwig Roemheld, 1871-1938, German)

ROGER SYNDROME, hypersecretion of saliva caused by esophageal cancer or esophageal irritation.
1. Roger LE, Poster FW, Sidbury JB Jr: J Pediatr 74:494-504, 1969

ROKITANSKY DISEASE, see Budd syndrome. (Karl F. von Rokitansky, 1804-1878, Austrian pathologist)

ROKITANSKY SYNDROME, ROKITANSKY-KÜSTER-HAUSER SYNDROME, see Mayer-Rokitansky-Küster syndrome. (Karl F. von Rokitansky)

ROLANDIC VEIN SYNDROME, hemiplegia resulting from interference with the cerebral venous circulation.
1. Dorland's Medical Dictionary. 28th ed. Philadelphia: WB Saunders, 1994

ROMAÑA SIGN, ROMAÑO SIGN, swelling of the eyelids, regional lymph glands, and conjunctivitis are features; an indication of Chagas disease. (Cecilio Romaña, Argentinian in Brazil)
1. Dorland's Medical Dictionary. 28th ed. Philadelphia: WB Saunders, 1994

ROMAÑO-WARD SYNDROME, hereditary prolongation of the Q-T interval on electrocardiography, usually in association with syncope and sudden death. An autosomal dominant trait transmitted without deafness. Cross-references: Ward- Ramaño syndrome. (Celilio Ramaño; O.C. Ward, Irish)
1. Romano C, Gemma G, Pongiglione R: Clin Pediatr 45:656-683, 1963
2. Ward OC: A new familial cardiac syndrome in children. J Irish Med Assoc 54:103-106, 1964
3. Zipes DP, Jalife J: Cardiac Electrophysiology: From Cell to Bedside. 2nd ed. Philadelphia: WB Saunders, 1995

ROMBERG SIGN, while standing with the feet together and eyes open, the patient sways or falls when the eyes close; a loss of proprioceptive control is indicated. Cross-reference: Branch-Romberg sign. (Moritz H. von Romberg, 1795-1873, German neurologist)
1. Baker AB, Baker LH: Clinical Neurology. Revised ed. Philadelphia: Harper & Row, 1982
2. Von Romberg MH: Lehrbuch der Nerven Krankheitan des Menschen. Berlin: Duncker, 1840-1846

ROMBERG SYNDROME, progressive hemifacial atrophy; consists of slowly progressive atrophy of the soft tissues of essentially half the face, accompanied most frequently by contralateral Jacksonian epilepsy, trigeminal neuralgia, and changes in the eyes and hair. Cross-references: Parry-Romberg syndrome; Progressive hemifacial atrophy syndrome. (Moritz H. von Romberg)
1. Parry CH: Collections From Unpublished Medical Writings. London: Underwood, 1825
2. Von Romberg MH: Trophoneurosen. Klinische Ergebnisse. Berlin: A Foerstner, 1846, pp 75-81

ROMMELAERE SIGN, low amounts of phosphate and sodium chloride in the urine of the patient with cancer cachexia. (Guillaume Rommelaere, 1836-1916, Belgian)
1. Casas EC: Diccionario Terminologico de Ciencias Medicas. 5th ed. Salvat Editores, SA, 1954

ROPE SIGN, acute angulation between the chin and the larynx because of weakness of the hyoid muscles; seen in the patient with bulbar poliomyelitis.
1. Dorland's Medical Dictionary. 28th ed. Philadelphia: WB Saunders, 1994

ROQUE SIGN, unilateral dilatation of the pupil and elevation of the upper eyelid caused by cervical sympathetic damage with lesioning of the apex of the lung.
1. Casas EC: Diccionario Terminologico de Ciencias Medicas. 5th ed. Salvat Editores, SA, 1954

RORSCHACH INK BLOT TEST, a measurement for evaluating personality via the use of patterns of ink blots. Also, a task that makes demands on intellectual and visuointegrative capacity. (Hermann Rorschach, 1884-1922, Swiss psychiatrist)
1. Baker AB, Baker LH: Clinical Neurology. Revised ed. Philadelphia: Harper & Row, 1982
2. Reitan RM: Validity of Rorschach test as a measure of psychological effects of brain damage. Arch Neurol Psychiatr 73:445, 1955

ROSAI-DORFMAN SYNDROME, an idiopathic histioproliferative disease affecting the lymph nodes. Massive lymphadenopathy, fever, and pallor are features. (Juan Rosai, U.S.)
1. Rosai J, Dorfman RF: Sinus histiocytosis with massive lymphadenopathy. A newly recognized benign clinicopathologic entity. Arch Pathol Lab Med 87:63, 1969

ROSE OPERATION, ablation of the gasserian ganglion.
1. Maffei WE: Os Fundamentos da Medicina. 2nd ed. Livraria Editora Artes Médicas Ltda, 1978

ROSEN NEURALGIA, tic douloureux of the chorda tympani.
1. Baker AB, Baker LH: Clinical Neurology. Revised ed. Philadelphia: Harper & Row, 1982
2. Rosen S: Tic douloureux of the chorda tympani: report of cases. Arch Neurol Psychiatr 69:375-378, 1953

ROSENBACH DISEASE, see Heberden nodes. (Anton J.F. Rosenbach, 1842-1923, German)

ROSENBACH SIGN, difficulty in obtaining the superficial abdominal reflexes. Reflex may be absent in acute abdominal conditions, obesity, abdominal distention, or bladder distention. (Ottomar Rosenbach, 1851-1907, German)
1. Baker AB, Baker LH: Clinical Neurology. Revised ed. Philadelphia: Harper & Row, 1982

ROSENBACH SYNDROME, paroxysmal tachycardia with gastric and respiratory complications. Cross-reference: Fox-Backer-Rosenbach disease. (Ottomar Rosenbach)
1. Rosenbach O: Dtsch Med Wochenschr 5:535-538, 1879

ROSENHEIM SIGN, a friction sound in the left hypochondrium; may be an indication of spondylitis.
1. Casas EC: Diccionario Terminologico de Ciencias Medicas. 5th ed. Salvat Editores, SA, 1954

ROSENTHAL SIGN, pain produced in the vertebral column with faradic current; an indication of spondylitis.
1. Casas EC: Diccionario Terminologico de Ciencias Medicas. 5th ed. Salvat Editores, SA, 1954

ROSENTHAL SYNDROME, a hereditary hemorrhagic disorder owing to factor XI deficiency; clinically similar to hemophilia. (Robert L. Rosenthal, U.S. hematologist)
1. Rosenthal RL: Proc Soc Exp Biol Med 82:171-174, 1953

ROSENTHAL-KLOEPFER SYNDROME, see Touraine-Solente-Golé syndrome.

ROSER SIGN, ROSER-BRAUN SIGN, lack of dural pulsation; an indication of a brain tumor or abscess. (Wilhelm Roser, 1817-1888, German surgeon; Heinrich Braun, 1847-1911, German surgeon)
1. Casas EC: Diccionario Terminologico de Ciencias Medicas. 5th ed. Salvat Editores, SA, 1954

ROSEWATER SYNDROME, see Reifenstein syndrome.

ROSS RIVER FEVER, polyarthritis caused by alphavirus and associated exclusively with a mild, undifferentiated disease mostly encountered in tropical and semitropical countries.
1. Bennett JC, Plum F (eds): Cecil Textbook of Medicine. 20th ed. Philadelphia: WB Saunders, 1996
2. Ritchie AC: Boyd's Textbook of Pathology. 9th ed. Philadelphia: Lea & Febiger, 1990

ROSS SYNDROME, see Adie syndrome (Alexander T. Ross, U.S.)

ROSSBACH DISEASE, hyperchlorhydria in the stomach. (Michael J. Rossbach, 1842-1894, German)
1. Rossbach MJ: Dtsch Arch Klin Med 35:383-401, 1884

ROSSELLI-GULIENETTI SYNDROME, a unique syndrome of woolly hair, cleft lip and palate, dystrophic nails, subungual keratosis, dystrophic facial skin, a papulofollicular dermatosis of the trunk, and hypoplasia or aplasia of the thumbs and popliteal pterygia. Cross-reference: Gross-Groh-Weppl syndrome.
1. Gorlin RJ, Cohen MM Jr, Levin LS: Syndromes of the Head and Neck. 3rd ed. New York: Oxford University Press, 1990
2. Rosselli D, Gulienetti R: Ectodermal dysplasia. Br J Plast Surg 14:190-204, 1961

ROSSOLIMO REFLEX, ROSSOLIMO SIGN, flexion of the toes elicited by tapping the ends of the toes. (Gregorij I. Rossolimo, 1860-1928, Russian neurologist)

1. Baker AB, Baker LH: Clinical Neurology. Revised ed. Philadelphia: Harper & Row, 1982
2. Grinker RR, Sahs AL: Neurology . 6th ed. Springfield: Charles C Thomas, 1966

ROSTRAL BASILAR ARTERY SYNDROME, a patient with occlusion of the rostral portion of the basilar artery who may experience extensive infarction of the mesencephalon, thalamus, hypothalamus, paramedian diencephalon, medial temporal lobes, and occipital lobes. Damage to these structures produces a variety of behavioral, neuro-ophthalmological, and motor signs.

1. Walsh FB, Hoyt EF, Miller NR: Clinical Neuro-Ophthalmology. 4th ed. Baltimore: Williams & Wilkins, 1982

ROTCH SIGN, a dull sound heard in the right 5th intercostal space; found in the patient with pericardial effusion. (Thomas M. Rotch, 1849-1914, U.S.)

1. Casas EC: Diccionario Terminologico de Ciencias Medicas. 5th ed. Salvat Editores, SA, 1954

ROTH [ROT]-BERNHARDT SYNDROME, see Bernhardt syndrome. (Vladimir Roth [Rot], 1848-1916, Russian neurologist)

ROTH SPOTS, oval retinal hemorrhages with clear pale centers associated with infective endocarditis. (Moritz von Roth, 1839-1914, Swedish pathologist)

1. Von Roth M: Dtsch Z Chir 1:471-484, 1872

ROTHMANN-MAKAI SYNDROME, a very rare variant of lobular panniculitis with numerous large lesions, affecting children; the lesions do not liquefy and healing usually occurs within 12 months. (Max Rothmann, 1868-1915, German pathologist; Endre Makai, Hungarian surgeon)

1. Makai E: Klin Wochenschr 7:2343-2346, 1928
2. Rothmann M: Virchow Arch Pathol Anat Physiol 136:156-159, 1894

ROTHMUND SYNDROME, ROTHMUND-THOMSON SYNDROME, congenital cutaneous dystrophy; a rare heritable disorder characterized by poikiloderma of the skin and frequently associated with juvenile cataracts and short stature. Cross-reference: Werner syndrome. (August Rothmund, 1830-1906, German ophthalmologist; Matthew S. Thomson, 1894-1969, British dermatologist)

1. Gorlin RJ, Cohen MM Jr, Levin LS: Syndromes of the Head and Neck. 3rd ed. New York: Oxford University Press, 1990
2. Rothmund A: Graefes Arch Ophthalmol 14:159-182, 1868
3. Thomson MS: Poikiloderma congenitale. Br J Dermatol 218:221-234, 1936
4. Werner CWO: Ueber Katarakt in Verbindung mit Sclerodermie. Inaug Disser Kiel, 1904

ROTHSCHILD SIGN, 1) flatness and immobility of the sternal angle; seen in the patient with tuberculosis; 2) lack of hair in the lateral one third of the eyebrow; seen in the patient with hypothyroidism.

1. Casas EC: Diccionario Terminologico de Ciencias Medicas. 5th ed. Salvat Editores, SA, 1954

ROTOR SYNDROME, inherited disorder of bilirubin metabolism. Occasional abdominal pain and mild fluctuating jaundice are characteristics. Autosomal recessive inheritance. (Arturo B. Rotor, Philippine)

1. Bennett JC, Plum F (eds): Cecil Textbook of Medicine. 20th ed. Philadelphia: WB Saunders, 1996
2. Ritchie AC: Boyd's Textbook of Pathology. 9th ed. Philadelphia: Lea & Febiger, 1990
3. Rotor AB, Manahan L, Florentin A: Familial non-hemolytic jaundice with direct van den Bergh reaction. Acta Med Philippina 5:37-49, 1948

ROUGE OPERATION, opening of the nasal sinuses through detachment of the upper lip and maxillary nasal cartilages.

1. Maffei WE: Os Fundamentos da Medicina. 2nd ed. Livraria Editora Artes Médicas Ltda, 1978

ROUGNON-HEBERDEN DISEASE, angina pectoris. (Nicholas Rougnon, 1727-1799, French physician; William Heberden, 1710-1801, British)

1. Heberden W: Trans R Coll Phys Lond 2:59-67, 1772

ROUSSEL SIGN, pain on percussion of the region between the clavicle and the 4th rib; an indication of incipient tuberculosis.

1. Casas EC: Diccionario Terminologico de Ciencias Medicas. 5th ed. Salvat Editores, SA, 1954

ROUSSY-LÉVY SYNDROME, a disorder affecting females with trisomy of the X chromosome; early deafness, mental deficiency, hypogonadism, and a possible block in androgen metabolism are features. Cross-reference: Lévy-Roussy syndrome. (Gustave Roussy, 1874-1948, French neuropathologist; G. Lévy, French neurologist)

1. Farmer TW: Pediatric Neurology. 2nd ed. Hagerstown: Harper & Row, 1975
2. Roussy G, Lévy G: Rev Neurol 33:427-450, 1926
3. Rowland LP (ed): Merritt's Textbook of Neurology. 9th ed. Baltimore: Williams & Wilkins, 1995

ROUTTE OPERATION, fixation of the great saphenous vein into the peritoneal cavity in order to drain ascites in the patient with liver cirrhosis.
1. Maffei WE: Os Fundamentos da Medicina. 2nd ed. Livraria Editora Artes Médicas Ltda, 1978

ROUX SIGN, lack of resistance in an empty cecum; seen in the patient with a suppurated appendix.
1. Casas EC: Diccionario Terminologico de Ciencias Medicas. 5th ed. Salvat Editores, SA, 1954

ROVIGHI SIGN, a trembling sensation felt on palpation and percussion of a superficial hydatid cyst of the liver. (Alberto Rovighi, 1856-1919, Italian)
1. Casas EC: Diccionario Terminologico de Ciencias Medicas. 5th ed. Salvat Editores, SA, 1954

ROVSING SIGN, pressure at the McBurney point causing pain in the right iliac fossa; seen in the patient with appendicitis only and not in other abdominal diseases. (Niels T. Rovsing, 1862-1927, Danish surgeon)
1. Campbell MF, Walsh PC: Campbell's Urology. 5th ed. Philadelphia: WB Saunders, 1986

ROVSING SYNDROME, characteristics include horseshoe kidney, nausea, abdominal discomfort, and pain on bending backward. Cross-reference: Symonds-Show syndrome. (Niels T. Rovsing)
1. Dorland's Medical Dictionary. 28th ed. Philadelphia: WB Saunders, 1994

ROWLAND DISEASE, see Hand-Schüller-Christian disease. (Russell S. Rowland, 1874-1938, U.S.)

ROWLEY-ROSENBERG SYNDROME, a metabolic disease with generalized aminoaciduria associated with growth retardation, muscular hypoplasia, pulmonary involvement, and right ventricular hypertrophy. (Peter T. Rowley, U.S.)
1. Rowley PT: Am J Med 31:187-204, 1961
2. Scriver CR, Rosenberg LE: Amino Acid Metabolism and Its Disorders. Philadelphia: WB Saunders, 1973

ROYAL FREE DISEASE, see Iceland disease.

RUAULT SIGN, a decrease in respiration amplitude of the lung vortex; seen in tuberculosis.
1. Casas EC: Diccionario Terminologico de Ciencias Medicas. 5th ed. Salvat Editores, SA, 1954

RUBELLA SYNDROME, see Congenital rubella syndrome.

RUBINSTEIN-TAYBI SYNDROME, consists of microcephaly with severe mental retardation, broad thumbs and toes, a beaked nose, and other anomalies. Cross-reference: Broad thumbs syndrome. (Jack H. Rubinstein, U.S. pediatrician; Hooshang Taybi, U.S. pediatrician/radiologist)
1. Atlas of Mental Retardation Syndromes. Washington, DC: Government Printing Office, 1969
2. Gorlin RJ, Cohen MM Jr, Levin LS: Syndromes of the Head and Neck. 3rd ed. New York: Oxford University Press, 1990
3. Rubinstein JH: The broad thumbs syndrome. Progress report 1968. Birth Defects 5:25, 1969
4. Rubinstein JH, Taybi H: Am J Dis Child 105:588-608, 1963

RUD SYNDROME, dwarfism-ichthyosiform erythroderma-mental deficiency; ichthyosis vulgaris, mental retardation, epilepsy, hypogonadism, chronic amenia, and arachnodactyly are characteristics. Cross-reference: Sjögren-Larsson syndrome. (Elnar Rud, Danish)
1. Ritchie AC: Boyd's Textbook of Pathology. 9th ed. Philadelphia: Lea & Febiger, 1990
2. Rud E: Hospitalstidende 70:505-538, 1927
3. Sjögren T, Larsson T: Acta Psychiatr Neurol Scand 32 (Suppl 113):1-112, 1957
4. York-More ME, Rundle AT: Rud's syndrome. J Ment Def Res 6:108-118, 1962

RÜDIGER SYNDROME, a lethal syndrome of somatic retardation, flexion contractures of the hands with thick, single palmar creases, small fingers and nails, unusual facies, and ureterovesical stenosis. Cross-reference: Ectrodactyly-ectodermal dysplasia-clefting syndrome. (Roswitha A. Rüdiger, German)
1. Gorlin RJ, Cohen MM Jr, Levin LS: Syndromes of the Head and Neck. 3rd ed. New York: Oxford University Press, 1990
2. Rüdiger RA, et al: Severe development failure with coarse facial features, distal limb hypoplasia, thickened palmar creases, bifid uvula and ureteral stenosis: a previously undescribed familial disorder with lethal outcome. J Pediatr 79:977-981, 1971

RUDIMENTARY OVARY SYNDROME, poorly defined entity of unknown etiology, said to be characterized by ovaries containing decreased numbers of follicles.
1. Gold JJ, Josimovich JB: Gynecologic Endocrinology. 3rd ed. New York: Plenum Medical, 1980, p 279

RUDIMENTARY TESTIS SYNDROME, despite testis less than 1 cm in greatest diameter, a small, well-formed penis is present. The testes consist of a few Leydig cells, small tubules containing Sertoli cells, and occasional spermatogonium. Wolffian derivatives are present; müllerian derivatives are

absent. No fertility. Cross-reference: Wilkins-Bergada syndrome.
1. Gold JJ, Josimovich JB: Gynecologic Endocrinology. 3rd ed. New York: Plenum Medical, 1980

RUGGI OPERATION, gastrojejunostomy with a double opening.
1. Maffei WE: Os Fundamentos da Medicina. 2nd ed. Livraria Editora Artes Médicas Ltda, 1978

RUMMO DISEASE, cardioptosis. (Gaetano Rummo, 1853-1917, Italian)
1. Casas EC: Diccionario Terminologico de Ciencias Medicas. 5th ed. Salvat Editores, SA, 1954

RUMPEL-LEEDE SIGN, RUMPEL-LEEDE TEST, RUMPEL-LEEDE PHENOMENON, small petechial hemorrhages appear on the arm after tourniquet placement; seen in the patient with scarlet fever and hemorrhagic diathesis. Cross-reference: Frugoni-Rumpel-Leede sign. (Theodor Rumpel, 1862-1923, German; Carl S. Leede, 1882-1964, U.S.)
1. Casas EC: Diccionario Terminologico de Ciencias Medicas. 5th ed. Salvat Editores, SA, 1954

RUMPF SIGN, tonic contractions and fibrillations; noted in the patient with traumatic neurosis.
1. Casas EC: Diccionario Terminologico de Ciencias Medicas. 5th ed. Salvat Editores, SA, 1954

RUNEBERG DISEASE, a form of progressive pernicious anemia. (Johann W. Runeberg, 1843-1918, Finnish)
1. Runeberg JW: Dtsch Arch Klin Med 28:499-520, 1880-1881

RUNTING SYNDROME, graft-vs.-host reaction characterized by diarrhea, dermatitis, hepato-splenomegaly, hemolytic anemia, and pancytopenia. Cross-reference: Wasting syndrome.
1. Dorland's Medical Dictionary. 28th ed. Philadelphia: WB Saunders, 1994

RUSSELL SYNDROME, RUSSELL EMACIATION SYNDROME, profound emaciation; anemia, blindness, nystagmus, and pallor of the skin are the chief manifestations of a diencephalic syndrome observed in infants and children from 2-6 months of age onward, in association with astrocytoma or some other type of glioma of the anterior hypothalamus. Cross-reference: Diencephalic syndrome. (Alexander R. Russell, British pediatrician)
1. Baker AB, Baker LH: Clinical Neurology. Revised ed. Philadelphia: Harper & Row, 1982
2. Russell A: A diencephalic syndrome of emaciation in infancy and childhood. Arch Dis Child 26:274, 1951

RUSSELL-SILVER SYNDROME, a congenital syndrome consisting of low birth weight despite a normal gestation period, short stature, lateral asymmetry, and a slight-to-moderate increase in excretion of gonadotropins, which may also be associated with in-curved 5th fingers, café-au-lait spots, syndactyly, a triangular face, turned down corners of the mouth, and precocious puberty. Cross-references: Partington syndrome; Silver-Russell syndrome. (Alexander R. Russell; Henry K. Silver, U.S. pediatrician)
1. Escobar V, Gleiser S, Weaver DD: Phenotypic and genetic analysis of Silver-Russell syndrome. Clin Genet 13:278, 1978
2. Russell A: Proc R Soc Med 47:1040-1044, 1954
3. Silver HK, Kiyasu W, George J, et al: Pediatrics 12:368-376, 1953

RUST PHENOMENON, the patient holds the head up with hands when getting up or lying down; seen in malignant disease of the cervical vertebrae. (Johann N. Rust, 1775-1840, Austrian surgeon)
1. Casas EC: Diccionario Terminologico de Ciencias Medicas. 5th ed. Salvat Editores, SA, 1954

RUST SYNDROME, lesions of the atlanto-occipital region secondary to tuberoclosis, syphilis, rigidity of the cervical spine, and drooping of the head. May be caused by inflammatory or neoplastic lesions. (Johann N. Rust)
1. Rust JN: Aufsätze und Abhändlungen aus dem Gebiete der Medizin. Chirurgie und Staatsarzneikunde. Berlin: Enslin, 1834

RUTHERFURD SYNDROME, relatively mild gingival enlargement, failure of tooth eruption, and corneal opacities are features. (Margaret E. Rutherfurd, 1910-1964, British dentist)
1. Gorlin RJ, Cohen MM Jr, Levin LS: Syndromes of the Head and Neck. 3rd ed. New York: Oxford University Press, 1990
2. Rutherfurd ME: Three generations of inherited dental defect. Br Med J 2:9-11, 1931

RUTHMUND-WERNER SYNDROME, scleroderma associated with juvenile cataract.
1. Maffei WE: Os Fundamentos da Medicina. 2nd ed. Livraria Editora Artes Médicas Ltda, 1978

RUVALCABA SYNDROME, hypoplastic alae nasi, small mouth, short metacarpal bones, mental deficiency, jovial personality, microcephaly, brachyphalangy, spondylodysplasia, polyposis colon, and pigmentary changes in the pelvis are features. Etiology unknown. (R.H.A. Ruvalcaba, U.S.)
1. Ruvalcaba RHA, Reichert A, Smith DW: J Pediatr 79:450-455, 1971

2. Smith DW, Jones KL: Recognizable Patterns of Human Malformations: Genetic, Embryologic, and Clinical Aspects. 3rd ed. Philadelphia: WB Saunders, 1982

RUVALCABA-MYHRE-SMITH SYNDROME, characterized by macrocephaly, hamartomatous polyps, and lipomas. Lipid storage myopathy has been reported in association with scoliosis and multiple joint contractures. (R.H.A. Ruvalcaba)

1. Gorlin RJ, Cohen MM Jr, Levin LS: Syndromes of the Head and Neck. 3rd ed. New York: Oxford University Press, 1990
2. Ruvalcaba RHA, Myhre S, Smith DW: Clin Genet 18:413-416, 1980

RUYSCH DISEASE, megacolon.

1. Casas EC: Diccionario Terminologico de Ciencias Medicas. 5th ed. Salvat Editores, SA, 1954

RYDYGIER OPERATION, splenopexy; surgical fixation of the spleen to a peritoneal pouch.

1. Maffei WE: Os Fundamentos da Medicina. 2nd ed. Livraria Editora Artes Médicas Ltda, 1978

RYUKYUAN HEREDITARY MOTOR NEUROPATHY, a unique autosomal disorder found only in the southern part of Japan. All patients are believed to be descendants of King Hokuzan from the 14th century. Facial and neck muscles are preserved and there is no bulbar weakness. Delayed walking sometimes until the 8th year, proximal weakness of the arms, depressed or absent tendon reflexes, pes cavus, scoliosis, and joint contractures are characteristics.

1. Kondo K, Tsubaki T, Sakamoto F: The Ryukyuan muscular atrophy. An obscure heritable neuromuscular disease found in the islands of southern Japan. J Neurol Sci 11:359-382, 1970

SABATHIE SIGN, dilatation or fullness of one or both jugular veins; seen in the patient with atherosclerosis or aneurysm of the aorta.

1. Casas EC: Diccionario Terminologico de Ciencias Medicas. 5th ed. Salvat Editores, SA, 1954

SABIN-FELDMAN SYNDROME, chorioretinitis and cerebral calcification similar to the manifestations of toxoplasmosis, but with all tests for toxoplasmosis negative. (Albert B. Sabin, U.S.; Henry A. Feldman, U.S. epidemiologist)

1. Sabin AB, Feldman HA: Chorioretinopathy associated with other evidence of cerebral damage in childhood: a syndrome of unknown etiology separable from congenital toxoplasmosis. J Pediatr 35:296-309, 1949

SACHS DISEASE, see Tay-Sachs disease.

SADDLEBACK FEVER, a distinctly biphasic illness that occurs in half the cases of Colorado tick fever.

1. Bennett JC, Plum F (eds): Cecil Textbook of Medicine. 20th ed. Philadelphia: WB Saunders, 1996

SAENGER SIGN, a slight retraction of the pupil after being in the dark for a while; seen in the patient with syphilis, but not in locomotor ataxia. (Alfred Saenger, 1861-1921, German neurologist)

1. Casas EC: Diccionario Terminologico de Ciencias Medicas. 5th ed. Salvat Editores, SA, 1954

SAETHRE-CHOTZEN SYNDROME, acrocephalosyndactyly type III; features include brachycephaly with a high forehead, cutaneous syndactyly, facial asymmetry, hypertelorism, and mild to moderate brachydactyly. Autosomal dominant inheritance. Cross-reference: Chotzen syndrome. (Haakon Saethre, Norwegian; F. Chotzen, German psychiatrist)

1. Chotzen F: Monatsschr Kinderheilkd 55:97-122, 1932
2. Friedman JM, Hanson JW, Graham CB, et al: Saethre-Chotzen syndrome: a broad and variable pattern of skeletal malformations. J Pediatr 91:929, 1977
3. Saethre H: Dtsch Z Nervenheilkd 117:533-555, 1931
4. Smith DW, Jones KL: Recognizable Patterns of Human Malformations: Genetic, Embryologic, and Clinical Aspects. 3rd ed. Philadelphia: WB Saunders, 1982

SAINT ANTHONY'S FIRE, erysipelas; an acute ß-hemolytic streptococcal infection of the skin, mostly of the face and head although infection can occur elsewhere. A portal of entry by an abrasion or a surgical procedure is common. Cross-references: Milian sign; Santa Antonio disease.

1. Ballenger JJ: Diseases of the Nose, Throat, Ear, Head and Neck. 12th ed. Philadelphia: Lea & Febiger, 1977

SAINT GERMAIN OPERATION, dilatation of prepuce in phimosis.

1. Maffei WE: Os Fundamentos da Medicina. 2nd ed. Livraria Editora Artes Médicas Ltda, 1978

SAINT LOUIS ENCEPHALITIS, caused by a member of the *Flavivirus* genus of the family *Togaviridae*, which shares a close antigenic relationship with the Japanese, Murray Valley, and West Nile viruses. The virus has been responsible for up to 80% of all reported cases of encephalitis of known etiology in the U.S. A total of 4824 cases were reported between 1955 and 1978.

1. Bennett JC, Plum F (eds): Cecil Textbook of Medicine. 20th ed. Philadelphia: WB Saunders, 1996

SAINT VITUS DANCE DISEASE, see Sydenham chorea.

SAKATI-NYHAN SYNDROME, SAKATI-NYHAN-TISDALE SYNDROME, acrocephalopoly-syndactyly type III; short limbs, congenital heart defect, ear anomalies, and skin defects are characteristics. (Nadia Sakati, U.S. pediatrician; William Nyhan, U.S. pediatrician)

1. Gorlin RJ, Cohen MM Jr, Levin LS: Syndromes of the Head and Neck. 3rd ed. New York: Oxford University Press, 1990
2. Sakati N, Nyhan WL, Tisdale WK: A new syndrome with acrocephalopolysyndactyly, cardiac disease, and distinctive defects of the ear skin and lower limbs. J Pediatr 79:104-109, 1971

SALDINO SYNDROME, see Achondrogenesis syndrome.

SALDINO-NOONAN SYNDROME, short rib-polydactyly syndrome type I; characterized by micromelia, a narrow chest and protuberant abdomen, postaxial polydactyly, remarkably short ribs, abnormally contoured ilia, peg-shaped or pointed femora, notched tibiae, general ossification deficiencies of the short tubular bones with poor corticomedullary demarcation, and various visceral anomalies. (Ronald M. Saldino, U.S. radiologist; Jacqueline A. Noonan, U.S. pediatric cardiologist)

1. Saldino RM, Noonan CC: Am J Roentgenol 114:257, 1972

SALINAS SYNDROME, a sporadic instance of multiple anomalies confined to the head and face. Coloboma and hypoplastic midface with cleft lip and/or palate are features.

1. Gorlin RJ, Cohen MM Jr, Levin LS: Syndromes of the Head and Neck. 3rd ed. New York: Oxford University Press, 1990
2. Salinas CF, et al: Case report 38: colobomas of lower lids, malar hypoplasia, antimongoloid slant and clefting. Syndrome Ident 4(1):5-6, 1976
3. Schwartz WB, et al: A syndrome of renal sodium loss and hyponatremia probably resulting from inappropriate secretion of antidiuretic hormone. Am J Med 23:259, 1957

SALISBURY-MELVIN SIGN, blood in retinal vessels does not circulate and is fragmented; an indication of imminent death.

1. Casas EC: Diccionario Terminologico de Ciencias Medicas. 5th ed. Salvat Editores, SA, 1954

SALMON SIGN, unilateral dilatation of the pupil in a patient with ruptured ectopic pregnancy.

1. Casas EC: Diccionario Terminologico de Ciencias Medicas. 5th ed. Salvat Editores, SA, 1954

SALONEN-HERVA-NORIO SYNDROME, see Hydrolethalus syndrome.

SALONICA DISEASE, see Trench fever.

SALT DEPLETION SYNDROME, SALT LOSING SYNDROME, mental confusion as a result of hyponatremia due to excessive loss of sodium in urine or from excessive water in the blood.

1. Ballenger JJ: Diseases of the Nose, Throat, Ear, Head and Neck. 12th ed. Philadelphia: Lea & Febiger, 1977

SALUS SIGN, the retinal veins appear like "bayonets"; seen in the patient with optic atrophy. (Robert Salus, Austrian ophthalmologist)

1. Bordas LB (ed): Neurologia Fundamental. 2nd ed. Toray, 1968

SALZE OPERATION, 1) resection of the first division of the trigeminal nerve; 2) suture of the Poupart ligament (inguinal ligament) to the pectineal aponeurosis for the radical cure of femoral hernia.

1. Maffei WE: Os Fundamentos da Medicina. 2nd ed. Livraria Editora Artes Médicas Ltda, 1978

SAN BLAS DISEASE, angina tonsillaris.

1. Casas EC: Diccionario Terminologico de Ciencias Medicas. 5th ed. Salvat Editores, SA, 1954

SAN ERASMO DISEASE, colic.

1. Casas EC: Diccionario Terminologico de Ciencias Medicas. 5th ed. Salvat Editores, SA, 1954

SAN FIACRO DISEASE, hemorrhoids.

1. Casas EC: Diccionario Terminologico de Ciencias Medicas. 5th ed. Salvat Editores, SA, 1954

SAN FRANCISCO SYNDROME, craniosynostosis, midface hypoplasia, ptosis of the eyelids, a bulbous nose, and small ears are characteristics.

1. Gorlin RJ, Cohen MM Jr, Levin LS: Syndromes of the Head and Neck. 3rd ed. New York: Oxford University Press, 1990

SAN GERVASIO DISEASE, rheumatism.

1. Casas EC: Diccionario Terminologico de Ciencias Medicas. 5th ed. Salvat Editores, SA, 1954

SAN GIL DISEASE, leprosy and cancer.

1. Casas EC: Diccionario Terminologico de Ciencias Medicas. 5th ed. Salvat Editores, SA, 1954

SAN HUBERTO DISEASE, rabies.
1. Casas EC: Diccionario Terminologico de Ciencias Medicas. 5th ed. Salvat Editores, SA, 1954

SAN JOAQUIM VALLEY DISEASE, coccidioidomycosis.
1. Casas EC: Diccionario Terminologico de Ciencias Medicas. 5th ed. Salvat Editores, SA, 1954

SAN JOB DISEASE, syphilis.
1. Casas EC: Diccionario Terminologico de Ciencias Medicas. 5th ed. Salvat Editores, SA, 1954

SAN LAZARO DISEASE, leprosy.
1. Casas EC: Diccionario Terminologico de Ciencias Medicas. 5th ed. Salvat Editores, SA, 1954

SAN MODESTO DISEASE, chorea.
1. Casas EC: Diccionario Terminologico de Ciencias Medicas. 5th ed. Salvat Editores, SA, 1954

SAN VALENTIN DISEASE, epilepsy.
1. Casas EC: Diccionario Terminologico de Ciencias Medicas. 5th ed. Salvat Editores, SA, 1954

SAN ZACARIAS DISEASE, mutism.
1. Casas EC: Diccionario Terminologico de Ciencias Medicas. 5th ed. Salvat Editores, SA, 1954

SANDERS SIGN, epigastric pulsation; seen in the patient with pericardial adhesions. (J. Sanders, 1777-1843, British)
1. Casas EC: Diccionario Terminologico de Ciencias Medicas. 5th ed. Salvat Editores, SA, 1954

SANDERS SYNDROME, epidemic keratoconjunctivitis. (Murray Sanders, U.S. bacteriologist)
1. Sanders M: Arch Ophthalmol 28:581-586, 1942

SANDFLY FEVER, see Pappataci fever.

SANDHOFF DISEASE, G_{M2} gangliosidosis type II; a glycogen storage disorder in which there is an accumulation not only of G_{M2} ganglioside and the corresponding trihexosylceramide, but also globoside since the terminal N-acetylgalactosamine of this component cannot be removed. Diagnosis is made by specific enzyme assay. The disease is a Tay-Sachs variant; the enzyme defect differs from that in Tay-Sachs disease in that both components A and B of hexosaminidase are deficient. (K. Sandhoff, German biochemist)
1. Baker AB, Baker LH: Clinical Neurology. Revised ed. Philadelphia: Harper & Row, 1982
2. Okada S, McCrea M, O'Brien JS: Sandhoff's disease (G_{M2} type 2): clinical, chemical, and enzyme studies in five patients. Pediatr Res 6:606, 1972

SANDIFER SYNDROME, dystonia of the heart and neck with gastroesophageal reflux and hiatal hernia. (Paul Sandifer, British radiologist)
1. Kinsbourne M: Lancet 1:1058-1062, 1964

SANFILIPPO SYNDROME, mucopolysaccharidosis type III; this syndrome can be produced by a deficiency of at least four different enzymes, all of which participate in degradation of heparan sulfate. Sleep disturbance may be an early manifestation in childhood. Behavior disturbances, hyperactivity, visceromegaly, mental retardation, and sensorineural deafness are features. (Sylvester Sanfilippo, U.S. pediatrician)
1. Bennett JC, Plum F (eds): Cecil Textbook of Medicine. 20th ed. Philadelphia: WB Saunders, 1996
2. Farmer TW: Pediatric Neurology. 2nd ed. Hagerstown: Harper & Row, 1975
3. Sanfilippo SJ, Padosin R, Langer LO Jr, et al: J Pediatr 63:837-838, 1963

SANGER OPERATION, see Müller operation.

SANSOM SIGN, a dull sound parasternally between the 2nd and 3rd interspaces; found in the patient with pericardial effusion. (Arthur E. Sansom, 1838-1907, British)
1. Casas EC: Diccionario Terminologico de Ciencias Medicas. 5th ed. Salvat Editores, SA, 1954

SANTA AGUEDA DISEASE, mammillitis.
1. Casas EC: Diccionario Terminologico de Ciencias Medicas. 5th ed. Salvat Editores, SA, 1954

SANTA ANTONIO DISEASE, see Saint Anthony's fire.

SANTA APOLONIA DISEASE, toothache.
1. Casas EC: Diccionario Terminologico de Ciencias Medicas. 5th ed. Salvat Editores, SA, 1954

SANTAVUORI DISEASE, a variant of neuronal ceroid lipofuscinosis; begins at about 8 months of age with progressive visual loss, loss of developmental milestones, myoclonic jerks, and microcephaly.

Optic atrophy, macular and retinal degeneration, and no response in the electroretinogram are features. Progression is rapid but infants may survive several years. (Pirkko Santavuori, Finnish)

1. Rowland LP (ed): Merritt's Textbook of Neurology. 9th ed. Baltimore: Williams & Wilkins, 1995
2. Santavuori P, Haltia M, Rapola J: Infantile type of so-called neuronal ceroid-lipofuscinosis. Dev Med Child Neurol 16:644-653, 1974

SANTINI SIGN, a booming sound of a hydatid cyst heard on percussion.

1. Casas EC: Diccionario Terminologico de Ciencias Medicas. 5th ed. Salvat Editores, SA, 1954

SAÕ PAULO DISEASE, a Brazilian fever transmitted by *Amblyomma cajennense*.

1. Casas EC: Diccionario Terminologico de Ciencias Medicas. 5th ed. Salvat Editores, SA, 1954

SARBÓ SIGN, analgesia of the peroneal nerve and locomotor ataxia. (Arthur von Sarbó, Hungarian neurologist)

1. Casas EC: Diccionario Terminologico de Ciencias Medicas. 5th ed. Salvat Editores, SA, 1954

SATOYOSHI DISEASE, phosphohexoisomerase deficiency; described in family members who experience muscle pain and stiffness with exercise. (Ejiro Satoyoshi, Japanese)

1. Baker AB, Baker LH: Clinical Neurology. Revised ed. Philadelphia: Harper & Row, 1982
2. Satoyoshi E, Kowa H: A myopathy due to glycolytic abnormality. Arch Neurol 17:248-256, 1967

SATTLER SIGN, elevation of the right leg causes pain with the patient in a seated position; seen in appendicitis.

1. Casas EC: Diccionario Terminologico de Ciencias Medicas. 5th ed. Salvat Editores, SA, 1954

SAUERBRUCH OPERATION, paravertebral thoracoplasty and resection of a portion of each rib from the transverse apophysis for treating pulmonary tuberculosis and empyema. (Ernst F. Sauerbruch, 1875-1951, German surgeon)

1. Maffei WE: Os Fundamentos da Medicina. 2nd ed. Livraria Editora Artes Médicas Ltda, 1978

SAUNDERS SIGN, hand flexion and extension of the wrist with opening of the mouth. (Edward W. Saunders, 1854-1927, U.S.)

1. Casas EC: Diccionario Terminologico de Ciencias Medicas. 5th ed. Salvat Editores, SA, 1954

SAUTER OPERATION, vaginal hysterectomy with the ovaries and fallopian tubes not removed.

1. Maffei WE: Os Fundamentos da Medicina. 2nd ed. Livraria Editora Artes Médicas Ltda, 1978

SAVAGE SYNDROME, hypergonadotropic amenorrhea in association with histologically normal ovarian follicular apparatus. This group of patients may have an ovarian cell membrane receptor defect, described literally in the expression "ovarian insensitivity syndrome." Cross-reference: Resistant ovary syndrome.

1. Gold JJ, Josimovich JB: Gynecologic Endocrinology. 3rd ed. New York: Plenum Medical, 1980, p 279
2. Jones GS, De Moraes-Ruehsen M: Am J Obstet Gynecol 104:597-600, 1969

SAVILL SYNDROME, epidemic exfoliative dermatitis. (Thomas D. Savill, 1856-1910, British)

1. Savill TD: Br Med J 2:1197-1202, 1891

SAY-BARBER SYNDROME, describes the symptoms of short stature, developmental delay, microcephaly, craniosynostosis (in one), a sloping forehead, beaked nose with high nasal bridge, highly arched palate, micrognathia, large protruding ears, flexion contractures, anal stenosis, hypoplastic patellae, scoliosis, small testes, and decreased subcutaneous fat; described in two brothers. (Burhan Say, U.S.)

1. Gorlin RJ, Cohen MM Jr, Levin LS: Syndromes of the Head and Neck. 3rd ed. New York: Oxford University Press, 1990
2. Say B, et al: Microcephaly, short stature, and developmental delay associated with a chemotactic defect and transient hypogammaglobulin anemia in two brothers. J Med Genet 23:355-359, 1986

SAY-MEYER TRIGONOCEPHALY SYNDROME, a familial syndrome of craniosynostosis, developmental delay, and short stature. (Burhan Say)

1. Cohen MM Jr: Craniosynostosis update 1987. Am J Med Genet Suppl 4:99-148, 1988
2. Say B, Meyer J: Am J Dis Child 135:711-712, 1981

SAY-POZNANSKI SYNDROME, cloverleaf skull, polydactyly of the hands and feet, grossly abnormal metacarpal and metatarsal bones, angular ulnae with probable fusion to the midportion of the radial bones, short, wide clavicles, winged scapulae, unusually shaped ribs with abnormal spacing between them and with prominent costovertebral junctions, and widely separated ischia are features.

1. Beighton P, et al: Osteoglophonic dwarfism. Pediatr Radiol 10:46-50, 1980
2. Gorlin RJ, Cohen MM Jr, Levin LS: Syndromes of the Head and Neck. 3rd ed. New York: Oxford University Press, 1990

SAYRE OPERATION, use of a plaster of Paris vest for the treatment of Pott disease. (Lewis A. Sayre, 1820-1900, U.S. surgeon)

1. Maffei WE: Os Fundamentos da Medicina. 2nd ed. Livraria Editora Artes Médicas Ltda, 1978

SCALDED-SKIN SYNDROME, exfoliative dermatitis of the newborn; *Staphylococcus aureus* is a common cause of cellulitis and the sole cause of this syndrome in neonates and young children. Cross-reference: Staphylococcal scalded-skin syndrome.

1. Ballenger JJ: Diseases of the Nose, Throat, Ear, Head and Neck. 12th ed. Philadelphia: Lea & Febiger, 1977
2. Krugman S, Katz SL: Infectious Diseases of Children. 7th ed. St Louis: CV Mosby, 1981
3. Lyell A: Br J Dermatol 68:355, 1956

SCALENUS ANTICUS SYNDROME, pain over the shoulder, often extending down the arm, due to compression of the nerves and vessels between a cervical rib and the scalenus anticus muscle. Cross-reference: Naffziger syndrome.

1. Grinker RR, Sahs AL: Neurology. 6th ed. Springfield: Charles C Thomas, 1966
2. Naffziger HC: Surg Gynecol Obstet 6:119-120, 1937

SCAPULOCOSTAL SYNDROME, pain in the superior or posterior aspect of the shoulder girdle and extending to contiguous regions, possibly as a result of a long-standing alteration in the relationship of the scapula and the posterior thoracic wall.

1. Michele AA: Scapulocostal syndrome: its mechanism and diagnosis. NY State J Med 55:2485-2493, 1955

SCAPULOPERONEAL SYNDROME, distal weakness in the legs resembling that of neurogenic peroneal muscular atrophy; however, sensory loss is lacking and there is proximal weakness in the shoulder girdle similar to that of facioscapulohumeral dystrophy.

1. Baker AB, Baker LH: Clinical Neurology. Revised ed. Philadelphia: Harper & Row, 1982
2. Bennett JC, Plum F (eds): Cecil Textbook of Medicine. 20th ed. Philadelphia: WB Saunders, 1996

SCARDINO-PRINCE OPERATION, SCARDINO VERTICAL FLAP PYELOPLASTY, pyeloureteroplasty using a vertical flap; described in 1953. (Peter Scardino, U.S. urologist)

1. Campbell MF, Walsh PC: Campbell's Urology. 5th ed. Philadelphia: WB Saunders, 1986

SCARF SYNDROME, *s*keletal abnormalities, *c*utis laxa and craniosynostosis, *a*mbiguous genitalia, *r*etardation, and *f*acial abnormalities (SCARF) are features.

1. Gorlin RJ, Cohen MM Jr, Levin LS: Syndromes of the Head and Neck. 3rd ed. New York: Oxford University Press, 1990
2. Koppe R, et al: Am J Med Genet 34:305-312, 1989

SCARPA DISEASE, exophthalmic goiter.

1. Casas EC: Diccionario Terminologico de Ciencias Medicas. 5th ed. Salvat Editores, SA, 1954

SCARPA OPERATION, 1) ligation of the femoral artery in the center of the Scarpa triangle (femoral trigone); 2) iridodialysis through the sclera. (Antonio Scarpa, 1747-1832, Italian anatomist, orthopedist/ophthalmologist)

1. Maffei WE: Os Fundamentos da Medicina. 2nd ed. Livraria Editora Artes Médicas Ltda, 1978

SCHAEFER REFLEX, a pyramidal tract response of the lower extremities; characterized by dorsiflexion of the toes and produced by deep pressure on the Achilles tendon. (Max Schaefer, 1852-1923, German neurologist)

1. Baker AB, Baker LH: Clinical Neurology. Revised ed. Philadelphia: Harper & Row, 1982
2. Pedro-Pons A: Patologia-y-Clinica Medicus. Salvat Editores, SA, 1952

SCHÄFER SYNDROME, pachyonychia congenita associated with retardation of physical and mental development, congenital cataracts, and microcephaly. (Erich Schäfer, German)

1. Schäfer E: Arch Dermatol Syph 148:425-432, 1925

SCHAMBERG DISEASE, progressive pigmentary dermatosis. (Jay F. Schamberg, 1870-1934, U.S. dermatologist)

1. Schamberg JFA: Br J Dermatol 13:1-5, 1901

SCHANZ SYNDROME, a series of symptoms indicating spinal weakness and consisting of a sense of fatigue, pain on pressure over the spinous processes, and pain on lying prone; caused by numerous forms of pathology affecting the spine. (Alfred Schanz, 1868-1931, German orthopedist)

1. Schanz A: Berl Klin Wochenschr 44:989-992, 1907

SCHAPIRO SIGN, when there is a slow pulse in the resting position, myocardial asthenia is indicated. (Heinrich Schapiro, 1852-1901, Russian)

1. Casas EC: Diccionario Terminologico de Ciencias Medicas. 5th ed. Salvat Editores, SA, 1954

SCHATSKI [SCHATZKI] RING, consists of a symmetrical, thin web located in the terminal esophagus. (Richard Schatski [Schatzki], 1901-1992, U.S. radiologist)
1. Schatzki R, Gary JE: Am J Roentgenol 70:911-922, 1956

SCHAUMANN SYNDROME, sarcoidosis. (Jörgen Schaumann, 1879-1953, Swedish dermatologist)

SCHAUMBERG DISEASE, see Addison disease. (H.H. Schaumberg, U.S. neuropathologist)

SCHEIE SYNDROME, a rare disorder due to a deficiency of α-L-iduronidase and characterized by severe corneal clouding, deformity of the hands, and aortic valve disease. A thickened dura may produce cervical myelopathy. Cross-reference: Spät-Hurler syndrome. (Harold G. Scheie, 1909-1990, U.S. ophthalmologist)
1. Farmer TW: Pediatric Neurology. 2nd ed. Hagerstown: Harper & Row, 1975
2. Scheie HBG, Hambrick GW Jr, Barness LA: Am J Ophthalmol 53:753-769, 1962

SCHELLONG-STRISOWER PHENOMENON, a reduction in systolic blood pressure on rising to the erect posture from the lying down position. (Fritz Schellong, 1891-1953, German)
1. Dorland's Medical Dictionary. 28th ed. Philadelphia: WB Saunders, 1994

SCHENCK DISEASE, see Beuermann disease. (Benjamin R. Schenck, 1873-1920, U.S.)

SCHEPELMANN SIGN, the patient has increased pain on bending toward the normal side; seen in cases of pleural effusion. (Emil Schepelmann, German)
1. Casas EC: Diccionario Terminologico de Ciencias Medicas. 5th ed. Salvat Editores, SA, 1954

SCHEUERMANN DISEASE, osteochondrosis of the vertebral epiphysis in juveniles. (Holger W. Scheuermann, 1877-1960, Danish surgeon)
1. Lumley JS, Clain A: Hamilton Bailey's Demonstration of Physical Signs in Clinical Surgery. 18th ed. London: Butterworth-Heinemann, 1997
2. Scheuermann HW: Ugeskr Laeger 82:385-93, 1920

SCHIASSI OPERATION, 1) anastomosis of epiploic vessels to achieve collateral circulation of portal blood; 2) treatment of leg varices by injection of an iodine solution; 3) wrapping the spleen with gauze soaked in a triiodomethane solution to achieve capsule formation and consequently decrease the volume of the organ.
1. Maffei WE: Os Fundamentos da Medicina. 2nd ed. Livraria Editora Artes Médicas Ltda, 1978

SCHICK SIGN, respiratory stridor in a child with bronchial lymph node tuberculosis. (Béla Schick, 1877-1967, Hungarian-born U.S. pediatrician)
1. Casas EC: Diccionario Terminologico de Ciencias Medicas. 5th ed. Salvat Editores, SA, 1954

SCHIEBE DISEASE, a congenital hereditary hearing loss. The malformation involves only the cochlea and saccule and is often accompanied by defects in pigmentation.
1. Ballenger JJ: Diseases of the Nose, Throat, Ear, Head and Neck. 12th ed. Philadelphia: Lea & Febiger, 1977

SCHILDER DISEASE, SCHILDER-FOIX DISEASE, cerebral sclerosis; a variant of multiple sclerosis. First described in the late 19th century. Cross-reference: Heubner-Schilder disease. (Paul Schilder, 1886-1940, German-born U.S. psychiatrist; Charles Foix, 1882-1927, French)
1. Baker AB, Baker LH: Clinical Neurology. Revised ed. Philadelphia: Harper & Row, 1982
2. Schilder P: Z Gesamte Neurol 15:359, 1913

SCHIMMELBUSCH DISEASE, cystic disease or intracystic papilliferous carcinoma of the breast. Cross-reference: Reclus disease. (Curt Schimmelbusch, 1860-1895, German surgeon)
1. Casas EC: Diccionario Terminologico de Ciencias Medicas. 5th ed. Salvat Editores, SA, 1954

SCHIMMELPENNING-FEUERSTEIN SYNDROME, see Epidermal nevus syndrome.

SCHINZEL-GIEDION SYNDROME, a syndrome of midface retraction, hirsutism, multiple skeletal anomalies, mental retardation, and seizures. (A. Schinzel, Swiss; Andreas Giedion, Swiss)
1. Al-Gazali LI, et al: The Schinzel-Giedion syndrome: clinical features and natural history. J Med Genet 25:275, 1988
2. Gorlin RJ, Cohen MM Jr, Levin LS: Syndromes of the Head and Neck. 3rd ed. New York: Oxford University Press, 1990
3. Schinzel A, Giedion A: Am J Med Genet 1:362-365, 1978

SCHIRMER SYNDROME, a variant of Sturge-Weber syndrome in which glaucoma occurs early in the course of the disease. (Rudolf Schirmer, 1831-1896, German ophthalmologist)
1. Schirmer RS: Graefes Arch Ophthalmol 7:119-121, 1860

SCHIRMER TEST, a test for lacrimation to check the integrity of the facial nerve proximal to the geniculate ganglion or greater superior petrosal nerve. Filter paper is placed hanging from the conjunctiva for 5 minutes. The result is considered abnormal if <25 mm wetness and/or <30% that of the normal side. (Otto W.A. Schirmer, 1864-1917, German ophthalmologist)
   1. Dorland's Medical Dictionary. 28th ed. Philadelphia: WB Saunders, 1994

SCHLANGE SIGN, a lack of peristalsis beyond the point of obstruction with dilatation of the bowels.
   1. Casas EC: Diccionario Terminologico de Ciencias Medicas. 5th ed. Salvat Editores, SA, 1954

SCHLATTER OPERATION, total ablation of the stomach to treat cancer.
   1. Maffei WE: Os Fundamentos da Medicina. 2nd ed. Livraria Editora Artes Médicas Ltda, 1978

SCHLATTER-OSGOOD DISEASE, see Osgood-Schlatter disease.

SCHLESINGER SIGN, extensor muscle spasm can be precipitated by flexing the hip and supporting the knee while in the supine position; seen in cases of tetanus. Cross-reference: Pool phenomenon. (Hermann Schlesinger, 1866-1934, Austrian)
   1. Casas EC: Diccionario Terminologico de Ciencias Medicas. 5th ed. Salvat Editores, SA, 1954

SCHLUNGE SIGN, see Schlange sign.

SCHMID METAPHYSEAL CHONDRODYSPLASIA SYNDROME, hereditary metaphyseal dysostosis; short stature, splaying of broad irregular metaphyses, tibial bowing, a waddling gait, and flaring of the lower rib cage are characteristics. Autosomal dominant inheritance.
   1. Schmid F: Beitrag zur Dysostosis enchondralis metaepiphysaria. Monatsschr Kinderheilkd 97:393-397, 1949
   2. Smith DW, Jones KL: Recognizable Patterns of Human Malformations: Genetic, Embryologic, and Clinical Aspects. 3rd ed. Philadelphia: WB Saunders, 1982

SCHMIDT SYNDROME, unilateral paralysis of a vocal cord, the velum palati, and the trapezius and sternocleidomastoid muscles. Cross-reference: Vagoaccessory syndrome. (Adolf Schmidt, 1865-1918, German)
   1. Grinker RR, Sahs AL: Neurology. 6th ed. Springfield: Charles C Thomas, 1966
   2. Schmidt A: Dtsch Med Wochenschr 18:606-608, 1892
   3. Wilson JD, Foster DW, Kronenberg HM, et al (eds): Williams Textbook of Endocrinology. 9th ed. Philadelphia: WB Saunders, 1998

SCHMORL DISEASE, chondroma of the intervertebral discs. (Christian G. Schmorl, 1861-1932, German pathologist)
   1. Schmorl CG: Fortschr Geb Roentgenol 38:265-279, 1928

SCHNECKENBECKEN DYSPLASIA, hypotonia, severe growth deficiency, a large cranium, short limbs with sausage-like fingers, and a narrow thorax with short ribs are features. Etiology unknown. Cross-reference: Thanatophoric dysplasia.
   1. Chemke J, Graff G, Lancet M: Familial thanatophoric dwarfism. Lancet 1:358, 1971
   2. Maroteau P, et al: Presse Med 75:2519-2524, 1967

SCHNITZLER SYNDROME, a progressive immunoproliferative disease with production of large amounts of a monoclonal macroglobulin (IgM). Chronic urticaria, fever of unknown origin, disabling bone pain, hyperostosis, an increased erythrocyte sedimentation rate, and macroglobulinemia are features. Cross-reference: Waldenström macroglobulinemia.
   1. Bennett JC, Plum F (eds): Cecil Textbook of Medicine. 20th ed. Philadelphia: WB Saunders, 1996
   2. Schnitzler L, Schubert B, Boasson M, et al: Bull Soc Fr Dermatol Syph 81:363, 1974
   3. Waldenström J: Acta Med Scand 117:216-247, 1944

SCHOLZ DISEASE, the juvenile form of metachromatic leukodystrophy; usually transmitted in a similar manner. (Willibald O. Scholz, German neurologist)
   1. Baker AB, Baker LH: Clinical Neurology. Revised ed. Philadelphia: Harper & Row, 1982

SCHÖNLEIN-HENOCH PURPURA, SCHÖNLEIN PURPURA, a necrotizing angiitis involving the small vessels, especially the capillaries in the upper dermis. Primarily affects children (boys more often than girls) and young adults. Cross-reference: Henoch-Schönlein purpura. (Johannes L. Schönlein, 1793-1864, German; Eduard H. Henoch, 1820-1910, German pediatrician)
   1. Henoch EH: Berl Klin Wochenschr 11:641-643, 1874
   2. Moschella SL, Hurley HJ: Dermatology. 2nd ed. Philadelphia: WB Saunders, 1985
   3. Ritchie AC: Boyd's Textbook of Pathology. 9th ed. Philadelphia: Lea & Febiger, 1990

SCHÖPF SYNDROME, oligodontia, hypotrichosis, palmoplantar hyperkeratosis, and apocrine hidrocystomas of the eyelid margins are features.

1. Gorlin RJ, Cohen MM Jr, Levin LS: Syndromes of the Head and Neck. 3rd ed. New York: Oxford University Press, 1990
2. Herbert SA, et al: Expression and inheritance of the Schöpf syndrome. Am J Med Genet (in press)
3. Schöpf E, et al: Syndrome of cystic eyelids, palmo-plantar keratosis, hypodontia and hypotrichosis as a possible autosomal recessive trait. Birth Defects 7(8):219-221, 1971

SCHOTTMÜLLER DISEASE, paratyphoid fever. Cross-reference: Brion-Kayser disease. (Hugo Schottmüller, 1867-1936, German)

1. Brion A, Kayser H: Munch Med Wochenschr 49:611-615, 1902
2. Schottmüller H: Dtsch Med Wochenschr 26:511-512, 1900

SCHRAMM OPERATION, injection of a corrosive solution directly on the carcinomatous tissue in cases of uterine carcinoma.

1. Maffei WE: Os Fundamentos da Medicina. 2nd ed. Livraria Editora Artes Médicas Ltda, 1978

SCHRAMM PHENOMENON, the ability of the examiner to visualize a funnel-shaped deformity of the entire posterior urethra; seen in spinal cord disease.

1. Dorland's Medical Dictionary. 28th ed. Philadelphia: WB Saunders, 1994

SCHRIDDE DISEASE, fetal hydrops. (Hermann A. Schridde, German pathologist)

1. Schridde HA: Munch Med Wochenschr 57:397-98, 1910

SCHRÖDER DISEASE, a deficiency of gonadotropin causing endometrial hypertrophy and hemorrhage. (Robert Schröder, 1884-1932, German gynecologist)

1. Casas EC: Diccionario Terminologico de Ciencias Medicas. 5th ed. Salvat Editores, SA, 1954

SCHRÖDER OPERATION, excision of the mucous membrane of the uterus in cases of chronic endometritis. (Robert Schröder)

1. Maffei WE: Os Fundamentos da Medicina. 2nd ed. Livraria Editora Artes Médicas Ltda, 1978

SCHRÖTTER DISEASE, hysterical coughing.

1. Casas EC: Diccionario Terminologico de Ciencias Medicas. 5th ed. Salvat Editores, SA, 1954

SCHRÖTTER SYNDROME, see Paget-Schrötter syndrome.

SCHUCHARDT OPERATION, paravaginal hysterectomy. (Karl Schuchardt, 1856-1901, German surgeon)

1. Maffei WE: Os Fundamentos da Medicina. 2nd ed. Livraria Editora Artes Médicas Ltda, 1978

SCHÜCKING OPERATION, method for vaginal hysterectomy in cases of prolapse of the uterus.

1. Maffei WE: Os Fundamentos da Medicina. 2nd ed. Livraria Editora Artes Médicas Ltda, 1978

SCHULE SIGN, a sad face with a wrinkle between the eyebrows.

1. Casas EC: Diccionario Terminologico de Ciencias Medicas. 5th ed. Salvat Editores, SA, 1954

SCHÜLLER PHENOMENON, due to an organic lesion, the patient walks sideways more easily toward the affected side than toward the healthy side; seen in the patient with hemiplegia. (Artur Schüller, 1874-1958, Austrian neurologist)

1. Dorland's Medical Dictionary. 28th ed. Philadelphia: WB Saunders, 1994

SCHÜLLER-CHRISTIAN DISEASE, see Hand-Schüller-Christian disease.

SCHULTZ SYNDROME, agranulocytic angioma. (Werner Schultz, 1878-1947, German internist)

1. Schultz W: Dtsch Med Wochenschr 48:1495-1496, 1922

SCHULTZE SIGN, SCHULTZE-CHVOSTEK SIGN, mechanical stimulation of the protruded tongue (i.e., tapping it with a percussion hammer) is followed by transient depression or dimpling at the site of stimulation. May be present in a patient with myotonia congenita or myotonic dystrophy. Cross-references: Chvostek sign; Tongue phenomenon. (Friedrich Schultze, 1848-1919, German gynecologist; Franz Chvostek, 1835-1884, Austrian surgeon)

1. Baker AB, Baker LH: Clinical Neurology. Revised ed. Philadelphia: Harper & Row, 1982
2. Bodechtel G: Diagnostico Diferencial de las Enfermedades Neurologicas. Madrid: Pas Montalvo Editorial, 1967

SCHWACHMAN SYNDROME, leukopenia, mild skeletal changes, pancreatic insufficiency, and bone marrow dysfunction are features. Presumed autosomal recessive inheritance. (Harry Schwachman, U.S.)

1. McLennan TW, Steinbach HL: Schwachman syndrome: the broad spectrum of bony abnormalities. Radiology 112:167, 1974
2. Schwachman H, et al: J Pediatr 63:835-837, 1963

SCHWALBE-ZIEHEN-OPPENHEIM DISEASE, see Oppenheim disease.

SCHWARTZ-BARTTER SYNDROME, see Inappropriate secretion of antidiuretic hormone, syndrome of. (William B. Schwartz, U.S.; Frederick C. Bartter, 1919-1983, U.S.)

SCHWARTZ-JAMPEL SYNDROME, SCHWARTZ-JAMPEL-ABERFELD SYNDROME, small stature, myotonia with fixed sad facies, limitation of motion in the hips, wrists, fingers, toes, and spine, pectus carinatum, a small high-pitched voice, and blepharophimosis are features. Autosomal recessive inheritance. (Oscar Schwartz, U.S. ophthalmologist; Robert S. Jampel, U.S. ophthalmologist)
1. Aberfeld DS, Hinterbuchner LP, Schneider M: Brain 88:313-322, 1965
2. Gorlin RJ, Cohen MM Jr, Levin LS: Syndromes of the Head and Neck. 3rd ed. New York: Oxford University Press, 1990
3. Schwartz O, Jampel RS: Arch Ophthalmol 68:52-57, 1962
4. Smith DW, Jones KL: Recognizable Patterns of Human Malformations: Genetic, Embryologic, and Clinical Aspects. 3rd ed. Philadelphia: WB Saunders, 1982

SCHWARTZE OPERATION, opening of the mastoid cells in cases of middle ear infection.
1. Maffei WE: Os Fundamentos da Medicina. 2nd ed. Livraria Editora Artes Médicas Ltda, 1978

SCHWARTZE SIGN, a normal eardrum, but with a pinkish blush seen on the promontory, especially with a translucent drumhead; indicative of a highly vascular otosclerotic focus.
1. Ballenger JJ: Diseases of the Nose, Throat, Ear, Head and Neck. 12th ed. Philadelphia: Lea & Febiger, 1977

SCHWARTZMANN-SANARELLI SYNDROME, a form of intravascular coagulopathy precipitated by Gram-negative sepsis.
1. Vannotti A: Clinique et Physiopathologie Médicales. Introduction a la Médecine Clinique. Libraire Maloine, SA, 1973

SCHWARZ-LÉLEK SYNDROME, consists of severe genu valgum and marked frontal bossing. Hyperostosis and sclerosis seen on radiographic findings.
1. Gorlin RJ, Cohen MM Jr, Levin LS: Syndromes of the Head and Neck. 3rd ed. New York: Oxford University Press, 1990
2. Lélek L: Camurati-Engelmannschee Erkrankung. Fortschr Roentgenstr 94:393-408, 1962
3. Schwarz E: Craniometaphyseal dysplasia. AJR 84:461-466, 1960

SCHWEDIAUER [SWEDIAUER] DISEASE, achillobursitis. (François X. Schwediauer [Swediauer], 1748-1824, Austrian)
1. Casas EC: Diccionario Terminologico de Ciencias Medicas. 5th ed. Salvat Editores, SA, 1954

SCHWENINGER-BUZZI DISEASE, anetoderma; macular atrophy occurs without any preceding inflammatory eruption. Large numbers of bluish-white macules appear suddenly, some of which are slightly protuberant. (Ernst Schweninger, 1850-1924, German dermatologist; Fausto Buzzi, German dermatologist)
1. Moschella SL, Hurley HJ: Dermatology. 2nd ed. Philadelphia: WB Saunders, 1985

SCIMITAR SYNDROME, SCIMITAR VEIN SYNDROME, a combination of hypoplasia of the right lung, dextroposition of the heart, and anomalous pulmonary venous drainage of the entire right lung is seen radiologically. The anomalous common venous trunk draining the right lung produces a curved shadow (like the blade of a scimitar) as it drains into the inferior vena cava below the diaphragm.
1. Cheitlin MD, Sokolow M: Clinical Cardiology. 5th ed. Norwalk, Conn: Appleton & Lange, 1993
2. Fowler NO: Cardiac Diagnosis and Treatment. 3rd ed. Cambridge: Harper & Row, 1980
3. Oakley D, Naik D, Verel D, et al: Scimitar vein syndrome: report of nine new cases. Am Heart J 107:596-598, 1984

SCLEROSTEOSIS SYNDROME, progressive thickening and overgrowth of bone; prominent asymmetric mandible with deafness, proptosis of eyes with blindness, and syndactyly of 2nd and 3rd fingers are features. Autosomal recessive inheritance. Cross-reference: Van Buchem syndrome.
1. Beighton P, Durr L, Hammersma H: The clinical features of sclerosteosis. Ann Intern Med 84:393, 1976
2. Smith DW, Jones KL: Recognizable Patterns of Human Malformations: Genetic, Embryologic, and Clinical Aspects. 3rd ed. Philadelphia: WB Saunders, 1982

SCOTT SYNDROME, resembles Saethre-Chotzen syndrome but differs by involving growth deficiency, moderate to severe mental retardation, and brachycephaly with absence of craniosynostosis. Cross-reference: Craniodigital syndrome. (C. Ronald Scott, U.S.)
1. Gorlin RJ, Cohen MM Jr, Levin LS: Syndromes of the Head and Neck. 3rd ed. New York: Oxford University Press, 1990

2. Lorenz P, Hinkel GH, Hoffmann C, et al: The craniodigital syndrome of Scott report of a second family. Am J Med Genet 37:224-226, 1990
3. Scott CR, Bryant JL, Graham CB: A new craniodigital syndrome with mental retardation. J Pediatr 78:658-663, 1971

SEABRIGHT BANTAM SYNDROME, see Albright syndrome.

SEASHORE TEST, a measurement of the sense of pitch, intensity, rhythm, and other components of innate musical ability.
1. Stedman's Medical Dictionary. 26th ed. Baltimore: Williams & Wilkins, 1995

SECKEL SYNDROME, nanocephalic dwarfism; characteristics are growth deficiency, mental deficiency, hypoplasia of facies, clinodactyly of the 5th finger, dislocation of the hip, and only 11 pairs of ribs. Probable autosomal recessive inheritance. Cross-reference: Virchow-Seckel syndrome. (Helmut P.G. Seckel, 1900-1960, Swiss pediatrician)
1. Seckel HPG: Bird-Headed Dwarfs: Studies in Developmental Anthropology Including Human Proportions. Springfield: Charles C Thomas, 1960, p 241
2. Smith DW, Jones KL: Recognizable Patterns of Human Malformations: Genetic, Embryologic, and Clinical Aspects. 3rd ed. Philadelphia: WB Saunders, 1982

SECOND-SET PHENOMENON, the rapid rejection by the recipient of a second tissue graft from the same donor as a consequence of the primary immune response induced by the first graft.
1. Dorland's Medical Dictionary. 28th ed. Philadelphia: WB Saunders, 1994

SECRÉTAN DISEASE, post-traumatic edema of the dorsum of the hand. (Henri Secrétan, 1856-1916, Swiss surgeon)
1. Casas EC: Diccionario Terminologico de Ciencias Medicas. 5th ed. Salvat Editores, SA, 1954

SEDLÁCKOVÁ SYNDROME, see Shprintzen syndrome.

SEELIGMÜLLER SIGN, facial neuralgia with a dilated ipsilateral pupil. (Otto L.G.A. Seeligmüller, 1837-1912, German neurologist)
1. Casas EC: Diccionario Terminologico de Ciencias Medicas. 5th ed. Salvat Editores, SA, 1954

SEGAWA DISEASE, progressive hereditary dystonia, with fluctuations during the daytime and remedied by sleeping. Most common in females under 5 years of age. (M. Segawa, Japanese)
1. Segawa M, et al: Adv Neurol 14:215-233, 1976

SEGMENTARY SYNDROME, a syndrome produced by an intramedullary lesion of the spinal cord and marked by weakness and wasting in the affected segment. Cross-reference: Metameric syndrome.
1. Dorland's Medical Dictionary. 28th ed. Philadelphia: WB Saunders, 1994

SEIDEL SIGN, a sickle-shaped arcuate scotoma extending at ends; appears as an upward or downward extension of a blind spot. (Erich Seidel, 1882-1946, German surgeon)
1. Casas EC: Diccionario Terminologico de Ciencias Medicas. 5th ed. Salvat Editores, SA, 1954

SEIP SYNDROME, see Berardinelli syndrome. (Martin F. Seip, Norwegian)

SEITELBERGER DISEASE, in the orthochromatic type, there is a greater amount of sudanophilic material in the macrophages. A variant of the Pelizaeus-Merzbacher disease. (Franz Seitelberger, Austrian neuropathologist)
1. Baker AB, Baker LH: Clinical Neurology. Revised ed. Philadelphia: Harper & Row, 1982
2. Scheithauer BW, Forno LS, Dorfman LJ, et al: Neuroaxonal dystrophy (Seitelberger's disease) with late onset, protracted course and myoclonic epilepsy. J Neurol Sci 36:247-258, 1978
3. Seitelberger F: Wien Zschr Nervenheilkd 9:228-289, 1954

SEITZ SIGN, a bronchial respiratory sound; an indication of cavitation in the lung. (Eugene Seitz, 1817-1899, German)
1. Casas EC: Diccionario Terminologico de Ciencias Medicas. 5th ed. Salvat Editores, SA, 1954

SELTER DISEASE, SELTER-SWIFT-FEER DISEASE, see Swift disease. (Paul Selter, 1866-1941, German pediatrician; Harry Swift, 1858-1937, Australian; Emil Feer-Sulzer, 1864-1955, Swiss pediatrician)

SELYE SYNDROME, see General adaptation syndrome. (Hans Selye, 1907-1982, French-Canadian physiologist)

SEMB OPERATION, extrafascial apicolytic thoracoplasty in cases of tuberculosis.
1. Maffei WE: Os Fundamentos da Medicina. 2nd ed. Livraria Editora Artes Médicas Ltda, 1978

SEMLIKI FOREST DISEASE, first isolated in 1942 from a suspension of *Aedes abnormalis* mosquitoes captured in the Semliki Forest of Uganda. Although the virus has not been associated with human disease, neutralizing antibodies have been detected in adult sera in Tongaland, Brazil, East Africa, and Portugal.

1. Baker AB, Baker LH: Clinical Neurology. Revised ed. Philadelphia: Harper & Row, 1982

SEMMOLA DISEASE, muscular pseudohypertrophy.

1. Casas EC: Diccionario Terminologico de Ciencias Medicas. 5th ed. Salvat Editores, SA, 1954

SEMON SIGN, a decrease in mobility of the vocal cords; seen in the patient with malignant tumor of the larynx. (Sir Felix Semon, 1849-1921, British laryngologist)

1. Casas EC: Diccionario Terminologico de Ciencias Medicas. 5th ed. Salvat Editores, SA, 1954

SENEAR-USHER SYNDROME, pemphigus erythematosus; a variant of pemphigus foliaceus in which the patient develops a characteristic malar butterfly dermatitis, suggestive of lupus erythematosus, and seborrhea-like lesions in other locations. (Francis E. Senear, 1889-1958, U.S. dermatologist; Barney D. Usher, 1899-1978, Canadian dermatologist)

1. Senear F, Usher B: Arch Dermatol Syph 13:761-781, 1926

SENN OPERATION, intestinal anastomosis using osseous plates.

1. Maffei WE: Os Fundamentos da Medicina. 2nd ed. Livraria Editora Artes Médicas Ltda, 1978

SENTER SYNDROME, a congenital syndrome of atypical ichthyosiform erythrokeratodermia, palmoplantar keratosis, and sensorineural hearing loss. Etiology unknown. Cross-reference: KID syndrome.

1. Senter TP, Jones KL, Sakati N, et al: Atypical ichthyosiform erythroderma and congenital sensorineural deafness—a distinct syndrome. J Pediatr 92:68, 1978
2. Smith DW, Jones KL: Recognizable Patterns of Human Malformations: Genetic, Embryologic, and Clinical Aspects. 3rd ed. Philadelphia: WB Saunders, 1982

SEPTIC SHOCK SYNDROME, sepsis is presumed to result from the effects of an endotoxin. Organisms that are considered normal flora, as well as highly virulent bacteria, are capable of causing sepsis.

1. Bennett JC, Plum F (eds): Cecil Textbook of Medicine. 20th ed. Philadelphia: WB Saunders, 1996

SEPTO-OPTIC DYSPLASIA SYNDROME, visual impairment, atrophic optic head, partial or complete pituitary growth hormone deficiency, absence of the septum pellucidum, and pendular nystagmus are features. Cross-reference: Gilford-Burnier syndrome.

1. Blethen SL, et al: Hypopituitarism and septo-optic dysplasia in first cousins. Am J Med Genet 21:123-129, 1985

SERESEWSKI-TURNER SYNDROME, see Turner syndrome.

SERTOLI-CELL-ONLY SYNDROME, a poorly understood developmental or structural defect of the testis leading to infertility. May encompass histological findings that can result from several etiologies. Cross-reference: Del Castillo syndrome. (Enrico Sertoli, 1842-1910, Italian histologist)

1. Del Castillo E, Trabucco A, de la Balze FA: J Clin Endocrinol 7:493-502, 1947
2. Wilson JD, Foster DW, Kronenberg HM, et al (eds): Williams Textbook of Endocrinology. 9th ed. Philadelphia: WB Saunders, 1998

SERUM HYPERVISCOSITY SYNDROME, manifested clinically by visual impairment, retinal vein enlargement, dizziness, nystagmus, hearing loss, vertigo, mucous membrane bleeding, and congestive heart failure.

1. Ballenger JJ: Diseases of the Nose, Throat, Ear, Head and Neck. 12th ed. Philadelphia: Lea & Febiger, 1977

SETLEIS SYNDROME, a familial syndrome with symptoms of bitemporal scarring that resembles forceps marks, periorbital puffiness with wrinkling of facial skin, abnormalities of the eyebrows and lashes, a flat nasal bridge with bulbous nasal tip, and increased mobility of facial skin associated with severe redundancy of soft tissues. (Howard Setleis, U.S.)

1. Gorlin RJ, Cohen MM Jr, Levin LS: Syndromes of the Head and Neck. 3rd ed. New York: Oxford University Press, 1990
2. Marion RW, et al: Autosomal recessive inheritance in the Setleis bitemporal "forceps marks" syndrome. Am J Dis Child 41:895-897, 1987
3. Setleis H, Kramer B, Valcarcel M, et al: Pediatrics 32:540-548, 1963

SETTING-SUN SIGN, see Collier sign.

SEVER DISEASE, epiphysitis of the calcaneum; a traction injury of the epiphyseal cartilage. Occurs most often in boys 8-12 years of age. (James W. Sever, 1878-1964, U.S. orthopedic surgeon)

1. Sever JW: NY Med State J 95:1027-1029, 1912

SÉZARY SYNDROME, a cutaneous lymphoma of helper T-cell origin, closely related to mycosis fungoides. Symptoms include pruritic erythroderma, lymphomatous skin infiltration, and large circulating mononuclear activated T-cells. (Albert Sézary, 1880-1956, French dermatologist)
1. Ritchie AC: Boyd's Textbook of Pathology. 9th ed. Philadelphia: Lea & Febiger, 1990
2. Sézary A, Bouvrain: Bull Soc Fr Dermatol Syph 45:254-260, 1938

SHAVER DISEASE, bauxite lung; interstitial pulmonary fibrosis occurring in workers engaged in the manufacture of corundum. (Cecil G. Shaver, Canadian)
1. Shaver CG, Ridell AR: J Indust Hyg 129:145-147, 1947

SHEEHAN SYNDROME, postpartum pituitary necrosis; an endocrine disorder associated with failure of lactation, caused by vascular injury to the pituitary during childbirth. Cross-references: Glinski-Simmonds syndrome; Postpartum pituitary necrosis syndrome; Reye-Sheehan syndrome; Simmonds syndrome; Thyrohypophysial syndrome. (Harold L. Sheehan, 1900-1988, British)
1. Grinker RR, Sahs AL: Neurology. 6th ed. Springfield: Charles C Thomas, 1966
2. Sheehan HL: J Pathol Bacteriol Lond 45:189-214, 1937
3. Simmonds M: Dtsch Med Wochenschr 40:322-323, 1914

SHELLY SIGN, fever blisters.
1. Casas EC: Diccionario Terminologico de Ciencias Medicas. 5th ed. Salvat Editores, SA, 1954

SHELVING OPERATION, see Koenig operation.

SHENSTONE OPERATION, occlusion of a bronchial fistula using an intercostal muscle.
1. Maffei WE: Os Fundamentos da Medicina. 2nd ed. Livraria Editora Artes Médicas Ltda, 1978

SHIBLEY SIGN, on auscultation, "e" is heard as "ah" over an area of consolidation or above pulmonary effusion. (Gerald S. Shibley, 1890-1981, U.S.)
1. Casas EC: Diccionario Terminologico de Ciencias Medicas. 5th ed. Salvat Editores, SA, 1954

SHIMAMUSHI DISEASE, see Tsutsugamushi disease.

SHIN BONE FEVER, see Trench fever.

SHORT FIRST METATARSAL SYNDROME, see Morton syndrome.

SHORT BOWEL SYNDROME, short gut syndrome. To maintain normal absorption, at least 90 cm of jejunum is needed; if less is available because of such causes as impaction or Crohn disease, the absorption of fat, calcium, and folic acid is impaired.
1. Ritchie AC: Boyd's Textbook of Pathology. 9th ed. Philadelphia: Lea & Febiger, 1990
2. Weset E, Urban E: Short bowel syndrome, in Haubrich WS, Schaffner F, Berk JE (eds): Bockus Gastroenterology. 5th ed. Philadelphia: WB Saunders, 1995, pp 1063-1071

SHORT SYNDROME, *s*hort stature, *h*yperextensibility of joints/hernia, *o*cular depression, *R*ieger anomaly, and *t*eething delay (SHORT).
1. Gorlin RJ, et al: Rieger anomaly and growth retardation (the S-H-O-R-T syndrome). Birth Defects 11(2):46-48, 1975
2. Lipson A, Cowell C, Gorlin RJ: The SHORT syndrome: further delineation and natural history. J Med Genet 26:473-475, 1989

SHOULDER-HAND SYNDROME, a symptom complex comprising stiffness or pain in the shoulder associated with pain and swelling of the hand. Cross-references: Hand-shoulder syndrome; Steinbrocker syndrome.
1. Grinker RR, Sahs AL: Neurology. 6th ed. Springfield: Charles C Thomas, 1966
2. Steinbrocker O: Ann Rheum Dis 6:80-84, 1947

SHPRINTZEN SYNDROME, mild intellectual impairment, small stature, conductive hearing loss, cleft of secondary palate, slender hypotonic and hyperextensible hands and fingers, and a ventricular septal defect are characteristics. Probable autosomal dominance, with X-linked dominance not excluded. Cross-references: Sedláčková syndrome; Velocardiofacial syndrome. (Robert J. Shprintzen, U.S. genealogist)
1. Gorlin RJ, Cohen MM Jr, Levin LS: Syndromes of the Head and Neck. 3rd ed. New York: Oxford University Press, 1990
2. Shprintzen RJ, et al: A new syndrome involving cleft palate, cardiac anomalies, typical facies, and learning disabilities: velo-cardio-facial syndrome. Cleft Palate J 15:56-62, 1978
3. Smith DW, Jones KL: Recognizable Patterns of Human Malformations: Genetic, Embryologic, and Clinical Aspects. 3rd ed. Philadelphia: WB Saunders, 1982

SHWACHMAN SYNDROME, SHWACHMAN-DIAMOND SYNDROME, metaphyseal chondrodysplasia associated with malabsorption and neutropenia. (Harry Shwachman, 1910-1986, U.S. pediatrician; Louis K. Diamond, U.S. pediatrician)
1. McKusick VA: Heritable Disorders of Connective Tissue. 4th ed. St Louis: CV Mosby, 1972
2. Shwachman H, Diamond LK, Oski FA, et al: J Pediatr 63:835-843, 1963; J Pediatr 65:645-663, 1964

SHY-DRAGER SYNDROME, multiple system atrophy; a specific neuronal degeneration involving the preganglionic sympathetic neurons, basal ganglia, cerebellum, and other regions of the central nervous system. Most common in middle-aged men. Cross-reference: Shy-Magee-Drager syndrome. (George M. Shy, 1919-1967, U.S. neurologist; Glenn A. Drager, 1917-1967, U.S. neurologist)
1. Fowler NO: Cardiac Diagnosis and Treatment. 3rd ed. Cambridge: Harper & Row, 1980
2. Rowland LP (ed): Merritt's Textbook of Neurology. 9th ed. Baltimore: Williams & Wilkins, 1995
3. Shy GM, Drager GA: A neurological syndrome associated with orthostatic hypotension. Arch Neurol 2:511-527, 1960

SHY-GONATAS SYNDROME, characteristics include progressive ptosis, external ophthalmoplegia, retinitis pigmentosa, ataxia, absent deep reflexes, elevated levels of cerebrospinal fluid protein, and histological features compatible with Refsum disease or Hurler syndrome. (George M. Shy)
1. Baker AB, Baker LH: Clinical Neurology. Revised ed. Philadelphia: Harper & Row, 1982
2. Gonatas NK: Am J Med 42:169-178, 1967
3. Shy GM, Silberberg DH, Appel SM, et al: Am J Med 42:163-169, 1967

SHY-MAGEE-DRAGER SYNDROME, see Shy-Drager syndrome.

SIAM DISEASE, yellow fever.
1. Casas EC: Diccionario Terminologico de Ciencias Medicas. 5th ed. Salvat Editores, SA, 1954

SIBERIAN TICK TYPHUS, north Asian tick-borne rickettsiosis; first recognized as a clinical entity distinct from other rickettsioses in the mid to late 1930s. Several species of ixodid ticks have been implicated as vectors.
1. Bennett JC, Plum F (eds): Cecil Textbook of Medicine. 20th ed. Philadelphia: WB Saunders, 1996

SICAR SIGN, metallic resonance heard on percussion with two coins on the front of the chest and auscultation at the back; found in effusion within the pleura. Cross-references: Heubner sign; Sieur sign.
1. Dorland's Medical Dictionary. 28th ed. Philadelphia: WB Saunders, 1994

SICARD SIGN, dorsiflexion of the great toe while an examination is being performed; increases the stretching of the tibial portion of the sciatic nerve and aggravates the patient's pain.
1. Baker AB, Baker LH: Clinical Neurology. Revised ed. Philadelphia: Harper & Row, 1982
2. Bordas LB (ed): Neurologia Fundamental. 2nd ed. Toray, 1968

SICARD SYNDROME, see Collet syndrome.

SICCA SYNDROME, a form of Sjögren syndrome in which the patient does not have a collagen disorder.
1. Deutsch HJ: Sjögren syndrome and pseudolymphoma. Ann Otol 76:1074-1084, 1967
2. Ritchie AC: Boyd's Textbook of Pathology. 9th ed. Philadelphia: Lea & Febiger, 1990

SICK BUILDING SYNDROME, respiratory symptoms, dryness, and itching of the face seen in a person occupying a poorly ventilated building. Cross-reference: Tight building syndrome.
1. Gravesen S, et al: Allergy 41:520-525, 1986

SICK EUTHYROID SYNDROME, see Silvestrini-Corda syndrome.

SICK SINUS SYNDROME, see Bradycardia syndrome.

SICKLE CELL ANEMIA, hemolytic anemia seen almost exclusively in Blacks and due to the inheritance of a gene for a structurally abnormal ß global chain subunit of adult hemoglobin, the ß5 chain of hemoglobin S. May present as recurrent abdominal pain stroke-like symptoms.
1. Bennett JC, Plum F (eds): Cecil Textbook of Medicine. 20th ed. Philadelphia: WB Saunders, 1996
2 Herrick JB: Arch Intern Med 6:517-521, 1910

SIEBOLD OPERATION, see Gigli operation.

SIEGAL-CATTAN-MAMOU SYNDROME, resembles Reimann syndrome with the addition of arthralgia; found among Jewish and Armenian populations and sometimes occurring with malaria. (Sheppard Siegal, U.S.)
1. Maffei WE: Os Fundamentos da Medicina. 2nd ed. Livraria Editora Artes Médicas Ltda, 1978

SIEGERT SIGN, the 5th finger is short and curved inward; seen in a mongoloid person. (Ferdinand Siegert, 1865-1946, German pediatrician)
1. Casas EC: Diccionario Terminologico de Ciencias Medicas. 5th ed. Salvat Editores, SA, 1954

SIEMENS SYNDROME, see Christ-Siemens-Touraine syndrome.

SIEUR SIGN, see Sicar sign.

SIGAULT OPERATION, symphysiotomy.
1. Maffei WE: Os Fundamentos da Medicina. 2nd ed. Livraria Editora Artes Médicas Ltda, 1978

SIGNORELLI SIGN, pain on pressure at the retromandibular area; seen in the patient with meningitis. (Augusto Signorelli, 1876-1952, Italian)
1. Casas EC: Diccionario Terminologico de Ciencias Medicas. 5th ed. Salvat Editores, SA, 1954

SILENGO SYNDROME, asymmetric crying facies, microcephaly, mental retardation, atrial septal defect, and patent ductus arteriosus are features.
1. Rimoin DL, et al: Principles and Practice of Medical Genetics. 3rd ed. Philadelphia: Churchill-Livingstone, 1996

SILEX SIGN, scar lines radiating from the mouth; occurs in cases of congenital syphilis. (Paul Silex, 1858-1929, German ophthalmologist)
1. Casas EC: Diccionario Terminologico de Ciencias Medicas. 5th ed. Salvat Editores, SA, 1954

SILFVERSKIÖLD SYNDROME, a form of eccentric osteochondrodysplasia in which the skeletal changes are chiefly in the extremities and which is inherited as a dominant characteristic. A Morquio syndrome variant.
1. Silfverskiöld N: A forme fruste of chondrodystrophia, with changes simulating several of the known local malacias. Acta Radiol 4:44-57, 1925

SILO FILLER DISEASE, pulmonary damage caused by nitric oxide and nitrogen dioxide formed during fermentation of silage. The nitrogen oxides may reach dangerous concentrations in the silo and a person who enters the silo may collapse and die.
1. Ritchie AC: Boyd's Textbook of Pathology. 9th ed. Philadelphia: Lea & Febiger, 1990

SILVER SYNDROME, SILVER-RUSSELL SYNDROME, see Russell-Silver syndrome.

SILVESTRINI-CORDA SYNDROME, a syndrome indicative of abnormally high estrogen activity, due to failure of the liver to inactivate the circulating estrogen; anorexia, asthenia with an eunuchoid body type in which there is absence of body hair, deficient libido, atrophy of the testes, sterility, and gynecomastia are features. Cross-references: Euthyroid sick syndrome; Sick euthyroid syndrome. (R. Silvestrini, Italian)
1. Corda C, Sulla CD: Minerva Med 5:1067-1069, 1925
2. Docter R, Krenning EP, DeJong M, et al: The sick euthyroid syndrome: changes in thyroid hormone serum parameters and hormone metabolism. Clin Endocrinol 39:499-510, 1993
3. Silvestrini R: Riforma Med 42:701-704, 1926

SIMMONDS DISEASE, a profound pituitary insufficiency resulting when the anterior lobe of the pituitary is destroyed. (Morris Simmonds, 1855-1925, German)
1. Baker AB, Baker LH: Clinical Neurology. Revised ed. Philadelphia: Harper & Row, 1982
2. Haymaker W: Bing's Local Diagnosis in Neurological Diseases. 15th ed. St Louis: CV Mosby, 1969
3. Simmonds M: Dtsch Med Wochenschr 4:322-323, 1914

SIMMONDS SYNDROME, SIMMONDS-SHEEHAN SYNDROME, see Sheehan syndrome.

SIMMONDS TEST, with the patient lying prone, the calf is squeezed transversely. If the tendon is intact or incompletely ruptured, the foot, which should project beyond the end of the examining table, is seen to undergo plantar flexion. If the tendon is completely ruptured, the foot remains still. (Franklin A. Simmonds, British orthopedic surgeon)
1. Lumley JS, Clain A: Hamilton Bailey's Demonstration of Physical Signs in Clinical Surgery. 18th ed. London: Butterworth-Heinemann, 1997

SIMON OPERATION, 1) colpocleisis or Marckwald operation. (G. Simon); 2) surgery to correct a perineal rupture. (J. Simon)
1. Maffei WE: Os Fundamentos da Medicina. 2nd ed. Livraria Editora Artes Médicas Ltda, 1978

SIMON SIGN, 1) dissociation of motion between the thorax and abdomen in meningitis (Sir John Simon, 1816-1904, British surgeon); 2) retraction or fixation of the umbilicus during peritonitis. (Charles E. Simon, 1866-1929, German ophthalmologist).
1. Casas EC: Diccionario Terminologico de Ciencias Medicas. 5th ed. Salvat Editores, SA, 1954

SIMON SYNDROME, breast cancer with pituitary metastases.

1. Casas EC: Diccionario Terminologico de Ciencias Medicas. 5th ed. Salvat Editores, SA, 1954

SIMOPOULOS SYNDROME, cerebral malformations and hydrocephalus as well as renal malformation.

1. Campbell MF, Walsh PC: Campbell's Urology. 5th ed. Philadelphia: WB Saunders, 1986

SIMPSON-GOLABI-BEHMEL SYNDROME, mental retardation and overgrowth; pre- and postnatal growth deficiency, intellectual impairment, characteristic facies, and other anomalies are features. Cross-references: Bulldog syndrome; Golabi-Rosen syndrome; Mental retardation-overgrowth syndrome. (J.L. Simpson, U.S)

1. Behmel A, Ploechl E, Rosenkranz W: Am J Med Genet 30:275-285, 1988
2. Golabi M, Rosen L: A new X-linked mental retardation: overgrowth syndrome. Am J Med Genet 17:345-358, 1984
3. Gorlin RJ, Cohen MM Jr, Levin LS: Syndromes of the Head and Neck. 3rd ed. New York: Oxford University Press, 1990
4. Simpson JL, Landey S, New M, et al: Birth Defects Orig Art Ser 11:18-24, 1975

SIMS OPERATION, surgical treatment of uterine anteflexion; consists of the creation of a communication between the uterine neck and the vaginal cul de sac. (James M. Sims, 1813-1870, U.S. gynecologist)

1. Maffei WE: Os Fundamentos da Medicina. 2nd ed. Livraria Editora Artes Médicas Ltda, 1978

SINDBIS DISEASE, symptoms are a low fever, with malaise, myalgia, and arthralgia, together with a striking maculopapular rash on the trunk which often becomes vesicular. The alphavirus that causes this virus is found in Europe, Africa, and Australia. (Named after the village in Egypt where first isolated.)

1. Ritchie AC: Boyd's Textbook of Pathology. 9th ed. Philadelphia: Lea & Febiger, 1990

SINDING-LARSEN-JOHANSSON SYNDROME, a frequently occurring avulsion injury to the proximal and distal poles of the patella; should be considered a chronic repetitive ligamentous injury. (Christian M.F. Sinding-Larsen, 1866-1930, Norwegian surgeon; Sven J. Johansson, Swedish surgeon)

1. Campbell WC, Crenshaw AH: Campbell's Operative Orthopaedics. 7th ed. St Louis: CV Mosby, 1987
2. Johansson S: Hygeia 84:161-166, 1922
3. Sinding-Larsen CMF: Acta Radiol 1:171-173, 1921

SINGAPORE EAR, see Hong Kong ear.

SINGLETON-MERTEN SYNDROME, consists of calcification of the aortic arch and aortic valve, hypoplastic tooth buds, and osteoporosis and widening of the metacarpal, carpal, and phalangeal bones. (Edward B. Singleton, U.S.)

1. Gay BB Jr, Kuhn JP: A syndrome of widened medullary cavities of bone, aortic calcification, abnormal dentition and muscular weakness (the Singleton-Merten syndrome). Radiology 118:389-395, 1976
2. Gorlin RJ, Cohen MM Jr, Levin LS: Syndromes of the Head and Neck. 3rd ed. New York: Oxford University Press, 1990
3. Singleton EB, Merten DF: An unusual syndrome of widened medullary cavities of the matacarpals and dentition. Pediatr Radiol 1:2-7, 1973

SINKLER PHENOMENON, in an extremity with spastic paralysis, sharp flexion of the toe may be followed by flexion of the knee and hip.

1. Dorland's Medical Dictionary. 28th ed. Philadelphia: WB Saunders, 1994

SINUS TARSI SYNDROME, pain in the tarsal sinus persists for many months after a sprain of the ankle.

1. Brown JE: Sinus tarsi syndrome. Clin Orthop 18:231-233, 1969
2. Campbell WC, Crenshaw AH: Campbell's Operative Orthopaedics. 7th ed. St Louis: CV Mosby, 1987

SIPPLE SYNDROME, multiple endocrine neoplasia type II; characterized by pheochromocytoma, neural tumors, and medullary carcinoma of the thyroid. Occurs in families as an expression of two distinct traits, each with autosomal dominant transmission. (John H. Sipple, U.S. respiratory physician)

1. Bennett JC, Plum F (eds): Cecil Textbook of Medicine. 20th ed. Philadelphia: WB Saunders, 1996
2. Fowler NO: Cardiac Diagnosis and Treatment. 3rd ed. Cambridge: Harper & Row, 1980
3. Sipple JH: Am J Med 31:163-166, 1961

SISTO SIGN, persistent crying in an infant with congenital syphilis. (Genaro Sisto, 1870-1923, Argentine pediatrician)

1. Casas EC: Diccionario Terminologico de Ciencias Medicas. 5th ed. Salvat Editores, SA, 1954

SIXTH DISEASE, see Zahorsky disease.

SJÖGREN SYNDROME, an autoimmune disease involving the salivary glands and characterized by keratoconjunctivitis sicca, xerostomia, and a connective tissue disease (usually rheumatoid arthritis). Cross-references: Dry eye syndrome; Gougerot-Houwer-Sjögren syndrome. (Henrik S.C. Sjögren, 1899-1989, Swedish ophthalmologist)
  1. Gougerot H: Bull Soc Fr Derm Syph 32:376-379, 1925
  2. Houwer AW: Ned Tijdschr Geneeskd 1:2299-2301, 1927
  3. Manthorpe R, Frost-Larsen K, Isager H, et al: Sjögren syndrome. Allergy 36:139, 1980
  4. Sjögren HSC: Acta Ophthalmol Suppl 2:1-151, 1933

SJÖGREN-LARSSON SYNDROME, see Rud syndrome. (Karl G.T. Sjögren, Swedish psychiatrist; Tage Larsson, Swedish)

SKEER SIGN, a small circle in the iris of both eyes; seen in the patient with tuberculous meningitis.
  1. Casas EC: Diccionario Terminologico de Ciencias Medicas. 5th ed. Salvat Editores, SA, 1954

SKEVAS-ZERFUS DISEASE, disease of sponge fishermen in Greece.
  1. Casas EC: Diccionario Terminologico de Ciencias Medicas. 5th ed. Salvat Editores, SA, 1954

SKODA SIGN, increased resonance of the upper part of the lung while compressing the inferior part of the lung; heard in the patient with pneumonia. (Josef P. Skoda, 1805-1881, Austrian)
  1. Casas EC: Diccionario Terminologico de Ciencias Medicas. 5th ed. Salvat Editores, SA, 1954

SKUTSCH OPERATION, technique for salpingostomy (creating an opening into a uterine tube).
  1. Maffei WE: Os Fundamentos da Medicina. 2nd ed. Livraria Editora Artes Médicas Ltda, 1978

SLEEP APNEA SYNDROME, episodes of cessation of breathing occurring at the transition from nonrapid eye movement to rapid eye movement (REM) sleep, with repeated awakening and excessive daytime sleepiness; occurs most frequently in middle-aged, obese males and is thought to have several causes, one being collapse or obstruction of the airway with the diminution of muscle tone that characterizes REM sleep. Cross-reference: Central sleep apnea syndrome.
  1. Tilkian AG, Guilleminault C, Schroeder KL, et al: Sleep induced apnea syndrome: prevalence of cardiac arrhythmias and their reversal after tracheostomy. Am J Med 63:348-358, 1977

SLEEP-RELATED GASTROESOPHAGEAL REFLUX SYNDROME, a patient with gastroesophageal reflux awakened from sleep with burning substernal pain (heartburn), a sour taste, coughing, choking, and even respiratory stridor.
  1. Rowland LP (ed): Merritt's Textbook of Neurology. 9th ed. Baltimore: Williams & Wilkins, 1995

SLIPPING RIB SYNDROME, see Cyriax syndrome.

SLONE DISEASE, a rare and painful familial illness that causes the pancreas to literally digest itself during attacks. (Described in Kentucky, afflicts generations of families.)
  1. Wall Street Journal, August 15, 1996, p B1

SLOTNICK-GOLDFARB SYNDROME, secondary amenorrhea, a lack of secondary sexual characteristics, normal stature, and eunuchoid habitus are features. Cross-reference: Streaked ovary syndrome.
  1. Neves-E-Castro, et al: Streaked ovary syndrome, Slotnick-Goldfarb syndrome. Obstet Gynecol 47:86-89, 1976
  2. Slotnick EA, Goldfarb AF: Obstet Gynecol 39:269-273, 1972

SLOW CEREBRATION SIGN, the patient is asked a question, does not respond for approximately 10-30 seconds, but then answers deliberately and accurately.
  1. Mazion JM: Illustrated Manual of Neurological Reflexes/Signs/Tests of Office Procedure. 2nd ed. Orlando: Daniels Publishing, 1980

SLUDER NEURALGIA, sphenopalatine neuralgia. (Greenfield Sluder, 1865-1925, U.S. otorhinolaryngologist)
  1. Sluder G: NY State Med J 87:989-990, 1908

SLUDER OPERATION, ablation of the tonsils together with their capsules. (Greenfield Sluder)
  1. Maffei WE: Os Fundamentos da Medicina. 2nd ed. Livraria Editora Artes Médicas Ltda, 1978

SLY SYNDROME, see Glucuronidase deficiency mucopolysaccharidosis. (William S. Sly, U.S.)

SMITH FRACTURE, the reverse of a Colles fracture; occurs much less commonly. The distal fragment of the radius is displaced toward the volar aspect instead of dorsally. (Robert W. Smith, 1807-1873, Irish surgeon)

1. Lumley JS, Clain A: Hamilton Bailey's Demonstration of Physical Signs in Clinical Surgery. 18th ed. London: Butterworth-Heinemann, 1997

SMITH SIGN, a bruit heard in the sternum of a patient lying supine; an indication of bronchial lymph node hypertrophy. Cross-reference: Eustace Smith sign. (Eustace Smith, 1835-1914, British)
1. Casas EC: Diccionario Terminologico de Ciencias Medicas. 5th ed. Salvat Editores, SA, 1954

SMITH-FINEMAN-MYERS SYNDROME, a rare hereditary syndrome with features of unusual facial appearance, short stature, and mental retardation. (Richard D. Smith, U.S.)
1. Gorlin RJ, Cohen MM Jr, Levin LS: Syndromes of the Head and Neck. 3rd ed. New York: Oxford University Press, 1990
2. Smith RD, Fineman RM, Myers GG: Short stature, psychomotor retardation, and unusual facial appearance in two brothers. Am J Med Genet 7:5-9, 1980

SMITH-LEMLI-OPITZ SYNDROME, microcephaly, epicanthal folds, horizontal upper palmar creases, and short thumb and toes are features. Cross-reference: Dysmorphic syndrome. (David Smith, 1926-1981, U.S. pediatrician; Luc Lemli, U.S. pediatrician; John M. Opitz, U.S. genealogist)
1. Farmer TW: Pediatric Neurology. 2nd ed. Hagerstown: Harper & Row, 1975
2. Opitz JM, Penchaszadeh VB, Holt MC, et al: Smith-Lemli-Opitz (RSM) syndrome bibliography. Am J Med Genet 28:745-750, 1987
3. Smith DW, Lemli L, Opitz JM: Newly recognized syndrome of multiple congenital anomalies. J Pediatr 64:210-217, 1964

SMITH-STRANG DISEASE, a hereditary defect in methionine absorption, in which the urine has a characteristic odor resembling that of the interior of an oasthouse due to á-hydroxybutyric acid formed by bacterial action on the unabsorbed methionine; marked by white hair, mental retardation, convulsions, and attacks of hyperpnea. (Allan J. Smith, British; Leonard B. Strang, British)
1. Smith AJ, Strang LB: Arch Dis Child 33:109-113, 1958

SMITHWISK OPERATION, lumbodorsal splenectomy through a transdiaphragmatic extrapleural incision, with resection of the great splanchnic nerve and the sympathetic ganglia from the 9th thoracic to the 1st lumbar vertebrae, for the treatment of arterial hypertension.
1. Maffei WE: Os Fundamentos da Medicina. 2nd ed. Livraria Editora Artes Médicas Ltda, 1978

SNEDDON SYNDROME, a syndrome of stroke and livedo reticularis; visual loss and dementia are seen in some patients. Immunosuppressive therapy is warranted. Etiology uncertain. (Ian B. Sneddon, British dermatologist)
1. Scully RE, et al: Case records of the Massachusetts General Hospital. N Engl J Med 332:452-459, 1995
2. Sneddon IB: Br J Dermatol 77:180-185, 1965

SNELLEN OPERATION, surgery for ectropion. (Hermann Snellen, 1834-1908, Dutch ophthalmologist)
1. Maffei WE: Os Fundamentos da Medicina. 2nd ed. Livraria Editora Artes Médicas Ltda, 1978

SNELLEN SIGN, see Riesman sign. (Hermann Snellen)

SOAVE OPERATION, a pediatric procedure for Hirschsprung disease by endorectal pull-through. (F. Soave, French-Italian pediatric surgeon)
1. Schwartz SI: Principles of Surgery. 4th ed. New York, McGraw-Hill, 1983

SOCIAL BREAKDOWN SYNDROME, symptoms of mentally ill patients due to the effects of long-term institutionalization, rather than to the primary illness; includes excessive passivity, assumption of the chronic sick role, and atrophy of work and social skills.
1. Dorland's Medical Dictionary. 28th ed. Philadelphia: WB Saunders, 1994

SOCIN OPERATION, enucleation of a thyroid tumor.
1. Maffei WE: Os Fundamentos da Medicina. 2nd ed. Livraria Editora Artes Médicas Ltda, 1978

SOFT SIGN, a series of tests for gross and fine motor function, subtle sensory deficits, visual motor abilities, and a variety of conceptual abilities.
1. Farmer TW: Pediatric Neurology. 2nd ed. Hagerstown: Harper & Row, 1975
2. Touwen BCL, Heinz FR: Clinics in Developmental Medicine, #38, Spastics International Medical Publications. Philadelphia: JB Lippincott, 1970
3. US Public Health Service, Pub. #2015, Washington DC, 1969

SOHVAL-SOFFER SYNDROME, a congenital syndrome consisting of male hypogonadism associated with multiple skeletal abnormalities of the cervical spine and ribs and mental retardation.

(Arthur R. Sohval, 1904-1985, U.S. internist; Louis J. Soffer, U.S. internist)
1. Dorland's Medical Dictionary. 28th ed. Philadelphia: WB Saunders, 1994

SOMNOLENCE SYNDROME, a transient condition of drowsiness, lethargy, anorexia, and irritability with electroencephalographic changes; occurs in children with acute leukemia or non-Hodgkin lymphoma after irradiation of the head.
1. Freeman JE, et al: Br Med J 4:523-525, 1973

SONNEBERG OPERATION, excision of the inferior mandibular nerve in the angle of the mandible.
1. Maffei WE: Os Fundamentos da Medicina. 2nd ed. Livraria Editora Artes Médicas Ltda, 1978

SORESI SIGN, with the patient lying supine and hip flexed, hepatic palpation causes pain at the McBurney point when the patient coughs; seen in appendicitis.
1. Casas EC: Diccionario Terminologico de Ciencias Medicas. 5th ed. Salvat Editores, SA, 1954

SORSBY SYNDROME, a congenital condition consisting of bilateral macular coloboma associated with apical dystrophy of the hands and feet; also frequently noted are brachydactyly confined to the distal two phalanges and the absence of big toes. (Arnold Sorsby, 1900-1980, British ophthalmologist)
1. Sorsby A: Congenital coloboma of the macula; together with an account of the familial occurrence of bilateral macular coloboma in association with apical dystrophy of hands and feet. Br Ophthalmol 19:65-90, 1935

SOTO-HALL SIGN, with the patient lying flat, flexion of the spine beginning at the neck and going downward; pain is felt at the site of the lesion in back abnormalities. (Ralph Soto-Hall, U.S.)
1. Evans RC: Illustrated Essentials in Orthopedic Physical Assessment. St Louis: Mosby Yearbook, 1994

SOTOS SYNDROME, cerebral gigantism; includes intrauterine overgrowth, generalized edema at birth, accelerated osseous maturation, dolichocephaly, large extremities, clumsiness, retarded motor and speech development, severe muscular hypotonia, contracture of the feet, wrist drop, and clinodactyly. Children with this syndrome are usually above the 90th percentile for length and weight at birth and continue to grow rapidly for the first few years of life. Autosomal recessive inheritance. Cross-reference: Nevo syndrome. (Juan F. Sotos, U.S.)
1. Cole TRP, Hughes HE: Sotos syndrome. J Med Genet 27:571-576, 1990
2. Rowland LP (ed): Merritt's Textbook of Neurology. 9th ed. Baltimore: Williams & Wilkins, 1995
3. Sotos JF, Dodge PR, Muirhead D, et al: Cerebral gigantism in childhood, a syndrome of excessively rapid growth with acromegalic features and a nonprogressive neurologic disorder. N Engl J Med 271:109-116, 1964

SOTTEAU OPERATION, occlusion of the inguinal canal using a double fold of the scrotum in cases of inguinal hernia.
1. Maffei WE: Os Fundamentos da Medicina. 2nd ed. Livraria Editora Artes Médicas Ltda, 1978

SOUQUES PHENOMENON, see Finger phenomenon. (Alexandre A. Souques, 1860-1944, French neurologist)

SOUQUES SIGN, when a patient sitting in a chair is suddenly thrown back, the lower extremities do not extend normally or otherwise attempt to counteract the loss of balance; an indication of advanced striatal disease. (Alexandre A. Souques)
1. Mazion JM: llustrated Manual of Neurological Reflexes/Signs/Tests of Office Procedure. 2nd ed. Orlando: Daniels Publishing, 1980

SOURDILLE OPERATION, fenestration surgery to re-establish hearing in cases of otosclerosis. A fistula in the horizontal semicircular canal is formed and covered by a cutaneous graft sutured to the tympanum.
1. Maffei WE: Os Fundamentos da Medicina. 2nd ed. Livraria Editora Artes Médicas Ltda, 1978

SOUTH AFRICAN TICK-BITE FEVER, a tick-borne infection in South Africa, due to *Rickettsia conorii*, the etiological agent of boutonneuse. Cross-reference: Nuftal-Santana disease.

SPACE ADAPTATION SYNDROME, a form of motion sickness occurring with loss of gravity during space flight; symptoms include nausea, vomiting, anorexia, headache, malaise, drowsiness, and lethargy.
1. Dorland's Medical Dictionary. 28th ed. Philadelphia: WB Saunders, 1994

SPAETH OPERATION, a block procedure that aims at avoiding the inconsistencies of the O'Brien block by injecting over the mandibular condyle and thereby catching the facial nerve before it divides.
1. Spaeth GL: Ophthalmic Surgery. Principles and Practice. Philadelphia: WB Saunders, 1982

SPALDING SIGN, radiological finding of overlap of the skull bones in a fetus; an indication of fetal death. Cross-reference: Horner sign. (Alfred B. Spalding, 1874-1942, U.S. obstetrician/gynecologist)
1. Casas EC: Diccionario Terminologico de Ciencias Medicas. 5th ed. Salvat Editores, SA, 1954

SPASTIC SYNDROME, clinical disturbances resulting from a lesion involving the pyramidal tract known collectively as the spastic syndrome.
1. Haymaker W: Bing's Local Diagnosis in Neurological Diseases. 15th ed. St Louis: CV Mosby, 1969

SPÄT-HURLER SYDNROME, see Scheie syndrome.

SPEAR-MICLE SYNDROME, soft-tissue tumors in the frontal area of the scalp together with unilateral coronal synostosis and plagiocephaly, facial anomalies, lumbar meningomyelocele, thoracic kyphoscoliosis, hip dislocation, and foot and elbow deformities.
1. Gorlin RJ, Cohen MM Jr, Levin LS: Syndromes of the Head and Neck. 3rd ed. New York: Oxford University Press, 1990

SPENCER DISEASE, see Bradley disease.

SPENS SYNDROME, see Adams-Stokes syndrome. (Thomas Spens, 1769-1842, Scottish)

SPHENOCAVERNOUS SYNDROME, an unruptured giant aneurysm of the middle cerebral artery may compress the venous outflow of the cavernous sinus, thus producing unilateral ophthalmoplegia, ipsilateral proptosis, and even ipsilateral visual loss with evidence of optic neuropathy.

SPHEROPHAKIA-BRACHYMORPHIA SYNDROME, see Weil-Marchesani syndrome.

SPIEGELBERG SIGN, a "sticky" sensation at the neck of the uterus when there is malignancy of the uterus.
1. Casas EC: Diccionario Terminologico de Ciencias Medicas. 5th ed. Salvat Editores, SA, 1954

SPIELMEYER-VOGT-SJÕGREN DISEASE, myoclonus in juvenile neuronal ceroid lipofuscinosis. Features can include sporadic myoclonic jerks, low-amplitude myoclonus involving the face and later the hands, and more severe myoclonus of the extremities that may precede a seizure. Cross-reference: Vogt-Spielmeyer disease. (Walter Spielmeyer, 1879-1935, German; Oskar Vogt, 1870-1959, German)
1. Spielmeyer W: Nissls Beitr Nerv Geistes Krkh, 1908
2. Vogt H: Monatsschr Psychiatr 18:161-171, 1905

SPIGELIAN HERNIA, abnormal hernia through the linea semilunaris, usually a few centimeters above the inguinal ligament. Difficult to clinically differentiate from interstitial hernia or lumbar hernia. (Adrian van der Spieghel [Spigelius], 1578-1625, Italian anatomist)
1. Lumley JS, Clain A: Hamilton Bailey's Demonstration of Physical Signs in Clinical Surgery. 18th ed. London: Butterworth-Heinemann, 1997

SPILLER SYNDROME, ascending paralysis with a possibly epidural mass lesion. Cross-reference: Erb-Charcot syndrome.
1. Spiller WG: Rev Neurol Psychiatr 9:494-498, 1911

SPILLMAN SIGN, expansion of the lungs can be impeded; seen in the patient with emphysema, but not in rib abscess.
1. Casas EC: Diccionario Terminologico de Ciencias Medicas. 5th ed. Salvat Editores, SA, 1954

SPINAL BLOCK SYNDROME, see Froin syndrome.

SPINAL SIGN, tonic contraction of the spinal muscles on the diseased side in a patient with pleurisy.
1. Dorland's Medical Dictionary. 28th ed. Philadelphia: WB Saunders, 1994

SPINAL TUMOR SYNDROME, a circumscribed tuberculous focus, usually arising from the posterior aspect of the vertebral body. Clinical picture resembles that of an intraspinal tumor.
1. Campbell WC, Crenshaw AH: Campbell's Operative Orthopaedics. 7th ed. St Louis: CV Mosby, 1987

SPINE SIGN, the disinclination to flex the spine anteriorly because of pain; occurs in the patient with poliomyelitis.
1. Dorland's Medical Dictionary. 28th ed. Philadelphia: WB Saunders, 1994

SPIVACK OPERATION, method of gastrostomy.
1. Maffei WE: Os Fundamentos da Medicina. 2nd ed. Livraria Editora Artes Médicas Ltda, 1978

SPLENIC FLEXURE SYNDROME, discomfort in the left upper abdominal quadrant, which may give rise to pain in the precordium and left shoulder and arm, simulating angina.

1. Payr E: Verh Dtsch Kongr Inn Med 27:276-305, 1910

SPLIT-BRAIN SYNDROME, an association of symptoms such as visual fields and limbs of one side do not coordinate with the corresponding other side produced by disruption of or interference with the connection between the hemispheres of the brain.

1. Geschwind N: Disconnection syndromes in animals and man. Brain 88:237-294, 1965

SPONDYLOEPIPHYSEAL DYSPLASIA CONGENITAL SYNDROME, growth deficiency, variable flat facies, cleft palate, myopia, kyphoscoliosis, lumbar lordosis, a barrel chest, lag in mineralization of epiphyses of limbs, and muscle weakness are features. Autosomal dominant inheritance.

1. Smith DW, Jones KL: Recognizable Patterns of Human Malformations: Genetic, Embryologic, and Clinical Aspects. 3rd ed. Philadelphia: WB Saunders, 1982
2. Spranger J, Langer LO: Spondyloepiphyseal dysplasia congenita. Radiology 94:313-322, 1970

SPRANGER SYNDROME, mucolipidosis type I; the childhood form of sialidosis (neuraminidase deficiency). Life span is somewhat reduced, but most patients survive into the 4th and 5th decades. (Jürgen W. Spranger, German)

1. Gorlin RJ, Cohen MM Jr, Levin LS: Syndromes of the Head and Neck. 3rd ed. New York: Oxford University Press, 1990
2. Spranger J: Mucolipidosis I: phenotype and nosology. Perspect Inherit Metab Dis 4:303-315, 1981
3. Spranger JW, Filbert EF, Tuffli GA, et al: Lancet 2:97-98, 1960

SPRENGEL DEFORMITY, characterized by congenital elevation and rotation of the scapulae; frequently associated with Klippel-Feil syndrome, cervical ribs, and syringomyelia. (Otto Sprengel, 1852-1915, German surgeon)

1. Green WT: The surgical correction of congenital elevation of the scapula (Sprengel deformity). J Bone Joint Surg (Am) 39:1439, 1957
2. Sprengel O: Arch Klin Chir Berl 41:545-549, 1891

SPRINZ-DUBIN SYNDROME, SPRINZ-NELSON SYNDROME, see Dubin-Johnson syndrome. (Helmuth Sprinz, German-born U.S. pathologist; Isidore Dubin, 1913-1981, U.S. pathologist; R.S. Nelson, U.S.)

SPURLING SIGN, nerve stretching tests; all modifications of the Lasègue maneuver in which either the foot or the great toe undergoes dorsiflexion.

1. Baker AB, Baker LH: Clinical Neurology. Revised ed. Philadelphia: Harper & Row, 1982

SPURWAY-EDDOWES SYNDROME, see Osteogenesis imperfecta syndrome type I. (John Spurway, British; Alfred Eddowes, 1850-1946, British)

SQUIRE SIGN, alternating myosis and mydriasis; seen in the patient with basilar meningitis. (Truman H. Squire, 1823-1899, U.S. surgeon)

1. Casas EC: Diccionario Terminologico de Ciencias Medicas. 5th ed. Salvat Editores, SA, 1954

STACKE OPERATION, formation of a single cavity containing the antrum, attic, tympanum, and external canal.

1. Maffei WE: Os Fundamentos da Medicina. 2nd ed. Livraria Editora Artes Médicas Ltda, 1978

STAIRS SIGN, difficulty descending a stairway; occurs in the patient with tabes dorsalis.

1. Dorland's Medical Dictionary. 28th ed. Philadelphia: WB Saunders, 1994

STAMM OPERATION, method of gastrostomy in which a cone from the gastric wall is taken through an incision in the left rectus muscle of the abdomen. The vertex of the cone is then perforated and a rubber tube is introduced and sutured.

1. Maffei WE: Os Fundamentos da Medicina. 2nd ed. Livraria Editora Artes Médicas Ltda, 1978

STANESCU SYNDROME, STANESCU OSTEOSCLEROSIS SYNDROME, short stature, brachycephaly, hypoplastic midface, ocular proptosis, micrognathia, brachydactyly, and dense cortices of the long bones are features. (V. Stanescu, Romanian)

1. Dipierri JE, Guzman JD: A second family with autosomal dominant osteosclerosis-type Stanescu. Am J Med Genet 18:13-18, 1984
2. Gorlin RJ, Cohen MM Jr, Levin LS: Syndromes of the Head and Neck. 3rd ed. New York: Oxford University Press, 1990
3. Stanescu V, Maximilian C, Poenaru S, et al: Rev Fr Endocrinol Clin 4:219-231, 1963

STANTON DISEASE, melioidosis; an acute infectious disease transmitted by rodents and a result

of *Pseudomonas pseudomallei.*
1. Whitmore A, Krishnaswami CS: Indian Med Gaz 47:262-267, 1912

STAPHYLOCOCCAL SCALDED-SKIN SYNDROME, see Scalded-skin syndrome

STAPHYLOCOCCAL TOXIC SHOCK SYNDROME, see Toxic shock syndrome.

STARTLE DISEASE, a stereotyped movement in response to an unexpected stimulus and consists of facial grimacing, blinking, head movement, hunching of the shoulder, bending of the elbows, forearm pronation, abdominal contraction, forward movement of the trunk, and knee flexion. Enhanced by anxiety, fatigue, and sleep deprivation.

STEELE-RICHARDSON-OLSZEWSKI SYNDROME, progressive supranuclear palsy; a rare condition usually seen in men over 50 years of age. (John Steele, Canadian neurologist; John C. Richardson, Canadian neurologist; Jerzy Olszewski, 1913-1966, Canadian neurologist)
1. Steele J, Richardson JC, Olszewski J: Arch Neurol 10:333-359, 1964

STEELL MURMUR, see Graham Steell murmur.

STEELY-HAIR SYNDROME, see Menkes syndrome.

STEIN-LEVENTHAL SYNDROME, see Polycystic ovary syndrome. (Irving F. Stein, U.S. gynecologist; Michael L. Leventhal, 1901-1971, U.S. obstetrician)

STEINACH OPERATION, ligature and resection of the ductus deferens in order to cause atrophy of the spermatogenic apparatus and proliferation of interstitial tissue; the production of gonadal hormones.
1. Maffei WE: Os Fundamentos da Medicina. 2nd ed. Livraria Editora Artes Médicas Ltda, 1978

STEINBERG THUMB SIGN, a relatively narrow palm of the hand, together with a long thumb and loose-jointedness. The thumb held across the palm extends well beyond the ulnar margin of the hand; seen in the patient with Marfan syndrome.
1. McKusick VA: Heritable Disorders of Connective Tissue. 4th ed. St Louis: CV Mosby, 1972

STEINBROCKER SYNDROME, see Shoulder-hand syndrome. (Otto Steinbrocker, U.S.)

STEINER SYNDROME, see Curtius syndrome. (L. Steiner, German)

STEINERT DISEASE, myotonic dystrophy; the distal extremities and the muscles of the face, jaw, neck, and eyelids become weak and wasted. Males and females are affected in this progressive familial disorder with early onset. Cross-references: Curschmann-Steinert disease; Nogues-Siral disease. (Hans Steinert, German)
1. Rowland LP (ed): Merritt's Textbook of Neurology. 9th ed. Baltimore: Williams & Wilkins, 1995

STEINERT SYNDROME, myotonic dystrophy; muscle degeneration, cataracts, testicular atrophy, amenorrhea or dysmenorrhea, ovarian cyst, and conduction defects with arrhythmias are features. Autosomal dominant inheritance. (Hans Steinert)
1. Aicardi J, Conti D, Goutieres F: Aspects dystrophie myotonique de Steinert. J Genet Hum 23 (Suppl 146):1975
2. Smith DW, Jones KL: Recognizable Patterns of Human Malformations: Genetic, Embryologic, and Clinical Aspects. 3rd ed. Philadelphia: WB Saunders, 1982
3. Steinert H: Dtsch Z Nervenheilkd 37:58-104, 1909

STEINHARDT SIGN, progressive discoloration of the soft palate from yellowish to pinkish; occurs in the patient with syphilis.
1. Casas EC: Diccionario Terminologico de Ciencias Medicas. 5th ed. Salvat Editores, SA, 1954

STEINMANN SIGN, flexion of the knee joint causes point tenderness from over the anterior joint line medially toward the collateral ligament; extension of the knee produces the reverse.
1. Evans RC: Illustrated Essentials in Orthopedic Physical Assessment. St Louis: Mosby Yearbook, 1994
2. Mazion JM: Illustrated Manual of Orthopedic Signs/Tests/Maneuvers for Office Procedure. 2nd ed. Orlando: Daniels Publishing, 1980

STELLWAG SIGN, apparent widening of the palpebral fissure; seen in the patient with exophthalmic goiter. (Carl von Carion Stellwag, 1823-1904, Austrian ophthalmologist)
1. Bodechtel G: Diagnostico Diferential de las Enfermedades Neurologicas. Madrid: Pas Montalvo Editorial, 1967

STERLES SIGN, auscultatory increase in sounds in the cardiac region; seen in the patient with intrathoracic tumor.
1. Casas EC: Diccionario Terminologico de Ciencias Medicas. 5th ed. Salvat Editores, SA, 1954

STERLING SIGN, in hemiplegia, active adduction of the shoulder on the normal side against resistance is accompanied by adduction of the shoulder on the paretic side.
1. Baker AB, Baker LH: Clinical Neurology. Revised ed. Philadelphia: Harper & Row, 1982

STERNBERG CELLS, STERNBERG-REED CELLS, see Reed cells. (Carl von Sternberg, 1872-1935, Austrian pathologist)

STERNBERG SIGN, pain on palpation of the shoulder muscles; seen in the patient with pleurisy. (Carl von Sternberg)
1. Casas EC: Diccionario Terminologico de Ciencias Medicas. 5th ed. Salvat Editores, SA, 1954

STEVENS-JOHNSON SYNDROME, generally recognized as a severe form of erythema multiforme major and carries significant mortality and morbidity. Frequently stated that rash, conjunctivitis, oral ulcers and vesicles, and systemic toxicity must be present before the diagnosis can be made. The trunk and face are also usually afflicted. Cross-references: Fiessinger-Rendu syndrome; Johnson-Stevens syndrome; Ocular-mucous membrane syndrome. (Albert M. Stevens, 1884-1945, U.S. pediatrician; Frank C. Johnson, 1894-1934, U.S. pediatrician)
1. Ballenger JJ: Diseases of the Nose, Throat, Ear, Head and Neck. 12th ed. Philadelphia: Lea & Febiger, 1977
2. Ritchie AC: Boyd's Textbook of Pathology. 9th ed. Philadelphia: Lea & Febiger, 1990
3. Stevens AM, Johnson FC: Am J Dis Child 24:526-533, 1922

STEWART-HOLMES SIGN, see Holmes sign. (Purves Stewart, 1869-1949, British; Eric G. Holmes, 1876-1965, British neurologist)

STIERLIN SIGN, a radiological finding of an empty cecum while the colon and ilium retain contrast material; seen in ileocecal tuberculosis. (Eduard Stierlin, 1878-1919, German surgeon)
1. Casas EC: Diccionario Terminologico de Ciencias Medicas. 5th ed. Salvat Editores, SA, 1954

STEWART-MOREL SYNDROME, see Morel syndrome. (Sir James P. Stewart, 1869-1949, British neurologist; Bénédikt A. Morel, 1809-1873, French psychiatrist)

STEWART-TREVES SYNDROME, see Paget disease (def. 2). (Fred W. Stewart, U.S.; Norman Treves, U.S.)

STICKLER SYNDROME, hereditary arthro-ophthalmopathy; flat facies, mandibular hypoplasia, iris atrophy, deafness, dental anomalies, myopia, retinal detachment and/or cataracts, hypotonia, and hyperextensible joints are features. Autosomal dominant inheritance. Cross-references: Marshall-Stickler syndrome; Wagner-Stickler syndrome. (Gunnar B. Stickler, U.S. pediatrician)
1. Smith DW, Jones KL: Recognizable Patterns of Human Malformations: Genetic, Embryologic, and Clinical Aspects. 3rd ed. Philadelphia: WB Saunders, 1982
2. Stickler GB, Belau PG, Farrell FJ, et al: Hereditary progressive arthro-ophthalmopathy. Mayo Clin Proc 40:433-455, 1965

STICKY PLATELET SYNDROME, seen in a patient with ischemic cerebrovascular disease who has increased platelet aggregation. Symptoms identical to that seen in a stroke patient.
1. Walsh FB, Hoyt FF, Miller NR: Clinical Neuro-Ophthalmology. 4th ed. Baltimore: Williams & Wilkins, 1982

STIEDA SYNDROME, STIEDA-PELLEGRINI SYNDROME, see Pellegrini disease.

STIFF-MAN SYNDROME, see Isaacs syndrome.

STIFF SKIN SYNDROME, congenital fascial dystrophy; very firm skin and limitation of jointer motion are features. Histochemically, the dermis shows abnormal amounts of hyaluronidase-digestible acid mucopolysaccharide.
1. Esterly NB, McKusick VA: Stiff skin syndrome. Pediatrics 47:360-369, 1971
2. McKusick VA: Heritable Disorders of Connective Tissue. 4th ed. St Louis: CV Mosby, 1972

STILL DISEASE, chronic juvenile rheumatoid arthritis. (George Still, 1868-1941, British)
1. Campbell WC, Crenshaw AH: Campbell's Operative Orthopaedics. 7th ed. St Louis: CV Mosby, 1987

STILLER SIGN, the 10th rib becomes loose; seen in gastric ptosis.
1. Casas EC: Diccionario Terminologico de Ciencias Medicas. 5th ed. Salvat Editores, SA, 1954

STILLING-TÜRK-DUANE SYNDROME, see Duane syndrome.

STOCKER SIGN, in typhoid fever, an activity (such as changing the sheet) does not irritate the patient, whereas in tuberculous meningitis, the patient complains vehemently with the slightest motion.
1. Casas EC: Diccionario Terminologico de Ciencias Medicas. 5th ed. Salvat Editores, SA, 1954

STOFFEL OPERATION, resection of a portion of the nerve trunk fascicles innervating a spastic, paralyzed muscle. (Adolph Stoffel, 1880-1937, German orthopedic surgeon)
1. Maffei WE: Os Fundamentos da Medicina. 2nd ed. Livraria Editora Artes Médicas Ltda, 1978

STOKES SIGN, intense pain to the right of the umbilicus; seen in the patient with acute enteritis.
1. Casas EC: Diccionario Terminologico de Ciencias Medicas. 5th ed. Salvat Editores, SA, 1954

STOKES-ADAMS ATTACK, deafness which may be associated with various skin changes. Widely spaced medial canthi with confluent eyebrows, depigmentation of the skin with leopard-like spots, atopic dermatitis, and hyperkeratosis may be present. Can result in sudden death or with skeletal defects such as the congenital absence of one or both tibias. (William Stokes, 1804-1878, Irish; Robert Adams, 1791-1875, Irish)
1. Bennett JC, Plum F (eds): Cecil Textbook of Medicine. 20th ed. Philadelphia: WB Saunders, 1996
2. Farmer TW: Pediatric Neurology. 2nd ed. Hagerstown: Harper & Row, 1975

STOKES-ADAMS SYNDROME, see Adams-Stokes syndrome. (William Stokes; Robert Adams)

STOKVIS DISEASE, enterogenous cyanosis. (Barend J.E. Stokvis, 1834-1902, Dutch)
1. Stokvis BJ: Ned Tschr Geneesk 38:678-693, 1902

STOLTZ OPERATION, surgery for vaginal cystocele.
1. Maffei WE: Os Fundamentos da Medicina. 2nd ed. Livraria Editora Artes Médicas Ltda, 1978

STRACHAN SYNDROME, STRACHAN-SCOTT SYNDROME, amblyopia with central visual scotoma, oral ulceration, dermatitis of perioral or anal skin, and painful distal neuropathy are features. Originally described in women working in the Jamaican sugarcane fields. The corners of the mouth, prepuce, anus, and vulva were excoriated. (William H.W. Strachan, 1857-1921, British)
1. Baker AB, Baker LH: Clinical Neurology. Revised ed. Philadelphia: Harper & Row, 1982
2. Dyck PJ: Peripheral Neuropathy. 3rd ed. Philadelphia: WB Saunders, 1993
3. Strachan H: Practitioner 59:477-484, 1897

STRAIGHT BACK SYNDROME, flat chest syndrome; loss of the normal degree of kyphosis of the upper thoracic spine often associated with a decrease in the anteroposterior diameter of the chest and associated with some unusual features during clinical and radiological examination that may incorrectly suggest a cardiac etiology.
1. Fowler NO: Cardiac Diagnosis and Treatment. 3rd ed. Cambridge: Harper & Row, 1980
2. McKusick VA: Heritable Disorders of Connective Tissue. 4th ed. St Louis: CV Mosby, 1972
3. Rawlings MS: The "straight back" syndrome: a new cause of pseudoheart disease. Am J Cardiol 5:333-338, 1960

STRAIGHT LEG RAISING TEST, see Lasègue sign.

STRAUS SIGN, the injection of pilocarpine in central facial paralysis does not change the sweating pattern, whereas pilocarpine causes a difference in peripheral paralysis. (Isadore Straus, 1845-1896, French)
1. Casas EC: Diccionario Terminologico de Ciencias Medicas. 5th ed. Salvat Editores, SA, 1954

STRAUSS SIGN, an increase in fat following the ingestion of fatty foods; seen in the patient with lymph ascites. (Hermann Strauss, 1868-1944, German)
1. Casas EC: Diccionario Terminologico de Ciencias Medicas. 5th ed. Salvat Editores, SA, 1954

STREAKED OVARY SYNDROME, see Slotnick-Goldfarb syndrome.

STROKE SYNDROME, caused by acute vascular lesions of the brain, such as hemorrhage, embolism, thrombosis, or ruptured aneurysm, which may be marked by hemiplegia or hemiparesis, vertigo, numbness, aphasia, and dysarthria; often followed by permanent neurological damage.
1. Dorland's Medical Dictionary. 28th ed. Philadelphia: WB Saunders, 1994

STRØM-ZOLLINGER-ELLISON SYNDROME, see Zollinger-Ellison syndrome. (Roar Strøm, Norwegian)

STRÖMBECK OPERATION, reduction mammoplasty which uses a horizontal dermal and parenchymal pedicle to transport the nipple-areolar complex.
1. Schwartz SI: Principles of Surgery. 4th ed. New York: McGraw-Hill, 1983

STROMEYER-LITTLE OPERATION, drainage of a liver abscess using a cannula.
1. Maffei WE: Os Fundamentos da Medicina. 2nd ed. Livraria Editora Artes Médicas Ltda, 1978

STRÜMPELL SIGN, 1) the inability to close the fist without marked dorsal extension of the wrist. Cross-reference: Radialis sign; 2) passive flexion of the forearm caused by pronation; seen in the

patient with hemiplegia. Cross-reference: Pronation sign; 3) sharp voluntary flexion of the thigh on the abdomen and of the leg on the thighs followed by involuntary dorsiflexion and adduction of the paretic hip and knee, without dorsiflexion of the foot. Cross-references: Anterior tibial sign; Tibialis sign. (Ernst Adolf von Strümpell, 1853-1925, German)
1. Baker AB, Baker LH: Clinical Neurology. Revised ed. Philadelphia: Harper & Row, 1982
2. Pedro Pons A: Patologia y Clinica Medicus. Salvat Editores, SA, 1952

STRÜMPELL-LEICHTENSTERN DISEASE, acute primary hemorrhagic encephalitis. (Ernst Adolf von Strümpell; Otto Leichtenstern, 1845-1900, German)
1. Bodechtel G: Diagnostico Diferential de las Enfermedades Neurologicas. Madrid: Pas Montalvo Editorial, 1967
2. Leichtenstern O: Dtsch Med Wochenschr 18:39-40, 1892
3. Von Strümpell A: Dtsch Arch Klin Med 47:53-74, 1890

STRÜMPELL-LORRAIN DISEASE, familial spastic paraplegia. (Ernst Adolf von Strümpell)
1. Bordas LB (ed): Neurologia Fundamental. 2nd ed. Toray, 1968
2. Lorrain M: Contribution a la l'Etude Paraplégie Spasmodique Familiale. Paris: Steinheil, 1898 (Thesis)
3. Von Strümpell A: Arch Psychiatr 10:676-717, 1880

STRÜMPELL-MARIE DISEASE, see Marie-Strümpell spondylitis.

STRUNSKY SIGN, forceful flexion of the fingers causing pain in the patient with inflammation. (Max Strunsky, 1873-1957, U.S. orthopedic surgeon)
1. Evans RC: Illustrated Essentials in Orthopedic Physical Assessment. St Louis: Mosby Yearbook, 1994

STUHMER DISEASE, balanitis causing obstruction of the urethra.
1. Casas EC: Diccionario Terminologico de Ciencias Medicas. 5th ed. Salvat Editores, SA, 1954

STURGE-KALISCHER-WEBER SYNDROME, STURGE-WEBER SYNDROME, neuro-oculocutaneous angiomatosis; a port wine nevus on the upper portion of the scalp and other anomalies including gyriform calcifications of the cerebral cortex and seizures. Cross-references: Dimitri disease; Encephalotrigeminal vascular syndrome; Jahnke syndrome; Kalischer disease; Klippel-Trenaunay-Weber syndrome; Lawford syndrome; Neurocutaneous syndrome; Sturge-Kalischer-Weber disease; Weber-Dimitri disease. (William A. Sturge, 1850-1919, British; Siegfried Kalischer, German; Frederick Parkes Weber, 1863-1962, British)
1. Dimitri V: Rev Assoc Med Argentina 36:1029, 1923
2. Kalischer S: Arch Psychiatr 34:171-180, 1901
3. Sturge WA: Trans Clin Soc Lond 12:162-167, 1879
4. Weber FP: J Neurol Psychopath 3:134-139, 1922

SUBCLAVIAN STEAL SYNDROME, if occlusion occurs in the proximal portion of one of the subclavian arteries, a cervical arterial collateral network develops and may cause retrograde flow of blood through the ipsilateral vertebral artery producing dizziness with exercise of the corresponding arm and nystagmus. The radial pulse on the affected side is usually diminished and there is a difference in blood pressure between the two arms. Described by Bosniak in 1964.
1. Baker AB, Baker LH: Clinical Neurology. Revised ed. Philadelphia: Harper & Row, 1982
2. Fowler NO: Cardiac Diagnosis and Treatment. 3rd ed. Cambridge: Harper & Row, 1980

SUDDEN INFANT DEATH SYNDROME, crib death; apneas occur during nonrapid eye movement sleep leading to cardiac arrest of child. Usually occurs between birth to first 6 months of life. Often unexplained.
1. Beckwith JB, Bergman AG: The sudden death syndrome of infancy. Hosp Pract 2:44-52, 1967
2. Krugman S, Katz SL: Infectious Diseases of Children. 7th ed. St Louis: CV Mosby, 1981
3. Ritchie AC: Boyd's Textbook of Pathology. 9th ed. Philadelphia: Lea & Febiger, 1990

SUDDEN UNEXPLAINED DEATH SYNDROME, night death; death of a person 2 years old or older of Southwest Asian origin for which no underlying cause can be found.
1. Parrish G, Downes D: JAMA 255:2893, 1986

SUDECK ATROPHY, posttraumatic osteoporosis. (Paul Sudeck, 1866-1938, German surgeon)
1. Lumley JS, Clain A: Hamilton Bailey's Demonstration of Physical Signs in Clinical Surgery. 18th ed. London: Butterworth-Heinemann, 1997
2. Sudeck P: Arch Klin Chir 62:147-156, 1900

SUKER SIGN, the patient cannot abduct the eye for a prolonged period; seen in exophthalmic goiter. (George F. Suker, U.S. ophthalmologist)
1. Casas EC: Diccionario Terminologico de Ciencias Medicas. 5th ed. Salvat Editores, SA, 1954

SULZBERGER PHENOMENON, SULZBERGER-CHASE PHENOMENON, absence of dermal contact hypersensitivity to sensitizing agents produced by prior oral feeding of the agent. Cross-reference: Chase phenomenon. (Marion B. Sulzberger, U.S. dermatologist)
1. Dorland's Medical Dictionary. 28th ed. Philadelphia: WB Saunders, 1994

SULZBERGER-GARBE SYNDROME, exudative discoid and lichenoid dermatitis. (Marion B. Sulzberger; William Garbe, Canadian dermatologist)
1. Sulzberger MB, Garbe W: Arch Dermatol Syph 36:247-278, 1937

SUMNER SIGN, induration and rigidity of the abdominal muscles in the iliac fossa; may be an indication of appendicitis, a ureteral stone, or torsion of the ovarian cyst. (F.W. Sumner, British surgeon)
1. Casas EC: Diccionario Terminologico de Ciencias Medicas. 5th ed. Salvat Editores, SA, 1954

SUPERIOR CEREBELLAR ARTERY SYNDROME, with involvement of the brachium conjunctivum and spinothalamic and trigeminothalamic tracts, results from occlusion of the branches of the cerebellar artery in the brain stem.
1. Baker AB, Baker LH: Clinical Neurology. Revised ed. Philadelphia: Harper & Row, 1982

SUPERIOR MESENTERIC ARTERY SYNDROME, compression of the third (or transverse) portion of the duodenum against the aorta by the superior mesenteric artery, resulting in complete or partial obstruction that may be chronic, intermittent, or acute. Symptoms range from mild to severe, including nausea and vomiting, pain, and extreme distention of the stomach and duodenum. Cross-reference: Wilkie syndrome.
1. Haymaker W: Bing's Local Diagnosis in Neurological Diseases. 15th ed. St Louis: CV Mosby, 1969

SUPERIOR RED NUCLEUS SYNDROME, due to involvement of the red nucleus, rubrothalamic tract, and inferior caudal thalamus; characterized by ipsilateral hemiasynergia and intention tremor without extraocular palsy or sensory deficit. The 3rd cranial nerve may also be affected, in which case oculomotor palsy occurs.
1. Haymaker W: Bing's Local Diagnosis in Neurological Diseases. 15th ed. St Louis, Mo: CV Mosby, 1969

SUPERIOR SULCUS TUMOR SYNDROME, see Pancoast syndrome.

SUPERIOR VENA CAVA SYNDROME, SUPERIOR/INFERIOR VENA CAVA SYNDROME, a partial or total obstruction of the superior vena cava or edema of the face, neck, or upper arms due to increased venous pressure related to compression of the superior vena cava. May be caused by primary bronchial tumors or metastatic mediastinal lymph nodes in lung cancer.
1. Dorland's Medical Dictionary. 28th ed. Philadelphia: WB Saunders, 1994

SUPRARUBRAL SYNDROME, results from occlusions of interpeduncular median arteries arborizing in the region of the rostral part of the red nucleus, the rubrothalamic pathway, and the prerectal area.
1. Baker AB, Baker LH: Clinical Neurology. Revised ed. Philadelphia: Harper & Row, 1982

SUPRASPINATUS SYNDROME, a term describing lesions that directly or indirectly affect the supraspinatus tendon.
1. Campbell WC: Crenshaw PC: Campbell's Operative Orthopaedics. 7th ed. St Louis: CV Mosby, 1987

SURINAM DISEASE, elephantiasis; described among Arabs.
1. Casas EC: Diccionario Terminologico de Ciencias Medicas. 5th ed. Salvat Editores, SA, 1954

SURMAY OPERATION, jejunostomy.
1. Maffei WE: Os Fundamentos da Medicina. 2nd ed. Livraria Editora Artes Médicas Ltda, 1978

SUTTON DISEASE, a severe form of recurrent ulcers on the oral mucosa, involving large ulcers that require months to heal and do so with scarring. (Richard L. Sutton, Jr., 1878-1952, U.S. dermatologist)
1. Ballenger JJ: Diseases of the Nose, Throat, Ear, Head and Neck. 12th ed. Philadelphia: Lea & Febiger, 1977
2. Sutton RL Jr: JAMA 117:175-176, 1941

SUTTON-GULL DISEASE, see Gull-Sutton disease.

SWEAT RETENTION SYNDROME, see Adie syndrome.

SWEATY SOCK SYNDROME, a deficiency of isovaleryl-CoA dehydrogenase. Seizures, lethargy, hepatosplenomegaly, and a peculiar "sweaty sock" body odor occur. Believed to be inherited as an autosomal recessive trait.
1. Farmer TW: Pediatric Neurology. 2nd ed. Hagerstown: Harper & Row, 1975

2. McKusick VA: Mendelian Inheritance in Man. Baltimore: Johns Hopkins University Press, 1983

SWEDIAUER DISEASE, see Schwediauer disease.

SWEET SYNDROME, neutrophilic dermatosis; a distinct entity characterized by one or more edematous, red, tender, or spontaneously painful plaques located predominantly on the upper body of middle-aged women. Has characteristic histopathological features and is usually accompanied by fever, peripheral leukocytosis, and a variety of constitutional symptoms. (Robert D. Sweet, British dermatologist)
  1. Sweet RD: Br J Dermatol 76:349-356, 1964

SWIFT DISEASE, SWIFT-FEER DISEASE, acrodynia. Cross-references: Feer disease; Selter disease. (Harry Swift, 1858-1937, Australian; Emil Feer-Sulzer, 1864-1955, Swiss pediatrician)
  1. Feer-Sulzer E: Erg Inn Med 23:100-122, 1923
  2. Selter P: Verh Ges Kinderheilkd 20:45-50, 1903
  3. Swift H: Lancet l:611, 1918

SWINGING FLASHLIGHT SIGN, see Marcus Gunn pupillary sign.

SWYER SYNDROME, testicular feminization; XY gonadal dysgenesis. Chromosomally competent forms of gonadal failure with XY karyotypes are infrequent but important because of the high risk of dysgenetic ridge tumor and the occasional diagnostic confusion with forms of androgen insensitivity syndromes.
  1. Gold JJ, Josimovich JB: Gynecologic Endocrinology. 3rd ed. New York: Plenum Medical, 1980
  2. Swyer GIM: Br Med J 2:709-712, 1955

SWYER-JAMES SYNDROME, SWYER-JAMES-MACLEOD SYNDROME, unilateral hyperlucent lung; a relatively rare disorder generally discovered radiographically. Cross-references: Hyperlucent lung syndrome; Macleod syndrome. (Paul R. Swyer, Canadian; G.C.W. James, U.S.; William M. MacLeod, 1911-1977, British)
  1. Ritchie AC: Boyd's Textbook of Pathology. 9th ed. Philadelphia: Lea & Febiger, 1990
  2. Swyer PR, James GCW: Thorax 8:133-136, 1953

SYDENHAM CHOREA, an acute chorea encountered primarily during childhood, with the greatest incidence between ages 5 and 15. Often associated with rheumatic fever. Cross-reference: Saint Vitus dance disease. (Thomas Sydenham, 1624-1689, British)
  1. Bennett JC, Plum F (eds): Cecil Textbook of Medicine. 20th ed. Philadelphia: WB Saunders, 1996
  2. Nausieda PA, et al: Sydenham chorea: an update. Neurology 39:331, 1980
  3. Sydenham T: Schedula Monitoria de Novae Febris Ingressu. London: Kettilby, 1686

SYLVEST DISEASE, see Bornholm disease. (Ejnar Sylvest, 1880-1931, Norwegian)

SYLVIAN SYNDROME, SYLVIAN AQUEDUCT SYNDROME, consists of combinations of ocular signs: impaired vertical gaze, vertical nystagmus, convergence nystagmus, convergence spasm, retraction nystagmus, extraocular palsy, and poor pupillary constriction to light in adjustments to close vision. Cross-reference: Koerber-Salus-Elschnig syndrome.
  1. Elschnig A: Med Klin 9:8-11, 1913
  2. Koerber H: Ophthalmol Klin 7:65-67, 1903
  3. Rowland LP (ed): Merritt's Textbook of Neurology. 9th ed. Baltimore: Williams & Wilkins, 1995
  4. Salus R: Arch Augenheilkd 68:61-76, 1911

SYMONDS-SHOW SYNDROME, see Rovsing syndrome.

SYMPHALANGISM-BRACHYDACTYLY SYNDROME, see Facio-audio-symphalangism syndrome.

SZABO SIGN, sensory changes in the skin below the lateral malleolus; seen in the patient with sciatic pain. (Dionys Szabo, 1856-1918, Hungarian)
  1. Casas EC: Diccionario Terminologico de Ciencias Medicas. 5th ed. Salvat Editores, SA, 1954

SZYMANOWSKY OPERATION, various methods for correction of hypospadia, urethral fistula, ectropion, and blepharoplasty.
  1. Maffei WE: Os Fundamentos da Medicina. 2nd ed. Livraria Editora Artes Médicas Ltda, 1978

TABYI SYNDROME, see Otopalatodigital syndrome.

TAENZER DISEASE, ulerythema ophryogenes. (Paul R. Taenzer, 1858-1919, German)
  1. Casas EC: Diccionario Terminologico de Ciencias Medicas. 5th ed. Salvat Editores, SA, 1954

TAGLIACOTIAN OPERATION, a method of rhinoplasty once used in Italy. (Gasparo Tagliacozzi, 1546-1599, Italian surgeon)
1. Maffei WE: Os Fundamentos da Medicina. 2nd ed. Livraria Editora Artes Médicas Ltda, 1978

TAIT OPERATION, see Lawson-Tait operation.

TAKAYASU DISEASE, see Aortic arch syndrome. (Mikito Takayasu, 1860-1938, Japanese ophthalmologist)

TAKEJONESCU DISEASE, aortitis believed to be caused by typhus.
1. Casas EC: Diccionario Terminologico de Ciencias Medicas. 5th ed. Salvat Editores, SA, 1954

TALMA DISEASE, acquired myotonia. (Sape Talma, 1847-1948, Dutch)
1. Talma S: Ned Tschr Geneesk 28:321-328, 1892

TALMA OPERATION, omentopexy.
1. Maffei WE: Os Fundamentos da Medicina. 2nd ed. Livraria Editora Artes Médicas Ltda, 1978

TANGIER DISEASE, a familial lipoprotein deficiency. The patient presents in childhood with an absence of high-density lipoprotein and extremely low levels of the apoproteins AI and AIL. (Named for an island in the Chesapeake Bay where the first cases were described.)
1. Bennett JC, Plum F (eds): Cecil Textbook of Medicine. 20th ed. Philadelphia: WB Saunders, 1996
2. Moschella SL, Hurley HJ: Dermatology. 2nd ed. Philadelphia: WB Saunders, 1985

TANSINI OPERATION, resection of a breast followed by mammoplasty.
1. Maffei WE: Os Fundamentos da Medicina. 2nd ed. Livraria Editora Artes Médicas Ltda, 1978

TANSINI SIGN, cancer of the pylorus causes abdominal depression; if there is bowel obstruction, the abdomen is distended.
1. Casas EC: Diccionario Terminologico de Ciencias Medicas. 5th ed. Salvat Editores, SA, 1954

TANYOL SIGN, the umbilicus is displaced upward by a swelling arising from the pelvis or downward by ascites. (Hasib Tanyol, U.S.)
1. Lumley JS, Clain A: Hamilton Bailey's Demonstration of Physical Signs in Clinical Surgery. 18th ed. London: Butterworth-Heinemann, 1997

TAPIA SYNDROME, unilateral paralysis of the muscles of the tongue and of the vocal cord and soft palate are the main features caused by extra-axial lesions at the base of the skull. (Antonio G. Tapia, 1875-1950, Spanish)
1. Gorlin RJ, Cohen MM Jr, Levin LS: Syndromes of the Head and Neck. 3rd ed. New York: Oxford University Press, 1990
2. Tapia AG: Arch Int Laryngol 22:780-785, 1906
3. Tapia AG: Siglo Med Madrid 52:211-213, 1905

TARNIER SIGN, the disappearance of the angle between the superior and inferior segments; an indication of imminent abortion. (Etienne S. Tarnier, 1828-1897, French obstetrician)
1. Casas EC: Diccionario Terminologico de Ciencias Medicas. 5th ed. Salvat Editores, SA, 1954

TARSAL TUNNEL SYNDROME, characterized by paresis or paralysis of the intrinsic muscles of the foot, numbness and paresthesia over the sole, and burning pain; features are similar to carpal tunnel syndrome and acroparesthesia. Cross-reference: Jogger foot syndrome.
1. Bennett JC, Plum F (eds): Cecil Textbook of Medicine. 20th ed. Philadelphia: WB Saunders, 1996
2. Keck C: The tarsal tunnel syndrome. J Bone Joint Surg (Am) 44:180-182, 1962
3. Riccciardi-Pollini PT, Moneta MR, et al: The tarsal tunnel syndrome: a report of eight cases. Foot Ankle 6:146-149, 1985

TARUI DISEASE, glycogen storage disease type VII; the disease is characterized by muscle phosphofructokinase deficiency. The patient experiences decreased exercise tolerance and fatigues easily during childhood. (Seiichiro Tarui, Japanese)
1. Baker AB, Baker LH: Clinical Neurology. Revised ed. Philadelphia: Harper & Row, 1982
2. Tarui S, Okuno G, Ikura Y, et al: Phosphofructokinase deficiency in skeletal muscle. A new type of glycogenesis. Biochem Biophys Res Commun 19:517-523, 1965

TAUSSIG OPERATION, see Blalock-Taussig operation.

TAUSSIG-BING MALFORMATION, in the Taussig-Bing heart, the ventricular septal defects bear a close relation to the pulmonary valve rather than to the aorta. (Helen B. Taussig, 1898-1986, U.S. pediatrician; Richard J. Bing, U.S.)
1. Braunwald E: Heart Disease: A Textbook of Cardiovascular Medicine. 4th ed. Philadelphia: WB Saunders, 1992

2. Taussig HB, Bing RJ: Am Heart J 37:551-559, 1949

TAY SIGN, a reddish spot in the retina; seen in the patient with Tay-Sachs disease. (Warren Tay, 1843-1927, British ophthamologist)

1. Casas EC: Diccionario Terminologico de Ciencias Medicas. 5th ed. Salvat Editores, SA, 1954

TAY-SACHS DISEASE, G_{M2} gangliosidosis type I or amaurotic familial idiocy; a form of cerebral poliodystrophy with onset during early infancy, with a highly consistent pattern of clinical evolution terminating in death between ages 2 and 3. Largely confined to children of Ashkenazi Jewish ancestry derived from Eastern Europe; only rarely has it appeared in Caucasians. Cross-reference: Sachs disease. (Warren Tay; Bernard Sachs, 1858-1944, U.S. neurologist)

1. Kase NG, Weingold AB: Principles and Practice of Clinical Gynecology. New York: John Wiley & Sons, 1983
2. Sachs B: J Nerv Ment Dis 19:603-607, 1892; 23:475-479, 1896; 30:1-13, 1903
3. Tay W: Trans Ophthalmol Soc 1:57, 1881

TAYLOR DISEASE, see Pick-Herxheimer disease. (Robert W. Taylor, 1842-1908, U.S. dermatologist)

TEGMENTAL SYNDROME, see Benedikt syndrome.

TELLAIS SIGN, pigmentation of the eyelid; seen in the patient with exophthalmic goiter.

1. Casas EC: Diccionario Terminologico de Ciencias Medicas. 5th ed. Salvat Editores, SA, 1954

TEMPORAL LOBE SYNDROME, lesions of the temporal lobes produce no elementary findings except for a right upper quadrant field defect in some cases. Lesions in the posterior part of the left superior temporal gyrus lead to Wernicke aphasia. Bilateral destruction of the medial temporal lobes on both sides leads to Korsakoff syndrome. Destruction of the left medial temporal region leads to memory loss, predominantly verbal. Unilateral right medial temporal lesions should theoretically lead to memory loss for nonverbal stimuli.

1. Bennett JC, Plum F (eds): Cecil Textbook of Medicine. 20th ed. Philadelphia: WB Saunders, 1996

TEMPOROMANDIBULAR JOINT SYNDROME temporomandibular neuralgia infrequently found in individuals who, by virtue of alterations of the bite, develop severe pain in the face. Cross-references: Costen syndrome; Mandibular pain dysfunction syndrome.

1. Costen JB: Ann Otol Rhinol Laryngol 43:1-15, 1934
2. Grinker RR, Sahs AL: Neurology. 6th ed. Springfield, Ill: Charles C Thomas, 1966

TEN HORN SIGN, stretching the right spermatic cord causes pain; an indication of appendicitis. (C. ten Horn, Dutch surgeon)

1. Casas EC: Diccionario Terminologico de Ciencias Medicas. 5th ed. Salvat Editores, SA, 1954

TENDON SHEATH SYNDROME, see Brown syndrome.

TERRILON OPERATION, excision of hydatic cysts through squeezing by elastic ligatures.

1. Maffei WE: Os Fundamentos da Medicina. 2nd ed. Livraria Editora Artes Médicas Ltda, 1978

TERRY SYNDROME, retrolental fibroplasia. (Theodore Terry, 1899-1946, U.S. ophthalmologist)

1. Terry TL: Am J Ophthalmol 25:203-204, 1942

TERSON SYNDROME, vitreous hemorrhage associated with subarachnoid hemorrhage. May occur in one or both eyes and be so severe as to obscure all fundus detail. (Albert Terson, 1867-1935, French ophthalmologist)

1. Castren GA: Pathogenesis and treatment of Terson's syndrome. Acta Ophthalmol 41:430-434, 1963
2. Terson A: Ann Oculist 147:410-417, 1912

TESTICULAR FEMINIZATION SYNDROME, an extreme form of male pseudohermaphroditism, with female external development, including secondary sex characteristics, but with the presence of testes and the absence of a uterus and fallopian tubes; due to end-organ resistance to the action of 5α-testosterone. The patient with this syndrome has elevations in serum gonadotropins but is a gonadal male. Cross-references: Congenital androgen insensitivity syndrome; Goldberg-Maxwell syndrome.

1. Gold JJ, Josimovich JB: Gynecologic Endocrinology. 3rd ed. New York: Plenum Medical, 1980

TESTIVIN SIGN, a urine test to check for infectious disease. (G. Testivin, French chemist)

1. Casas EC: Diccionario Terminologico de Ciencias Medicas. 5th ed. Salvat Editores, SA, 1954

TETHERED CORD SYNDROME, patient presents with neurological deficits involving the lower extremities and/or bladder; the condition improves following section of a thick, tight filum terminale discovered by magnetic resonance imaging and at laminectomy. May be associated with spina bifida occulta. Cross-reference: Filum terminale syndrome.

1. Garceau GJ: J Bone Joint Surg 35A:711, 1953

TETRAPLOIDY SYNDROME, relatively common in embryos lost spontaneously during the first trimester and rare in live-born infants. Living examples have exhibited severe mental retardation, low birth weight, and microcephaly.

1. Gorlin RJ, Cohen MM Jr, Levin LS: Syndromes of the Head and Neck. 3rd ed. New York: Oxford University Press, 1990
2. Lafer CZ, Neu RL: A liveborn infant with tetraploidy. Am J Med Genet 31:375-378, 1988

TETRASOMY (9p) SYNDROME, includes psychomotor retardation and (in 50% or more of the cases) hypotonia, microcephaly, hydrocephaly, wide sutures and fontanels, hypertelorism, enophthalmos, epicanthal folds, strabismus, a bulbous-beaked nose, low-set malformed pinnae, down-slanting mouth, retromicrognathia, and a short neck. Extremely rare.

1. Calvalcanti DP, et al: Tetrasomy 9p caused by idic(9)(pter-q13-pter). Am J Med Genet 27:497-503, 1987
2. Gorlin RJ, Cohen MM Jr, Levin LS: Syndromes of the Head and Neck. 3rd ed. New York: Oxford University Press, 1990

TEXTOR OPERATION, disarticulation of the knee using a curved and transverse incision.

1. Maffei WE: Os Fundamentos da Medicina. 2nd ed. Livraria Editora Artes Médicas Ltda, 1978

THALAMIC SYNDROME, see Déjerine-Roussy syndrome.

THANATOPHORIC DYSPLASIA, see Schneckenbecken dysplasia.

THANOS SYNDROME, see Proteus syndrome.

THEIMICH LIP SIGN, percussion of the orbicularis oris muscle produces pouting of the lips. (Martin Theimich, German pediatrician)

1. Casas EC: Diccionario Terminologico de Ciencias Medicas. 5th ed. Salvat Editores, SA, 1954

THEOBALD OPERATION, subconjunctival strabotomy.

1. Maffei WE: Os Fundamentos da Medicina. 2nd ed. Livraria Editora Artes Médicas Ltda, 1978

THERMIC SIGN, see Kashida sign.

THIBIERGE-WEISSENBACH DISEASE, cutaneous and muscular calcification apparently similar to scleroderma. (Georges Thibierge, 1856-1926, French; Raymond Weissenbach, 1885-1963, French)

1. Bodechtel G: Diagnostico Diferential de las Enfermedades Neurologicas. Madrid: Pas Montalvo Editorial, 1967

THIELE SYNDROME, tenderness and pain in the region of the lower portion of the sacrum and coccyx, or in contiguous soft tissues and muscles. (George H. Thiele, U.S. proctologist)

1. Dorland's Medical Dictionary. 28th ed. Philadelphia: WB Saunders, 1994

THIEMANN SYNDROME, acrodysplasia epiphysaria; a disease of adolescence with features of painful fusiform swelling of the proximal interphalangeal joints, most frequently the middle fingers. (H. Thiemann, German)

1. Thiemann H: Fortschr Roentgenol 14:79-87, 1909/1910

THOMAS OPERATION, colpotomy.

1. Maffei WE: Os Fundamentos da Medicina. 2nd ed. Livraria Editora Artes Médicas Ltda, 1978

THOMAS SIGN, a fixed flexion deformity of the hip joint can be masked by increased normal lordosis. Observing the patient lying down may be deceiving because the entire limb lies flat. Cross-reference: Hugh Owen Thomas sign. (Hugh Owen Thomas, 1834-1891, British orthopedic surgeon)

1. Casas EC: Diccionario Terminologico de Ciencias Medicas. 5th ed. Salvat Editores, SA, 1954

THOMAYER SIGN, in peritonitis, the mesentery contracts and deviates the bowels to the right, producing more tympanic sound on the right than the left.

1. Casas EC: Diccionario Terminologico de Ciencias Medicas. 5th ed. Salvat Editores, SA, 1954

THOMSEN DISEASE, myotonia congenita; a rare disorder present from early childhood and characterized by difficulty in relaxing skeletal muscle after forceful contraction. (Asmus J. Thomsen, 1815-1896, Danish)

1. Rowland LP (ed): Merritt's Textbook of Neurology. 9th ed. Baltimore: Williams & Wilkins, 1995.
2. Thomsen AJ: Arch Psychiatr 6:706-718, 1875-1876

THOMSON SIGN, see Pastia sign. (Frederick H. Thomson, 1867-1938, British)

THORACIC OUTLET SYNDROME, compression of nerves and vessels in the outlet of the thorax and the costoclavicular area or between the clavicle and the first rib. Paresthesias of the fingers were formerly frequently attributed to compression of the brachial plexus by a cervical rib or a tight anterior scalene muscle. Most such patients have either nerve root compression from a cervical disc or carpal tunnel syndrome. Cross-references: Cervical rib syndrome; Costoclavicular syndrome; Outlet syndrome; Scalenus anticus syndrome.
> 1. Campbell WC: Crenshaw PC: Campbell's Operative Orthopaedics. 7th ed. St Louis: CV Mosby. 1987
> 2. Rowland LP (ed): Merritt's Textbook of Neurology. 9th ed. Baltimore: Williams & Wilkins, 1995

THORNTON SIGN, deep pain in the paralumbar area; seen in cases of renal stones. (Knowsley Thornton, 1845-1904, British)
> 1. Casas EC: Diccionario Terminologico de Ciencias Medicas. 5th ed. Salvat Editores, SA, 1954

THROMBOCYTOPENIA SYNDROME, see Wiskott-Aldrich syndrome.

THROMBOCYTOPENIA-ABSENT RADIUS SYNDROME, see Radial aplasia-thrombocytopenia syndrome.

THROMBOEMBOLIC SYNDROME, the association between formation of thrombi in the deep veins of the leg and pulmonary embolism.
> 1. Dorland's Medical Dictionary. 28th ed. Philadelphia: WB Saunders, 1994

THURSTON HOLLAND SIGN, type II epiphyseal fractures have a metaphyseal spike attached to the separated epiphysis, with the separation extending through the epiphyseal plate.
> 1. Campbell WC, Crenshaw AH: Campbell's Operative Orthopedics. 7th ed. St Louis: CV Mosby, 1987

THURSTON SYNDROME, median cleft of the vermilion border of the upper lip and postaxial polydactyly of the hands and feet. All reports have been from India.
> 1. Gorlin RJ, Cohen MM Jr, Levin LS: Syndromes of the Head and Neck. 3rd ed. New York: Oxford University Press, 1990
> 2. Thurston EO: A case of median hare-lip associated with other malformations. Lancet 2:996-997, 1909

THYROHYPOPHYSIAL SYNDROME, see Sheehan syndrome.

TIBIALIS SIGN, see Strümpell sign, def. 3.

TIEGEL OPERATION, method for suturing a tracheal wound.
> 1. Maffei WE: Os Fundamentos da Medicina. 2nd ed. Livraria Editora Artes Médicas Ltda, 1978

TIETZE SYNDROME, a rare autosomal dominant disorder with a total absence of melanin in the skin and hair, complete deafness, and hypoplastic eyebrows in the presence of normal eye color. (Walter Tietze, U.S.)
> 1. Braunwald E: Heart Disease: A Textbook of Cardiovascular Medicine. 4th ed. Philadelphia: WB Saunders, 1992
> 2. Kayser HL: Tietze syndrome: a review of literature. Am J Med 21:982-989, 1956
> 3. Tietze W: Am J Hum Genet 15:259-264, 1963

TIGHT BUILDING SYNDROME, see Sick building syndrome.

TILLAUX DISEASE, thelitis. Cross-reference: Phocas disease. (Paul J. Tillaux, 1834-1904, French)
> 1. Casas EC: Diccionario Terminologico de Ciencias Medicas. 5th ed. Salvat Editores, SA, 1954

TILLAUX OPERATION, cholecystenterostomy.
> 1. Maffei WE: Os Fundamentos da Medicina. 2nd ed. Livraria Editora Artes Médicas Ltda, 1978

TILTED DISC SYNDROME, a spectrum of optic disc anomalies in which the disc is asymmetrically abnormal in shape and is associated with a variably abnormal vascular pattern.
> 1. Young SE, et al: Am J Ophthalmol 82:16-23, 1976

TIMME SYNDROME, insufficiency of multiple endocrine organs. (Walter Timme, 1874-1956, U.S.)
> 1. Timme W: Endocrinology 2:209-240, 1918

TINEL SIGN, distal tingling on percussion; tapping or pressing on a nerve evokes pain or paresthesias in the distal portion of the area innervated. The point at which that stimulus fails to have an effect is presumed to be the most distal point the growing axons have reached. Cross-reference: DTP sign. (Jules Tinel, 1879-1952, French neurologist)
> 1. Campbell WC, Crenshaw AH: Campbell's Operative Orthopedics. 7th ed. St Louis: CV Mosby, 1987
> 2. Grinker RR, Sahs AL: Neurology. 6th ed. Springfield: Charles C Thomas, 1966

TIRED HOUSEWIFE SYNDROME, a form of mild hypothyroidism characterized by mild lassitude, fatigue, mild anemia, constipation, apathy, slight cold intolerance, menstrual irregularities, inability to conceive, dry skin, some hair loss, and slight to moderate weight gain.

1. Dorland's Medical Dictionary. 28th ed. Philadelphia: WB Saunders, 1994

TOBEY-AYER TEST, a comparison of the rise in cerebrospinal fluid pressure with the alternating compression of one or both jugular veins; a test for occlusion of the lateral sinus. (George L. Tobey, 1881-1947, U.S. ear, nose, throat surgeon; James B. Ayer, U.S. neurologist)

1. Ballenger JJ: Diseases of the Nose, Throat, Ear, Head and Neck. 12th ed. Philadelphia: Lea & Febiger, 1977
2. Pedro-Pons A: Patologia-y-Clinica Medicus. Salvat Editores, SA, 1952

TODD PARALYSIS, transitory monoparesis or hemiparesis ranging from a few hours to one or two days, following an epileptic seizure. (Robert B. Todd, 1809-1860, British)

1. Baker AB, Baker LH: Clinical Neurology. Revised ed. Philadelphia: Harper & Row, 1982
2. Todd RB: Clinical Lectures on Paralysis, Certain Disease of the Brain. 2nd ed. London: Churchill, 1856

TODD SYNDROME, see Alice in Wonderland syndrome.

TOLOSA-HUNT SYNDROME, painful ophthalmoplegia with lesions of the orbit, orbital apex, superior orbital fissure, and cavernous sinus with an extensive array of pathological processes. Cross-reference: Rochon-Duvigneaud syndrome. (Eduardo Tolosa, Spanish neurosurgeon; William E. Hunt, U.S. neurosurgeon)

1. Gorlin RJ, Cohen MM Jr, Levin LS: Syndromes of the Head and Neck. 3rd ed. New York: Oxford University Press, 1990
2. Hunt WE, Meacher JN, Le Fever HE, et al: Painful ophthalmoplegia: its relation to indolent inflammation of the cavernous sinus. Neurology 11:56-62, 1961
3. Rochon-Duvigneaud A: Arch Ophthalmol 16:746-760, 1896
4. Tolosa E: J Neurol Neurosurg Psychiatry 17:300-302, 1954
5. Zachariades N, Vairaktaris E, Papavassiliou D, et al: Orbital apex syndrome. Int J Oral Maxillofac Surg 16:352-354, 1987

TOMA SIGN, while lying on the back, percussion of the right side is tympanic and the left side is dull; seen in the patient with ascites.

1. Casas EC: Diccionario Terminologico de Ciencias Medicas. 5th ed. Salvat Editores, SA, 1954

TOMMASELLI SYNDROME, fever and hematuria caused by quinine ingestion. (Salvatore Tommaselli, 1834-1906, Italian)

1. Casas EC: Diccionario Terminologico de Ciencias Medicas. 5th ed. Salvat Editores, SA, 1954

TOMMASI SIGN, alopecia near the gastrocnemius muscle; seen in the patient with gout.

1. Casas EC: Diccionario Terminologico de Ciencias Medicas. 5th ed. Salvat Editores, SA, 1954

TONGUE PHENOMENON, see Schultze sign.

TORNWALDT DISEASE, a chronic inflammation of the pharyngeal bursa. (Gustavas L. Tornwaldt, 1843-1910, German)

1. Ballenger JJ: Diseases of the Nose, Throat, Ear, Head and Neck. 12th ed. Philadelphia: Lea & Febiger, 1977

TORRE SYNDROME, TORRE-MUIR SYNDROME, see Muir-Torre syndrome.

TOURAINE-SOLENTE-GOLÉ SYNDROME, pachydermoperiostosis; characterized by coarsening of the facial features with thickening and furrowing of the face, forehead, and scalp, and clubbing of the digits with new periosteal bone formation. Autosomal dominant inheritance. Cross-references: Cutis verticis gyrata syndrome; Pachydermoperiostosis syndrome; Rosenthal-Kloepfer syndrome. (Albert Touraine, 1883-1961, French dermatologist; G. Solente, French; L. Golé, French)

1. Friedreich N: Hyperostoses des Gesamte Skeletts. Virchow Arch Pathol Anat 43:83-87, 1868
2. Hochmuth WP, et al: Touraine-Solente-Golé syndrome. Med Klin 70:146-150, 1975
3. Rosenthal JW, Kloepfer HW: An acromegaloid cutis verticis gyrata, corneal leukopa syndrome. A new medical entity. Arch Ophthalmol 68:722-726, 1962
4. Touraine A, Solente G, Golé L: Presse Med 42:1820-1824, 1935

TOURETTE SYNDROME, see Gilles de la Tourette syndrome.

TOURNAY SIGN, pupillary dilatation of the eye on extreme lateral gaze. Cross-reference: Gianelli sign. (Auguste Tournay, 1878-1969, French ophthalmologist)

1. Casas EC: Diccionario Terminologico de Ciencias Medicas. 5th ed. Salvat Editores, SA, 1954

TOWNES-BROCKS SYNDROME, a syndrome of sensorineural hearing loss, imperforate anus, "lop" ears, abnormal thumbs, pes planus, and anomalies of the metacarpal and metatarsal bones, and the digits. Autosomal dominant inheritance with complete penetrance and variable expressivity.

1. Gorlin RJ, Cohen MM Jr, Levin LS: Syndromes of the Head and Neck. 3rd ed. New York: Oxford University Press, 1990
2. Smith DW, Jones KL: Recognizable Patterns of Human Malformations: Genetic, Embryologic, and Clinical Aspects. 3rd ed. Philadelphia: WB Saunders, 1982

TOWNSEND OPERATION, arthrodesis of the astragalonavicular articulation with anterior tibial tendon transposition and widening of the Achilles tendon for the treatment of pes planus.

1. Maffei WE: Os Fundamentos da Medicina. 2nd ed. Livraria Editora Artes Médicas Ltda, 1978

TOXIC SHOCK SYNDROME, *Staphylococcus aureus* infection with multisystem organ involvement and in severe cases organ failure. Cross-reference: Staphylococcal toxic shock syndrome.

1. Hoeprich PD, Jordan MC: Infectious Diseases. 4th ed. Philadelphia: JB Lippincott, 1989
2. Krugman S, Katz SL: Infectious Diseases of Children. 7th ed. St Louis: CV Mosby, 1981

TRAM TRACK SIGN, extravasation of contrast medium into parallel veins which accompany the middle meningeal artery produces this sign characteristic of an epidural bleed.

1. Baker AB, Baker LH: Clinical Neurology. Revised ed. Philadelphia: Harper & Row, 1982

TRANSFUSION SYNDROME, see Placental transfusion syndrome.

TRANSLOCATION DOWN SYNDROME, Down syndrome in which the excess chromosomal material (the long arm of chromosome 21) is translocated to another acrocentric chromosome (in standard trisomy 21, there is an additional chromosome 21). A carrier of the translocation chromosome has 45 chromosomes including the translocation chromosome and may be at increased risk of having a child with Down syndrome.

1. Dorland's Medical Dictionary. 28th ed. Philadelphia: WB Saunders, 1994

TRAUBE SIGN, a double sound is audible in the femoral artery; found in the patient with aortic insufficiency. (Ludwig Traube, 1818-1876, German)

1. Casas EC: Diccionario Terminologico de Ciencias Medicas. 5th ed. Salvat Editores, SA, 1954

TRAUBE-HERVING WAVES SIGN, rhythmic waves of increased intracranial pressure extending over several respiratory cycles.

TREACHER COLLINS SYNDROME, TREACHER COLLINS-FRANCESCHETTI SYNDROME, mandibulofacial dysostosis. In addition to microtia, this combination of anomalies includes atresia of the external auditory canal, malformation of the malleus and incus, a short deformed mandible, downward-slanting eyes with notched lower lids, and involvement of the malar bone and maxilla. Occurrence is usually bilateral. Cross-reference: Franceschetti-Klein syndrome. (Edward Treacher Collins, 1862-1932, British neurologist)

1. Ballenger JJ: Diseases of the Nose, Throat, Ear, Head and Neck. 12th ed. Philadelphia: Lea & Febiger, 1977
2. Franceschetti A, Klein D: Acta Ophthalmol 27:143-224, 1949
3. Treacher Collins E: Case with symmetrical congenital notches in outer part of each lower lid, and defective development of molar bones. Trans Ophthalmol Soc UK 20:190-192, 1900

TRÉLAT SIGN, yellow spots near tuberculous ulcers in the mouth; an indication of miliary abscesses. (Ulysse Trélat, 1828-1890, French surgeon)

1. Casas EC: Diccionario Terminologico de Ciencias Medicas. 5th ed. Salvat Editores, SA, 1954

TRENCH FEVER, a self-limiting febrile disease transmitted by the body louse *Pediculus humanus corporis;* characterized by headache, fever, and severe pain in the bones, joints, and muscles. Fatalities are rare but the disease is characterized in most patients by a relapsing course. Cross-references: His-Werner disease; Ikwa disease; Moosa fever; Quintan fever; Salonica fever; Shin bone fever; Volhynia fever; Werner-His disease.

1. Bennett JC, Plum F (eds): Cecil Textbook of Medicine. 20th ed. Philadelphia: WB Saunders, 1996

TRENCH FOOT, immersion foot; characterized by painful swollen feet or hands due to prolonged exposure of the extremities to water. Manifestations of muscle necrosis, ulcerations, and gangrene may eventually result.

1. Bennett JC, Plum F (eds): Cecil Textbook of Medicine. 20th ed. Philadelphia: WB Saunders, 1996

TRENCH MOUTH, see Vincent angina.

TRENDELENBURG SIGN, the pelvis is displaced to the side opposite dislocation; seen in the patient with paralysis of the gluteus maximus muscle. (Friedrich Trendelenburg, 1844-1924, German surgeon)

1. Bodechtel G: Diagnostico Diferential de las Enfermedades Neurologicas. Madrid: Pas Montalvo Editorial, 1967
2. Lumley JS, Clain A: Hamilton Bailey's Demonstration of Physical Signs in Clinical Surgery. 18th ed. London:

Butterworth-Heinemann, 1997

TREPIDATION SIGN, patellar clonus.

1. Dorland's Medical Dictionary. 28th ed. Philadelphia: WB Saunders, 1994

TRESILIAN SIGN, a reddish appearance at the opening of the Stensen duct; seen in the patient with mumps. (Frederick J. Tresilian, 1862-1926, British)

1. Dorland's Medical Dictionary. 28th ed. Philadelphia: WB Saunders, 1994

TREVES OPERATION, opening of a Pott disease abscess through the lumbar region followed by curettage of the bone and abscess sac.

1. Maffei WE: Os Fundamentos da Medicina. 2nd ed. Livraria Editora Artes Médicas Ltda, 1978

TRICHODENTO-OSSEOUS SYNDROME, amelogenesis imperfecta, taurodontism, curly and kinky hair, square jaw and brittle nails, and, at times, sclerotic bones are features.

1. Crawford JL: Concomitant taurodontism and amelogenesis imperfecta in the American Caucasian. J Dent Child 37:171-175, 1970
2. Lichtenstein J, Warson R, Jorgenson R, et al: The tricho-dento-osseous (T.D.O.) syndrome. Am J Hum Genet 24:569-582, 1972
3. Shapiro SD, Quattromani FL, Jorgenson RJ, et al: Tricho-dento-osseous syndrome: heterogeneity or clinical variability. Am J Med Genet 16:225-226, 1983

TRICHO-ONYCHO-DENTAL SYNDROME, characteristics include curly hair that is relatively sparse and easily detachable, decreased facial, axillary, and pubic hair, hard and thin enamel, and dysplastic dentin that fills the pulp. A tendency toward precocious eruption of teeth, taurodontism, and short open roots, but no tendency for permanent teeth to be impacted.

1. Fuks AB, Levin S, Grinbaum M, et al: Multiple taurodontism associated with osteoporosis. J Pedodont 7(1):68-74, 1982
2. Gorlin RJ, Cohen MM Jr, Levin LS: Syndromes of the Head and Neck. 3rd ed. New York: Oxford University Press, 1990

TRICHORHINOPHALANGEAL SYNDROME, see Langer-Giedion syndrome.

TRIMBLE SIGN, pigment lesions around the mouth; an indication of secondary syphilis.

1. Casas EC: Diccionario Terminologico de Ciencias Medicas. 5th ed. Salvat Editores, SA, 1954

TRIPIER SIGN, vibration of the thoracic wall by flicking; seen in the patient with abundant pleural effusion.

1. Casas EC: Diccionario Terminologico de Ciencias Medicas. 5th ed. Salvat Editores, SA, 1954

TRIPLOIDY SYNDROME, the presence of 69 chromosomes or three full sets in humans; growth deficiency, syndactyly of 3rd and 4th fingers, and congenital heart defects and brain anomalies are characteristics.

1 Niebuhr E: Triploidy in man. Hum Genet 21:103-125, 1974
2. Smith DW, Jones KL: Recognizable Patterns of Human Malformations: Genetic, Embryologic, and Clinical Aspects. 3rd ed. Philadelphia: WB Saunders, 1982

TRIPOD SIGN, with the patient's legs dangling over the edge of the examining table, full knee extension is tested. The sign is present if the patient extends the trunk and leans back on the upper extremities when the knees are bilaterally extended. Indicates tightness of the hamstring muscles.

1. Mazion JM: Illustrated Manual of Orthopedic Signs/Tests/Maneuvers for Office Procedure. 2nd ed. Orlando: Daniels Publishing, 1980

TRISMUS-PSEUDOCAMPYLODACTYLY SYNDROME, limited ability to open the mouth and curvature of the fingers at all interphalangeal joints on dorsiflexion of the wrists, due to shortened flexor muscle-tendon units. Cross-reference: Hecht syndrome.

1. Beals R, Hecht F: J Bone Joint Surg 53A:987-993, 1971
2. Mabry CC, Barnett IS, Hutcheson MH, et al: Trismus camptomelic syndrome. Dutch-Kentucky syndrome. J Pediatr 85:503-508, 1974
3. Robertson RD, et al: Linkage analysis with the trismus-pseudocamptodactyly syndrome. Am J Med Genet 12: 115-120, 1982

TRISOMY 4p SYNDROME, characteristic facies, severe mental deficiency with or without seizures, and growth deficiency are features.

1. Crane J, Sujanski W, Smith A: 4q Trisomy syndrome: report of 4 additional cases and segregation analysis of 21 families with different translocation. Am J Med Genet 4:219, 1979
2. Smith DW, Jones KL: Recognizable Patterns of Human Malformations: Genetic, Embryologic, and Clinical Aspects.

3rd ed. Philadelphia: WB Saunders, 1982

TRISOMY 8 SYNDROME, characteristic features are thick lips, deep set eyes, prominent ears, and camptodactyly.
1. Smith DW, Jones KL: Recognizable Patterns of Human Malformations: Genetic, Embryologic, and Clinical Aspects. 3rd ed. Philadelphia: WB Saunders, 1982

TRISOMY 9 MOSAIC SYNDROME, joint contractures, congenital heart defects, and low-set malformed ears are features.
1. Okatsuka A, et al: Trisomy 9 mosaicism with punctate mineralization in developing cartilages. Eur J Pediatr 131:271, 1979
2. Smith DW, Jones KL: Recognizable Patterns of Human Malformations: Genetic, Embryologic, and Clinical Aspects. 3rd ed. Philadelphia: WB Saunders, 1982

TRISOMY 9 SYNDROME, psychomotor retardation is present in all patients; the majority have low birth weight and/or failure to thrive and neurological impairment. Most die before 4 months of age. Not appreciably different in phenotype from the trisomy 9 mosaic syndrome.
1. Gorlin RJ, Cohen MM Jr, Levin LS: Syndromes of the Head and Neck. 3rd ed. New York: Oxford University Press, 1990
2. Levy I, et al: Gastrointestinal abnormalities in the syndrome of mosaic trisomy 9. J Med Genet 26:280-281, 1989

TRISOMY 13 SYNDROME, defects of the eyes, nose, lip, and forebrain of the holoprosencephaly type; polydactyly, narrow hyperconvex fingernails, and skin defects of the posterior scalp are features. Cross-references: Patau syndrome; Trisomy D syndrome.
1. Patau K, Smith DW, Therman E: Lancet 1:1980-1983, 1960
2. Smith DW, Jones KL: Recognizable Patterns of Human Malformations: Genetic, Embryologic, and Clinical Aspects. 3rd ed. Philadelphia: WB Saunders, 1982
3. Warburg M, Mikkelsen M: A case of 13-15 trisomy or Bartholin-Patau syndrome. Acta Ophthalmol 41:321, 1963

TRISOMY 14 SYNDROME, features include frequent polyhydramnios and severely retarded postnatal growth and psychomotor development. Characteristic facies, body and facial asymmetry, and congenital heart anomaly are also found. Has been reported in spontaneously aborted fetuses; most living examples are mosaic.
1. Gorlin RJ, Cohen MM Jr, Levin LS: Syndromes of the Head and Neck. 3rd ed. New York: Oxford University Press, 1990

TRISOMY 18 SYNDROME, characteristics include clenched hand, short sternum, and low-arched dermal ridge patterning on fingertips. Cross-references: Edwards syndrome; Trisomy E syndrome.
1. Smith DW, Jones KL: Recognizable Patterns of Human Malformations: Genetic, Embryologic, and Clinical Aspects. 3rd ed. Philadelphia: WB Saunders, 1982
2. Turleau C, de Grouchy J: Trisomy 18 qter and trisomy mapping of chromosome 18. Clin Genet 12:361, 1977

TRISOMY 20 SYNDROME, blepharophimosis, large and poorly formed ears, and cubitus valgus are features.
1. Schinzel A: Trisomy 20pter-q11 in a malformed boy from a t(13;20) (p11;q11) translocation carrier mother. Hum Genet 53(2):169, 1980
2. Smith DW, Jones KL: Recognizable Patterns of Human Malformations: Genetic, Embryologic, and Clinical Aspects. 3rd ed. Philadelphia: WB Saunders, 1982

TRISOMY 21 SYNDROME, see Down syndrome.

TRISOMY 22 SYNDROME, a degree of somatic and mental retardation, normal birth weight, and a microcephalic head; the facies is not extremely dysmorphic, with a flat nasal tip due to a short septum as well as craniofacial asymmetry.
1. Gorlin RJ, Cohen MM Jr, Levin LS: Syndromes of the Head and Neck. 3rd ed. New York: Oxford University Press, 1990
2. Lin AE, et al: Congenital heart disease in supernumerary der(22), t(11;22) syndrome. Clin Genet 29:269-275, 1986

TRISOMY C SYNDROME, trisomy for any chromosome of group C, most frequently number 8.
1. Pfeiffer RA: Trisomy 8, in Yunis JJ (ed): New Chromosomal Syndromes. New York: Academic Press, 1977, p 219

TRISOMY D SYNDROME, see Trisomy 13 syndrome.

TRISOMY E SYNDROME, see Trisomy 18 syndrome.

TROELL-JUNET SYNDROME, acromegaly, diabetes mellitus, and hyperostosis of the skull; occurs in females. (Nils A. Troell, 1881-1914, Swedish)
1. Junet R: Helvet Med Acta 22:167-183, 1955

2. Moore S: Troell-Junet syndrome. Acta Radiol 39:485-493, 1953
3. Troell A: Sven Lak Tidn 35:763-811, 1938

TROISIER SIGN, enlargement of left supraclavicular lymph nodes due to carcinoma of the stomach or lung. Some lymph nodes receive lymph from the thoracic duct. If a carcinoma is present, tumor emboli are released into the thoracic duct and can lodge in a supraclavicular lymph node, causing early metastasis which may be the first evidence of abdominal tumor. (Charles E. Troisier, 1844-1919, French pathologist)

1. Ritchie AC: Boyd's Textbook of Pathology. 9th ed. Philadelphia: Lea & Febiger, 1990

TROISIER SYNDROME, TROISIER-HANOT-CHAUFFARD SYNDROME, see Hanot-Chauffard syndrome. (Charles E. Troisier)

TRÖMNER SIGN, with the thumb and index finger of one hand, the examiner holds the patient's hand by grasping either the proximal or the middle phalanx of the partly flexed middle finger. With the middle finger of the other hand, the examiner taps the volar surface of the distal phalanx of the middle finger (see Hoffmann sign). (Ernest L.O. Trömner, 1868-1949, German neurologist)

1. Baker AB, Baker LH: Clinical Neurology. Revised ed. Philadelphia: Harper & Row, 1982

TROPICAL SPLENOMEGALY SYNDROME, in malaria-endemic areas, many children have slight or moderate enlargement of the spleen, but this regresses as malarial immunity is acquired. However, in such areas adult patients are sometimes encountered who have massive enlargement of the spleen for which no infective or neoplastic cause can be found. Common in some parts of New Guinea. Cross-reference: Malarial hyperreactive spleen syndrome.

1. Bennett JC, Plum F (eds): Cecil Textbook of Medicine. 20th ed. Philadelphia: WB Saunders, 1996
2. Musgrave WE, et al: Bull Johns Hopkins Hosp 17:28, 1906

TROTTER SYNDROME, usual characteristics include metastasis involving neoplastic growth with invasion directly from a palatal or maxillary sinus tumor, and the presence of deafness. (Wilfred Trotter, 1872-1939, British)

1. Ballenger JJ: Diseases of the Nose, Throat, Ear, Head and Neck. 12th ed. Philadelphia: Lea & Febiger, 1977
2. Gorlin RJ, Cohen MM Jr, Levin LS: Syndromes of the Head and Neck. 3rd ed. New York: Oxford University Press, 1990
3. Trotter W: Br Med J 2:1057-1059, 1911

TROUSSEAU SIGN, carpal spasm is induced by tightening a blood pressure cuff around the arm. Inflation of the cuff should be maintained for 4 minutes before concluding that the test is negative; an indication of latent tetany. (Armand Trousseau, 1801-1867, French)

1. Baker AB, Baker LH: Clinical Neurology. Revised ed. Philadelphia: Harper & Row, 1982
2. Grinker RR, Sahs AL: Neurology. 6th ed. Springfield: Charles C Thomas, 1966

TROUSSEAU SYNDROME, spontaneous venous thrombosis of the upper and/or lower extremities in association with visceral carcinoma. (Armand Trousseau)

1. Durham RH: Arch Intern Med 96:380-386, 1955

TROYER SYNDROME, a recessive form of infantile spastic paraplegia associated with dysarthria and distal wasting.

1. Cross HE, McKusick VA: Mental retardation and neurologic disorders in a genetic isolate, in Barbeau, Brunette JR (eds): Progress in Neuro-Genetics. Amsterdam: Excerpta Medica International Congress Series No. 175, 1969, p 759
2. Farmer TW: Pediatric Neurology. 2nd ed. Hagerstown: Harper & Row, 1975

TSUTSUGAMUSHI DISEASE, an acute febrile typhus-like disease of rural Asia, transmitted by the bite of larval trombiculid mites (chiggers) and caused by *Rickettsia tsutsugamushi*. The site of infection is often marked by an eschar accompanied by regional lymphadenitis. Cross-references: Barme-Birmania-Burma disease; Japanese disease; Kedani disease; Megaw disease; Shimamushi disease.

1. Baker AB, Baker LH: Clinical Neurology. Revised ed. Philadelphia: Harper & Row, 1982
2. Bennett JC, Plum F (eds): Cecil Textbook of Medicine. 20th ed. Philadelphia: WB Saunders, 1996

TUBEROUS SCLEROSIS SYNDROME, see Bourneville disease.

TUFFIER OPERATION, apicolysis.

1. Maffei WE: Os Fundamentos da Medicina. 2nd ed. Livraria Editora Artes Médicas Ltda, 1978

TUMOR LYSIS SYNDROME, a constellation of metabolic abnormalities consisting of severe hyperphosphatemia, hyperkalemia, hyperuricemia, and hypocalcemia occurring after effective induction of chemotherapy in cases of rapidly growing malignant neoplasms; thought to be due to release of intracellular products after cell lysis.

1. Bennett JC, Plum F (eds): Cecil Textbook of Medicine. 20th ed. Philadelphia: WB Saunders, 1996

TUOMAALA-HAAPANEN SYNDROME, a familial syndrome with characteristics of brachymeta-pody, anodontia, hypotrichosis, and albinism. (Paavo Tuomaala, Finnish ophthalmologist)
1. Gorlin RJ, Cohen MM Jr, Levin LS: Syndromes of the Head and Neck. 3rd ed. New York: Oxford University Press, 1990
2. Tuomaala P, Haapanen E: Three siblings with similar anomalies in the eyes, bones, and skin. Acta Ophthalmol 46:365-371, 1968

TÜRCK DISEASE, secondary parenchymatous degeneration of the spinal cord. (Ludwig Türck, 1810-1868, Austrian neurologist)
1. Casas EC: Diccionario Terminologico de Ciencias Medicas. 5th ed. Salvat Editores, SA, 1954

TURCOT SYNDROME, TURCOT-DESPRÉS-ST. PIERRE SYNDROME, represents the rare association of adenomas of the colon with a variety of tumors of the central nervous system. The polyps have a high frequency of malignant transformation. Cross-reference: Glioma-polyposis syndrome. (Jacques Turcot, Canadian surgeon)
1. Bennett JC, Plum F (eds): Cecil Textbook of Medicine. 20th ed. Philadelphia: WB Saunders, 1996
2. Turcot J, Després MP, St. Pierre F: Malignant tumors of central nervous system associated with familial polyposis of colon: report of two cases. Dis Colon Rectum 2:465-468, 1959

TURGENSEN SIGN, crepitus; seen in the patient with tuberculous pleurisy.
1. Casas EC: Diccionario Terminologico de Ciencias Medicas. 5th ed. Salvat Editores, SA, 1954

TURNER SIGN, see Grey Turner sign. (George Grey Turner, 1877-1951, British surgeon)

TURNER SYNDROME, gonadal dysgenesis; a syndrome of sexual infantilism, short stature, muscu-loskeletal abnormalities, and streak gonads associated with abnormalities of sex chromosome number or morphology. Affected patients have just 45 chromosomes, the loss of one X chromosome producing an XO chromosome. The phenotype is female. Cross-references: Morgagni-Turner-Albright syndrome; Seresewski-Turner syndrome; XO syndrome. (Henry H. Turner, 1892-1970, U.S. endocrinologist)
1. Farmer TW: Pediatric Neurology. 2nd ed. Hagerstown: Harper & Row, 1975
2. Hurst JW, Schlant RC, Alexander RW: The Heart: Arteries and Veins. 8th ed. New York: McGraw-Hill, 1994
3. Turner HH: Endocrinology 23:566-574, 1938

TURYN SIGN, dorsiflexion of the big toe causing pain in the gluteal region; seen in the patient with sciatica. (Felix Turyn, Polish)
1. Casas EC: Diccionario Terminologico de Ciencias Medicas. 5th ed. Salvat Editores, SA, 1954

TWIN-TO-TWIN TRANSFUSION SYNDROME, unbalanced placental circulation in twin preg-nancy; develops in 20% of monochorionic twin pregnancies. If the syndrome is severe, one twin is small, pale, and anemic, while the other is heavier, edematous, and polycythemic.
1. Ritchie AC: Boyd's Textbook of Pathology. 9th ed. Philadelphia: Lea & Febiger, 1990

TWORT-D'HERELLE PHENOMENON, bacteriophagia; the phenomenon of transmissible bacte-rial lysis. Cross-reference: D'Herelle phenomenon. (Frederick W. Twort, 1877-1950, British bacteri-ologist; Feliz H. D'Herelle, 1873-1949, French bacteriologist)
1. Dorland's Medical Dictionary. 28th ed. Philadelphia: WB Saunders, 1994

TYNDALL PHENOMENON, a transverse beam of light is rendered visible via being broken up by solid particles suspended in a liquid or gas. (John Tyndall, 1820-1893, British physicist)
1. Dorland's Medical Dictionary. 28th ed. Philadelphia: WB Saunders, 1994

TYSON GLANDS, bilateral sebaceous glands that produce smegma, situated on either side of the frenum and communicating, not with the urethra, but with the preputial sac. (Edward Tyson, 1650-1708, British anatomist)
1. Bennett JC, Plum F (eds): Cecil Textbook of Medicine. 20th ed. Philadelphia: WB Saunders, 1996
2. Lumley JS, Clain A: Hamilton Bailey's Demonstration of Physical Signs in Clinical Surgery. 18th ed. London: Butterworth-Heinemann, 1997

UHTHOFF SIGN, transient visual impairment due to heat exposure or exertion; seen in the patient with multiple sclerosis. (Wilhelm Uhthoff, 1853-1927, German ophthalmologist)
1. Casas EC: Diccionario Terminologico de Ciencias Medicas. 5th ed. Salvat Editores, SA, 1954

ULLRICH SYNDROME, ULLRICH-TURNER SYNDROME, see Male Turner syndrome. (Otto Ullrich, 1894-1957, German pediatrician)

ULLRICH-FEICHTIGER SYNDROME, a condition of micrognathia, hexadactyly, and genital abnormalities, with a depressed nose, small eyes, hypertelorism, and protuberant ears, as well as other defects. (Otto Ullrich; H. Feichtiger, German)

1. Feichtiger H: Ein Neuer, Typischer, Vorwiegend der Akren Betreffender Fehlbindungskomples. Rostock, 1943 (Thesis)
2. Ullrich O: Ergebn Inn Med Kinderheilkd NF 2:412-420, 1951

ULNAR TUNNEL SYNDROME, results from compression of the ulnar nerve within a tight, triangular, fibro-osseous tunnel about 1.5 cm long; located at the carpus.
1. Campbell WC, Crenshaw AH: Campbell's Operative Orthopaedics. 7th ed. St Louis: CV Mosby, 1987
2. Lotem M, et al: Plast Reconstr Surg 52:553-556, 1973

UMBERT OPERATION, excision of the epididymis.
1. Maffei WE: Os Fundamentos da Medicina. 2nd ed. Livraria Editora Artes Médicas Ltda, 1978

UNDERWOOD DISEASE, sclerema neonatorum. (Michael Underwood, 1737-1820, British pediatrician)
1. Underwood M: A Treatise on the Diseases of Children. London: Mathews, 1784

UNILATERAL INTERNUCLEAR OPHTHALMOPLEGIA SYNDROME, see Bielschowsky-Lutz-Cogan syndrome.

UNILATERAL NEVOID TELANGIECTASIA SYNDROME, generalized essential telangiectasia activated from a dormant vascular nevus that becomes manifest under the possible influence of estrogens (pregnancy or menarche) or increased venous pressure (liver disease).
1. Dorland's Medical Dictionary. 28th ed. Philadelphia: WB Saunders, 1994

UNNA DISEASE, seborrheic eczema. (Paul G. Unna, 1850-1929, German dermatologist)
1. Unna PG: Monatsschr Prakt Dermatol 6:827-846,1887

UNSCHULD SIGN, gastrocnemius muscle cramps; an early indication of diabetes. (Paul Unschuld, 1835-1905, German internist)
1. Casas EC: Diccionario Terminologico de Ciencias Medicas. 5th ed. Salvat Editores, SA, 1954

UNVERRICHT DISEASE, UNVERRICHT-LUNDBORG PROGRESSIVE MYOCLONUS EPILEPSY (PME), see Lafora disease. (Heinrich Unverricht, 1853-1912, German; Herman Lundborg, 1868-1943, Swedish)

URBACH-WIETHE DISEASE, cutaneous-mucosal hyalinosis; a rare, hereditary metabolic disorder characterized by hyalin-like infiltrates in virtually every organ of the body. Thickened, beaded eyelids and a husky voice from birth permit easy recognition. (Erich Urbach, 1893-1946, dermatologist; Camillo Wiethe, 1888-1949, Austrian otologist)
1. Urbach E: Arch Dermatol Vener 159:451-466, 1929
2. Wiethe C: Z Hals Nas Ohrenheilkd 10:359-362, 1924

URETHRAL SYNDROME, an entity in which a patient suffers from urinary hesitance, frequency, urgency, dysuria, and, at times, suprapubic pain and back pain in the absence of objective urological findings. While usually termed the female urethral syndrome, there is no reason to believe that a similar condition does not occur in males or in children of either sex. Cross-reference: Female urethral syndrome.
1. Campbell MF, Walsh PC: Campbell's Urology. 5th ed. Philadelphia: WB Saunders, 1986

URIOLLA SIGN, hemolytic malaria; malaria with blackish urine. Cross-reference: Blackwater fever.
1. Casas EC: Diccionario Terminologico de Ciencias Medicas. 5th ed. Salvat Editores, SA, 1954

UROFACIAL SYNDROME, hydronephrosis, hydroureter, and unusual facies are features. Facial grimacing is evident only when crying or smiling. Cross-reference: Ochoa syndrome.
1. Gorlin RJ, Cohen MM Jr, Levin LS: Syndromes of the Head and Neck. 3rd ed. New York: Oxford University Press, 1990

USHER SYNDROME, a hereditary disorder characterized by sensorineural deafness and retinitis pigmentosa. (Charles H. Usher, 1865-1942, British ophthalmologist)
1. Usher CH: R Lund Ophth Hosp Rep 19:130-236, 1914

UTERINE HERNIA SYNDROME, hernial protrusion of the uterus.
1. Kase NG, Weingold AB: Principles and Practice of Clinical Gynecology. New York: John Wiley & Sons, 1983

UVEOMENINGITIS SYNDROME, see Harada syndrome.

VAGABOND DISEASE, VAGRANT DISEASE, see Greenhow disease.

VAGOACCESSORY SYNDROME, see Schmidt syndrome.

VALLAS OPERATION, osteotomy of the hyoid bone.
1. Maffei WE: Os Fundamentos da Medicina. 2nd ed. Livraria Editora Artes Médicas Ltda, 1978

VALSALVA MANUEVER, a test of the patency of eustachian tubes. The patient is asked to pinch the nose, close the mouth, and blow. The patient signals with the free hand when he/she feels "something give." If a tube is blocked, a point in favor of otitis media as it forms part of the middle ear cleft, the crackle on that side is absent. (Antonio M. Valsalva, 1666-1723, Italian anatomist)
1. Lumley JS, Clain A: Hamilton Bailey's Demonstration of Physical Signs in Clinical Surgery. 18th ed. London: Butterworth-Heinemann, 1997

VALSUANI DISEASE, pernicious anemia in puerperal women. (Emilio Valsuani, Italian)
1. Casas EC: Diccionario Terminologico de Ciencias Medicas. 5th ed. Salvat Editores, SA, 1954

VAN BOGAERT-BERTRAND SYNDROME, spongy degeneration of the white matter in infants, with encephalitis and myoclonic genus dementia. Etiology related to the measles virus. (Ludo van Bogaert, Belgian neuropathologist; Ivan G. Bertrand, French neuropathologist)
1. Van Bogaert L: J Neurol 8:1010-120, 1945

VAN BOGAERT-SCHERER-EPSTEIN SYNDROME, cerebrotendinous xanthomatosis; bilateral cataracts, a progressive and slow cerebellar syndrome, and mental retardation are features. (Ludo van Bogaert)
1. Nelson WE, Vaughan VC, McKay RJ: Tratado de Pediatria. 6th ed. Salvat Editores, SA, 1971
2. Van Bogaert L, Scherer HJ, Epstein E: Une Forme Cérébrale de Cholestérinose Généralisée. Paris: Masson, 1937

VAN BUCHEM DISEASE, see Sclerosteosis syndrome. (Francis S. van Buchem, 1898-1979, Dutch)

VAN DER HOEVE SYNDROME, see Osteogenesis imperfecta syndrome type I. (Jan van der Hoeve, 1878-1952, Dutch ophthalmologist)

VAN DER MUELEN OPERATION, a multistage urethroplasty repair; described in 1964 and 1982.
1. Campbell MF, Walsh PC: Campbell's Urology. 5th ed. Philadelphia: WB Saunders, 1986

VAN DER WOUDE SYNDROME, consists of cleft lip and/or cleft palate occurring in association with cysts of the lower lip and hypodontia. Autosomal dominance inheritance. (Anne Van der Woude, U.S.)
1. Smith DW, Jones KL: Recognizable Patterns of Human Malformations: Genetic, Embryologic, and Clinical Aspects. 3rd ed. Philadelphia: WB Saunders, 1982
2. Van der Woude A: Am J Hum Genet 6:244-256, 1954

VAN HOOK OPERATION, see Hook operation.

VAN LAERE SYNDROME, progressive sensory neural deafness with paralysis of other cranial nerves caused by cancer of the skull base. (J. Van Laere, Belgian)
1. Casas EC: Diccionario Terminologico de Ciencias Medicas. 5th ed. Salvat Editores, SA, 1954

VAN LINT OPERATION, an infiltrative block with local anesthesia for cataract removal. Can anesthetize the facial nerve branches to the orbicularis muscle as they run over the periosteum just lateral to the orbit.
1. Spaeth GL: Ophthalmic Surgery. Principles and Practice. Philadelphia: WB Saunders, 1982

VANISHING TESTIS SYNDROME, XY agonadism, rudimentary testis syndrome, and congenital anorchia are characteristics. Results from cessation of testicular function during the critical stages of male sexual differentiation (i.e., at 8-14 weeks of gestational age). Cross-reference: Embryonic testicular regression syndrome.
1. Abeyaratue MR, Aherne WA, Scott JES: The vanishing testis. Lancet 2:822-826, 1969

VANZETTI SIGN, a horizontal pelvis; seen in the patient with sciatic pain and scoliosis. (Tito Vanzetti, 1809-1888, Italian surgeon)
1. Casas EC: Diccionario Terminologico de Ciencias Medicas. 5th ed. Salvat Editores, SA, 1954

VAQUEZ DISEASE, VAQUEZ-OSLER DISEASE, see Osler disease.

VÁRADI SYNDROME, polydactyly, cleft lip/palate, lingual lump, and cerebellar anomalies are found. Cross-reference: Joubert-Boltshauser syndrome. (V. Váradi, Hungarian)
1. Gorlin RJ, Cohen MM Jr, Levin LS: Syndromes of the Head and Neck. 3rd ed. New York: Oxford University Press, 1990
2. Váradi V, Szabo L, Papp Z: Syndrome of polydactyly, cleft lip/palate or lingual lump, and psychomotor retardation in endogamic gypsies. J Med Genet 17:119-122, 1980

VARELA SIGN, alteration of the psoas muscle shadow on x-ray.
1. Casas EC: Diccionario Terminologico de Ciencias Medicas. 5th ed. Salvat Editores, SA, 1954

VARIOT DISEASE, microsphygmia.
1. Casas EC: Diccionario Terminologico de Ciencias Medicas. 5th ed. Salvat Editores, SA, 1954

VASQUEZ-HURST-SOTOS-SYNDROME, gynecomastia but not hypotonia.
1. Kase NG, Weingold AB: Principles and Practice of Clinical Gynecology. New York: John Wiley & Sons, 1983
2. Vasquez SB, Hurst DI, Sotos JF: Pediatrics 83:280-284, 1979

VEDDER SIGN, slight pressure on the calf muscles causing pain; seen in cases of beri-beri. (Edward B. Vedder, 1878-1952, U.S. surgeon)
1. Casas EC: Diccionario Terminologico de Ciencias Medicas. 5th ed. Salvat Editores, SA, 1954

VEIT OPERATION, embryotomy by evisceration and traction of the fetus.
1. Maffei WE: Os Fundamentos da Medicina. 2nd ed. Livraria Editora Artes Médicas Ltda, 1978

VELEZ SIGN, inversion of the leukocyte count in tuberculosis.
1. Casas EC: Diccionario Terminologico de Ciencias Medicas. 5th ed. Salvat Editores, SA, 1954

VELOCARDIOFACIAL SYNDROME, see Shprintzen syndrome.

VELPEAU OPERATION, resection of the maxilla through an incision from the angle of the mouth to the midpoint of the zygoma.
1. Maffei WE: Os Fundamentos da Medicina. 2nd ed. Livraria Editora Artes Médicas Ltda, 1978

VELPEAU SIGN, deformity of the distal end of the wrist; seen in the case of a distal radius fracture.
1. Casas EC: Diccionario Terminologico de Ciencias Medicas. 5th ed. Salvat Editores, SA, 1954

VENTRUTO SYNDROME, brachydactyly, aplastic or hypoplastic nails, symphalangism, carpal and tarsal fusion, dysplastic hip joints, and craniosynostosis are features.
1. Gorlin RJ, Cohen MM Jr, Levin LS: Syndromes of the Head and Neck. 3rd ed. New York: Oxford University Press, 1990
2. Ventruto V, Di Girolamo R, Festa B, et al: Family study of inherited syndrome with multiple congenital deformities: symphalangism, carpal and tarsal fusion, brachydactyly, craniosynostosis, strabismus, hip osteochondritis. J Med Genet 13:394-398, 1976

VERCO SIGN, hemorrhagic spots on the hands and feet; hemorrhagic striae and erythema nodosum are features.
1. Casas EC: Diccionario Terminologico de Ciencias Medicas. 5th ed. Salvat Editores, SA, 1954

VERGER-DÉJERINE SYNDROME, an alteration in localization sense, with abnormal behavior, lack of tactile discrimination, and astereognosis. Cross-reference: Riddoch syndrome. (H. Verger; Joseph J. Déjerine, 1849-1917, French neurologist)
1. Bordas LB (ed): Neurologia Fundamental. 2nd ed. Toray, 1968
2. Déjerine J, Mouzon J: Rev Neurol 28:1265, 1914/1915
3. Verger H: Rev Neurol 2:1201-1205, 1902

VERHOEFF OPERATION, posterior sclerotomy followed by multiple electrolytic punctures in cases of retinal detachment. (Frederick Verhoeff, 1874-1968, U.S. ophthalmologist)
1. Maffei WE: Os Fundamentos da Medicina. 2nd ed. Livraria Editora Artes Médicas Ltda, 1978

VERMEL SIGN, visible pulsation of the temporal artery and hypertension with ipsilateral headache.
1. Casas EC: Diccionario Terminologico de Ciencias Medicas. 5th ed. Salvat Editores, SA, 1954

VERMOOTEN SIGN, in males, the diagnosis of a complete intrapelvic rupture of the urethra is certain if, on introducing the finger into the rectum, the prostate cannot be felt but in its position there is an indefinite doughy swelling (blood and urine), or if the prostate is felt but is displaced upward. This sign is not present consistently; its absence does not rule out urethral rupture. (Vincent Vermooten, 1897-1969, U.S. urologist)
1. Lumley JS, Clain A: Hamilton Bailey's Demonstration of Physical Signs in Clinical Surgery. 18th ed. London: Butterworth-Heinemann, 1997

VERNER-MORRISON SYNDROME, watery diarrhea, hypokalemia, and death due to renal failure associated with islet cell tumor are characteristics. Cross-references: Diarrheogenic syndrome; Pancreatic cholera syndrome; WDHA syndrome. (John V. Verner, U.S.; Ashton B. Morrison, U.S.)
1. Verner JV, Morrison AB: Am J Med 25:374-380, 1958
2. Wilson JD, Foster DW, Kronenberg HM, et al (eds): Williams Textbook of Endocrinology. 9th ed. Philadelphia: WB Saunders, 1998

VERNET SYNDROME, see Jugular foramen syndrome. (Maurice Vernet, French neurologist)

VERNEUIL DISEASE, syphilitic bursopathy. (Aristide Verneuil, 1823-1895, French surgeon)
   1. Casas EC: Diccionario Terminologico de Ciencias Medicas. 5th ed. Salvat Editores, SA, 1954

VERNEUIL OPERATION, iliac colotomy through a vertical incision, suturing the intestine to the edges of the wound.
   1. Maffei WE: Os Fundamentos da Medicina. 2nd ed. Livraria Editora Artes Médicas Ltda, 1978

VERSE DISEASE, intervertebral calcinosis.
   1. Casas EC: Diccionario Terminologico de Ciencias Medicas. 5th ed. Salvat Editores, SA, 1954

VERTICAL RETRACTION SYNDROME, the main clinical features include limitation of movement of the affected eye on elevation or depression associated with a retraction of the globe and narrowing of the palpebral fissure.
   1. Walsh FB, Hoyt EF, Miller NR: Clinical Neuro-Ophthalmology. 4th ed. Baltimore: Williams & Wilkins, 1982

VERVET MONKEY DISEASE, see Marburg virus disease.

VIALETTO-VAN LAERE SYNDROME, presents during the 2nd decade with facial weakness, dysphagia, and dysarthria, often preceded by bilateral deafness of the sensorineural type. Affects the lower six cranial nerves.
   1. Dyck PJ: Peripheral Neuropathy. 3rd ed. Philadelphia: WB Saunders, 1993

VICQ D'AZYR OPERATION, cricothyrotomy. (Felix Vicq d'Azyr, 1748-1794, French anatomist)
   1. Maffei WE: Os Fundamentos da Medicina. 2nd ed. Livraria Editora Artes Médicas Ltda, 1978

VIDAL DISEASE, neurodermatitis. (Jean B.E. Vidal, 1825-1893, French dermatologist)
   1. Casas EC: Diccionario Terminologico de Ciencias Medicas. 5th ed. Salvat Editores, SA, 1954

VIDAL OPERATION, subcutaneous venous ligation in cases of varicocele.
   1. Maffei WE: Os Fundamentos da Medicina. 2nd ed. Livraria Editora Artes Médicas Ltda, 1978

VIEUSSENS DISEASE, aortic insufficiency. (Raymond de Vieussens, 1641-1715, French anatomist)
   1. Casas EC: Diccionario Terminologico de Ciencias Medicas. 5th ed. Salvat Editores, SA, 1954

VIGOUROUX SIGN, the electrical resistance of the skin is lowered in exophthalmic goiter. Cross-reference: Charcot-Vigouroux sign.
   1. Pedro-Pons A: Patologia-y-Clinica Medicus. Salvat Editores, SA, 1952

VILLARET SIGN, in lesions of the sciatic nerve, checking the ankle reflex produces flexion of the hallux.
   1. Casas EC: Diccionario Terminologico de Ciencias Medicas. 5th ed. Salvat Editores, SA, 1954

VILLARET SYNDROME, a condition caused by trauma, neoplasm, or infection resulting in ipsilateral paralysis of the last four cranial nerves plus involvement of the cervical sympathetic chain, precipitating Horner syndrome. Cross-reference: Retroparotid space syndrome. (Maurice Villaret, 1877-1946, French neurologist)
   1. Gorlin RJ, Cohen MM Jr, Levin LS: Syndromes of the Head and Neck. 3rd ed. New York: Oxford University Press, 1990
   2. Villaret M: Rev Neurol 23:188-190, 1916

VINCENT ANGINA, pseudomembranous angina; a *Spirillum* associated with a fusiform bacillus found in certain forms of ulcerative tonsillitis and gingivitis. Most frequently found in young people. Cross-reference: Trench mouth. (John H. Vincent, 1862-1950, French)
   1. Ballenger JJ: Diseases of the Nose, Throat, Ear, Head and Neck. 12th ed. Philadelphia: Lea & Febiger, 1977

VINCENT DISEASE, see Plaut-Vincent disease. (John H. Vincent)

VINCENT SIGN, see Argyll Robertson pupil.

VINSON SYNDROME, see Plummer-Vinson syndrome.

VIPOND SIGN, generalized adenopathy with concurrent fever; seen in various exanthemas of children.
   1. Casas EC: Diccionario Terminologico de Ciencias Medicas. 5th ed. Salvat Editores, SA, 1954

VIRCHOW DISEASE, leontiasis ossea or megalocephaly. (Rudolf Virchow, 1821-1902, German pathologist)
   1. Casas EC: Diccionario Terminologico de Ciencias Medicas. 5th ed. Salvat Editores, SA, 1954

VIRCHOW-SECKEL SYNDROME, see Seckel syndrome. (Rudolf Virchow)

VLADIMIROFF-MIKULICZ OPERATION, see Mikulicz operation, def. 2. (Alexander Vladimiroff, 1837-1903, Russian surgeon; Johann von Mikulicz-Radecki, 1850-1905, Polish surgeon)

VOGT SYNDROME, congenital chorea; spastic cerebral diplegia. (Cécile Vogt, 1875-1962, French-born German; Oskar Vogt, 1870-1959, German neurologist)
1. Vogt C, Vogt O: J Psychol Neurol 25:627-846, 1920

VOGT-KOYANAGI-HARADA SYNDROME, characterized by depigmentation of the skin and hair, inflammatory ocular lesions (usually consisting of iridocyclitis or exudative retinal detachment), and meningitis. (Alfred Vogt, 1879-1943, Swiss ophthalmologist; Yoshizo Koyanagi, 1880-1954, Japanese ophthalmologist; Einosuke Harada, 1892-1947, Japanese ophthalmologist)
1. Grinker RR, Sahs AL: Neurology. 6th ed. Springfield: Charles C Thomas, 1966
2. Harada E: Nippon Ganka Gakkai Zasshi 301:356-361, 1926
3. Koyanagi Y: Klin Monatsbl Augenheilkd 82:194-211, 1929
4. Vogt A: Klin Monatsbl Augenheilkd 44:228-242, 1906

VOGT-SPIELMEYER DISEASE, see Spielmeyer-Vogt-Sjögren disease. (Heinrich Vogt, German)

VOLHYNIA FEVER, see Trench fever.

VOLKMANN ISCHEMIC CONTRACTURE SYNDROME, refers to contractures of the muscles of the hand and the volar aspect of the forearm, and the crippling deformities to which they give rise and that follow fractures in the region of the elbow, particularly supracondylar fractures of the humerus. (Richard von Volkmann, 1830-1889, German surgeon)
1. Von Volkmannn R: Zbl Chir 8:801-803, 1881

VOLKMANN OPERATION, incision of the tunica vaginalis in cases of hydrocele.
1. Maffei WE: Os Fundamentos da Medicina. 2nd ed. Livraria Editora Artes Médicas Ltda, 1978

VOLKOVITSCH SIGN, recurrent, chronic appendicitis with right iliac fossa mass.
1. Casas EC: Diccionario Terminologico de Ciencias Medicas. 5th ed. Salvat Editores, SA, 1954

VOLTOLINI SIGN, see Heryng sign. (Friedrich E.R. Voltolini, 1819-1889, German otorhinolaryngologist)

VON BASEDOW DISEASE, see Graves disease. (Karl A. von Basedow, 1799-1854, German)

VON BECHTEREW SYNDROME, ankylosing spondylitis in which there is prominent involvement of the spinal articulations, sacroiliac joints, and paravertebral soft tissues. (Vladimir M. von Bechterew, 1857-1927, Russian neurologist)
1. Bennett JC, Plum F (eds): Cecil Textbook of Medicine. 20th ed. Philadelphia: WB Saunders, 1996

VON ECONOMO DISEASE, encephalitis lethargica; rarely encountered since the 1920s. (Constantin von Economo, 1876-1931, Austrian neurologist)
1. Krugman S, Katz SI: Infectious Diseases of Children. 7th ed. St Louis: CV Mosby, 1981
2. Von Economo C: Wien Klin Wochenschr 30:581-585, 1917

VON GIERKE DISEASE, glycogen storage disease type I; an inborn glycogen metabolism disorder due to glucose-6-phosphatase deficiency. The prototype of the hepatic forms of glycogen storage disease. (Edgar von Gierke, 1877-1945, German pathologist)
1. Sidbury JB: The Genetics of the Glycogens Affecting Muscles: Exploratory Concepts in Muscular Dystrophy and Related Disorders. Amsterdam: Excerpta Medica, International Congress Series No. 147, 1967
2. Von Gierke E: Beitr Pathol Anat 82:497-513, 1929

VON GRAEFE SIGN, the patient is asked to follow the examiner's finger, which is moved up and down several times (but not too slowly). A positive result is persistent lagging of the upper eyelid behind the corneoscleral limbus. (Albrecht F.W.E.A. von Graefe, 1828-1870, German ophthalmologist)
1. Lumley JS, Clain A: Hamilton Bailey's Demonstration of Physical Signs in Clinical Surgery. 18th ed. London: Butterworth-Heinemann, 1997

VON GRAEFE SYNDROME, chronic progressive ophthalmoplegia and myopathy. Cross-reference: Graefe disease. (Albrecht F.W.E.A. von Graefe)
1. Thomas HM: Congenital facial paralyses. J Nerv Ment Dis 25:571-593, 1898
2. Von Graefe A: Berl Klin Wochenschr 5:127, 1868

VON HACKER OPERATION, see Hacker operation.

VON HIPPEL-LINDAU SYNDROME, angioma of the retina and cerebellar hemangioblastoma. Autosomal dominant inheritance. Cross-references: Hippel syndrome; Lindau disease. (Eugen von

Hippel, 1867-1939, German ophthalmologist; Arvid Lindau, 1892-1958, Swiss pathologist)

1. Lindau A: Studien über Kleinhineystem. Acta Pathol Microbiol Scand (Suppl) 1:1-128, 1926
2. Smith DW, Jones KL: Recognizable Patterns of Human Malformations: Genetic, Embryologic, and Clinical Aspects. 3rd ed. Philadelphia: WB Saunders, 1982
3. Von Hippel E: Versammlung Ophthalmol Ges 24:269, 1895

VON JAKSCH DISEASE, anemia infantum pseudoleukemica.

1. Dorland's Pocket Medical Dictionary. 22nd ed. Philadelphia: WB Saunders, 1977

VON MONAKOW SYNDROME, see Monakow syndrome.

VON NOORDEN DISEASE, scleroderma in the genitalia.

1. Casas EC: Diccionario Terminologico de Ciencias Medicas. 5th ed. Salvat Editores, SA, 1954

VON RECKLINGHAUSEN DISEASE, generalized neurofibromatosis; characterized by various tumor formations connected with the nervous system, although tumors arising from the covering cells of the peripheral nervous system are the most common. A congenital disease, often hereditary. Autosomal dominant inheritance. Cross-reference: Neurofibromatosis syndrome. (Friedrich von Recklinghausen, 1833-1910, German histologist/pathologist)

1. Cheitlin MD, Sokolow M: Clinical Cardiology. 5th ed. Norwalk, Conn: Appleton & Lange, 1993
2. D'Agostino AN, Soule EH, Miller RH, et al: Primary malignant neoplasms of nerves (malignant neurilemomas) in patients without manifestations of multiple neurofibromatosis (von Recklinghausen's disease). Cancer 16:1003-1027, 1963
3. Mulvihill JJ, et al: Neurofibromatosis 1 (Recklinghausen disease) and neurofibromatosis 2 (bilateral acoustic neurofibromatosis): an update. Ann Intern Med 113:39-52, 1990
4. Von Recklinghausen FD: Fortschr R Virchows, 1891

VON WILLEBRAND DISEASE, due to deficiency of a plasma protein required for the normal adherence of platelets to the site of vascular injury and possibly for the formation of platelet aggregates. Cross-reference: Minot-von Willebrand disease. (Erik A. von Willebrand, 1870-1949, Finnish)

1. Baker AB, Baker LH: Clinical Neurology. Revised ed. Philadelphia: Harper & Row, 1982
2. Bennett JC, Plum F (eds): Cecil Textbook of Medicine. 20th ed. Philadelphia: WB Saunders, 1996
3. Von Willebrand EA: Fin Lakaresal Handl 68:87, 1926

VORONOFF OPERATION, transplantation of monkey testicles to man.

1. Maffei WE: Os Fundamentos da Medicina. 2nd ed. Livraria Editora Artes Médicas Ltda, 1978

VROLIK DISEASE, osteogenesis imperfecta; la maladie de Lobstein in the French-speaking portion of the medical world. "Ivar the Boneless," the mastermind behind the Scandinavian invasion of England in the last quarter of the ninth century, probably suffered from this. He is said to have had cartilage where bones should have been. He could not walk and was carried onto the battlefields. Cross-references: Eddowes syndrome; Van der Hoeve disease. (Willem Vrolik, 1801-1863, Dutch anatomist)

1. McKusick VA: Heritable Disorders of Connective Tissue. 4th ed. St Louis: CV Mosby, 1972
2. Vrolik W: Tabulae ad Illustrandam Embryogenes in Hominis et Mammalium, tam Naturalem quan Abnormen. Lipsiae: Weigel, 1854

VROLIK SYNDROME, see Osteogenesis imperfecta syndrome type II.

V-Y OPERATION, see Wharton-Jones operation.

W SYNDROME, a multiple congenital anomaly-mental retardation syndrome; median cleft of the upper lip, mental retardation, and pugilistic facies are found.

1. Gorlin RJ, Cohen MM Jr, Levin LS: Syndromes of the Head and Neck. 3rd ed. New York: Oxford University Press, 1990
2. Pallister PD, Hermann J, Springer JW, et al: The W syndrome. Birth Defects 10(7):51-60, 1974

WAARDENBURG SYNDROME, increased interocular distance, heterochromia iridis, congenital deafness, white forelock, and aberrant mid upper face development are characteristics. Hypertrichosis of the eyebrows tending to join at midline is also present. Cross-reference: Klein-Waardenburg syndrome. (Petras J. Waardenburg, 1886-1979, Dutch ophthalmologist)

1. Farmer TW: Pediatric Neurology. 2nd ed. Hagerstown: Harper & Row, 1975
2. Smith DW, Jones KL: Recognizable Patterns of Human Malformations: Genetic, Embryologic, and Clinical Aspects. 3rd ed. Philadelphia: WB Saunders, 1982
3. Waardenburg PJ: A new syndrome combining developmental anomalies of the eyelids, eyebrows and nose root with pigmentary defects of the iris and head and with congenital deafness. Am J Hum Genet 3:195-253, 1951

WACHENHEIM-REDER SIGN, a rectal examination causes pain in the patient with appendicitis.

1. Casas EC: Diccionario Terminologico de Ciencias Medicas. 5th ed. Salvat Editores, SA, 1954

WAGNER OPERATION, osteoplastic craniotomy.

1. Maffei WE: Os Fundamentos da Medicina. 2nd ed. Livraria Editora Artes Médicas Ltda, 1978

WAGNER-STICKLER SYNDROME, see Stickler syndrome.

WAHL SIGN, 1) tympanic sound elicited by percussion above a bowel obstruction; 2) bruit in a vessel following trauma.

1. Casas EC: Diccionario Terminologico de Ciencias Medicas. 5th ed. Salvat Editores, SA, 1954

WALDENSTRÖM MACROGLOBULINEMIA, see Schnitzler syndrome. (Jan G. Waldenstrom, Swedish)

WALDENSTRÖM UVEOPAROTITIS SYNDROME, see Heerfordt syndrome. (Jan G. Waldenström)

WALDHAUSEN OPERATION, a subclavian flap technique used in infants with coarctation.

1. Schwartz SI: Principles of Surgery. 4th ed. New York: McGraw-Hill, 1983

WALKER-MURDOCH WRIST SIGN, a sign that reflects both a thin wrist and long digits; the thumb and 5th finger, when clasped around the wrist, usually overlap appreciably in patients with Marfan syndrome.

1. McKusick VA: Heritable Disorders of Connective Tissue. 4th ed. St Louis: CV Mosby, 1972

WALKER-WARBURG SYNDROME, the association of lissencephaly, hydrocephalus, severe cerebellar abnormality, and ocular malformation. May present clinically in a number of dissimilar ways. Autosomal recessive inheritance. Cross-references: Chemke syndrome; HARD+E syndrome; Warburg syndrome. (Arthur Earl Walker, 1907-1995, U.S. neurosurgeon; Mette Warburg, Danish ophthalmologist)

1. Gorlin RJ, Cohen MM Jr, Levin LS: Syndromes of the Head and Neck. 3rd ed. New York: Oxford University Press, 1990
2. Walker AE: Lissencephaly. Arch Neurol Psych 48:13-29, 1942
3. Warburg M: Birth Defects 7:136-154, 1971

WALLENBERG SYNDROME, a syndrome resulting from ischemia in the area supplied by the posterior inferior cerebellar artery. Symptoms include ipsilateral ataxia without tremor, vagus nerve paralysis, loss of pain and temperature sensation in the face, and Horner syndrome. Cross-references: Lateral bulbar syndrome; Lateral medullary syndrome; Posterior inferior cerebellar artery syndrome. (Adolf Wallenberg, 1862-1949, German neurologist)

1. Rowland LP (ed): Merritt's Textbook of Neurology. Philadelphia: Lea & Febiger, 1989
2. Wallenberg A: Acute bulbaraffection (Embolie der Art. Cerebellar post. inf. sinistr.) Arch Psychiatr Nervenkr 27:504-540, 1895

WALTON OPERATION, cuneiform resection of the lesser curvature of the stomach followed by gastroenterostomy, for treatment of ulcers.

1. Maffei WE: Os Fundamentos da Medicina. 2nd ed. Livraria Editora Artes Médicas Ltda, 1978

WARBURG SYNDROME, see Walker-Warburg syndrome.

WARD-ROMANO SYNDROME, see Romano-Ward syndrome.

WARDROP DISEASE, malignant onychia. (James Wardrop, British surgeon)

1. Wardrop J: Med Chir Trans Lond 5:129-143, 1814

WARDROP OPERATION, peripheral or distal ligation of an artery in cases of an aneurysm. (James Wardrop)

1. Maffei WE: Os Fundamentos da Medicina. 2nd ed. Livraria Editora Artes Médicas Ltda, 1978

WARLOMONT OPERATION, modification of the Fraefe method for cataract extraction.

1. Maffei WE: Os Fundamentos da Medicina. 2nd ed. Livraria Editora Artes Médicas Ltda, 1978

WARTENBERG SIGN, the examiner places his/her middle and index fingers across the tips of the patient's slightly bent four fingers and then taps the examiner's own fingers lightly with a percussion hammer to ensure flexion of the patient's four fingers. Flexion of the thumb is positive for a pyramidal tract lesion. (Robert Wartenberg, 1887-1956, U.S. neurologist)

1. Bordas LB (ed): Neurologia Fundamental. 2nd ed. Toray, 1968
2. Haymaker W: Bing's Local Diagnosis in Neurological Diseases. 15th ed. St Louis: CV Mosby, 1969

WARTENBERG SYNDROME, involuntary movements similar to those trying to catch a ball or wipe the face. Wartenberg "migrant sensory neuritis" is a recurrent/remitting multifocal sensory neuropathy characterized by pain of sudden onset in the distribution of a cutaneous sensory nerve. (Robert Wartenberg)

1. Bodechtel G: Diagnostico Diferential de las Enfermedades Neurologicas. Madrid: Pas Montalvo Editorial, 1967
2. Thomas PK, et al: Hereditary neuralgic amyotrophy associated with a relapsing multifocal sensory neuropathy. J Neurol Neurosurg Psychiatry 56:107-109, 1993

WARTHIN SIGN, exaggeration of pulmonary sounds; seen in the patient with acute pericarditis. (Alfred S. Warthin, 1866-1931, U.S. pathologist)

1. Casas EC: Diccionario Terminologico de Ciencias Medicas. 5th ed. Salvat Editores, SA, 1954

WARTHIN TUMOR, parotid adenolymphoma, generally soft and sometimes fluctuant; tends to occur in white males and is seen only after the 40th year. (Alfred S. Warthin)

1. Warthin AS: J Cancer Res 13:116-125, 1929

WASSILIEFF DISEASE, see Weil disease.

WASTING SYNDROME, see Runting syndrome.

WATERHOUSE-FRIDERICHSEN SYNDROME, acute vascular collapse with adrenal hemorrhage associated with severe systemic infection, especially with meningococcus. Cross-reference: Friderichsen syndrome. (Rupert Waterhouse, 1873-1958, British; Carl Friderichsen, Danish pediatrician)

1. Friderichsen C: Jahrb Kinderheilkd 87:109-125, 1918
2. Grinker RR, Sahs AL: Neurology. 6th ed. Springfield: Charles C Thomas, 1966
3. Krugman S, Katz SL: Infectious Diseases of Children. 7th ed. St Louis: CV Mosby, 1981
4. Waterhouse R: Lancet 1:577-578, 1911

WATTS OPERATION, see Freeman operation. (James W. Watts, 1904-1994, U.S.)

WDHA SYNDROME, watery diarrhea, hypokalemia, and achlorhydria (WDHA); see Verner-Morrison syndrome.

WEAVER SYNDROME, WEAVER-SMITH SYNDROME, accelerated skeletal maturation. Etiology unknown. (David D. Weaver, U.S.)

1. Smith DW, Jones KL: Recognizable Patterns of Human Malformations: Genetic, Embryologic, and Clinical Aspects. 3rd ed. Philadelphia: WB Saunders, 1982
2. Weaver DD, Graham CB, Thomas IT, et al: A new overgrowth syndrome with accelerated skeletal maturation, unusual facies and camptodactyly. J Pediatr 84:547-552, 1974

WEBER DISEASE, WEBER-CHRISTIAN DISEASE, relapsing nodular panniculitis; a group of syndromes characterized by subcutaneous nodules and inflammation in the fat lobules. Termed this disease when cutaneous lesions are associated with systemic complaints. Cross-reference: Christian-Weber disease. (Frederick Parkes Weber, 1863-1962, British; Henry A. Christian, 1876-1951, U.S. internist)

1. Bennett JC, Plum F (eds): Cecil Textbook of Medicine. 20th ed. Philadelphia: WB Saunders, 1996
2. Moschella SL, Hurley HJ: Dermatology. 2nd ed. Philadelphia: WB Saunders, 1985

WEBER SYNDROME, a lesion situated in the basis pedunculi produces complete hemiplegia of the contralateral side by affecting fibers involved in movements of the limbs, face, and tongue; there is paralysis of the extraocular muscles of the ipsilateral side due to interruption of the 3rd cranial nerve. (Sir Hermann D. Weber, 1823-1918, British)

1. Haymaker W: Bing's Local Diagnosis in Neurological Diseases. 15th ed. St Louis: CV Mosby, 1969

WEBER TEST, a measurement of hearing; place a vibrating tuning fork on the center of the patient's forehead. Normally, the sound is appreciated by both ears equally and, if the patient occludes one external auditory meatus with a finger, the sound becomes louder on that side. Similarly, in unilateral middle-ear deafness, the sound is lateralized to the affected side. If the sound is lateralized to the good ear, it suggests that deafness in the affected ear is perceptive. (Friedrich E. Weber, 1832-1891, German otologist)

1. Lumley JS, Clain A: Hamilton Bailey's Demonstration of Physical Signs in Clinical Surgery. 18th ed. London: Butterworth-Heinemann, 1997

WEBER-COCKAYNE SYNDROME, localized epidermolysis bullosa simplex. Cross-reference: Goldscheider syndrome. (Frederick Parkes Weber; Edward A. Cockayne, 1880-1956, British)

1. Cockayne EA: Br J Dermatol 50:358-362, 1938
2. Weber FP: Proc R Soc Med 19:72, 1926

WEBER-DIMITRI DISEASE, see Sturge-Kalischer-Weber syndrome.

WEBER-FERGUSSON OPERATION, for carcinoma of the maxillary sinus, with removal of the eye.

1. Cummings C: Otolaryngology. Head and Neck Surgery. 6th ed. St Louis: CV Mosby, 1986
2. Schwartz SI: Principles of Surgery. 4th ed. New York: McGraw-Hill, 1983

WEBSTER OPERATION, see Baldy operation.

WECKER OPERATION, tattooing of the cornea to conceal leukomatous spots.

1. Maffei WE: Os Fundamentos da Medicina. 2nd ed. Livraria Editora Artes Médicas Ltda, 1978

WEDENSKY PHENOMENON, if a nerve is repeatedly and rapidly stimulated, the muscles contract in response to the first stimulus and then fail to respond further; if the stimuli are repeated at a slower rate, the muscles respond to every stimulus. (Nikolai Y. Wedensky, 1852-1922, Russian neurologist)

1. Dorland's Medical Dictionary. 28th ed. Philadelphia: WB Saunders, 1994

WEGENER GRANULOMATOSIS, characterized by the classic clinicopathological features of necrotizing granulomatous vasculitis involving the upper and lower respiratory tracts, glomerulonephritis, and varying degrees of systemic, small-vessel vasculitis. (Friedrich Wegener, 1907-1990, German pathologist)

1. Baker AB, Baker LH: Clinical Neurology. Revised ed. Philadelphia: Harper & Row, 1982
2. Wegener F: Beitr Pathol Anat 102:36-68, 1939
3. Wegener F: Verhandl Dtsch Pathol Ges 29:202-210, 1936

WEGNER SIGN, a dense radiological shadow representing an accumulating calcified matrix may be visible in the epiphyseal line; seen in osteochondritis. (Friedrich R. Wegner, 1843-1917, German pathologist)

WEIL DISEASE, leptospirosis, often with cardiac involvement. Findings include petechiae or large foci of hemorrhage in the epicardium. Involvement of the arterioventricular conduction system may be a prominent feature. Commonly seen in conjunction with ST segment and T-wave changes, atrial and ventricle arrhythmias, and sinus bradycardia. Cross-references: Lancereaux-Mathieu disease; Larrey-Weil disease; Wassilieff disease. (Adolf Weil, 1848-1916, German)

1. Braunwald E: Heart Disease: A Textbook of Cardiovascular Medicine. 4th ed. Philadelphia: WB Saunders, 1992
2. Weil A: Dtsch Arch Klin Med 39:209-232, 1886

WEILL SIGN, the lack of expansion in the subclavicular region of the affected side; seen in infantile pneumonia. (Edmond Weill, 1858-1924, French pediatrician)

1. Dorland's Medical Dictionary. 28th ed. Philadelphia: WB Saunders, 1994

WEILL-MARCHESANI SYNDROME, dystrophia mesodermalis congenita hyperplastica; a congenital disorder of connective tissue transmitted as an autosomal dominant or recessive trait and characterized by brachycephaly, brachydactyly, short stature with a broad chest and heavy musculature, reduced joint mobility, spherophakia, ectopia lentis, myopia, and glaucoma. Cross-references: Marchesani syndrome; Spherophakia-brachymorphia syndrome. (Georges Weill, 1866-1952, French ophthalmologist; Oswald Marchesani, 1900-1952, German ophthalmologist)

1. Fowler NO: Cardiac Diagnosis and Treatment. Cambridge: Harper & Row, 1980
2. Marchesani O: Klin Monatsbl Augenheilkd 103:392-406, 1939
3. Smith DW, Jones KL: Recognizable Patterns of Human Malformations: Genetic Embryologic, and Clinical Aspects. Philadelphia: WB Saunders, 1982
4. Weill G: Ann Ocul 169:21-44, 1932

WEINGARTEN DISEASE, tropical eosinophilia. (R.J. Weingarten, German who worked in India)

1. Weingarten RJ: Lancet 1:103-105, 1943

WEINGARTEN SYNDROME, tropical eosinophilia producing recurring bouts of cough and pulmonary symptoms. (R.J. Weingarten)

1. Weingarten RJ: Lancet 1:103-105, 1943

WEIR MITCHELL DISEASE, see Mitchell disease.

WEISS SIGN, see Chvostek sign.

WELLS SYNDROME, eosinophilic cellulitis; a recurrent, usually itchy, occasionally painful, papulovesicular eruption which in severe cases may be associated with fever, arthralgia, and malaise. (G.C. Wells, British)

1. Bennett JC, Plum F (eds): Cecil Textbook of Medicine. 20th ed. Philadelphia: WB Saunders, 1996
2. Wells GC: Trans St Johns Hosp Dermatol Soc 37:46-56, 1971

WEPFER DISEASE, cerebral hemorrhage.

1. Casas EC: Diccionario Terminologico de Ciencias Medicas. 5th ed. Salvat Editores, SA, 1954

WERDNIG-HOFFMANN DISEASE, infantile progressive muscular atrophy; a familial disorder. Autosomal recessive gene transmission. (Guido Werdnig, 1844-1919, neurologist; Johann Hoffmann, 1857-1919, German neurologist)
1. Campbell WC, Crenshaw AH: Campbell's Operative Orthopaedics. 7th ed. St Louis: CV Mosby, 1987
2. Hoffmann J: Dtsch Zschr Nervenheilkd 1:95-120, 1891
3. Werdnig G: Arch Psychiatr 22:437-480, 1891

WERMER SYNDROME, multiple endocrine neoplasia type I; the familial occurrence of multiple tumors of the pituitary, parathyroid glands, and pancreatic islet cell associated with a high incidence of peptic ulcer. (Paul Wermer, 1898-1975, U.S. internist)
1. Bennett JC, Plum F (eds): Cecil Textbook of Medicine. 20th ed. Philadelphia: WB Saunders, 1996
2. Wermer P: Am J Med 16:363-371, 1954

WERNER SCHULTZ DISEASE, see Schultz syndrome. (Werner Schultz, 1878-1947, German internist)

WERNER SYNDROME, see Rothmund syndrome. (C.W. Otto Werner, 1879-1936, U.S.)

WERNER-HIS DISEASE, see Trench fever. (Heinrich Werner, 1874-1946, German; Wilhelm His, Jr., 1863-1934, German)

WERNICKE APHASIA, sensory aphasia; comprehension of both spoken and written language is severely impaired and repetition of spoken and written language is poor. Most commonly, no hemiplegia or other elementary neurological signs. Results from a lesion in the Wernicke area (i.e., the posterior portion of the superior temporal gyrus). (Karl Wernicke, 1848-1905, German neurologist)
1. Ritchie AC: Boyd's Textbook of Pathology. 9th ed. Philadelphia: Lea & Febiger, 1990
2. Wernicke K: Der Aphasische Symptomenkomplex. Breslau: Cohn, Weigert, 1874

WERNICKE SIGN, pupillary reaction due to damage of the optic tract; seen in hemianopsia. (Karl Wernicke)
1. Dorland's Medical Dictionary. 28th ed. Philadelphia: WB Saunders, 1994

WERNICKE SYNDROME, a manifestation of thiamin deficiency; of particular importance in alcoholics, involving ocular abnormalities and psychosis. Peripheral neuritis is frequently associated. Cross-references: Gayet disease; Meynert syndrome. (Karl Wernicke)
1. Gayet M: Arch Physiol Norm Pathol 2:341-351, 1875
2. Korsakoff SS: Vest Psikhrat 4:1887
3. Rowland LP (ed): Merritt's Textbook of Neurology. Philadelphia: Lea & Febiger, 1989
4. Wernicke K: Lehrbuch der Gehirnkrankeiten fur Aerzte und Studierende. Kassel: J Fisher, 1881

WERNICKE-KORSAKOFF SYNDROME, the coexistence of the Wernicke syndrome with the Korsakoff syndrome (organic amnesia). (Karl Wernicke; Sergei S. Korsakoff, 1854-1900, Russian neurologist)
1. Haymaker W: Bing's Local Diagnosis in Neurological Diseases. 15th ed. St Louis: CV Mosby, 1969

WERTHEIM OPERATION, a procedure for hysterectomy with pelvic lymphadenectomy; primarily performed for cancer of the cervix. (Ernst Wertheim, 1864-1920, Austrian gynecologist)
1. Schwartz SI: Principles of Surgery. 4th ed. New York: McGraw-Hill, 1983

WERTHEIM-SCHAUTA OPERATION, interposition of the uterus between the urinary bladder and the anterior wall of the vagina in cases of cystocele. (Ernst Wertheim; Friedrich Schauta, 1849-1919, Austrian gynecologist)
1. Maffei WE: Os Fundamentos da Medicina. 2nd ed. Livraria Editora Artes Médicas Ltda, 1978

WESSELBRON DISEASE, caused by a *Flavivirus* that commonly infects sheep in Africa. Infection transmitted by mosquitoes; occasionally the virus causes a febrile illness in humans. (Named for a town in South Africa where the agent was first isolated.)
1. Ritchie AC: Boyd's Textbook of Pathology. 9th ed. Philadelphia: Lea & Febiger, 1990

WEST NILE FEVER, an acute, febrile, mosquito-borne viral illness marked by headache, myalgia, lymphadenopathy, and rash. Generally self-limiting, although occasionally death results from encephalitis in the elderly. Caused by a small ribonucleic acid-containing virus (family Togaviridae, genus *Flavivirus*). (Reported in Uganda, Egypt, South Africa, Israel, and India.)
1. Bennett JC, Plum F (eds): Cecil Textbook of Medicine. 20th ed. Philadelphia: WB Saunders, 1996

WEST SYNDROME, tuberous sclerosis when skin lesions are associated with infantile spasms, hyperarrhythmia, and mental retardation. (W.J. West, British)

1. Rowland LP (ed): Merritt's Textbook of Neurology. Philadelphia: Lea & Febiger, 1989
2. West WJ: On a peculiar form of infantile convulsions. Lancet 1:724-725, 1840/41

WESTBERG DISEASE, a disorder causing whitish spots on the skin.

1. Casas EC: Diccionario Terminologico de Ciencias Medicas. 5th ed. Salvat Editores, SA, 1954

WESTERMARK SIGN, avascularity of the normal radiological shadow of pulmonary tissue distal to a pulmonary embolism. (Neil Westermark, German radiologist)

1. Braunwald E: Heart Disease: A Textbook of Cardiovascular Medicine. 4th ed. Philadelphia: WB Saunders, 1992

WESTPHAL SIGN, absence of the knee jerk reflex; seen in the patient with locomotor ataxia. Cross-reference: Erb-Westphal sign. (Karl F.O. Westphal, 1833-1890, German neurologist)

1. Bodechtel G: Diagnostico Diferencial de las Enfermedades Neurologicas. Madrid, 1967

WESTPHAL-PILTZ PHENOMENON, see Piltz sign. (Alexander K.O. Westphal, 1863-1941, German neurologist)

WESTPHAL-STRÜMPELL DISEASE, hepatolenticular degeneration. Cross-reference: Wilson disease. (Karl F.O. Westphal; Ernst A. von Strümpell, 1853-1925, German)

1. Von Strümpell EA: Dtsch Zschr Nervenheilkd 12:114-149, 1898
2. Westphal KFO: Arch Psychiatr 14:87-134, 1883
3. Wilson SAK: Brain 34:295-509, 1912

WEYERS SYNDROME, acrodental dysostosis involving postaxial hexadactyly, bony cleft of the mandibular symphysis, and anomalies of the incisors and oral vestibule are features. Cross-reference: Curry-Hall syndrome. (Helmut Weyers, German)

1. Gorlin RJ, Cohen MM Jr, Levin LS: Syndromes of the Head and Neck. 3rd ed. New York: Oxford University Press, 1990
2. Weyers H: Fortschr Roentgenol 77:562-567, 1952
3. Weyers H: Zur Kenntnis der Chondroektodermaldyplasie (Ellis-van-Creveld). Z Kinderheilkd 78:111-129, 1956

WHARTON DUCT, the submandibular duct, which runs anteriorly between the mylohyoid, hyoglossus, and genioglossus muscles and the sublingual gland to open in the caruncula sublingualis. (Thomas Wharton, 1614-1673, English anatomist)

1. Ballenger JJ: Diseases of the Nose, Throat, Ear, Head and Neck. 12th ed. Philadelphia: Lea & Febiger, 1977

WHARTON-JONES OPERATION, surgery for ectropion in which a V-shaped incision is made on the inferior eyelid and is transformed into a Y-shape via sutures. Cross-reference: V-Y operation.

1. Maffei WE: Os Fundamentos da Medicina. 2nd ed. Livraria Editora Artes Médicas Ltda, 1978

WHEELHOUSE OPERATION, perineal urethrotomy; seen in urethral stricture. (Claudius Wheelhouse, 1826-1909, British surgeon)

1. Maffei WE: Os Fundamentos da Medicina. 2nd ed. Livraria Editora Artes Médicas Ltda, 1978

WHELAN SYNDROME, facial asymmetry, pseudocleft lip, lobulated tongue, and hydronephrosis are found.

1. Gorlin RJ, Cohen MM Jr, Levin LS: Syndromes of the Head and Neck. 3rd ed. New York: Oxford University Press, 1990
2. Whelan DT, et al: The oro-facial-digital syndrome. Clin Genet 8:205-212, 1975

WHIPLASH SHAKE SYNDROME, a constellation of injuries to the brain and eye that may occur when a small child is shaken vigorously while being held by the trunk or limbs with the head unsupported. This stretching and tearing of the cerebral vessels and brain substance may lead to subdural hematomas and retinal hemorrhages and is sometimes associated with cerebral contusion. May result in paralysis, blindness and other visual disturbances, convulsions, and death. Cross-reference: Battered child syndrome.

1. Kempe HC: JAMA 181:17-24, 1962

WHIPPLE DISEASE, lipophagic intestinal granulomatosis or intestinal lipodystrophy; there is heavy infiltration of the intestinal wall and lymphatic system by macrophages filled with glycoprotein. A generalized disease with steatorrhea as its principal feature, occurring predominantly in males in the 4th and 7th decades. (George Whipple, 1878-1976, U.S. pathologist)

1. Hurst JW, Schlant RC, Alexander RW: The Heart: Arteries and Veins. 8th ed. New York: McGraw-Hill, 1994
2. Whipple GH: Bull Johns Hopkins Hosp 18:382-391, 1907

WHIPPLE OPERATION, partial pancreatectomy; a procedure used to treat pancreatic lesions. (Allen O. Whipple, 1881-1963, U.S. surgeon)

1. Schwartz SI: Principles of Surgery. 4th ed. New York: McGraw-Hill, 1983

WHISTLING FACE SYNDROME, WHISTLING FACE-WINDMILL VANE HAND SYN-DROME, see Freeman-Sheldon syndrome.

WHITE DISEASE, see Darier-White disease. (James C. White, 1833-1916, U.S.)

WHITMORE DISEASE, melioidosis; a glanders-like disease of rodents, transmissible to humans and caused by *Pseudomonas pseudomallei*. (Alfred Whitmore, 1876-1946, British surgeon)
  1. Whitmore A: Indian Med Gaz 47:262-267, 1912

WHYTT DISEASE, tuberculous meningitis associated with hydrocephalus. (Robert Whytt, 1714-1766, Scottish)
  1. Whytt R: Observations on Dropsy of the Brain. Edinburgh: Balfour, 1768

WICHMANN DISEASE, laryngeal stridor. (Johann Wichmann, 1740-1802, German)
  1. Casas EC: Diccionario Terminologico de Ciencias Medicas. 5th ed. Salvat Editores, SA, 1954

WIDAL SYNDROME, see Hayem-Widal syndrome. (Georges F.I. Widal, 1862-1929, French)

WIDAL-ABRAMI DISEASE, see Abrami disease. (Georges F.I. Widal)

WIDMER SIGN, the right axillary temperature is greater than the left; seen in appendicitis.
  1. Casas EC: Diccionario Terminologico de Ciencias Medicas. 5th ed. Salvat Editores, SA, 1954

WIDOWITZ SIGN, diphtheritic paralysis with slow motion on blinking the eyes; seen in diphtheric paralysis. (Jannak Widowitz, Polish)
  1. Casas EC: Diccionario Terminologico de Ciencias Medicas. 5th ed. Salvat Editores, SA, 1954

WIEDEMANN-BECKWITH SYNDROME, see Beckwith syndrome. (Hans R. Wiedemann)

WIEDEMANN-RAUTENSTRAUCH SYNDROME, an aged facies is present from birth. Birth size is small, growth is slow, and mental and motor development are usually deficient; there is frontal and biparietal bossing. (Hans R. Wiedemann)
  1. Gorlin RJ, Cohen MM Jr, Levin LS: Syndromes of the Head and Neck. 3rd ed. New York: Oxford University Press, 1990
  2. Rautenstrauch T, Snigula F, Krieg T, et al: Progeria: a cell culture study and clinical report of familial incidence. Eur J Pediatr 124:101-111, 1977
  3. Wiedemann HR: An identified neonatal progeroid syndrome. Follow-up report. Eur J Pediatr 130:65-70, 1979

WIES OPERATION, full thickness transverse tarsotomy with marginal rotation.
  1. Spaeth GL: Ophthalmic Surgery. Principles and Practice. Philadelphia: WB Saunders, 1982

WILDER SIGN, nystagmus on lateral gaze; an early indication of exophthalmic goiter. (William H. Wilder, 1860-1935, U.S. ophthalmologist)
  1. Casas EC: Diccionario Terminologico de Ciencias Medicas. 5th ed. Salvat Editores, SA, 1954

WILDERVANCK SYNDROME, features are fused cervical vertebrae, sensorineural hearing loss, and abducens palsy with retracted globe. Inheritance is poorly understood. Cross-reference: Cervico-oculo-acoustic syndrome.(L.S. Wildervanck, Dutch)
  1. Gorlin RJ, Cohen MM Jr, Levin LS: Syndromes of the Head and Neck. 3rd ed. New York: Oxford University Press, 1990
  2. Wildervanck LS: Klippel-Feil syndrome associated with abducens paralysis, bulbar retraction and deaf-mutism. Ned Tijdschr Geneeskd 96:2751-2756, 1952

WILDERVANCK-SMITH SYNDROME, see Miller syndrome.

WILFRED-HARRIS SYNDROME, glossopharyngeal neuralgia.
  1. Pedro-Pons A: Patologia-y-Clinica Medicus. Salvat Editores, SA, 1952

WILKIE SYNDROME, see Superior mesenteric artery syndrome.

WILKINS-BERGADA SYNDROME, see Rudimentary testis syndrome.

WILKS DISEASE, chronic parenchymatous dermatitis. (Samuel Wilks, 1824-1911, British)
  1. Wilks S: Guys Hosp Rep 8:263-265, 1862

WILLIAMS SIGN, a muffled tympanic sound; seen in the patient with pleural effusion. (Charles J.B. Williams, 1805-1889, British)
  1. Casas EC: Diccionario Terminologico de Ciencias Medicas. 5th ed. Salvat Editores, SA, 1954

WILLIAMS SYNDROME, characteristics are supravalvular aortic stenosis, atypical facies (broad prominent forehead, flattened bridge of the nose, epicanthal folds, and long upper lip), mild mental retardation, and low-pitched voice. Children with this syndrome are particularly friendly and converse

easily. Cross-reference: Elfin facies syndrome. (J.C.P. Williams, New Zealand cardiologist)
1. Braunwald E: Heart Disease: A Textbook of Cardiovascular Medicine. 4th ed. Philadelphia: WB Saunders, 1992
2. Williams JC, Barratt-Boyes BG, Lowe JB: Circulation 24:1311-1318, 1961

WILLIAMS-CAMPBELL SYNDROME, bronchiectasis due to congenital bronchomalacia owing to the absence of annular cartilage distal to the first division of the peripheral bronchi. (Howard Williams, Australian; Peter E. Campbell, Australian)
1. Williams H, Campbell P: Arch Dis Child 35:185-191, 1960

WILLIAMSON SIGN, the blood pressure in the leg is lower than the arm on the same side of the body; seen in the patient with pneumothorax and pleural effusion. (Oliver K. Williamson, 1866-1941, British)
1. Casas EC: Diccionario Terminologico de Ciencias Medicas. 5th ed. Salvat Editores, SA, 1954

WILLISIANA PHENOMENON, Willis paracusis; the ability to hear better in a noisy place, such as in a moving train, than in quiet surroundings. (Thomas Willis, 1621-1675, British)
1. Haymaker W: Bing's Local Diagnosis in Neurological Diseases. 15th ed. St Louis: CV Mosby, 1969
2. Shapiro SL: Paracusis Willisiana. Eye Ear Nose Throat Month 46:622-625, 1967

WILMS OPERATION, resection of the ribs causing inward depression of the thoracic wall and lung compression in cases of tuberculosis.
1. Maffei WE: Os Fundamentos da Medicina. 2nd ed. Livraria Editora Artes Médicas Ltda, 1978

WILMS TUMOR, a sharply demarcated and usually encapsulated solitary tumor occurring in the kidney. (Max Wilms, 1867-1918, German surgeon)
1. Campbell WC, Crenshaw AH: Campbell's Urology. 5th ed. Philadelphia: WB Saunders, 1986
2. Wilms M: Die Mischgeschwülste. Leipzig, 1899

WILSON DISEASE, see Westphal-Strümpell disease. (Samuel A.K. Wilson, 1878-1937, British neurologist)

WILSON SIGN, while lying down, the affected knee is flexed to a right angle and the leg is fully internally rotated. The knee is then gradually extended while in the rotated position. If the patient complains of pain over the anterior aspect of the medial femoral condyle and it is relieved at this point on external rotation of the leg, it is a sign of osteochondritis of the knee. (Samuel A.K. Wilson)
1. Evans RC: Illustrated Essentials in Orthopedic Physical Assessment. St Louis: Mosby Yearbook, 1994

WILSON TYPE II SYNDROME, incomplete male pseudohermaphroditism, with pseudovaginal perineoscrotal hypospadias. The patient is usually classified as female at birth. Autosomal recessive inheritance.
1. Gold JJ, Josimovich JB: Gynecologic Endocrinology. 3rd ed. New York: Plenum Medical, 1980

WILSON-BROCQ DISEASE, exfoliative dermatitis. (Anne J.L. Brocq, 1856-1928, French dermatologist)
1. Casas EC: Diccionario Terminologico de Ciencias Medicas. 5th ed. Salvat Editores, SA, 1954

WILSON-MIKITY SYNDROME, hyperpnea and cyanosis during the 1st month of life, with abdominal distention; vomiting, diarrhea, and eosinophilia are features. Cross-reference: Pulmonary dysmaturity syndrome. (Miriam G. Wilson, U.S. pediatrician; Victor G. Mikity, U.S. radiologist)
1. Nelson WE, Vaughan VC, McKay RJ: Tratado de Pediatria. 6th ed. 1971
2. Wilson MG, Mikity VG: Am J Dis Child 99:489-499, 1960

WIMBERGER SIGN, a radiolucent area in the medial aspect of the proximal tibial metaphyses; characteristic of an infant with congenital syphilis. (Heinrich Wimberger, German radiologist)
1. Krugman S, Katz SL: Infectious Disease of Children. 7th ed. St Louis: CV Mosby, 1981

WINCHESTER SYNDROME, fibro-osteolytic dwarfism; a nonlysosomal connective tissue disorder inherited as an autosomal recessive trait and characterized by dwarfism, multiple contractures, joint destruction simulating that of advanced rheumatoid arthritis, corneal opacities, osteolysis of carpal and tarsal bones, severe osteoporosis, and gargoyle-like facies.
1. Winchester P, Grossman H, Lim WN, et al: AJR 106:121-128, 1969

WINCKEL DISEASE, a fatal disease of the newborn, with jaundice, hemoglobinuria, bloody urine, hemorrhage, cyanosis, and convulsions. (Franz K.L.W. von Winckel, 1837-1911, German)
1. Von Winckel F: Dtsch Med Wochenschr, 1879

WINDSCHEID DISEASE, nervous system symptoms in arteriosclerosis.
1. Casas EC: Diccionario Terminologico de Ciencias Medicas. 5th ed. Salvat Editores, SA, 1954

WINDSOCK SYNDROME, a ventricular septal aneurysm producing subpulmonary obstruction.

1. Fowler NO: Cardiac Diagnosis and Treatment. Cambridge: Harper & Row, 1980

WINIWARTER DISEASE, see Buerger disease. (Felix von Winiwarter, 1852-1931, German surgeon)

WINIWARTER OPERATION, cholecystenterostomy.
1. Maffei WE: Os Fundamentos da Medicina. 2nd ed. Livraria Editora Artes Médicas Ltda, 1978

WINKEL OPERATION, vaginal hysterectomy.
1. Maffei WE: Os Fundamentos da Medicina. 2nd ed. Livraria Editora Artes Médicas Ltda, 1978

WINKELMAN DISEASE, progressive degeneration of the globus pallidus. (Nathaniel Winkelman, 1891-1956, U.S. neurologist)
1. Casas EC: Diccionario Terminologico de Ciencias Medicas. 5th ed. Salvat Editores, SA, 1954

WINKLER DISEASE, a painful, nodular growth on the auricle; an interesting but rare tumor occurring on the top of the helix. Consists of tiny arteriovenous anastomoses with many nerve endings; similar to a glomus body. Seen mainly in men and is of unknown origin. (Max Winkler, 1875-1952, Swiss)
1. Ballenger JJ: Diseases of the Nose, Throat, Ear, Head and Neck. 12th ed. Philadelphia: Lea & Febiger, 1977
2. Winkler M: Arch Derm Syph 121:278-285, 1915/1916

WINTER SYNDROME, a congenital syndrome consisting of renal hypoplasia or aplasia, anomalies of the internal genitalia (especially vaginal atresia), and anomalous ossicles of the middle ear producing deafness. (Jeremy S.D. Winter, U.S.)
1. Winter JSD, et al: J Pediatr 72:88-93, 1968

WINTERBOTTOM SIGN, swelling of the posterior cervical lymph nodes; characteristic of African trypanosomiasis. (Thomas M. Winterbottom, 1765-1859, British)
1. Dorland's Medical Dictionary. 28th ed. Philadelphia: WB Saunders, 1994

WINTRICH SIGN, if the sound heard on percussion changes with the mouth open and then closed, a cavitary lesion of the lung is indicated. (Anton Wintrich, 1812-1882, German)
1. Casas EC: Diccionario Terminologico de Ciencias Medicas. 5th ed. Salvat Editores, SA, 1954

WISCONSIN SYNDROME, craniosynostosis, mental deficiency, up-slanting palpebral fissures, microtia, and short fourth metatarsals with recessed fourth toes are features.
1. Gorlin RJ, Cohen MM Jr, Levin LS: Syndromes of the Head and Neck. 3rd ed. New York: Oxford University Press, 1990

WISKOTT-ALDRICH SYNDROME, cutaneous lesions associated with malignancy (reticuloendothe-lial), excematous lesions of the scalp, face, flexures, and buttocks, and purpura on the skin and mucous membranes. Sex-linked recessive inheritance. Cross-references: Aldrich syndrome; Thrombocytopenia syndrome; X-linked syndrome. (Alfred Wiskott, 1898-1978, German pediatrician; Robert A. Aldrich, U.S. pediatrician)
1. Aldrich RA, Steinberg AG, Campbell DC: Pediatrics 13:133-139, 1954
2. Smith DW, Jones KL: Recognizable Patterns of Human Malformations: Genetic, Embryologic, and Clinical Aspects. 3rd ed. Philadelphia: WB Saunders, 1982
3. Wiskott A: Familiärer angeborener Morbus Werlhoffi. Monatsschr Kinderheilkd 68:212-216, 1937

WITHDRAWAL SYNDROME, occurs when a drug or alcohol is no long available to a person addicted to that particular substance. Cross-reference: Abstinence syndrome.
1. Bennett JC, Plum F (eds): Cecil Textbook of Medicine. 20th ed. Philadelphia: WB Saunders, 1996

WITKOP SYNDROME, see Mucoepithelial dysplasia syndrome. (Carl J. Witkop, Jr., U.S.)

WITKOP-VON SALLMANN SYNDROME, see Hereditary benign intraepithelial dyskeratosis syn-drome. (Carl J. Witkop, Jr.)

WOILLEZ DISEASE, acute idiopathic congestion of the lungs. (Eugene J. Woillez, 1811-1882, French)
1. Woillez EJ: Arch Gen Med Par 3:385-400, 1854

WOLCOTT-RALLISON SYNDROME, see Mauriac syndrome. (C.D. Wolcott, U.S.)

WOLF-HIRSCHHORN SYNDROME, the low-birth-weight infant is characteristically hypotonic, with severe psychomotor and growth retardation, mild microcephaly, craniofacial asymmetry, a high forehead, wide nasal bridge with prominent glabella, nasal beaking, hypertelorism, and epicanthal folds. Cross-reference: Del(4p) syndrome.
1. Gorlin RJ, Cohen MM Jr, Levin LS: Syndromes of the Head and Neck. 3rd ed. New York: Oxford University Press, 1990

2. Martsolf JT, et al: Familial transmission of Wolf syndrome resulting from specific deletion 4p16 from t(48) (p16;p21) mat. Clin Genet 31:366-369, 1987

3. Wolf U, et al: Deletions on short arms of a B chromosome without "cri-du-chat" syndrome. Lancet 1:769, 1965

WOLFE OPERATION, transplantation of rabbit conjunctiva in cases of symblepharon.

1. Maffei WE: Os Fundamentos da Medicina. 2nd ed. Livraria Editora Artes Médicas Ltda, 1978

WOLFF-PARKINSON-WHITE SYNDROME, the most common variety of pre-excitation syndrome, resulting from an accessory atrioventricular pathway (the bundle of Kent). (Louis Wolff, U.S.; John Parkinson, British; Paul D. White, 1886-1973, U.S.)

1. Bennett JC, Plum F (eds): Cecil Textbook of Medicine. 20th ed. Philadelphia: WB Saunders, 1996

2. Cheitlin MD, Sokolow M: Clinical Cardiology. 5th ed. Norwalk, Conn: Appleton & Lange, 1993

3. Wolff L, Parkinson J, White PD: Am Heart J 5:685-704, 1930

WOLFLER SIGN, when there is pyloric obstruction, liquids pass easily and solids do not.

1. Casas EC: Diccionario Terminologico de Ciencias Medicas. 5th ed. Salvat Editores, SA, 1954

WOLFRAM SYNDROME, the hereditary association of diabetes mellitus, diabetes insipidus, optic atrophy, and neural deafness. (Donald J. Wolfram, U.S.)

1. Wolfram DJ, Wagener HP: Diabetes mellitus and simple optic atrophy among siblings: report of four cases. Mayo Clin Proc 13:715-718, 1938

WOLMAN DISEASE, primary familial xanthomatosis with adrenal involvement. Infants are normal at birth, but in the first few weeks of life have severe vomiting, abdominal distention, diarrhea, poor weight gain, jaundice, and unexplained fever. Hepatosplenomegaly may be massive and there may be a papulovesiculopustular rash on the face, neck, shoulders, and chest. Autosomal recessive lipidosis. Cross-reference: Kahana disease. (Moshe Wolman, Israeli neuropathologist)

1. Kahana D, Berant M, Wolman M: Primary familial xanthomatosis with adrenal involvement (Wolman disease). Report of a further case with nervous system involvement and pathogenetic considerations. Pediatrics 42:70-76, 1968

2. Wolman M: Pediatrics 28:742-757, 1961

3. Young ER, Patrick AD: Deficiency of acid esterase activity in Wolman's disease. Arch Dis Child 45:664-668, 1970

WOOD OPERATION, occlusion of urinary bladder exstrophy using a cutaneous graft from the abdominal wall.

1. Maffei WE: Os Fundamentos da Medicina. 2nd ed. Livraria Editora Artes Médicas Ltda, 1978

WOOD SIGN, a divergent gaze and relaxed orbicularis oculi muscle; an indication of deep anesthesia. (Horatio C. Wood, 1874-1958, U.S. physicist)

1. Casas EC: Diccionario Terminologico de Ciencias Medicas. 5th ed. Salvat Editores, SA, 1954

WORINGER-KOLOPP DISEASE, pagetoid reticulosis; a solitary skin lesion of long duration and slow growth that shows a large number of abnormal mononuclear cells infiltrating the epidermis with an underlying reactive mixed dermal infiltrate. (M.M. Fredéric Woringer, 1903-1964, French dermatologist; P. Kolopp, French dermatologist)

1. Woringer F, Kolopp P: Ann Derm Syph 10:945-948, 1939

WOSS SIGN, the venous hum disappears upon percussion of the neck; seen in the patient with thrombosis of the lateral sinus.

1. Casas EC: Diccionario Terminologico de Ciencias Medicas. 5th ed. Salvat Editores, SA, 1954

WREDEN SIGN, a gelatinous substance coming out of the ears; an indication of fetal death.

1. Casas EC: Diccionario Terminologico de Ciencias Medicas. 5th ed. Salvat Editores, SA, 1954

WRIGHT OPERATION, arthrectomy of the knee through an anterior transverse and curved incision; cataract extraction through a corneal incision.

1. Maffei WE: Os Fundamentos da Medicina. 2nd ed. Livraria Editora Artes Médicas Ltda, 1978

WRIGHT SYNDROME, see Hyperabduction syndrome. (Irving S. Wright, U.S.)

WÜTZER OPERATION, radical cure of inguinal hernia through invagination of the scrotum into the canal.

1. Maffei WE: Os Fundamentos da Medicina. 2nd ed. Livraria Editora Artes Médicas Ltda, 1978

WYBURN-MASON SYNDROME, consists of an arteriovenous aneurysm of the midbrain, a unilateral malformation of the retinal vessels, and a nevus flammeus in the region of the affected eye. (Roger Wyburn-Mason, British)

1. Krayenbühl HA, Yasargil MG: Cerebral Angiography. Stuttgart: Thieme Medical, 1982

2. Moschella SL, Hurley HJ: Dermatology. 2nd ed. Philadelphia: WB Saunders, 1985

3. Wyburn-Mason R: Brain 66:163-203, 1943

WYETH OPERATION, a method for disarticulation of the hip.
1. Maffei WE: Os Fundamentos da Medicina. 2nd ed. Livraria Editora Artes Médicas Ltda, 1978

WYLIE OPERATION, shortening of the round ligaments through perforation and suturing in cases of retroflexion of the uterus. Cross-reference: Gill-Wylie operation.
1. Maffei WE: Os Fundamentos da Medicina. 2nd ed. Livraria Editora Artes Médicas Ltda, 1978

WYNTER SIGN, lack of abdominal respiration; seen in the patient with acute peritonitis.
1. Casas EC: Diccionario Terminologico de Ciencias Medicas. 5th ed. Salvat Editores, SA, 1954

X-LINKED HYDROCEPHALUS SYNDROME, hydrocephalus, short flexed thumbs, and mental deficiency are features. X-linked recessive trait.
1. Fairre J, et al: X-linked hydrocephalus. Childs Brain 2:226, 1976
2. Smith DW, Jones KL: Recognizable Patterns of Human Malformations: Genetic, Embryologic, and Clinical Aspects. 3rd ed. Philadelphia: WB Saunders, 1982

X-LINKED LYMPHOPROLIFERATIVE SYNDROME, characterized by defective cellular or humoral immune response to the Epstein-Barr virus (EBV). Fulminant infectious mononucleosis, fatal B cell malignancies, or hypogammaglobulinemia can result from the EBV infection.
1. Dorland's Medical Dictionary. 28th ed. Philadelphia: WB Saunders, 1994

X-LINKED SPONDYLOEPIPHYSEAL DYSPLASIA SYNDROME, flattened vertebrae presenting in mid-childhood, small iliac wings, and short femoral neck are features. X-linked recessive trait.
1. Bannerman RM, Ingall GB, Mohn JF: X-linked spondyloepiphyseal dysplasia tarda. J Med Genet 8:291, 1971
2. Smith DW, Jones KL: Recognizable Patterns of Human Malformations: Genetic, Embryologic, and Clinical Aspects. 3rd ed. Philadelphia: WB Saunders, 1982

X-LINKED SYNDROME, see Wiskott-Aldrich syndrome.

XERODERMA PIGMENTOSA SYNDROME, undue sensitivity to sunlight, atrophic and pigmentary skin changes, and actinic skin tumors are features. Autosomal recessive inheritance.
1. Rook A, Wilkinson DS, Ebling FJG (eds): Textbook of Dermatology. Oxford: Blackwell Scientific, 1968
2. Smith DW, Jones KL: Recognizable Patterns of Human Malformations: Genetic, Embryologic, and Clinical Aspects. 3rd ed. Philadelphia: WB Saunders, 1982

XO SYNDROME, see Turner syndrome.

XX SYNDROME, the 46,XX karyotype, resembles the Klinefelter syndrome, but smaller in stature. Patients have male psychosexual identification and relatively normal body habitus.
1. De la Chapelle A: Am J Hum Genet 24:71-105, 1972
2. Kase NG, Weingold AB: Principles and Practice of Clinical Gynecology. New York: John Wiley & Sons, 1983

XXX SYNDROME, the genetic presence of three X chromosomes; one girl in 1000 is born with trisomy XXX. Most develop normally physically and mentally, although some are mentally retarded.
1. Jacobs PA, et al: Lancet 2:423-425, 1959
2. Smith DW, Jones KL: Recognizable Patterns of Human Malformations: Genetic, Embryologic, and Clinical Aspects. 3rd ed. Philadelphia: WB Saunders, 1982

XXXX SYNDROME, the genetic presence of four X chromosomes; other than mental deficiency, other features have been variable.
1. Gardner RJM, Veale AMO, Sands VE: XXXX syndrome: case report, and a note on genetic counselling and fertility. Humangenetik 17:323, 1973
2. Smith DW, Jones KL: Recognizable Patterns of Human Malformations: Genetic, Embryologic, and Clinical Aspects. 3rd ed. Philadelphia: WB Saunders, 1982

XXXXX SYNDROME, see Penta-X syndrome.

XXXY AND XXXXY SYNDROMES, hypogenitalism, limited elbow pronation, and a low dermal ridge count on the fingertips are features.
1. Braunwald E: Heart Disease: A Textbook of Cardiovascular Medicine. 4th ed. Philadelphia: WB Saunders, 1992
2. Smith DW, Jones KL: Recognizable Patterns of Human Malformations: Genetic, Embryologic, and Clinical Aspects. 3rd ed. Philadelphia: WB Saunders, 1982

XXY SYNDROME, see Klinefelter syndrome.

YANKAUER OPERATION, surgical treatment of chronic suppuration of the middle ear consisting of rubberizing the bone of the eustachian tube and blocking the pathway of the infection.
1. Maffei WE: Os Fundamentos da Medicina. 2nd ed. Livraria Editora Artes Médicas Ltda, 1978

YELLOW NAIL SYNDROME, a syndrome associated with lymphedema, especially of the legs, consisting of a yellowish to greenish discoloration of the nails, which may be smooth, thickened, excessively curved on the long axis, and slow growing. The nails may become loose and be shed.

1. Samman PD, White WF: The "yellow nail" syndrome. Br J Dermatol 76:153-157, 1964

YELLOW VERNIX SYNDROME, YELLOW VERNIX AND DYSMATURITY SYNDROME, see Placental dysfunction syndrome.

YERGASON SIGN, the elbow is flexed to a right angle and the forearm is pronated by the patient. The clinician grasps the patient's wrist and then requests the patient to supinate the forearm against resistance, thus bringing the biceps muscle into action. When pain is localized to the anteromedial aspect of the shoulder, the sign is positive. (Robert M. Yergason, 1885-1949, U.S. orthopedic surgeon)

1. Lumley JS, Clain A: Hamilton Bailey's Demonstration of Physical Signs in Clinical Surgery. 18th ed. London: Butterworth-Heinemann, 1997

YOUNG SYNDROME, obstructive azoospermia and chronic sinopulmonary infections. Cross-reference: Barry-Perkins-Young syndrome. (Donald Young)

1. Young D: Surgical treatment of male fertility. J Reprod Fertil 23:541-542, 1970

YUNIS-VARÓN SYNDROME, consists of pre- and postnatal deficiency, hypoplastic clavicles, absence of thumbs and first metatarsal bones, and distal aphalangia. (Emilio Yunis, Colombian)

1. Gorlin RJ, Cohen MM Jr, Levin LS: Syndromes of the Head and Neck. 3rd ed. New York: Oxford University Press, 1990
2. Yunis E, Varón H: Cleidocranial dysostosis, severe micrognathism, bilateral absence of thumbs and first metatarsal bone, and distal aphalangia. Am J Dis Child 134:649-653, 1980

ZAHORSKY DISEASE, exanthema subitum or roseola infantum. An acute, benign viral illness seen in infants and young children. Three to five days of high fever, either sustained or spiking, is followed by a morbilliform rash that appears either as the fever resolves or shortly thereafter. Cross-reference: Sixth disease. (John Zahorsky, 1871-1963, U.S.)

1. Krugman S, Katz SL: Infectious Diseases of Children. 7th ed. St Louis: CV Mosby, 1981
2. Zahorsky J: Pediatrics 22:60-64, 1810

ZAUFAL SIGN, a saddle-shaped nose; a characteristic of syphilis. (Emanuel Zaufal, 1833-1910, Czech rhinologist)

1. Casas EC: Diccionario Terminologico de Ciencias Medicas. 5th ed. Salvat Editores, SA, 1954

ZEIS GLANDS, the ciliary glands or the sebaceous glands of the eyelids. (Eduard Zeis, 1807-1868, German ophthalmologist)

1. Lumley JS, Clain A: Hamilton Bailey's Demonstration of Physical Signs in Clinical Surgery. 18th ed. London: Butterworth-Heinemann, 1997

ZELENY SIGN, a bird-like sound in the left iliac fossa; found in the patient with typhoid fever.

1. Casas EC: Diccionario Terminologico de Ciencias Medicas. 5th ed. Salvat Editores, SA, 1954

ZELLER OPERATION, autoplasty in syndactyly.

1. Maffei WE: Os Fundamentos da Medicina. 2nd ed. Livraria Editora Artes Médicas Ltda, 1978

ZELLWEGER SYNDROME, an autosomal recessive disorder consisting of craniofacial abnormalities, hypotonia, hepatomegaly, polycystic kidney, jaundice, and death in early infancy. Associated with the absence of peroxisomes in the liver and kidneys. Cross-reference: Cerebrohepatorenal syndrome. (Hans Zellweger, Swiss-born U.S. pediatrician)

1. Bowen P, Lee CSN, Zellweger H, et al: A familial syndrome of multiple congenital defects. Bull Johns Hopkins Hosp 114:402-414, 1964
2. Campbell MF, Walsh PC: Campbell's Urology. 5th ed. Philadelphia: WB Saunders, 1986
3. Smith DW, Jones KL: Recognizable Patterns of Human Malformations: Genetic, Embryologic, and Clinical Aspects. 3rd ed. Philadelphia: WB Saunders, 1982

ZENKER DIVERTICULUM, pharyngoesophageal diverticulum. Not anatomically an esophageal diverticulum, as its neck is above the upper scriptions of esophageal diverticula. An epiphrenic diverticulum usually occurs on the right side of the esophagus, just above the lower esophageal sphincter. (Friedrich A. von Zenker, 1825-1898, German pathologist)

1. Bennett JC, Plum F (eds): Cecil Textbook of Medicine. 20th ed. Philadelphia: WB Saunders, 1996

ZERI SIGN, synchrony of the heart and respiration; seen in the patient with Adam-Stokes syndrome.

1. Casas EC: Diccionario Terminologico de Ciencias Medicas. 5th ed. Salvat Editores, SA, 1954

ZIEMAN SIGN, when seeking a palpable pulse, the index finger lies over the indirect, the middle finger over the direct, and the ring finger over the femoral site. (Stephen A. Zieman, 1898-1973, U.S. surgeon)

1. Lumley JS, Clain A: Hamilton Bailey's Demonstration of Physical Signs in Clinical Surgery. 18th ed. London: Butterworth-Heinemann, 1997

ZIEVE SYNDROME, alcoholic hyperlipidemia; hemolytic anemia and fatty necrosis of the liver are features. (Leslie Zieve, U.S.)

1. Vannotti A: Clinique et Physiopathologie Médicales. Introduction a la Médecine Clinique. Libraire Maloine, SA, 1973
2. Zieve L: Ann Intern Med 48:471-496, 1958

ZIMMERMAN-LABAND SYNDOME, see Laband syndrome.

ZINSSER-ENGMAN-COLE SYNDROME, dyskeratosis congenita; reticular skin hyperpigmentation, nail dystrophy, lacrimal duct obstruction, leukoplakia of the mucous membranes, bone marrow hypofunction, and a predisposition to malignancy are characteristics. Cross-reference: Dyskeratosis congenita syndrome. (Ferdinand Zinsser, 1865-1952, German dermatologist; Martin Engman, 1869-1966, U.S. dermatologist; Harold N. Cole, 1884-1966, U.S. dermatologist)

1. Addison J, Rice MS: The association of dyskeratosis congenita and Fanconi's anemia. Med J Aust 1:797, 1965
2. Cole HN, Rauschkolb JE, Toomey J: Arch Dermatol Syph 21:71-95, 1930
3. Engman MF: Arch Dermatol Syph Suppl 13:685-687, 1926
4. Zinsser F: Ikonogr Dermatol (Kyoto) 5:219-223, 1906

ZOLLINGER-ELLISON SYNDROME, severe peptic ulcerations of the stomach, duodenum, and jejunum, associated with a pancreatic tumor are characteristics. Cross-reference: Strøm-Zollinger-Ellison syndrome. (Robert M. Zollinger, 1903-1992, U.S. surgeon; Edwin H. Ellison, 1918-1970, U.S. surgeon)

1. Baker AB, Baker LH: Clinical Neurology. Hagerstown: Harper & Row, 1982
2. Strøm A: Acta Chir Scand 104:252-260, 1952/53
3. Zollinger RM, Ellison EH: Ann Surg 142:709-728, 1955

ZUGSMITH SIGN, when the second rib space is percussed it has a sound like the liver; found in the patient with stomach cancer.

1. Casas EC: Diccionario Terminologico de Ciencias Medicas. 5th ed. Salvat Editores, SA, 1954

Timir Banerjee, MD, is a graduate of the University of Calcutta. He was trained at the Ohio State University by Dr. W. E. Hunt. He taught at Ohio State University and held positions at St. Mary and Elizabeth Hospital, Louisville, Kentucky, the University of North Carolina, and University of Wisconsin at Madison. Dr. Banerjee served as a medical volunteer in India, Brazil, and Africa; currently, he is in Nepal performing volunteer work. Dr. Banerjee served in the United States Navy as a commander.

Alvaro Augusto Domingues da Silva, MD, graduated from the Rio de Janeiro School of Medicine, Rio de Janeiro, Brazil. He is professor of neuroanatomy at Londrina State University, Londrina, and professor of neuroanatomy and neurology at North Parana University, Parana, Brazil. He has a great interest in the history of medicine.

AANS Publications Office
Lebanon, New Hampshire

Gay Palazzo
Researcher and Editor

Joanne Needham
Linda Dorr
Editors

Barbara Homeyer
Compositor

Kim DeVillers
Administrative Assistant